Basic and Clinical Science Course

Louis B. Cantor, MD, Indianapolis, Indiana, *Senior Secretary for Clinical Education*

Christopher J. Rapuano, MD, Philadelphia, Pennsylvania, *Secretary for Lifelong Learning and Assessment*

George A. Cioffi, MD, New York, New York, *BCSC Course Chair*

Section 2

Faculty

Lawrence M. Levine, MD, *Chair,* Jacksonville, Florida

Vikram S. Brar, MD, Richmond, Virginia

Michael H. Goldstein, MD, Boston, Massachusetts

Alon Kahana, MD, PhD, Ann Arbor, Michigan

William R. Katowitz, MD, Philadelphia, Pennsylvania

Simon K. Law, MD, Los Angeles, California

David A. Mackey, MD, Perth, Western Australia

The Academy wishes to acknowledge the following committees for review of this edition:

Committee on Aging: Hilary A. Beaver, MD, Houston, Texas

Vision Rehabilitation Committee: Thomas O'Donnell, MD, Memphis, Tennessee

Practicing Ophthalmologists Advisory Committee for Education: Edward K. Isbey III, MD, *Primary Reviewer* and *Chair,* Asheville, North Carolina; Hardeep S. Dhindsa, MD, Reno, Nevada; Robert G. Fante, MD, Denver, Colorado; Bradley D. Fouraker, MD, Tampa, Florida; Dasa V. Gangadhar, MD, Wichita, Kansas; James M. Mitchell, MD, Edina, Minnesota; James A. Savage, MD, Memphis, Tennessee; Robert E. Wiggins Jr, MD, Asheville, North Carolina

European Board of Ophthalmology: Peter J. Ringens, MD, PhD, FEBO, *EBO Chair,* Maastricht, the Netherlands; Wagih Aclimandos, MB BCh, DO, FEBO, *EBO Liaison,* London, United Kingdom; Costantino Bianchi, MD, FEBO, Milan, Italy

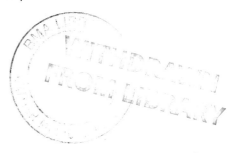

Financial Disclosures

Academy staff members who contributed to the development of this product state that within the 12 months prior to their contributions to this CME activity and for the duration of development, they have had no financial interest in or other relationship with any entity discussed in this course that produces, markets, resells, or distributes ophthalmic health care goods or services consumed by or used in patients, or with any competing commercial product or service.

The authors and reviewers state that within the 12 months prior to their contributions to this CME activity and for the duration of development, they have had the following financial relationships:*

Dr Beaver: Genzyme (L)

Dr Fouraker: Addition Technology (C, L), Alcon Laboratories (C, L), KeraVision (C, L), Ophthalmic Mutual Insurance Company (C, L)

Dr Goldstein: Eleven Biotherapeutics (C, O), Hemera Biosciences (O)

Dr Isbey: Allscripts (C), Medflow (C)

Dr Law: Allergan (L, S)

Dr Savage: Allergan (L)

Dr Wiggins: Medflow/Allscripts (C), Ophthalmic Mutual Insurance Company (C)

The other authors and reviewers state that within the 12 months prior to their contributions to this CME activity and for the duration of development, they have had no financial interest in or other relationship with any entity discussed in this course that produces, markets, resells, or distributes ophthalmic health care goods or services consumed by or used in patients, or with any competing commercial product or service.

*C = consultant fees, paid advisory boards, or fees for attending a meeting; L = lecture fees (honoraria), travel fees, or reimbursements when speaking at the invitation of a commercial sponsor; O = equity ownership/stock options of publicly or privately traded firms (excluding mutual funds) with manufacturers of commercial ophthalmic products or commercial ophthalmic services; P = patents and/or royalties that might be viewed as creating a potential conflict of interest; S = grant support for the past year (all sources) and all sources used for a specific talk or manuscript with no time limitation

Recent Past Faculty

> Balamurali K. Ambati, MD, PhD
> Hilary A. Beaver, MD
> K. V. Chalam, MD, PhD
> Sandeep Grover, MD
> Tony Wells, MB ChB

In addition, the Academy gratefully acknowledges the contributions of numerous past faculty and advisory committee members who have played an important role in the development of previous editions of the Basic and Clinical Science Course.

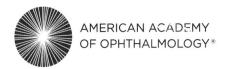

AMERICAN ACADEMY
OF OPHTHALMOLOGY®

Fundamentals and Principles of Ophthalmology

Last major revision 2014–2015

2018-2019

BCSC

Basic and Clinical
Science Course™

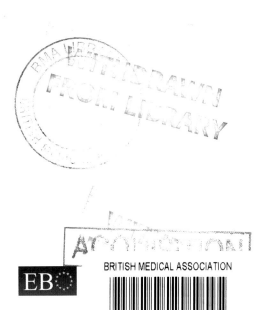

Protecting Sight. Empowering Lives.®

EB

The American Academy of Ophthalmology is accredited by the Accreditation Council for Continuing Medical Education (ACCME) to provide continuing medical education for physicians.

The American Academy of Ophthalmology designates this enduring material for a maximum of 15 *AMA PRA Category 1 Credits*™. Physicians should claim only the credit commensurate with the extent of their participation in the activity.

Originally released June 2014; reviewed for currency September 2017; CME expiration date: June 1, 2019. *AMA PRA Category 1 Credits*™ may be claimed only once between June 1, 2014, and the expiration date.

BCSC® volumes are designed to increase the physician's ophthalmic knowledge through study and review. Users of this activity are encouraged to read the text and then answer the study questions provided at the back of the book.

To claim *AMA PRA Category 1 Credits*™ upon completion of this activity, learners must demonstrate appropriate knowledge and participation in the activity by taking the posttest for Section 2 and achieving a score of 80% or higher. For further details, please see the instructions for requesting CME credit at the back of the book.

The Academy provides this material for educational purposes only. It is not intended to represent the only or best method or procedure in every case, nor to replace a physician's own judgment or give specific advice for case management. Including all indications, contraindications, side effects, and alternative agents for each drug or treatment is beyond the scope of this material. All information and recommendations should be verified, prior to use, with current information included in the manufacturers' package inserts or other independent sources, and considered in light of the patient's condition and history. Reference to certain drugs, instruments, and other products in this course is made for illustrative purposes only and is not intended to constitute an endorsement of such. Some material may include information on applications that are not considered community standard, that reflect indications not included in approved FDA labeling, or that are approved for use only in restricted research settings. **The FDA has stated that it is the responsibility of the physician to determine the FDA status of each drug or device he or she wishes to use, and to use them with appropriate, informed patient consent in compliance with applicable law.** The Academy specifically disclaims any and all liability for injury or other damages of any kind, from negligence or otherwise, for any and all claims that may arise from the use of any recommendations or other information contained herein.

AAO, AAOE, American Academy of Ophthalmology, Basic and Clinical Science Course, BCSC, EyeCare America, EyeNet, EyeSmart, EyeWiki, Femtocenter, Focal Points, IRIS, ISRS, OKAP, ONE, Ophthalmic Technology Assessments, *Ophthalmology, Ophthalmology Retina,* Preferred Practice Pattern, ProVision, The Ophthalmic News & Education Network, and the AAO logo (shown on cover) and tagline (Protecting Sight. Empowering Lives.) are, among other marks, the registered trademarks and trademarks of the American Academy of Ophthalmology.

Cover image: From BCSC Section 12, *Retina and Vitreous.* End-stage chorioretinal atrophy in pathologic myopia. *(Courtesy of Richard F. Spaide, MD.)*

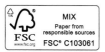

Printed in the United States of America.

American Academy of Ophthalmology Staff

Dale E. Fajardo, EdD, MBA, *Vice President, Education*

Beth Wilson, *Director, Continuing Professional Development*

Ann McGuire, *Acquisitions and Development Manager*

Stephanie Tanaka, *Publications Manager*

D. Jean Ray, *Production Manager*

Beth Collins, *Medical Editor*

Naomi Ruiz, *Publications Specialist*

American Academy of Ophthalmology
655 Beach Street
Box 7424
San Francisco, CA 94120-7424

Contents

General Introduction xvii

Objectives 1

PART I   Anatomy 3

1   Orbit and Ocular Adnexa 5
  Orbital Anatomy 5
    Orbital Volume 5
    Bony Orbit 5
    Orbital Margin 5
    Orbital Roof 5
    Medial Orbital Wall 6
    Orbital Floor 6
    Lateral Orbital Wall 7
    The Facial Skeleton and Aging 7
    Orbital Foramina, Ducts, Canals, and Fissures. 7
    Periorbital Sinuses 10
  Cranial Nerves 11
  Ciliary Ganglion 11
    Branches of the Ciliary Ganglion 11
    Short Ciliary Nerves 12
  Extraocular Muscles. 13
    Extraocular Muscle Insertions 13
    Extraocular Muscle Distribution in the Orbit 15
    Extraocular Muscle Origins 16
    Blood Supply to the Extraocular Muscles 17
    Innervation of the Extraocular Muscles 17
    Fine Structure of the Extraocular Muscles 18
  Eyelids 18
    Anatomy. 19
    Vascular Supply of the Eyelids 25
    Lymphatics of the Eyelids 27
    Accessory Eyelid Structures 27
  Lacrimal Gland and Excretory System 28
    Lacrimal Gland 28
    Accessory Glands 29
    Lacrimal Excretory System 29
  Conjunctiva 30
  Tenon Capsule 31

Vascular Supply and Drainage of the Orbit 32
  Posterior and Anterior Ciliary Arteries. 32
  Vortex Veins 35

2 The Eye **37**
Topographic Features of the Globe 37
Precorneal Tear Film 38
Cornea 38
  Characteristics of the Central and Peripheral Cornea 38
  Epithelium and Basal Lamina 39
  Nonepithelial Cells 40
  Bowman Layer 40
  Stroma. 40
  Descemet Membrane 41
  Endothelium 41
Sclera. 43
Limbus 44
Anterior Chamber 45
Trabecular Meshwork 48
  Uveal Trabecular Meshwork 49
  Corneoscleral Meshwork. 49
  Pericanalicular Connective Tissue 49
  Schlemm Canal. 50
  Collector Channels 51
Uveal Tract 53
Iris 53
  Stroma 54
  Vessels and Nerves 55
  Posterior Pigmented Layer 55
  Dilator Muscle 55
  Sphincter Muscle 56
Ciliary Body 57
  Ciliary Epithelium and Stroma 57
  Ciliary Muscle 58
Choroid 59
  Bruch Membrane 60
  Choriocapillaris 61
Lens 63
  Capsule 64
  Epithelium 64
  Fibers 64
  Zonular Fibers (Suspensory Ligaments) 66
Retina. 67
  Retinal Pigment Epithelium 67
  Neurosensory Retina 69
Macula 75
Ora Serrata 78
Vitreous. 78

3 Cranial Nerves: Central and Peripheral Connections **83**

Cranial Nerve I (Olfactory Nerve). 83
Cranial Nerve II (Optic Nerve) 83
    Intraocular Region 86
    Intraorbital Region 87
    Intracanalicular Region 89
    Intracranial Region 90
    Blood Supply of the Optic Nerve 90
    Chiasm 92
    Optic Tract 93
    Lateral Geniculate Body 93
    Optic Radiations 93
    Visual Cortex 93
Cranial Nerve III (Oculomotor Nerve) 93
    Pathways for the Pupil Reflexes 96
Cranial Nerve IV (Trochlear Nerve) 96
Cranial Nerve V (Trigeminal Nerve) 97
    Mesencephalic Nucleus 97
    Main Sensory Nucleus 97
    Spinal Nucleus and Tract 97
    Motor Nucleus 99
    Divisions of Cranial Nerve V 100
Cranial Nerve VI (Abducens Nerve) 101
Cranial Nerve VII (Facial Nerve) 102
Cavernous Sinus 105
Other Venous Sinuses 105
Circle of Willis 105

PART II Embryology **109**

4 Ocular Development **111**

General Principles 111
Eye Development 115
    Lens and Anterior Segment Formation 117
    Uvea 122
    Retina and Posterior Segment 122
    Sclera 124
    Orbit and Extraocular Muscles 124
Genetic Cascades and Morphogenic Gradients 126
    Homeobox Gene Program 126
    Growth Factors, Diffusible Ligands, and Morphogens 127
    Future Directions 127

PART III Genetics 129

Introduction 131
Terminology 131
Glossary 131

5 Molecular Genetics 147
Gene Structure 147
The Cell Cycle 148
Noncoding DNA 150
Gene Transcription and Translation:
   The Central Dogma of Genetics 151
    Intron Excision 152
    Alternative Splicing and Isoforms . . . 152
    Methylation 153
    X-Inactivation 153
    Imprinting 153
DNA Damage and Repair 154
    Repair 154
    Apoptosis 155
Mutations and Disease 155
    Mutations Versus Polymorphisms . . . 155
    Cancer Genes 156
Mitochondrial Disease 157
    Chronic Progressive External Ophthalmoplegia . . . 158
    Leber Hereditary Optic Neuropathy . . . 158
    Neuropathy, Ataxia, and Retinitis Pigmentosa . . . 158
    MELAS and MIDD 159
The Search for Genes in Specific Diseases . . . 159
    Genetic Markers 159
    Gene Dosage 159
    Linkage and Disease Association . . . 160
    Candidate Gene Approaches . . . 161
Mutation Screening 161
    Direct Sequencing 161
    Genome-Wide Association Studies . . . 163
Gene Therapy 169
    Replacement of Absent Gene Product in X-Linked
      and Recessive Disease 169
    Strategies for Dominant Diseases . . . 169

6 Clinical Genetics 171
Pedigree Analysis 172
Patterns of Inheritance 173
    Dominant Versus Recessive . . . 173
    Autosomal Recessive Inheritance . . . 174
    Autosomal Dominant Inheritance . . . 177

X-Linked Inheritance 178
Maternal Inheritance 181
Terminology: Hereditary, Genetic, Familial, Congenital 181
Genes and Chromosomes 184
Alleles 184
Mitosis 185
Meiosis 186
Segregation 186
Independent Assortment 187
Linkage 187
Chromosomal Analysis 187
Indications for Chromosome Analysis 188
Aneuploidy of Autosomes 189
Mosaicism 190
Ophthalmically Important Chromosomal Aberrations 192
Mutations 193
Polymorphisms 194
Genome, Genotype, Phenotype 194
Single-Gene Disorders 194
Anticipation 194
Penetrance 195
Expressivity 196
Pleiotropism 196
Racial and Ethnic Concentration of Genetic Disorders 196
Lyonization 197
Complex Genetic Disease:
Polygenic and Multifactorial Inheritance 200
Pharmacogenetics 201
Clinical Management of Genetic Disease 202
Accurate Diagnosis 202
Complete Explanation of the Disease 202
Treatment of the Disease Process 202
Genetic Counseling 204
Issues in Genetic Counseling 205
Reproductive Issues 206
Referral to Providers of Support for Persons With Disabilities 207
Recommendations for Genetic Testing of Inherited Eye Disease 207

PART IV Biochemistry and Metabolism **209**

Introduction **211**

7 Tear Film **213**
Lipid Layer 214
Aqueous Layer 215
Mucin Layer 217
Tear Secretion 217
Tear Dysfunction 220

8 Cornea **223**
Epithelium 224
Bowman Layer 225
Stroma 225
Descemet Membrane and Endothelium 227

9 Aqueous Humor, Iris, and Ciliary Body **229**
Introduction to the Aqueous Humor 229
Dynamics of the Aqueous Humor 229
Composition of the Aqueous Humor 230
    Inorganic Ions 232
    Organic Anions 232
    Carbohydrates 232
    Glutathione and Urea 232
    Proteins 233
    Growth-Modulatory Factors 234
    Vascular Endothelial Growth Factors 235
    Oxygen and Carbon Dioxide 235
Clinical Implications of Breakdown
    of the Blood–Aqueous Barrier 236
Introduction to the Iris and Ciliary Body 236
Eicosanoids 237
    Types and Actions 237
    Synthesis 238
    Prostaglandin Receptors 239
Ocular Receptors 240

10 Lens **241**
Structure of the Lens 241
    Capsule 241
    Epithelium 242
    Cortex and Nucleus 242
Chemical Composition of the Lens 243
    Membranes 243
    Lens Proteins 243
Physiologic Aspects of the Lens 245
Lens Metabolism and Formation of Sugar Cataracts 246
    Energy Production 246
    Carbohydrate Cataracts 246

11 Vitreous **249**
Composition 249
    Collagen 249
    Hyaluronan 250
    Soluble and Fibril-Associated Proteins 251
    Zonular Fibers and Low-Molecular-Weight Solutes 252

Biochemical Changes With Aging and Disease 252
   Vitreous Liquefaction and Posterior Vitreous Detachment 252
   Myopia 253
   Vitreous as an Inhibitor of Angiogenesis 253
   Physiologic Changes After Vitrectomy 254
   Injury With Hemorrhage and Inflammation 254
   Involvement of Vitreous in Macular Hole Formation 254
   Genetic Disease Involving the Vitreous 255
   Enzymatic Vitreolysis 255

12 Retina 257
Neural Retina—The Photoreceptors 257
   Rod Phototransduction 257
   Cone Phototransduction 261
   Rod-Specific Gene Defects 263
   Cone- and Rod-Specific Gene Defects 264
   Cone-Specific Gene Defects 264
   RPE-Specific Gene Defects 264
   Ubiquitously Expressed Genes Causing Retinal Degenerations 265
Inner Nuclear Layer 266
Retinal Electrophysiology 268

13 Retinal Pigment Epithelium 271
Anatomical Description 271
Biochemical Composition 273
   Proteins 273
   Lipids 274
   Nucleic Acids 274
Major Physiologic Roles of the RPE 274
   Visual Pigment Regeneration 274
   Phagocytosis of Shed Photoreceptor Outer-Segment Discs 276
   Transport 277
   Pigmentation 277
   Retinal Adhesion 278
The RPE in Disease 278

14 Free Radicals and Antioxidants 281
Cellular Sources of Active Oxygen Species 281
Mechanisms of Lipid Peroxidation 282
Oxidative Damage to the Lens 283
Vulnerability of the Retina to Free Radicals 285
Antioxidants in the Retina and RPE 286
   Selenium, Glutathione, Glutathione Peroxidase, and
      Glutathione-S-Transferase 287
   Vitamin E 287
   Superoxide Dismutase and Catalase 287
   Ascorbate 288
   Carotenoids 288

PART V   Ocular Pharmacology 291

15 Pharmacologic Principles 293
Introduction 293
    Pharmacokinetics 293
    Pharmacodynamics 293
    Pharmacotherapeutics 294
    Toxicity 294
    Pharmacologic Principles in Elderly Patients 295
Pharmacokinetics: The Route of Drug Delivery 295
    Topical Administration 295
    Local Administration 299
    Systemic Administration 300
    Methods of Ocular Drug Design and Delivery 301
Pharmacodynamics: The Mechanism of Drug Action 304

16 Ocular Pharmacotherapeutics 305
Legal Aspects of Medical Therapy 305
Compounding Pharmaceuticals 306
Cholinergic Drugs 307
    Muscarinic Drugs 308
    Nicotinic Drugs 314
Adrenergic Drugs 316
    α-Adrenergic Drugs 317
    β-Adrenergic Drugs 321
Carbonic Anhydrase Inhibitors 323
Prostaglandin Analogues 327
Combined Medications 328
Osmotic Drugs 328
    Actions and Uses 328
    Specific Osmotic Drugs 328
Anti-inflammatory Drugs 329
    Glucocorticoids 329
    Nonsteroidal Anti-inflammatory Drugs 334
    Antiallergic Drugs: Mast-Cell Stabilizers and Antihistamines 337
    Antifibrotic Drugs 340
Medications for Dry Eye 341
Ocular Decongestants 342
Antimicrobial Drugs 343
    Penicillins and Cephalosporins 343
    Other Antibacterial Drugs 346
    Antifungal Drugs 354
    Antiviral Drugs 356
    Medications for *Acanthamoeba* Infections 361
Local Anesthetics 362
    Overview 362
    Topical Anesthetics in Anterior Segment Surgery 365

Purified Neurotoxin Complex 366
Hyperosmolar Drugs 366
Irrigating Solutions 367
Diagnostic Agents 367
Viscoelastic Agents 368
Fibrinolytic Agents 369
Thrombin 369
Antifibrinolytic Agents 369
Vitamin Supplements and Antioxidants 370
Interferon 370
Growth Factors 371

Basic Texts 373
Related Academy Materials 375
Requesting Continuing Medical Education Credit 377
Study Questions 379
Answer Sheet for Section 2 Study Questions 385
Answers 387
Index 391

General Introduction

The Basic and Clinical Science Course (BCSC) is designed to meet the needs of residents and practitioners for a comprehensive yet concise curriculum of the field of ophthalmology. The BCSC has developed from its original brief outline format, which relied heavily on outside readings, to a more convenient and educationally useful self-contained text. The Academy updates and revises the course annually, with the goals of integrating the basic science and clinical practice of ophthalmology and of keeping ophthalmologists current with new developments in the various subspecialties.

The BCSC incorporates the effort and expertise of more than 90 ophthalmologists, organized into 13 Section faculties, working with Academy editorial staff. In addition, the course continues to benefit from many lasting contributions made by the faculties of previous editions. Members of the Academy Practicing Ophthalmologists Advisory Committee for Education, Committee on Aging, and Vision Rehabilitation Committee review every volume before major revisions. Members of the European Board of Ophthalmology, organized into Section faculties, also review each volume before major revisions, focusing primarily on differences between American and European ophthalmology practice.

Organization of the Course

The Basic and Clinical Science Course comprises 13 volumes, incorporating fundamental ophthalmic knowledge, subspecialty areas, and special topics:

1 Update on General Medicine
2 Fundamentals and Principles of Ophthalmology
3 Clinical Optics
4 Ophthalmic Pathology and Intraocular Tumors
5 Neuro-Ophthalmology
6 Pediatric Ophthalmology and Strabismus
7 Orbit, Eyelids, and Lacrimal System
8 External Disease and Cornea
9 Intraocular Inflammation and Uveitis
10 Glaucoma
11 Lens and Cataract
12 Retina and Vitreous
13 Refractive Surgery

In addition, a comprehensive Master Index allows the reader to easily locate subjects throughout the entire series.

References

Readers who wish to explore specific topics in greater detail may consult the references cited within each chapter and listed in the Basic Texts section at the back of the book.

These references are intended to be selective rather than exhaustive, chosen by the BCSC faculty as being important, current, and readily available to residents and practitioners.

Self-Assessment and CME Credit

Each volume of the BCSC is designed as an independent study activity for ophthalmology residents and practitioners. The learning objectives for this volume are given on page 1. The text, illustrations, and references provide the information necessary to achieve the objectives; the study questions allow readers to test their understanding of the material and their mastery of the objectives. Physicians who wish to claim CME credit for this educational activity may do so by following the instructions given at the end of the book.

Conclusion

The Basic and Clinical Science Course has expanded greatly over the years, with the addition of much new text, numerous illustrations, and video content. Recent editions have sought to place greater emphasis on clinical applicability while maintaining a solid foundation in basic science. As with any educational program, it reflects the experience of its authors. As its faculties change and medicine progresses, new viewpoints emerge on controversial subjects and techniques. Not all alternate approaches can be included in this series; as with any educational endeavor, the learner should seek additional sources, including Academy Preferred Practice Pattern Guidelines.

The BCSC faculty and staff continually strive to improve the educational usefulness of the course; you, the reader, can contribute to this ongoing process. If you have any suggestions or questions about the series, please do not hesitate to contact the faculty or the editors.

The authors, editors, and reviewers hope that your study of the BCSC will be of lasting value and that each Section will serve as a practical resource for quality patient care.

Objectives

Upon completion of BCSC Section 2, *Fundamentals and Principles of Ophthalmology,* the reader should be able to

- identify the bones making up the orbital walls and the orbital foramina

- identify the origin and pathways of cranial nerves I–VII

- identify the origins and insertions of the extraocular muscles

- describe the distribution of the arterial and venous circulations of the orbit and optic nerve

- summarize the structural-functional relationships of the outflow pathways for aqueous humor of the eye

- delineate the events of early embryogenesis that are important for the subsequent development of the eye and orbit

- identify the roles of growth factors, homeobox genes, and neural crest cells in the genesis of the eye

- describe the sequence of events in the differentiation of the ocular tissues during embryonic and fetal development of the eye

- draw a simple pedigree and recognize the main patterns of inheritance

- describe the organization of the human genome and the role of genetic mutations in health and disease

- demonstrate how appropriate diagnosis and management of genetic diseases can lead to better patient care

- understand the role of the ophthalmologist in the provision of genetic counseling as well as the indications for ordering genetic testing

- identify the biochemical composition of the various parts of the eye and the eye's secretions

- list the varied functions of the retinal pigment epithelium such as phagocytosis and vitamin A metabolism

- summarize the role of free radicals and antioxidants in the eye

- describe the features of the eye that facilitate or impede drug delivery

- understand the basic principles underlying the use of autonomic therapeutic agents in a variety of ocular conditions

- list the indications, contraindications, mechanisms of action, and adverse effects of various drugs used in the management of glaucoma

- describe the mechanisms of action of antibiotic, antiviral, and antifungal medications

- discuss the anesthetic agents used in ophthalmology

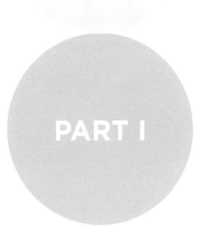

PART I

Anatomy

CHAPTER **1**

Orbit and Ocular Adnexa

Orbital Anatomy

Orbital Volume

Each eye lies within a bony orbit, the volume of which, in the adult, is slightly less than 30 cm^3. Each orbit is pear shaped; the optic nerve represents the stem. The orbital entrance averages approximately 35 mm in height and 45 mm in width. The maximum width is located approximately 1 cm behind the anterior orbital margin. In adults, the depth of the orbit varies from 40 to 45 mm from the orbital entrance to the orbital apex. Both race and sex affect each of these measurements.

Bony Orbit

Seven bones make up the bony orbit (Fig 1-1; also see Chapter 1 in BCSC Section 7, *Orbit, Eyelids, and Lacrimal System*):

1. frontal bone
2. zygomatic bone
3. maxilla (or maxillary bone)
4. ethmoid (or ethmoidal) bone
5. sphenoid bone
6. lacrimal bone
7. palatine bone

Orbital Margin

The orbital margin forms a quadrilateral spiral whose superior margin is formed by the frontal bone, which is interrupted medially by the supraorbital notch. The medial margin is formed above by the frontal bone and below by the posterior lacrimal crest of the lacrimal bone and the anterior lacrimal crest of the maxillary bone. The inferior margin derives from the maxillary and zygomatic bones. Laterally, the zygomatic and frontal bones complete the rim.

Orbital Roof

The orbital roof is formed from both the orbital plate of the frontal bone and the lesser wing of the sphenoid bone. The fossa for the lacrimal gland, lying anterolaterally behind

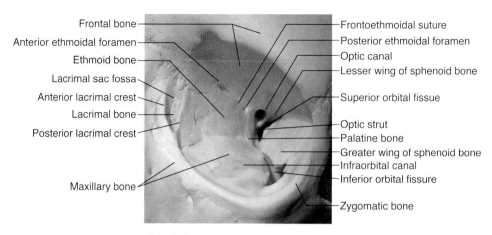

Frontal bone
Anterior ethmoidal foramen
Ethmoid bone
Lacrimal sac fossa
Anterior lacrimal crest
Lacrimal bone
Posterior lacrimal crest
Maxillary bone

Frontoethmoidal suture
Posterior ethmoidal foramen
Optic canal
Lesser wing of sphenoid bone
Superior orbital fissue
Optic strut
Palatine bone
Greater wing of sphenoid bone
Infraorbital canal
Inferior orbital fissure
Zygomatic bone

Figure 1-1 Anatomy of the left orbit in a human skull. *(Courtesy of Alon Kahana, MD, PhD.)*

the zygomatic process of the frontal bone, resides within the orbital roof. Medially, the trochlear fossa is located on the frontal bone approximately 4 mm from the orbital margin and is the site of the pulley of the superior oblique muscle, where the trochlea, a curved plate of hyaline cartilage, is attached.

Helveston EM, Merriam WW, Ellis FD, Shellhamer RH, Gosling CG. The trochlea. A study of the anatomy and physiology. *Ophthalmology.* 1982;89(2):124–133.

Medial Orbital Wall

The medial wall of the orbit is formed from 4 bones:

1. frontal process of the maxillary bone
2. lacrimal bone
3. orbital plate of the ethmoid bone
4. lesser wing of the sphenoid bone

The ethmoid bone makes up the largest portion of the medial wall. The lacrimal fossa is formed by the frontal process of the maxilla and the lacrimal bone. Below, the lacrimal fossa is continuous with the bony nasolacrimal canal, which extends into the inferior meatus (the space beneath the inferior turbinate) of the nose. The paper-thin structure of the medial wall of the ethmoid bone is reflected in its name, *lamina papyracea.*

Orbital Floor

The floor of the orbit, which is the roof of the maxillary antrum, or sinus, is composed of 3 bones:

1. maxillary bone
2. palatine bone
3. orbital plate of the zygomatic bone

The infraorbital groove traverses the floor and descends anteriorly into a canal. It exits as the infraorbital foramen, below the orbital margin of the maxillary bone. Arising from the floor of the orbit just lateral to the opening of the nasolacrimal canal is the inferior oblique muscle, the only extraocular muscle that does not originate from the orbital apex. The floor of the orbit slopes downward approximately 20° from posterior to anterior. Before puberty, the orbital floor bones are immature and more prone to "trapdoor"-type fractures.

> Egbert JE, May K, Kersten RC, Kulwin DR. Pediatric orbital floor fracture: direct extraocular muscle involvement. *Ophthalmology.* 2000;107(10):1875–1879.

Lateral Orbital Wall

The thickest and strongest of the orbital walls, the lateral wall of the orbit is formed from 2 bones: the zygomatic bone and the greater wing of the sphenoid bone. The lateral orbital tubercle *(Whitnall tubercle),* a small elevation of the orbital margin of the zygomatic bone, lies approximately 11 mm below the frontozygomatic suture. This important landmark is the site of attachment for the following structures:

- ligament of the lateral rectus muscle
- suspensory ligament of the eyeball (Lockwood suspensory ligament)
- lateral palpebral ligament
- aponeurosis of the levator palpebrae superioris muscle
- Whitnall ligament

The Facial Skeleton and Aging

Facial bones are believed to undergo various degrees of resorption in elderly individuals. This resorption can factor into the appearance of tissue descent.

> Mendelson B, Wong CH. Changes in the facial skeleton with aging: implications and clinical applications in facial rejuvenation. *Aesthetic Plast Surg.* 2012;36(4):753–760. Epub 2012 May 12.

Orbital Foramina, Ducts, Canals, and Fissures

Foramina

The *optic foramen* leads from the middle cranial fossa to the apex of the orbit. It is directed forward, laterally, and somewhat downward and conducts the optic nerve, the ophthalmic artery, and sympathetic fibers from the carotid plexus. The optic foramen passes through the lesser wing of the sphenoid bone. The *supraorbital foramen* (which, in some people, is a notch instead of a foramen) is located at the medial third of the superior margin of the orbit. It transmits blood vessels and the supraorbital nerve, which is a branch of the ophthalmic division (V_1) of cranial nerve V (CN V, the trigeminal nerve). The *anterior ethmoidal foramen* is located at the frontoethmoidal suture and transmits the anterior ethmoidal vessels and nerve. The *posterior ethmoidal foramen* lies at the junction of the roof and the medial wall of the orbit and transmits the posterior ethmoidal vessels and nerve through the frontal bone. The *zygomatic foramen* lies in the lateral aspect of the zygomatic bone and contains the zygomaticofacial and zygomaticotemporal branches of the zygomatic nerve and the zygomatic artery.

Nasolacrimal duct

The nasolacrimal duct travels inferiorly from the lacrimal fossa into the inferior meatus of the nose.

Infraorbital canal

The infraorbital canal continues anteriorly from the infraorbital groove and exits 4 mm below the inferior orbital margin. From here it transmits the infraorbital nerve, which is a branch of V_2 (the maxillary division of CN V).

Fissures

The *superior orbital fissure* (Fig 1-2; also see Fig 1-1) is located between the greater and lesser wings of the sphenoid bone and lies lateral to and partly above and below the optic foramen. It is approximately 22 mm long and is spanned by the common tendinous ring of the rectus muscles *(annulus of Zinn)*. Above the ring, the superior orbital fissure transmits the following structures (Fig 1-3):

- lacrimal nerve of CN V_1
- frontal nerve of CN V_1
- CN IV (trochlear nerve)
- superior ophthalmic vein

Within the ring or between the 2 heads of the rectus muscle are the following:

- superior and inferior divisions of CN III (the oculomotor nerve)
- nasociliary branch of CN V_1
- sympathetic roots of the ciliary ganglion
- CN VI (the abducens nerve)

The course of the inferior ophthalmic vein is variable, and it can travel within or below the ring as it exits the orbit.

The *inferior orbital fissure* lies just below the superior fissure between the lateral wall and the floor of the orbit, providing access to the pterygopalatine and inferotemporal fossae. Therefore, it is close to the foramen rotundum and the pterygoid canal. The inferior

Figure 1-2 Axial computed tomography scan of the orbits. The superior orbital fissure (SOF) passes above and below the plane of the optic canal (OC) and is commonly mistaken for the OC. The OC lies in the same plane as the anterior clinoid processes (AClin) and may be cut obliquely in scans so that the entire canal length does not always appear. *(Courtesy of William R. Katowitz, MD.)*

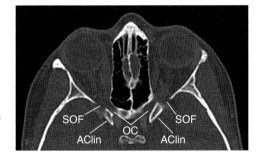

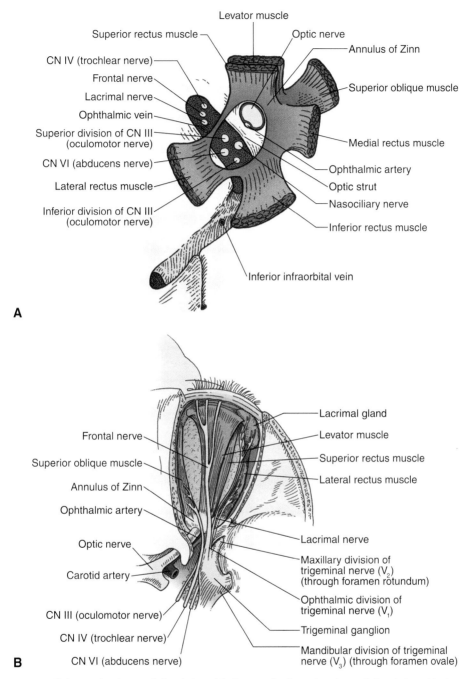

Figure 1-3 Schematic views of the right orbital apex. **A,** Anterior view of the right orbital apex showing the distribution of nerves as they enter through the superior orbital fissure and optic canal. **B,** Superior view of the right orbital apex. CN = cranial nerve. *(Reproduced with permission from Nerad JA.* Techniques in Ophthalmic Plastic Surgery. *Philadelphia: Saunders; 2010.)*

orbital fissure transmits the infraorbital and zygomatic branches of CN V_2, an orbital nerve from the pterygopalatine ganglion, and the inferior ophthalmic vein. The inferior ophthalmic vein connects with the pterygoid plexus before draining into the cavernous sinus.

Periorbital Sinuses

The periorbital sinuses have a close anatomical relationship with the orbits, which are located on either side of the root of the nose (Fig 1-4). The medial walls of the orbits, which border the nasal cavity anteriorly and the ethmoidal sinus and sphenoid sinus posteriorly, are almost parallel. In adults, the lateral wall of each orbit forms an angle of approximately 45° with the medial plane. The lateral walls border the middle cranial, temporal, and pterygopalatine fossae. Superior to the orbit are the anterior cranial fossa and the frontal sinus. The maxillary sinus and the palatine air cells are located inferiorly.

The periorbital sinuses offer a route for the spread of infection. Mucoceles occasionally arise from the sinuses and extend into the adjacent orbit; they may confuse the clinician in the differential diagnosis of orbital tumors. The inferomedial orbital strut is located along the inferonasal orbit, where the orbital bones slope from the floor to the medial wall. This region is significant because of its proximity to the ostium of the maxillary sinus (Fig 1-5).

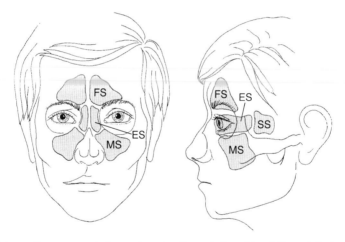

Figure 1-4 Schematic representations showing the relationship of the orbits to the paranasal sinuses. ES = ethmoidal sinus; FS = frontal sinus; MS = maxillary sinus; SS = sphenoid sinus.

Figure 1-5 Coronal computed tomography scan of the orbits and sinuses showing the relation of the middle inferomedial orbital strut (Strut) to the ostium of the maxillary sinus (Ost). The inferior bulla ethmoidalis (BE) marks the floor of the ethmoidal sinus. This region is referred to as the hiatus semilunaris. The fovea ethmoidalis is the roof of the ethmoidal sinus and is a lateral extension of the cribriform plate. *(Courtesy of William R. Katowitz, MD.)*

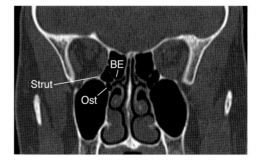

In addition, the *fovea ethmoidalis,* which forms the roof of the ethmoidal sinuses, is a lateral extension of the cribriform plate. It is important to identify this structure when planning lacrimal surgery to prevent inadvertent cerebral spinal fluid leakage as well as intracranial injury. The locations of the paranasal air sinuses and their relation to anatomical features of the skull are indicated in Fig 1-4 and discussed further in BCSC Section 7, *Orbit, Eyelids, and Lacrimal System.*

Doxanas MT, Anderson RL. *Clinical Orbital Anatomy.* Baltimore: Williams & Wilkins; 1984:232.

Kim JW, Goldberg RA, Shorr N. The inferomedial orbital strut: an anatomic and radiographic study. *Ophthal Plast Reconstr Surg.* 2002;18(5)355–364.

Zide BM. *Surgical Anatomy Around the Orbit: The System of Zones.* Philadelphia: Lippincott Williams & Wilkins; 2005.

Cranial Nerves

Six of the 12 cranial nerves (CN II–VII) directly innervate the eye and periocular tissues. Because certain tumors affecting CN I (the olfactory nerve) can give rise to important ophthalmic signs and symptoms, it is important for ophthalmologists to be familiar with the anatomy of this nerve. (Chapter 3 discusses the central and peripheral connections of CN I–VII; also see BCSC Section 7, *Orbit, Eyelids, and Lacrimal System.*)

Ciliary Ganglion

The ciliary ganglion is located approximately 1 cm in front of the annulus of Zinn, on the lateral side of the ophthalmic artery between the optic nerve and the lateral rectus muscle (Figs 1-6, 1-7). It receives 3 roots:

1. A long *sensory root* arises from the nasociliary branch of CN V_1. It is 10–12 mm long and contains sensory fibers from the cornea, the iris, and the ciliary body.
2. A short *motor root* arises from the inferior division of CN III, which also supplies the inferior oblique muscle. The fibers of the motor root synapse in the ganglion, and the postganglionic fibers carry parasympathetic axons to supply the iris sphincter.
3. A *sympathetic root* comes from the plexus around the internal carotid artery. It enters the orbit through the superior orbital fissure within the tendinous ring, passes through the ciliary ganglion without synapse, and innervates ocular blood vessels and the dilator muscles of the pupil.

Branches of the Ciliary Ganglion

Only the parasympathetic fibers synapse in the ciliary ganglion. The sympathetic fibers are postganglionic from the superior cervical ganglion and pass through it without synapse. Sensory fibers from cell bodies in the trigeminal ganglion carry sensation from the eye, orbit, and face. Together, the nonsynapsing sympathetic fibers; the sensory fibers;

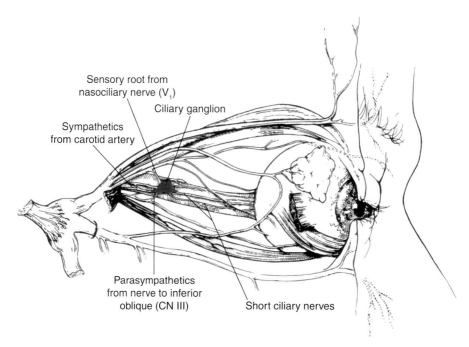

Sensory root from
nasociliary nerve (V₁)

Ciliary ganglion

Sympathetics
from carotid artery

Parasympathetics
from nerve to inferior
oblique (CN III)

Short ciliary nerves

Figure 1-6 Contributions to the ciliary ganglion. *(Reproduced with permission from Doxanas MT, Anderson RL. Clinical Orbital Anatomy. Baltimore: Williams & Wilkins; 1984.)*

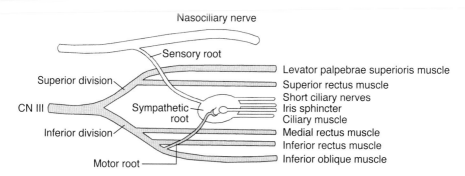

Nasociliary nerve

Sensory root

Superior division

CN III

Sympathetic
root

Inferior division

Motor root

Levator palpebrae superioris muscle
Superior rectus muscle
Short ciliary nerves
Iris sphincter
Ciliary muscle
Medial rectus muscle
Inferior rectus muscle
Inferior oblique muscle

Figure 1-7 Cranial nerve III and ciliary ganglion. The sympathetic fibers from the carotid artery are not shown (see Fig 1-6). *(Illustration by Sylvia Barker.)*

and the myelinated, fast-conducting postganglionic parasympathetic fibers form the short ciliary nerves.

Short Ciliary Nerves

Two groups of short ciliary nerves, totaling 6–10, arise from the ciliary ganglion (see Figs 1-6, 1-7). They travel on both sides of the optic nerve and, together with the long ciliary nerves, pierce the sclera around the optic nerve. They pass anteriorly between the choroid and the sclera into the ciliary muscle, where they form a plexus that supplies the cornea, the ciliary body, and the iris.

Extraocular Muscles

There are 7 extraocular muscles (Figs 1-8 through 1-11):

1. medial rectus
2. lateral rectus
3. superior rectus
4. inferior rectus
5. superior oblique
6. inferior oblique
7. levator palpebrae superioris

Extraocular Muscle Insertions

The 4 rectus muscles insert anteriorly on the globe. Starting at the medial rectus muscle and then proceeding to the inferior rectus, lateral rectus, and superior rectus muscles, the muscle insertions lie progressively farther from the limbus. An imaginary curve drawn through these insertions creates a spiral, which is called the *spiral of Tillaux* (Fig 1-12). The relationship

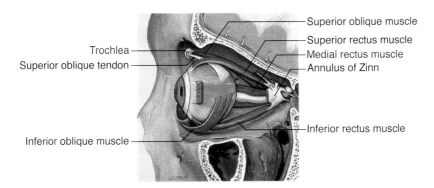

Figure 1-8   Extraocular muscles, lateral composite view of left eye. *(Reproduced with permission from Dutton JJ. Atlas of Clinical and Surgical Orbital Anatomy. Philadelphia: Saunders; 1994.)*

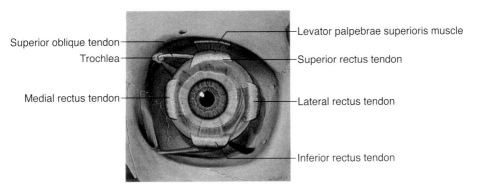

Figure 1-9   Extraocular muscles, frontal composite view of left eye. *(Reproduced with permission from Dutton JJ. Atlas of Clinical and Surgical Orbital Anatomy. Philadelphia: Saunders; 1994.)*

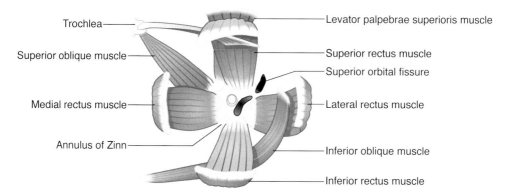

Trochlea
Superior oblique muscle
Medial rectus muscle
Annulus of Zinn

Levator palpebrae superioris muscle
Superior rectus muscle
Superior orbital fissure
Lateral rectus muscle
Inferior oblique muscle
Inferior rectus muscle

Figure 1-10 Extraocular muscles, frontal view, left eye, with globe removed. *(Reproduced with permission from Dutton JJ. Atlas of Clinical and Surgical Orbital Anatomy. Philadelphia: Saunders; 1994.)*

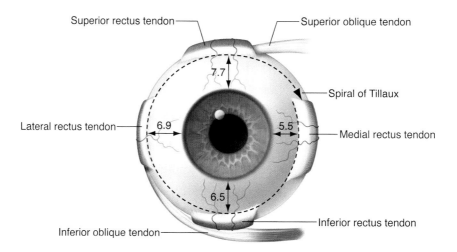

Medial rectus muscle

Superior oblique tendon

Annulus of Zinn
Inferior rectus muscle
Lateral rectus muscle

Superior rectus tendon

Figure 1-11 Extraocular muscles, superior composite view. *(Reproduced with permission from Dutton JJ. Atlas of Clinical and Surgical Orbital Anatomy. Philadelphia: Saunders; 1994.)*

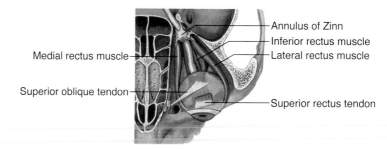

Superior rectus tendon
Superior oblique tendon
7.7
Spiral of Tillaux
Lateral rectus tendon
6.9
5.5
Medial rectus tendon
6.5
Inferior oblique tendon
Inferior rectus tendon

Figure 1-12 The medial rectus tendon is closest to the limbus, and the superior rectus tendon is farthest from it. By connecting the insertions of the tendons beginning with the medial rectus, then the inferior rectus, then the lateral rectus, and finally the superior rectus, a spiral (known as the *spiral of Tillaux*) is obtained. Measurements are in millimeters. *(Illustration by Christine Gralapp.)*

between the muscle insertions and the ora serrata is clinically important. A misdirected suture passed through the insertion of the superior rectus muscle could perforate the retina.

The superior oblique muscle, after passing through the trochlea in the superior nasal orbital rim, inserts onto the sclera superiorly, under the insertion of the superior rectus. The inferior oblique muscle inserts onto the sclera in the posterior inferior temporal quadrant (see Fig 1-12; Table 1-1).

Extraocular Muscle Distribution in the Orbit

Figures 1-10 and 1-11 show the arrangement of the extraocular muscles within the orbit. Note the relationship between the oblique extraocular muscles and the superior, medial, and

Table 1-1 Comparison of the Extraocular Muscles

Muscle	Origin	Insertion	Blood Supply	Size
Medial rectus	Annulus of Zinn	Medially, in horizontal meridian 5.5 mm from limbus	Inferior muscular branch of ophthalmic artery	40.8 mm long; tendon: 3.7 mm long, 10.3 mm wide
Inferior rectus	Annulus of Zinn at orbital apex	Inferiorly, in vertical meridian 6.5 mm from limbus	Inferior muscular branch of ophthalmic artery and infraorbital artery	40 mm long; tendon: 5.5 mm long, 9.8 mm wide
Lateral rectus	Annulus of Zinn spanning the superior orbital fissure	Laterally, in horizontal meridian 6.9 mm from limbus	Lacrimal artery	40.6 mm long; tendon: 8 mm long, 9.2 mm wide
Superior rectus	Annulus of Zinn at orbital apex	Superiorly, in vertical meridian 7.7 mm from limbus	Superior muscular branch of ophthalmic artery	41.8 mm long; tendon: 5.8 mm long, 10.6 mm wide
Superior oblique	Medial to optic foramen, between annulus of Zinn and periorbita	To trochlea, through pulley, at orbital rim, then hooking back under superior rectus, inserting posterior to center of rotation	Superior muscular branch of ophthalmic artery	40 mm long; tendon: 20 mm long, 10.8 mm wide
Inferior oblique	From a depression on orbital floor near orbital rim (maxilla)	Posterior inferior temporal quadrant at level of macula; posterior to center of rotation	Inferior branch of ophthalmic artery and infraorbital artery	37 mm long; no tendon: 9.6 mm wide at insertion

inferior rectus muscles. The location of the extraocular muscles within the orbit and their relationship to surrounding nerves and bone are illustrated in coronal, cross-sectional views (Figs 1-13 and 1-14) and in longitudinal, axial views (Figs 1-15 and 1-16).

Extraocular Muscle Origins

The annulus of Zinn consists of superior and inferior orbital tendons and is the origin of the 4 rectus muscles. The upper tendon gives rise to the entire superior rectus muscle, as

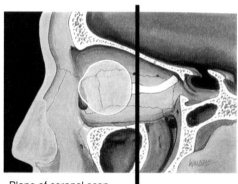

Figure 1-13 Location of the plane of the section shown in Figure 1-14. *(Reproduced with permission from Dutton JJ. Atlas of Clinical and Surgical Orbital Anatomy. Philadelphia: Saunders; 1994.)*

Plane of coronal scan

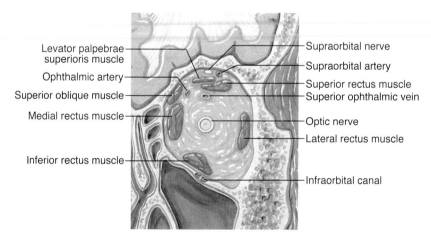

Levator palpebrae superioris muscle
Ophthalmic artery
Superior oblique muscle
Medial rectus muscle
Inferior rectus muscle

Supraorbital nerve
Supraorbital artery
Superior rectus muscle
Superior ophthalmic vein
Optic nerve
Lateral rectus muscle
Infraorbital canal

Figure 1-14 Coronal section through the central orbit just posterior to the globe. *(Reproduced with permission from Dutton JJ. Atlas of Clinical and Surgical Orbital Anatomy. Philadelphia: Saunders; 1994.)*

Figure 1-15 Location of the plane of the section shown in Figure 1-16. *(Reproduced with permission from Dutton JJ. Atlas of Clinical and Surgical Orbital Anatomy. Philadelphia: Saunders; 1994.)*

Plane of axial scan

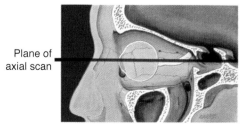

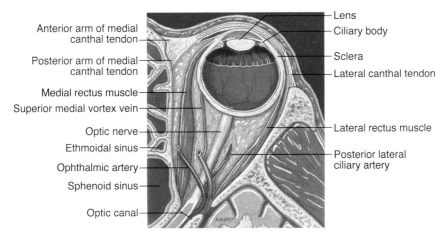

Figure 1-16 Axial section through the midorbit at the level of the optic nerve. The third portion of the ophthalmic artery crosses the nerve in the posterior orbit. *(Reproduced with permission from Dutton JJ. Atlas of Clinical and Surgical Orbital Anatomy. Philadelphia: Saunders; 1994.)*

well as portions of the lateral and medial rectus muscles. The inferior tendon gives rise to the entire inferior rectus muscle and portions of the medial and lateral rectus muscles. The levator palpebrae superioris muscle arises from the lesser wing of the sphenoid bone, at the apex of the orbit, just superior to the annulus of Zinn.

The superior oblique muscle originates from the periosteum of the body of the sphenoid bone, above and medial to the optic foramen. The inferior oblique muscle originates anteriorly, from a shallow depression in the orbital plate of the maxillary bone, at the anteromedial corner of the orbital floor, near the lacrimal fossa. From its origin, the inferior oblique muscle then extends posteriorly, laterally, and superiorly to insert into the globe.

Blood Supply to the Extraocular Muscles

The inferior and superior muscular branches of the ophthalmic artery, lacrimal artery, and infraorbital artery supply the extraocular muscles. The lateral rectus muscle is supplied by a single vessel derived from the lacrimal artery; the other rectus muscles receive 2 anterior ciliary arteries that communicate with the major arterial circle of the ciliary body via perforating scleral vessels. Vascular supply and venous drainage of orbital structures are discussed later in this chapter.

Innervation of the Extraocular Muscles

The lateral rectus muscle is innervated by CN VI (the abducens nerve); the superior oblique muscle is innervated by CN IV (the trochlear nerve); the levator palpebrae superioris, superior rectus, medial rectus, inferior rectus, and inferior oblique muscles are innervated by CN III (the oculomotor nerve). Cranial nerve III has superior and inferior divisions: the upper division innervates the levator palpebrae superioris and superior rectus muscles, and the lower division innervates the medial rectus, inferior rectus, and inferior oblique muscles.

Fine Structure of the Extraocular Muscles

In the extraocular muscles, the ratio of nerve fibers to muscle fibers is very high (1:3–1:5) compared with the ratio of nerve axons to muscle fibers in skeletal muscle (1:50–1:125). This high ratio enables precise control of ocular movements. The fibers of the extraocular muscles are a mixture of slow, tonic-type and fast, twitch-type fibers.

Tonic-type muscle fibers are unique to extraocular muscles. Smaller than twitch-type fibers, they contract slowly and smoothly and tend to be located more superficially in the muscle, nearer the orbital wall. Tonic-type fibers are innervated by multiple grapelike nerve endings *(en grappe)* and are useful for smooth pursuit movements.

Twitch-type fibers are more similar to skeletal muscle fibers. Larger than tonic-type fibers and located deeper in the muscle, they contract rapidly and have platelike nerve endings *(en plaque).* Twitch-type fibers aid in rapid saccadic movements of the eye. The fibers of the extraocular muscles can be further classified by contractile properties, histochemical profile, and myosin content.

Porter JD, Baker RS, Ragusa RJ, Brueckner JK. Extraocular muscles: basic and clinical aspects of structure and function. *Surv Ophthalmol.* 1995;39(6):451–484.

Spencer FR, Porter JD. Structural organization of the extraocular muscles. *Reviews in Oculomotor Research.* Amsterdam: Elsevier; 1988:33–79. In: Büttner-Ennever JA, ed. *Neuroanatomy of the Oculomotor System;* vol 2.

Eyelids

The *palpebral fissure* is the exposed zone between the upper and lower eyelids (Fig 1-17). Normally, the adult fissure is 27–30 mm long and 8–11 mm wide. The upper eyelid, which is more mobile than the lower, can be raised 15 mm by the action of the levator palpebrae superioris muscle alone. If the frontalis muscle of the brow is used, the palpebral fissure

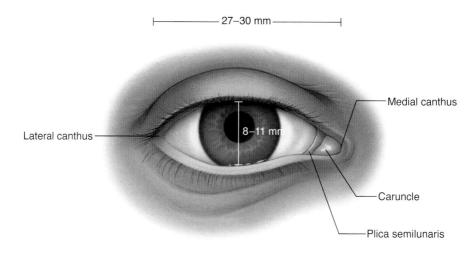

Figure 1-17   Landmarks of the external eye. *(Illustration by Christine Gralapp.)*

can be widened an additional 2 mm. The levator muscle is innervated by CN III. See also BCSC Section 7, *Orbit, Eyelids, and Lacrimal System.*

Anatomy

Although small in surface area, the eyelid is complex in its structure and function. When describing the anatomy of the upper eyelid, it is helpful to divide it into distinct segments from the dermal surface inward. These segments include the following structures (Figs 1-18 through 1-23):

1. skin
2. eyelid margin
3. subcutaneous connective tissue
4. orbicularis oculi muscle
5. orbital septum
6. levator palpebrae superioris muscle
7. Müller muscle
8. tarsus
9. conjunctiva

Eyelid skin

The eyelid skin, the thinnest in the body, contains fine hairs, sebaceous glands, and sweat glands. A superior eyelid fold is present near the upper border of the tarsus, where the levator aponeurosis establishes its first insertional attachments. (In many individuals of Asian descent, there are few attachments of the levator aponeurosis to the skin near the upper tarsal border, and the superior eyelid fold is minimal or absent.) The aponeurosis forms its firmest attachments on the anterior aspect of the tarsus, approximately 3 mm superior to the eyelid margin. Figure 1-20 depicts the 2 major racial variations in eyelid anatomy.

Eyelid margin

The eyelid margin contains several important landmarks (see Fig 1-22). A small opening, the punctum of the canaliculus, presents medially at the summit of each lacrimal papilla. The superior punctum, normally hidden by slight internal rotation, is located more medially. The inferior punctum is usually apposed to the globe and is not normally visible without eversion.

Along the entire length of the free margin of the eyelid is the delicate *gray line* (or *intermarginal sulcus*), which corresponds histologically to the most superficial portion of the orbicularis oculi muscle, the muscle of Riolan, and to the avascular plane of the eyelid. Anterior to this line, the eyelashes (or cilia) arise, and behind this line are the openings of the tarsal (or meibomian) glands just anterior to the mucocutaneous junction.

The eyelashes are arranged in 2 or 3 irregular rows along the anterior dermal edge of the eyelid margin. They are usually longer and more numerous on the upper eyelid than on the lower one. The margins contain the *glands of Zeis*, which are modified sebaceous glands associated with the cilia, and the *glands of Moll*, which are apocrine sweat glands in the skin (see Fig 1-21; Table 1-2).

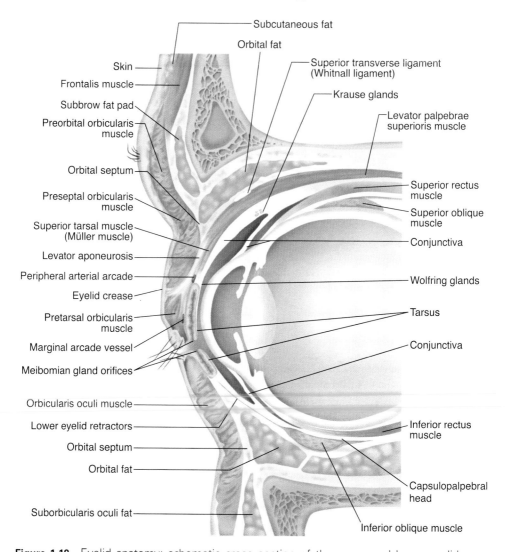

Subcutaneous fat

Orbital fat

Skin

Frontalis muscle

Subbrow fat pad

Preorbital orbicularis muscle

Orbital septum

Preseptal orbicularis muscle

Superior tarsal muscle (Müller muscle)

Levator aponeurosis

Peripheral arterial arcade

Eyelid crease

Pretarsal orbicularis muscle

Marginal arcade vessel

Meibomian gland orifices

Orbicularis oculi muscle

Lower eyelid retractors

Orbital septum

Orbital fat

Suborbicularis oculi fat

Superior transverse ligament (Whitnall ligament)

Krause glands

Levator palpebrae superioris muscle

Superior rectus muscle

Superior oblique muscle

Conjunctiva

Wolfring glands

Tarsus

Conjunctiva

Inferior rectus muscle

Capsulopalpebral head

Inferior oblique muscle

Figure 1-18 Eyelid anatomy: schematic cross section of the upper and lower eyelid areas. *(Modified from Stewart WB. Surgery of the Eyelid, Orbit, and Lacrimal System. Ophthalmology Monograph 8, vol 2. San Francisco: American Academy of Ophthalmology; 1994:23, 85. Illustration by Cyndie C.H. Wooley.)*

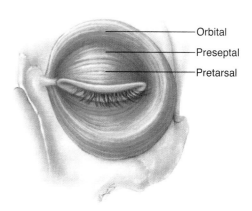

Orbital

Preseptal

Pretarsal

Figure 1-19 The 3 parts of the orbicularis oculi muscle. *(Reproduced with permission from Katowitz JA, ed. Pediatric Oculoplastic Surgery. Philadelphia: Springer-Verlag; 2002.)*

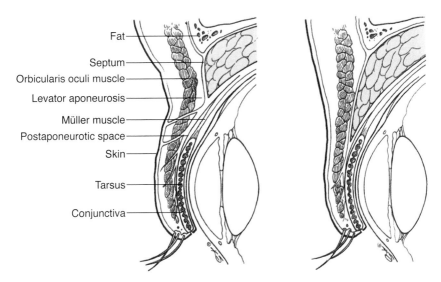

Fat
Septum
Orbicularis oculi muscle
Levator aponeurosis
Müller muscle
Postaponeurotic space
Skin
Tarsus
Conjunctiva

Figure 1-20 Racial variations in eyelid anatomy. Variant I *(left):* the orbital septum inserts onto the levator aponeurosis above the tarsus. Variant II (Asian, *right)*: the orbital septum inserts into the levator aponeurosis between the eyelid margin and the superior border of the tarsus, and there are fewer aponeurotic attachments to the skin. *(Reproduced with permission from Katowitz JA, ed. Pediatric Oculoplastic Surgery. Philadelphia: Springer-Verlag; 2002.)*

Subcutaneous connective tissue

The loose connective tissue of the eyelid contains no fat. Blood or other fluids can accumulate beneath the skin and cause rapid and dramatic swelling of the lids.

Orbicularis oculi muscle

The orbicularis oculi muscle is arranged in several concentric bands around the palpebral fissure and can be subdivided into orbital, preseptal, and pretarsal parts (see Fig 1-19). The muscle fibers are short and are connected by myomyous junctions. Of all the facial muscles, the orbicularis oculi muscle has fibers with the smallest diameter. Innervation occurs by the facial nerve (CN VII), and end plates are arranged in clusters over the entire length of the muscle. This arrangement may influence the action of botulinum A toxin, which is used in the treatment of blepharospasm. The orbital part inserts in a complex way into the medial canthal tendon and into other portions of the orbital rim and the corrugator supercilii muscle. The orbital part acts as a sphincter and functions solely as a voluntary muscle.

The palpebral part of the orbicularis oculi muscle functions both voluntarily and involuntarily in spontaneous and reflex blinking. The preseptal and pretarsal portions unite along the superior palpebral furrow. The pretarsal orbicularis muscle adheres firmly to the tarsus; a portion of it attaches to the anterior lacrimal crest and the posterior lacrimal crest (sometimes called the Horner muscle) and plays a role in tear drainage (see Fig 1-23).

Orbicularis fibers extend to the eyelid margin, where there is the small bundle of striated muscle fibers called the *muscle of Riolan.* Disinsertion of the lower eyelid retractors from the tarsus may cause laxity of the lower eyelid, followed by spastic entropion, an inward turning of the eyelid margin.

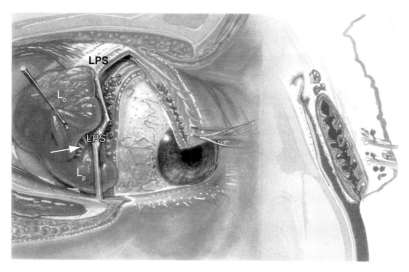

Figure 1-21 The lacrimal secretory system. The conjunctival and tarsal mucin-secreting goblet cells *(green)* produce a mucoprotein layer covering the epithelial surface of the cornea and conjunctiva. The accessory lacrimal exocrine glands of Krause and Wolfring are present in the subconjunctival tissues *(blue)* and contribute to the aqueous layer of the precorneal tear film. Oil-producing meibomian glands and palpebral glands of Zeis and Moll are shown in *pink*. The orbital lobe of the lacrimal gland (L$_o$) and the palpebral lobe of the lacrimal gland (L$_p$) are separated by the lateral horn of the levator palpebrae superioris muscle (LPS). The tear ducts *(arrow)* from the orbital portion traverse the palpebral portion. *(Reproduced with permission from Zide BM, Jelks GW. Surgical Anatomy of the Orbit. New York: Raven; 1985.)*

Figure 1-22 Anatomical landmarks of the lower eyelid margin. The gray line, or inter-marginal sulcus, is visible between the bases of the cilia and the orifices of the meibomian glands. The lower eyelid has been slightly everted to clearly expose the inferior lacrimal puncta. *(Illustration by Christine Gralapp.)*

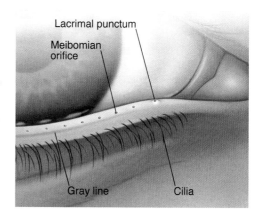

Lander T, Wirtschafter JD, McLoon LK. Orbicularis oculi muscle fibers are relatively short and heterogeneous in length. *Invest Ophthalmol Vis Sci.* 1996;37(9):1732–1739.

Orbital septum

A thin sheet of connective tissue called the orbital septum encircles the orbit as an extension of the periosteum of the roof and the floor of the orbit (see Fig 1-18). It also attaches to the anterior surface of the levator palpebrae superioris muscle. Posterior to the orbital

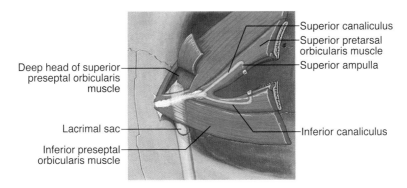

Figure 1-23 Lacrimal drainage system and the orbicularis oculi muscle. *(Reproduced with permission from Dutton JJ. Atlas of Clinical and Surgical Orbital Anatomy. Philadelphia: Saunders; 1994.)*

Table 1-2 Glands of the Eye and Adnexa

Glands	Location	Secretion	Content
Lacrimal	Orbital gland	Exocrine	Aqueous
	Palpebral gland	Exocrine	Aqueous
Accessory lacrimal	Plica, caruncle	Exocrine	Aqueous
Krause	Eyelid	Exocrine	Aqueous
Wolfring	Eyelid	Exocrine	Aqueous
Meibomian	Tarsus	Holocrine	Oily
Zeis	Follicles of cilia	Holocrine	Oily
	Eyelid, caruncle	Holocrine	Oily
Moll	Eyelid	Apocrine	Sweat
Goblet cell	Conjunctiva	Holocrine	Mucus
	Plica, caruncle	Holocrine	Mucus

septum is the orbital fat. In both the upper and lower eyelids, the orbital septum attaches to the aponeurosis. The orbital septum thus provides a barrier to anterior or posterior extravasation of blood or the spread of inflammation. The intermuscular orbital septa can be identified in coronal magnetic resonance imaging (MRI) studies with fat suppression and gadolinium enhancement.

Superiorly, the septum is attached firmly to the periosteum of the superior half of the orbital margin. It passes medially in front of the trochlea and continues along the medial margin of the orbit, along the margin of the frontal process of the maxillary bone, and onto the inferior margin of the orbit. Here, the septum also delimits the lateral spread of edema, inflammation, or blood trapped anterior to it and appears clinically as a dramatic barrier to these processes.

Levator palpebrae superioris muscle

The levator palpebrae superioris muscle originates from the lesser wing of the sphenoid bone (see Fig 1-18). The body of the levator muscle overlies the superior rectus as it travels anteriorly toward the eyelid. The Whitnall ligament is formed by a condensation of tissue surrounding the superior rectus and levator muscles. Near the Whitnall ligament, the levator muscle changes direction from horizontal to more vertical, and it divides anteriorly into the aponeurosis and posteriorly into the superior tarsal (Müller) muscle.

The aponeurosis inserts into the anterior surface of the tarsus and passes by the medial and lateral horns into the canthal tendons. The fibrous elements of the aponeurosis pass through the orbicularis oculi muscle and insert subcutaneously to produce the superior eyelid fold. The aponeurosis also inserts into the trochlea of the superior oblique muscle and into the fibrous tissue bridging the supraorbital notch. Aponeurotic attachments also exist with the conjunctiva of the upper fornix and the orbital septum.

Together, the levator muscle and tendon are 50–55 mm long. The muscle, which elevates the upper eyelid, is 40 mm long and is innervated by the superior division of CN III.

Müller muscle

The Müller muscle is a smooth (nonstriated), sympathetically innervated muscle that originates from the undersurface of the levator palpebrae superioris muscle in the upper eyelid. A similar smooth muscle arises from the capsulopalpebral head of the inferior rectus in the lower eyelid. The Müller muscle attaches to the upper border of the upper tarsus and to the conjunctiva of the upper fornix. The capsulopalpebral muscle, which is much weaker than the Müller muscle, attaches to the lower border of the lower tarsus (see Fig 1-18).

Tarsus

The *tarsal plates* consist of dense connective tissue, not cartilage. They are attached to the orbital margin by the medial and lateral palpebral ligaments. Although the upper and lower tarsal plates are similar in length (29 mm) and in thickness (1 mm), the upper tarsus is almost 3 times as wide vertically (11 mm) as the lower tarsus (4 mm).

The *tarsal (meibomian) glands* are modified holocrine sebaceous glands that are oriented vertically in parallel rows through the tarsus (Fig 1-24). Their distribution and number within the eyelid can be observed by infrared transillumination of the eyelid (Fig 1-25). A single row of 30–40 meibomian orifices is present in the upper eyelid, but there are only 20–30 orifices in the lower lid. Oil from these orifices forms a reservoir on the skin of the lid margin and is spread onto the tear film with each blink. Aging is associated with an alteration in the lipid profile of meibomian gland secretions and with meibomian gland loss in adults.

The hair bulbs of the cilia are located anterior to the tarsus and the meibomian gland orifices. Misdirection in the orientation of the eyelashes (trichiasis) or aberrant growth through the orifices of the meibomian glands (distichiasis) may occur as either a congenital defect or an acquired one; occasionally, these defects are hereditary.

Arita R, Itoh K, Inoue K, Amano S. Noncontact infrared meibography to document age-related changes of the meibomian glands in a normal population. *Ophthalmology.* 2008;115(5): 911–915.

Sullivan BD, Evans JE, Dana MR, Sullivan DA. Influence of aging on the polar and neutral lipid profiles in human meibomian gland secretions. *Arch Ophthalmol.* 2006;124(9):1286–1292.

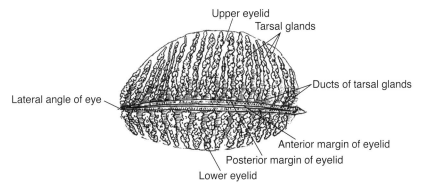

Figure 1-24 Posterior view of the eyelids with the palpebral fissure nearly closed. Note the tarsal glands with their short ducts and orifices. The palpebral conjunctiva has been removed to show the tarsal glands in situ. *(Reproduced with permission from Snell RS, Lemp MA. Clinical Anatomy of the Eye. Boston: Blackwell; 1989.)*

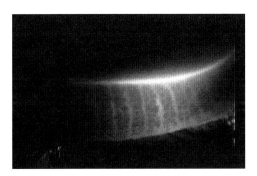

Figure 1-25 Distribution of the meibomian glands in the lower eyelid, as revealed by infrared transillumination. The glands appear as dark gray linear structures. *(Courtesy of William Mathers, MD.)*

Conjunctiva

The palpebral conjunctiva is a transparent vascularized membrane covered by a nonkeratinized epithelium that lines the inner surface of the eyelids. Continuous with the conjunctival fornices (cul-de-sacs), it merges with the bulbar conjunctiva before terminating at the limbus (Fig 1-26). The conjunctiva is discussed further later in the chapter.

Vascular Supply of the Eyelids

The blood supply of the eyelids is derived from the facial system, which arises from the external carotid artery, and the orbital system, which originates from the internal carotid artery along branches of the ophthalmic artery (Fig 1-27). The terminal branches of the ophthalmic artery anastomose with the terminal branches of the external carotid artery. The superficial and deep plexuses of arteries provide a vast blood supply to the upper and lower eyelids. The facial artery becomes the angular artery as it passes upward, forward, and lateral to the nose, where it serves as an important landmark in *dacryocystorhinostomy*.

The *marginal arterial arcade* is located 3 mm from the free border of the eyelid, just above the ciliary follicles. It is either between the tarsal plate and the orbicularis oculi muscle or within the tarsus. A smaller peripheral arcade runs along the upper

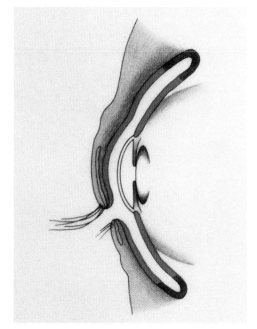

Figure 1-26 The conjunctiva consists of bulbar *(red)*, forniceal *(black)*, and palpebral *(blue)* portions.

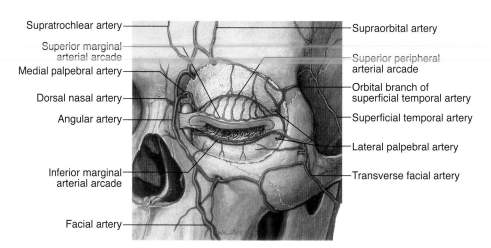

Supratrochlear artery —
Superior marginal arterial arcade —
Medial palpebral artery —
Dorsal nasal artery —
Angular artery —
Inferior marginal arterial arcade —
Facial artery —
— Supraorbital artery
— Superior peripheral arterial arcade
— Orbital branch of superficial temporal artery
— Superficial temporal artery
— Lateral palpebral artery
— Transverse facial artery

Figure 1-27 Periorbital and eyelid arteries, frontal view. *(Reproduced with permission from Dutton JJ. Atlas of Clinical and Surgical Orbital Anatomy. Philadelphia: Saunders; 1994.)*

margin of the tarsal plate within the Müller muscle. The superficial temporal artery is a terminal branch of the external carotid artery and is discussed in greater detail in BCSC Section 5, *Neuro-Ophthalmology*. The venous drainage system of the eyelids can be divided into 2 components: a superficial (or pretarsal) system, which drains into the internal and external jugular veins, and a deep (or posttarsal) system, which flows into the cavernous sinus.

Lymphatics of the Eyelids

Lymphatic vessels are present in the eyelids and conjunctiva, but neither lymphatic vessels nor nodes are present in the orbit. Lymphatic drainage from the eyelids parallels the course of the veins (Fig 1-28). Two groups of lymphatics exist:

1. a medial group that drains into the submandibular lymph nodes
2. a lateral group that drains into the superficial preauricular lymph nodes

Clinically, swelling of the lymph nodes is a diagnostic sign of several external eye infections, including adenoviral conjunctivitis and Parinaud oculoglandular syndrome.

Accessory Eyelid Structures

Caruncle

The caruncle is a small, fleshy, ovoid structure attached to the inferomedial side of the plica semilunaris (see Fig 1-17). As a piece of modified skin, it contains sebaceous glands and fine, colorless hairs. The surface is covered by nonkeratinized, stratified squamous epithelium.

Plica semilunaris

The plica semilunaris is a narrow, highly vascular, crescent-shaped fold of the conjunctiva located lateral to and partly under the caruncle (see Fig 1-17). Its lateral border is free and separated from the bulbar conjunctiva, which it resembles histologically. The epithelium of the plica is rich in goblet cells. The plica's stroma contains fat and some nonstriated muscle. The plica is a vestigial structure analogous to the nictitating membrane, or third eyelid, of dogs and other animals.

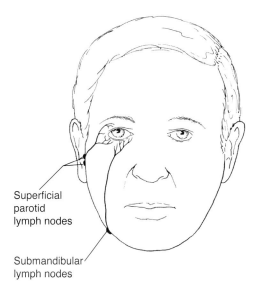

Superficial
parotid
lymph nodes

Submandibular
lymph nodes

Figure 1-28 The lymphatic drainage of the eyelids. *(Reproduced with permission from Snell RS, Lemp MA. Clinical Anatomy of the Eye. Boston: Blackwell; 1989.)*

Lacrimal Gland and Excretory System

Lacrimal Gland

The main lacrimal gland is located in a shallow depression within the orbital part of the frontal bone. The gland is separated from the orbit by fibroadipose tissue and is divided into 2 parts by a lateral expansion of the levator aponeurosis (see Fig 1-21). When the upper eyelid is everted, the smaller, palpebral part can be seen in the superolateral conjunctival fornix. An isthmus of glandular tissue may exist between the palpebral lobe and the main orbital gland.

A variable number of thin-walled excretory ducts, blood vessels, lymphatics, and nerves pass from the main orbital gland into the palpebral lacrimal gland. The ducts continue downward, and about 12 of them empty into the conjunctival fornix approximately 5 mm above the superior margin of the upper tarsus. Because the lacrimal excretory ducts pass through the palpebral portion of the gland, biopsy of the lacrimal gland is usually performed on the main part to avoid sacrificing the ducts.

The lacrimal glands are exocrine glands that produce a serous secretion. The body of each gland contains 2 cell types (Fig 1-29):

1. acinar cells, which line the lumen of the gland
2. myoepithelial cells, which surround the parenchyma and are covered by a basement membrane

The lacrimal gland undergoes structural and functional alterations with age, which may play a role in acquired dry-eye disease.

The lacrimal artery, a branch of the ophthalmic artery, supplies the gland with blood. The lacrimal gland receives secretomotor cholinergic, vasoactive intestinal polypeptide (VIP)-ergic, and sympathetic nerve fibers in addition to sensory innervation via

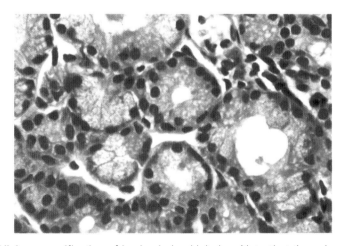

Figure 1-29 Higher magnification of lacrimal gland lobules. Note that the acinar cells forming the lobules are surrounded by myoepithelial cells that contain flattened nuclei (H&E, ×64). *(Courtesy of Thomas A. Weingeist, PhD, MD.)*

the lacrimal nerve (CN V$_1$). Cyclic adenosine monophosphate is the second messenger for VIP-ergic and β-adrenergic stimulation of the gland; cholinergic stimulation acts through inositol 1,4,5-triphosphate–activated protein kinase C. The gland also contains α$_1$-adrenergic receptors. The gland's extremely complex neuroanatomy governs both reflex and psychogenic stimulation (see BCSC Section 5, *Neuro-Ophthalmology*).

Rocha EM, Alves M, Rios JD, Dartt DA. The aging lacrimal gland: changes in structure and function. *Ocul Surf.* 2008;6(4):162–174.

Accessory Glands

The accessory lacrimal *glands of Krause* and *Wolfring* are located at the proximal lid borders or in the fornices and are cytologically identical to the main lacrimal gland; they receive similar innervation (see Fig 1-21). They account for approximately 10% of the total lacrimal secretory mass.

Lacrimal Excretory System

The lacrimal drainage system includes the upper and lower puncta, the lacrimal canaliculi, the lacrimal sac, and the nasolacrimal duct (Fig 1-30). The lacrimal papillae are located at the extreme nasal border of the eyelids at their junction with the inner canthus. The puncta are directed posteriorly into the tear lake at the inner canthus. Each tiny opening, or *lacrimal punctum*, has a diameter of approximately 0.3 mm. The inferior punctum is approximately 6.5 mm from the medial canthus; the superior punctum is 6.0 mm from it. The lower eyelid punctum sits closer to the corneal limbus due to the growth of the maxillary sinus, which draws the lower eyelid punctum laterally. These openings lead to the *lacrimal canaliculi,* the *lacrimal sac,* and finally the *nasolacrimal duct,* which, in turn,

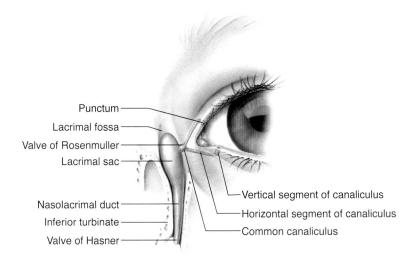

Figure 1-30 The lacrimal drainage system. *(Reproduced with permission from Katowitz JA, ed.* Pediatric Oculoplastic Surgery. *Philadelphia: Springer-Verlag; 2002.)*

leads to the nose. In 90% of people, the canaliculi join to form a common canaliculus. A persistent membrane over the valve of Hasner is often associated with tearing and discharge in infants.

The lacrimal puncta and the canaliculi are lined with stratified squamous nonkeratinized epithelium that merges with the epithelium of the eyelid margins. Near the lacrimal sac, the epithelium changes into 2 layers:

1. a superficial columnar layer
2. a deep, flattened cell layer

Goblet cells and occasionally cilia are present. In the canaliculi, the substantia propria consists of collagenous connective tissue and elastic fibers. The wall of the lacrimal sac resembles adenoid tissue and has a rich venous plexus and many elastic fibers.

For further discussion of the lacrimal system, see BCSC Section 7, *Orbit, Eyelids, and Lacrimal System.*

Cassady JV. Developmental anatomy of nasolacrimal duct. *AMA Arch Ophthalmol.* 1952; 47(2):141–158.

Conjunctiva

The conjunctiva can be divided into 3 geographic zones: palpebral, forniceal, and bulbar. The *palpebral conjunctiva* begins at the mucocutaneous junction of the eyelid and covers the lid's inner surface. This part adheres firmly to the tarsus. The tissue becomes redundant and freely movable in the fornices *(forniceal conjunctiva),* where it becomes enmeshed with fibrous elements of the levator aponeurosis and the Müller muscle in the upper eyelid. In the lower eyelid, fibrous expansions of the inferior rectus muscle sheath fuse with the inferior tarsal muscle, the equivalent of the Müller muscle. The conjunctiva is reflected at the cul-de-sac and attaches to the globe. The delicate *bulbar conjunctiva* is freely movable but fuses with the Tenon capsule and inserts into the limbus.

Anterior ciliary arteries supply blood to the bulbar conjunctiva. The tarsal conjunctiva is supplied by branches of the marginal arcades of the lids. The proximal arcade, running along the upper border of the lid, sends branches proximally to supply the forniceal conjunctiva and then the bulbar conjunctiva as the posterior conjunctival arteries. The limbal blood supply derives from the ciliary arteries through the anterior conjunctival arteries. The vascular watershed between the anterior and posterior territories lies approximately 3–4 mm from the limbus. The innervation of the conjunctiva is derived from the ophthalmic division of CN V.

The conjunctiva is a mucous membrane consisting of nonkeratinizing squamous epithelium with numerous goblet cells and a thin, richly vascularized substantia propria containing lymphatic vessels, plasma cells, macrophages, and mast cells. A lymphoid layer extends from the bulbar conjunctiva to the subtarsal folds of the lids. In places, specialized aggregations of *conjunctiva-associated lymphoid tissue (CALT)* correspond to *mucosa-associated lymphoid tissue (MALT)* elsewhere and comprise collections of T and B lymphocytes underlying a modified epithelium. These regions are concerned with antigen processing.

The thickness of the conjunctival epithelium varies from 2 to 5 cells. The basal cells are cuboidal and evolve into flattened polyhedral cells as they reach the surface. The goblet cells (unicellular mucous glands) are concentrated in the inferior and medial portions of the conjunctiva, especially in the region of the caruncle and plica semilunaris. They are sparsely distributed throughout the remainder of the conjunctiva and are absent in the limbal region.

Knop N, Knop E. Conjunctiva-associated lymphoid tissue in the human eye. *Invest Ophthalmol Vis Sci.* 2000;41(6):1270–1279.

Tenon Capsule

The Tenon capsule (the *fascia bulbi*) is an envelope of elastic connective tissue that fuses posteriorly with the optic nerve sheath and anteriorly with a thin layer of tissue called the *intermuscular septum,* which is located 3 mm posterior to the limbus. The Tenon capsule is the cavity within which the globe moves. It is composed of compactly arranged collagen fibers and a few fibroblasts.

The Tenon capsule is thickest in the area of the equator of the globe. Connections between the Tenon capsule and the periorbital tissues help suspend the globe in the orbit. The extraocular muscles penetrate this connective tissue approximately 10 mm posterior to their insertions. The connective tissues form sleeves around the penetrating extraocular muscles, creating pulleys suspended from the periorbita. These pulleys stabilize the position of the muscles relative to the orbit during eye movements. The pulleys are connected to one another and to the Tenon fascia by connective tissue bands containing collagen, elastin, and smooth muscle (Fig 1-31). Age-related connective tissue degeneration can lead to acquired strabismus.

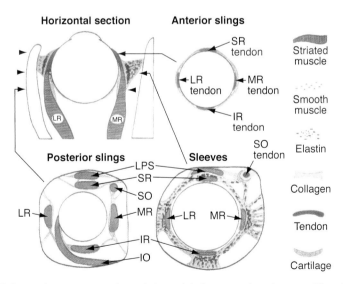

Figure 1-31 Schematic representation of the orbital connective tissues. IR = inferior rectus; LPS = levator palpebrae superioris; LR = lateral rectus; MR = medial rectus; SO = superior oblique; SR = superior rectus. *(Reproduced with permission from Demer JL, Miller JM, Pouken V, Vinters HV, Glasgow BJ. Evidence for fibromuscular pulleys of the recti extraocular muscles. Invest Ophthalmol Vis Sci. 1995;36(6): 1125. © Association for Research in Vision and Ophthalmology.)*

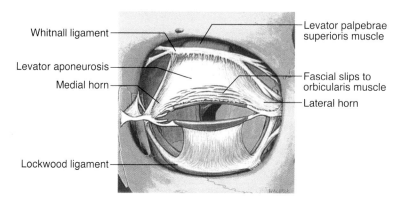

Whitnall ligament

Levator palpebrae
superioris muscle

Levator aponeurosis
Medial horn

Fascial slips to
orbicularis muscle
Lateral horn

Lockwood ligament

Figure 1-32 The upper and lower tarsal plates and their attachments to the levator aponeurosis and to the Whitnall ligament. *(Reproduced with permission from Dutton JJ.* Atlas of Clinical and Surgical Orbital Anatomy. *Philadelphia: Saunders; 1994.)*

The suspensory *ligament of Lockwood* is a fusion of the sheath of the inferior rectus muscle, the inferior tarsal muscle, and the check ligaments of the medial and lateral rectus muscles (Fig 1-32). It provides support for the globe and the anteroinferior orbit. The fusion of the sheath of the inferior rectus muscles, the Lockwood ligament, and the inferior tarsal muscle is an important consideration in surgery, because an operation on the inferior rectus muscle may be associated with palpebral fissure changes.

Demer JL. Mechanics of the orbita. *Dev Ophthalmol.* 2007;40:132–157.

Rutar T, Demer JL. "Heavy eye" syndrome in the absence of high myopia: a connective tissue degeneration in elderly strabismic patients. *J AAPOS.* 2009;13(1):36–44. Epub 2008 Oct 18.

Vascular Supply and Drainage of the Orbit

Posterior and Anterior Ciliary Arteries

Approximately 20 short posterior ciliary arteries and 10 short posterior ciliary nerves enter the globe in a ring around the optic nerve (Figs 1-33 through 1-35). Usually, 2 long ciliary arteries and nerves enter the sclera on either side of the optic nerve close to the horizontal meridian. The course of these vessels can usually be followed for a short distance in the suprachoroidal space. The posterior ciliary vessels originate from the ophthalmic artery and supply the whole uveal tract, the cilioretinal arteries, the sclera, the margin of the cornea, and the adjacent conjunctiva. Occlusion of the posterior ciliary vessels (as in giant cell arteritis) may have profound consequences for the eye, such as anterior ischemic optic neuropathy.

The anterior ciliary arteries also arise from the ophthalmic artery and usually supply (in pairs) the superior, medial, and inferior rectus muscles (Figs 1-36, 1-37). A single anterior ciliary vessel enters the lateral rectus muscle from the lacrimal artery. The anterior and posterior ciliary vessels usually anastomose with the long posterior ciliary vessels

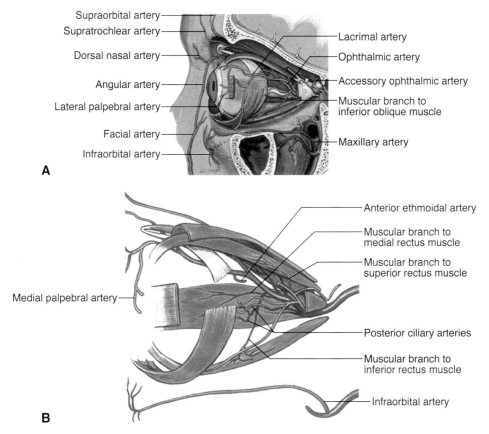

Supraorbital artery
Supratrochlear artery
Dorsal nasal artery
Angular artery
Lateral palpebral artery
Facial artery
Infraorbital artery

Lacrimal artery
Ophthalmic artery
Accessory ophthalmic artery
Muscular branch to
inferior oblique muscle
Maxillary artery

A

Anterior ethmoidal artery
Muscular branch to
medial rectus muscle
Muscular branch to
superior rectus muscle

Medial palpebral artery

Posterior ciliary arteries
Muscular branch to
inferior rectus muscle

Infraorbital artery

B

Figure 1-33 Orbital arteries. **A,** Lateral view with extraocular muscles, composite view. **B,** Central dissection. *(Reproduced with permission from Dutton JJ. Atlas of Clinical and Surgical Orbital Anatomy. Philadelphia: Saunders; 1994.)*

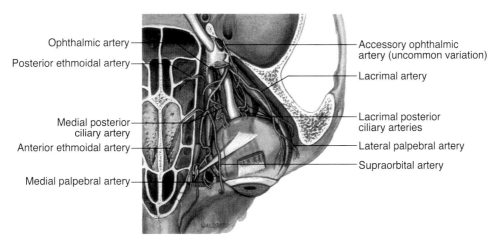

Ophthalmic artery
Posterior ethmoidal artery

Medial posterior
ciliary artery
Anterior ethmoidal artery

Medial palpebral artery

Accessory ophthalmic
artery (uncommon variation)
Lacrimal artery

Lacrimal posterior
ciliary arteries
Lateral palpebral artery
Supraorbital artery

Figure 1-34 Orbital arteries, superior composite view. *(Reproduced with permission from Dutton JJ. Atlas of Clinical and Surgical Orbital Anatomy. Philadelphia: Saunders; 1994.)*

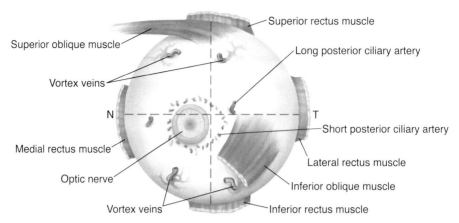

Figure 1-35 Posterior view of the right globe. N = nasal; T = temporal. *(Modified by Cyndie Wooley from illustration by Thomas A. Weingeist, PhD, MD.)*

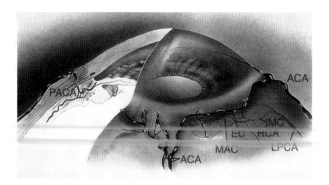

Figure 1-36 Three-dimensional representation of the multilevel collateral circulation in the primate anterior uvea in both surface and cutaway views. To the left, in cross section, perforating branches of the anterior ciliary artery are shown as they pass through the sclera to supply the intramuscular circle and major arterial circle. ACA = anterior ciliary artery; EC = episcleral circle; IMC = intramuscular circle; LPCA = long posterior ciliary artery; MAC = major arterial circle; PACA = posterior perforating anterior ciliary artery; RCA = recurrent ciliary artery. *(Reproduced with permission from Morrison JC, Van Buskirk EM. Anterior collateral circulation in the primate eye. Ophthalmology. 1983;90(6):707.)*

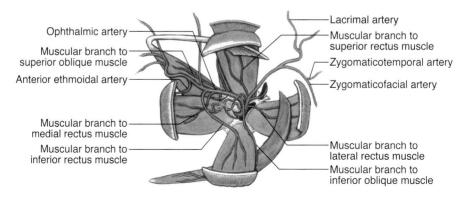

Figure 1-37 Orbital arteries, frontal view with extraocular muscles. *(Reproduced with permission from Dutton JJ. Atlas of Clinical and Surgical Orbital Anatomy. Philadelphia: Saunders; 1994.)*

via anastomoses that perforate the sclera anterior to the rectus muscle insertions. Within the eye, the posterior ciliary vessel forms the intramuscular circle of the iris, from which branches supply the major arterial circle (which is usually discontinuous). This circle lies within the apex of the ciliary muscle, which it supplies together with the iris. The iris vessels have a radial arrangement that is visible upon slit-lamp examination in lightly pigmented blue irises. This radial arrangement can be distinguished from the irregular new iris vessels formed in rubeosis iridis.

Vortex Veins

The vortex veins drain the venous system of the choroid, ciliary body, and iris (see Fig 1-35). Each eye contains 4–7 (or more) veins. One or more veins are usually located in each quadrant and exit 14–25 mm from the limbus between the rectus muscles. The ampullae of the vortex veins are 8–9 mm from the ora serrata and are visible by indirect ophthalmoscopy. A circle connecting these ampullae corresponds roughly to the equator and divides the central or posterior fundus from the peripheral portion. The vortex veins join the orbital venous system after leaving the eye (Fig 1-38).

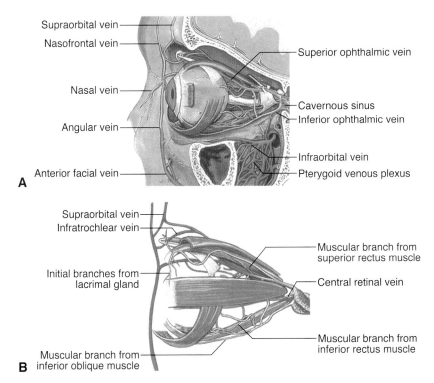

Figure 1-38 Orbital veins, lateral view. **A,** Composite view. **B,** Central dissection. *(Reproduced with permission from Dutton JJ. Atlas of Clinical and Surgical Orbital Anatomy. Philadelphia: Saunders; 1994.)*

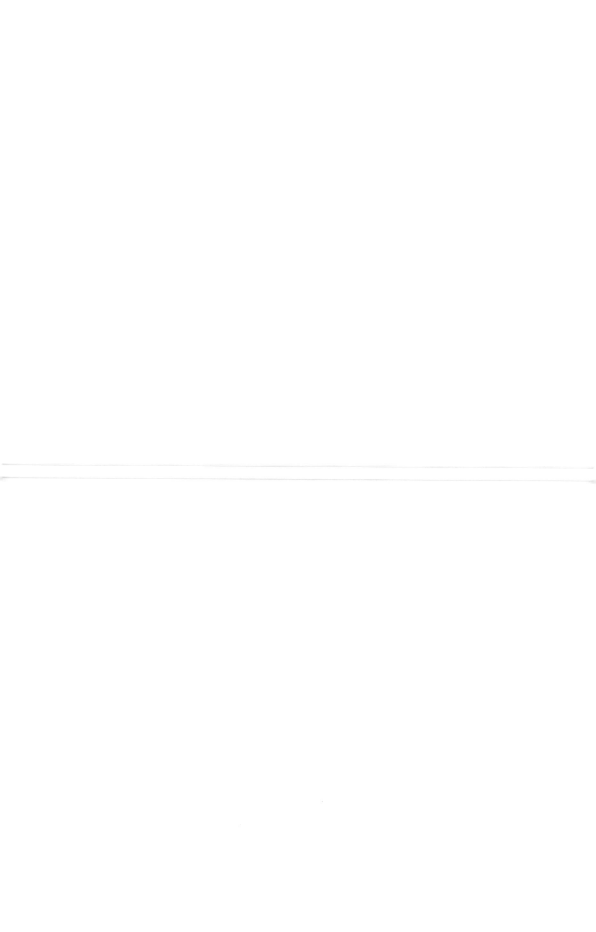

CHAPTER 2

The Eye

Topographic Features of the Globe

The eyeball, or globe, is not a true sphere. The radius of curvature of the cornea (8 mm) is smaller than that of the sclera (12 mm), making the shape of the globe an oblate spheroid (Fig 2-1). The anteroposterior diameter of the adult eye is approximately 23–25 mm. Myopic eyes tend to be longer, and hyperopic eyes tend to be shorter. The average transverse diameter of the adult eye is 24 mm.

The eye contains 3 compartments: the anterior chamber, the posterior chamber, and the vitreous cavity. The anterior chamber, the space between the iris and the cornea, is filled with aqueous fluid. It is approximately 3 mm deep and has an average volume of 200 μL. The posterior chamber is the anatomical portion of the eye posterior to the iris and anterior to the lens and vitreous face. It is also filled with aqueous fluid and has an average volume of 60 μL. The largest compartment is the vitreous cavity, which makes up

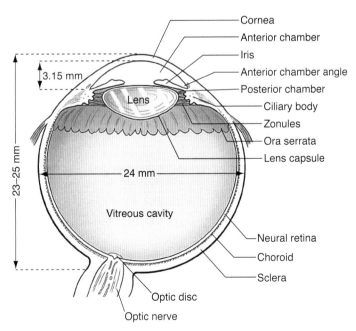

Figure 2-1 Sagittal section of eye with absent vitreous and major structures identified. Dimensions are approximate and are average for the normal adult eye. *(Illustration by Christine Gralapp.)*

more than two-thirds of the volume of the eye (5–6 mL) and contains the vitreous gel. The total volume of the average adult eye is approximately 6.5–7.0 mL.

The eyeball is composed of 3 concentric layers. The outermost layer consists of the clear *cornea* anteriorly and the opaque white *sclera* posteriorly. The outermost corneo-scleral layer is composed of tough and protective tissues.

The cornea occupies the center of the anterior pole of the globe. Because the sclera and conjunctiva overlap the cornea anteriorly, slightly more above and below than medi-ally and laterally, the cornea appears elliptical when viewed from the front. In adults, it measures about 12 mm in the horizontal meridian and about 11 mm in the vertical. From behind, when the cornea is viewed at its posterior landmark (the Schwalbe line—the ter-mination of the Descemet membrane), its circumference appears circular. The cornea is approximately 1 mm thick at its periphery and 0.5 mm thick centrally. The limbus, which borders the cornea and the sclera, is gray and translucent.

The middle layer of the globe is the *uvea*, which consists of the choroid, ciliary body, and iris. Highly vascular, it serves nutritive and supportive functions.

The innermost layer of the globe is the *retina*. This photosensitive layer contains the photoreceptors and neural elements that initiate the processing of visual information. Other important surface features of the globe, such as the vortex veins, the posterior cili-ary artery and nerves, and extraocular muscle insertions are discussed in Chapter 1; the optic nerve and its surrounding meningeal sheaths are discussed in Chapter 3.

Precorneal Tear Film

The exposed surfaces of the cornea and globe are covered by the precorneal tear film, which is composed conceptually of 3 layers:

1. a *superficial oily layer* produced predominantly by the meibomian glands
2. a *middle aqueous layer* produced by the main and accessory lacrimal glands
3. a *deep mucin layer* derived from the conjunctival goblet cells

Maintenance of the precorneal tear film is vital for normal corneal function. In addition to lubricating the surface of the cornea and conjunctiva, tears produce a smooth optical sur-face; allow for the diffusion of oxygen and other nutrients; and contain immunoglobulins, lysozyme, and lactoferrin. Aberrations in the tear film result from a variety of diseases (eg, dry eye, blepharitis) that can profoundly affect the integrity of the surface and conse-quently the patient's vision.

Cornea

Characteristics of the Central and Peripheral Cornea

The air–tear film interface at the surface of the cornea forms a positive lens of approxi-mately 43 diopters (D) in air and constitutes the main refractive element of the eye

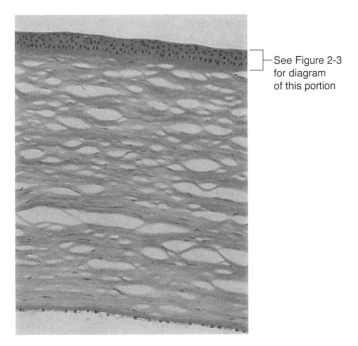

See Figure 2-3
for diagram
of this portion

Figure 2-2 Cornea. The empty spaces in the stroma are artifactitious (H&E ×32). *(Courtesy of Thomas A. Weingeist, PhD, MD.)*

(Fig 2-2). The central third of the cornea is nearly spherical and measures approximately 4 mm in diameter in the normal eye. Because the posterior surface of the cornea is more curved than the anterior surface, the central cornea is thinner (0.5 mm) than the peripheral cornea (1.0 mm). The cornea becomes flatter in the periphery, but the rate of flattening is not symmetric. Flattening is more extensive nasally and superiorly than temporally and inferiorly. This topography is important in contact lens fitting. BCSC Section 8, *External Disease and Cornea,* discusses the cornea in detail.

Epithelium and Basal Lamina

The anterior surface of the cornea is derived from surface ectoderm and is covered by a nonkeratinized, stratified squamous epithelium whose basal columnar layer is attached to a basal lamina by hemidesmosomes (Fig 2-3). The basal cells have a width of 12 μm and a density of approximately 6000 cells/mm². The occasional recurrence of corneal erosion following a traumatic corneal abrasion may be due to improper formation of hemidesmosomes after an epithelial abrasion.

Overlying the basal cell layer are 2 or 3 layers of polygonal "wing" cells. The superficial corneal epithelial cells are extremely thin (30 μm) and are attached to one another by occlusion of the zonular fibers (sometimes referred to as zonules). These zonular fibers confer the properties of a semipermeable membrane to the epithelium. Microplicae and microvilli make the apical surfaces of the wing cells highly irregular; however, the

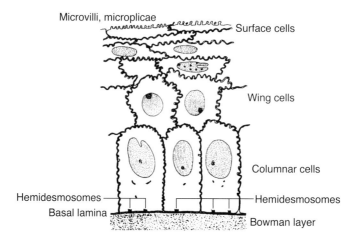

Figure 2-3 The corneal epithelium and Bowman layer, showing hemidesmosomes along the basal lamina. *(Illustration by Thomas A. Weingeist, PhD, MD.)*

precorneal tear film renders the surfaces optically smooth. Although the deeper epithelial cells are firmly attached to one another by desmosomes, they migrate continuously from the basal region toward the tear film, into which they are shed. They also migrate centripetally from their stem cell source at the limbus. Division of the slow-cycling stem cells gives rise to a progeny of daughter cells (transient amplifying cells), whose division serves to maintain the corneal epithelium. Diffuse damage to the limbal stem cells (eg, by chemical burns or trachoma) leads to chronic epithelial surface defects.

Fine BS, Yanoff M. *Ocular Histology: A Text and Atlas.* 2nd ed. Hagerstown, MD: Harper & Row; 1979:163–168.

Nonepithelial Cells

Nonepithelial cells may appear within the corneal epithelial layer. Wandering histiocytes, macrophages, lymphocytes, and pigmented melanocytes are usually components of the peripheral cornea. Antigen-presenting Langerhans cells are found peripherally and move centrally with age or in response to keratitis.

Bowman Layer

Beneath the basal lamina is the Bowman layer, or Bowman membrane, a tough layer consisting of randomly dispersed collagen fibrils. It is a modified region of the anterior stroma that is 8–12 µm thick. Unlike the Descemet membrane, it is not restored after injury but rather is replaced by scar tissue.

Stroma

The stroma constitutes approximately 90% of the total corneal thickness in humans (see Fig 2-5). It is composed of collagen-producing keratocytes, ground substance, and collagen lamellae. The collagen fibrils form obliquely oriented lamellae in the anterior third of the stroma (with some interlacing) and parallel lamellae in the posterior two-thirds. The corneal collagen fibrils extend across the entire diameter of the cornea, finally winding circumferentially around the limbus. The fibrils are remarkably uniform in size and separation, and this regularity helps determine the transparency of the cornea. Separation of the collagen fibrils by edema fluid leads to stromal clouding. The macroperiodicity of the fibrils (640 Å) is typical of collagen. The stroma's collagen types are I, III, V, and VI. Type VII forms the anchoring fibril of the epithelium.

The ground substance of the cornea consists of proteoglycans that run along and between the collagen fibrils. Their glycosaminoglycan components (eg, keratan sulfate) are highly charged and account for the swelling property of the stroma. The keratocytes lie between the corneal lamellae and synthesize both collagen and proteoglycans. Ultrastructurally, they resemble fibrocytes.

The cornea has approximately 2.4 million keratocytes, which occupy about 5% of the stromal volume; the density is higher anteriorly (1058 cells/mm^2) than posteriorly (771 cells/mm^2). Keratocytes are highly active cells rich in mitochondria, rough endoplasmic reticula, and Golgi apparatuses. They have attachment structures, communicate by gap junctions, and have unusual fenestrations in their plasma membranes. Their flat profile and even distribution in the coronal plane ensure a minimum disturbance of light transmission. Studies with vital dyes suggest that there may be at least 3 different types of keratocytes.

Müller LJ, Pels L, Vrensen GF. Novel aspects of the ultrastructural organization of human corneal keratocytes. *Invest Ophthalmol Vis Sci.* 1995;36(13):2557–2567.

Mustonen RK, McDonald MB, Srivannaboon S, Tan AL, Doubrava MW, Kim CK. Normal human corneal cell populations evaluated by in vivo scanning slit confocal microscopy. *Cornea.* 1998;17(5):485–492.

Descemet Membrane

The basal lamina of the corneal endothelium, the Descemet membrane, is periodic acid–Schiff (PAS) positive (Fig 2-4). It is a true basement membrane, and its thickness increases with age. At birth, the Descemet membrane is 3–4 μm thick; its thickness increases to 10–12 μm at adulthood. It is composed of an anterior banded zone that develops in utero and a posterior nonbanded zone that is laid down by the corneal endothelium throughout life (Fig 2-5). These zones provide a historical record of the synthetic function of the endothelium. Like other basal laminae, the Descemet membrane is rich in type IV collagen.

Peripheral excrescences of the Descemet membrane, known as *Hassall-Henle warts*, are common, especially among elderly people. Central excrescences (cornea guttae) also appear with increasing age.

Endothelium

The corneal endothelium is composed of a single layer of mostly hexagonal cells derived from the neural crest (Fig 2-6). Therefore, the corneal endothelium is of neuroectodermal origin. Approximately 500,000 cells are present, at a density of about 3000/mm^2.

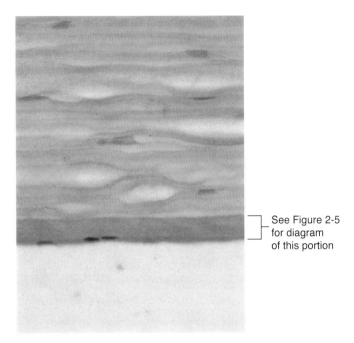

See Figure 2-5
for diagram
of this portion

Figure 2-4 Posterior cornea. Note the appearance of the Descemet membrane and the corneal endothelium (H&E ×64). *(Courtesy of Thomas A. Weingeist, PhD, MD.)*

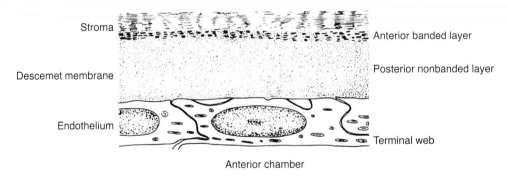

Figure 2-5 Corneal endothelium and the Descemet membrane. *(Illustration by Thomas A. Weingeist, PhD, MD.)*

The size, shape, and morphology of the endothelial cells can be observed by specular microscopy at the slit lamp. The apical surfaces of these cells face the anterior chamber; their basal surfaces abut the Descemet membrane. Typically, young endothelial cells have large nuclei and abundant mitochondria. The active transport of ions by these cells leads to the transfer of water from the corneal stroma and the maintenance of stromal deturgescence and transparency. Mitosis of the endothelium is rare in humans, and the overall number of endothelial cells decreases with age.

Adjacent endothelial cells interdigitate in a complex way and form a variety of adherent junctions, but desmosomes are never observed between normal cells. In cross section, pinocytotic vesicles and a terminal web (a meshwork of fine fibrils that increases the

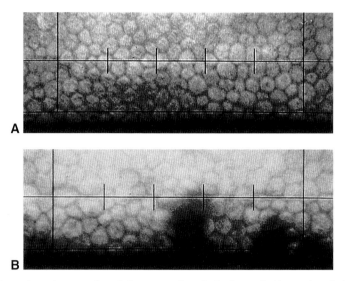

Figure 2-6 Specular micrographs of the corneal endothelium. **A,** Normal endothelium. **B,** Endothelium of a patient with Fuchs endothelial dystrophy, showing larger, more irregular cells (polymegethism); the 3 dark areas toward the bottom are cornea guttae. Both images were taken at the same magnification. *(Courtesy of David Palay, MD, and David Litoff, MD.)*

density of the cytoplasm) can be observed toward the apical surface of the cells. Junctional complexes are present at the overlapping apicolateral boundaries of contiguous cells. They form a significant but lesser barrier to ion and water flow than do the tight junctions of the epithelium.

Endothelial cell dysfunction and loss—through surgical injury, inflammation, or inherited disease (eg, Fuchs endothelial dystrophy)—may cause endothelial decompensation, stromal edema, and vision failure. In humans, endothelial mitosis is limited, and destruction of cells causes cell density to decrease and residual cells to spread and enlarge.

Foster CS, Azar DT, Dohlman CH. *Smolin and Thoft's The Cornea: Scientific Foundations and Clinical Practice.* 4th ed. Philadelphia: Lippincott Williams & Wilkins; 2004.

Sclera

The sclera covers the posterior four-fifths of the surface of the globe, with an anterior opening for the cornea and a posterior opening for the optic nerve. The tendons of the rectus muscles insert into the superficial scleral collagen. The Tenon capsule covers the sclera and rectus muscles anteriorly, and both are overlain by the bulbar conjunctiva. The capsule and conjunctiva fuse near the limbus.

The sclera is thinnest (0.3 mm) just behind the insertions of the rectus muscles and thickest (1.0 mm) at the posterior pole around the optic nerve head. It is 0.4–0.5 mm thick at the equator and 0.6 mm thick anterior to the muscle insertions. Because of the thinness of the sclera, strabismus and retinal detachment surgery require careful placement of sutures. Scleral rupture following blunt trauma can occur at several sites: in a circumferential arc parallel to the corneal limbus opposite the site of impact, at the insertion of the rectus muscles, or at the equator of the globe. The most common site is the superonasal quadrant near the limbus.

The sclera, like the cornea, is essentially avascular except for the superficial vessels of the episclera and the intrascleral vascular plexus located just posterior to the limbus. Numerous channels, or *emissaria,* penetrate the sclera, allowing for the passage of arteries, veins, and nerves. Extraocular extension of malignant melanoma of the choroid often occurs by way of the emissaria.

Branches of the ciliary nerves that supply the cornea sometimes leave the sclera to form loops posterior to the nasal and temporal limbus. These nerve loops, called *Axenfeld loops,* are sometimes pigmented and, consequently, have been mistaken for uveal tissue or malignant melanoma.

Anteriorly, the episclera consists of a dense vascular connective tissue that merges deeply with the superficial sclera and superficially with the Tenon capsule and the conjunctiva. The scleral stroma is composed of bundles of collagen, fibroblasts, and a moderate amount of ground substance. Collagen fibrils of the sclera vary in size and shape and taper at their ends, indicating that they are not continuous fibers as in the cornea. In general, the outer scleral collagen fibers have a larger diameter (1600 Å) than the inner collagen fibers have (1000 Å). The inner layer of the sclera *(lamina fusca)* blends imperceptibly with the suprachoroidal and supraciliary lamellae of the uveal tract. The collagen fibers in this portion of the sclera branch and intermingle with the outer ciliary body and choroid. The bundles of collagen fibers contain electron-dense bodies, fibroblasts, and melanocytes. The opaque, porcelain-white appearance of the sclera contrasts markedly with the transparency of the cornea and is primarily due to 2 factors: (1) the greater variation in fibril separation and diameter and (2) the greater degree of fibril interweaving in the sclera. In addition, the lack of vascular elements, such as the scleral emissaria, contributes to corneal clarity.

Limbus

The transition zone between the peripheral cornea and the anterior sclera, known as the limbus, is defined differently by anatomists, pathologists, and clinicians. Although not a distinct anatomical structure, the limbus is important for 2 reasons: (1) its relationship to the chamber angle and (2) its use as a surgical landmark. The following 5 structures are included in the limbus:

1. conjunctiva and limbal palisades
2. Tenon capsule
3. episclera
4. corneoscleral stroma
5. aqueous outflow apparatus

The transition from opaque sclera to clear cornea occurs gradually over 1.0–1.5 mm and is difficult to define histologically. The corneoscleral junction begins centrally in a plane connecting the end of the Bowman layer and the *Schwalbe line,* which is the termination of the Descemet membrane. Internally, its posterior limit is the anterior tip of the scleral

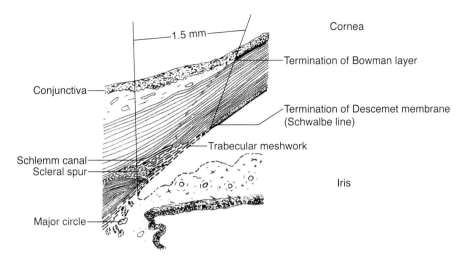

Figure 2-7 Anterior chamber angle and limbus, depicting the concept of the limbus. *Solid lines* represent the limbus as viewed by pathologists; the *green dotted line* represents the limbus as viewed by anatomists. *(Illustration by Thomas A. Weingeist, PhD, MD.)*

spur. Pathologists consider the posterior limit of the limbus to be formed by another plane perpendicular to the surface of the eye, approximately 1.5 mm posterior to the termination of the Bowman layer in the horizontal meridian and 2.0 mm posterior in the vertical meridian, where there is greater scleral overlap (Fig 2-7).

The surgical limbus can be divided conceptually into 2 equal zones: (1) an anterior bluish-gray zone overlying the clear cornea and extending from the Bowman layer to the Schwalbe line and (2) a posterior white zone overlying the trabecular meshwork and extending from the Schwalbe line to the scleral spur, or iris root.

Anterior Chamber

The anterior chamber is bordered anteriorly by the cornea and posteriorly by the iris diaphragm and the pupil. The anterior chamber angle, which lies at the junction of the cornea and the iris, consists of the following 5 structures (Fig 2-8):

1. Schwalbe line
2. Schlemm canal and trabecular meshwork
3. scleral spur
4. anterior border of the ciliary body (where its longitudinal fibers insert into the scleral spur)
5. iris

The depth of the anterior chamber varies. It is deeper in aphakia, pseudophakia, and myopia and shallower in hyperopia. In the normal adult emmetropic eye, the anterior chamber is approximately 3 mm deep at its center and reaches its narrowest point slightly

Figure 2-8 Semidiagrammatic representation of the structures of the angle of the anterior chamber and ciliary body. **A,** Composite gonioscopic and cross-sectional view of the anterior segment of the eye. **B,** Enlarged view. Note the superimposed trabecular sheets with intratrabecular spaces through which aqueous humor percolates to reach the Schlemm canal. C = cornea; CB = ciliary body; I = iris; IP = iris process; S = sclera; SC = Schlemm canal; SL = Schwalbe line; SS = scleral spur; TM = trabecular meshwork; Z = zonular fibers. *(Reproduced with permission from Tripathi RC, Tripathi BJ. Functional anatomy of the anterior chamber angle. In: Jakobiec FA, ed. Ocular Anatomy, Embryology, and Teratology. Philadelphia: Harper & Row; 1982.)*

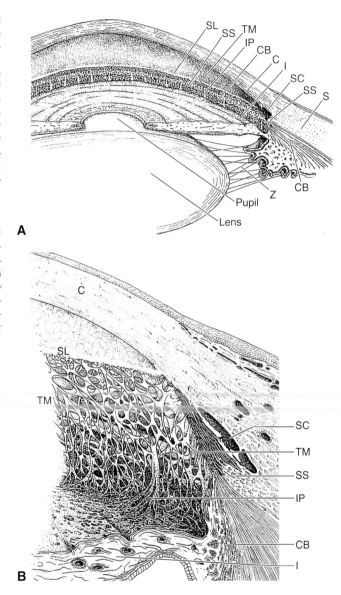

central to the angle recess. The volume of the anterior chamber is approximately 200 μL in the emmetropic eye.

The anterior chamber is filled with *aqueous humor,* which is produced by the ciliary epithelium in the posterior chamber. The fluid passes through the pupil aperture and drains chiefly by the conventional pathway through the trabecular meshwork into the Schlemm canal and partly by the nontrabecular uveoscleral drainage pathway, across the ciliary body into the supraciliary space. The uveoscleral pathway, thought to be influenced by age, accounts for up to 50% of aqueous outflow in young people. BCSC Section 10, *Glaucoma,* discusses the anterior chamber and aqueous humor in detail.

High-resolution ultrasound biomicroscopy provides detailed 2-dimensional views of the anterior segment of the eye and is performed in vivo (Fig 2-9), allowing the clinician to view the relationship of the structures in the anterior segment under different pathologic conditions.

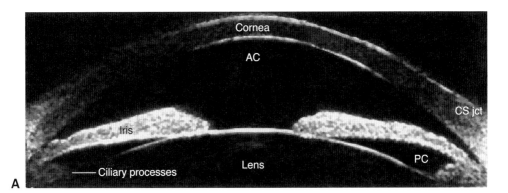

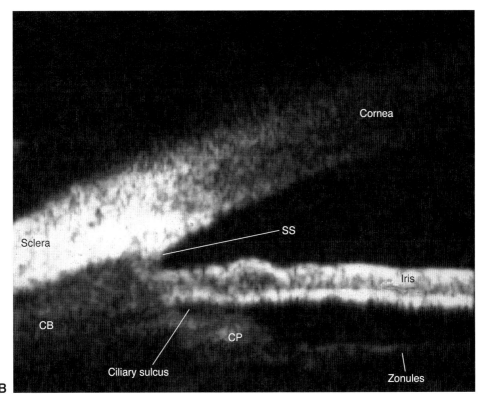

Figure 2-9 **A,** Ultrasound biomicroscopic composite image of the anterior segment, including the anterior chamber (AC). The iris is slightly convex, indicating mild pupillary block. The corneoscleral junction (CS jct), ciliary processes, and posterior chamber (PC) region are clearly imaged. The angle is narrow but open. Iris–lens contact is small. **B,** High-resolution ultrasound image of the anterior segment. Note the location of the ciliary sulcus. CB = ciliary body; CP = ciliary process; SS = scleral spur. *(Part A courtesy of Charles Pavlin, MD; part B courtesy of K. Nischal, MD.)*

The internal scleral sulcus accommodates the Schlemm canal externally and the trabecular meshwork internally. The Schwalbe line, the periphery of the Descemet membrane, forms the anterior margin of the sulcus; the scleral spur is its posterior landmark. The scleral spur receives the insertion of the longitudinal ciliary muscle, and contraction opens up the trabecular spaces. Contractile cells are found within the scleral spur, as are structures resembling mechanoreceptors, which receive a sensory innervation.

Myofibroblast-like scleral spur cells with contractile properties are disposed circumferentially within the scleral spur. They are connected by elastic tissue to the trabecular meshwork; in experiments, stimulation with vasoactive intestinal polypeptide (VIP) or calcitonin gene–related peptide (CGRP) causes an increase in outflow facility. Individual scleral spur cells are innervated by unmyelinated axons, the terminals of which contact the cell membranes of the spur cells without an intervening basal lamina. The nerve fibers in this region are immunoreactive for neuropeptide Y, substance P, CGRP, VIP, and nitrous oxide; therefore, they are mediated by sympathetic, sensory, and pterygopalatine nerve pathways. There are no cholinergic fibers in this region. Myelinated nerve fibers extending forward from the ciliary region to the inner aspect of the scleral spur yield branches to the meshwork and to club-shaped endings in the scleral spur. These endings have the morphologic features of mechanoreceptors found elsewhere in the body, such as in the carotid artery. The endings are incompletely covered by a Schwann cell sheath and make contact with extracellular matrix materials such as elastin. Various functions have been proposed for these endings, including (1) proprioception to the ciliary muscle, which inserts into the scleral spur, signaling contraction of the scleral spur cells, and (2) baroreception in response to changes in intraocular pressure.

Tamm ER, Koch TA, Mayer B, Stefani FH, Lütjen-Drecoll E. Innervation of myofibroblast-like scleral spur cells in human and monkey eyes. *Invest Ophthalmol Vis Sci.* 1995;36(8):1633–1644.

Trabecular Meshwork

The relationship of the trabecular meshwork (see Figs 2-7, 2-8) and the Schlemm canal to other structures is complex because the outflow apparatus is composed of tissue derived from the cornea, sclera, iris, and ciliary body (Fig 2-10). The trabecular meshwork is a circular spongework of connective tissue lined by trabeculocytes. These cells have contractile properties, which may influence outflow resistance. They also have phagocytic properties. The meshwork is roughly triangular in cross section; the apex is at the Schwalbe line, and the base is formed by the scleral spur and the ciliary body. Some trabecular tissue passes posterior to the spur. The trabecular meshwork can be divided into 3 layers (see BCSC Section 10, *Glaucoma,* Chapter 2, Fig 2-3):

1. uveal portion
2. corneoscleral meshwork
3. juxtacanalicular tissue, which is directly adjacent to the Schlemm canal

The uveal portion and the corneoscleral meshwork can be divided by an imaginary line drawn from the Schwalbe line to the scleral spur. The uveal meshwork lies internal and the corneoscleral meshwork external to this line.

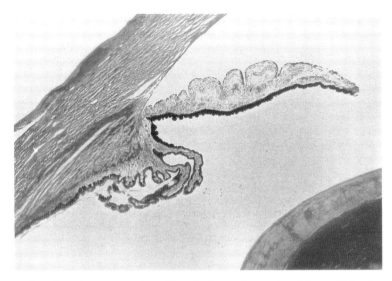

Figure 2-10 Anterior chamber angle, ciliary body, and peripheral lens. Note the triangular shape of the ciliary body. The muscle fibers appear red in contrast with the connective tissue. The scleral spur is clearly delineated from the ciliary muscle in the region of the trabecular meshwork. The lens is artifactually displaced posteriorly (Masson trichrome ×8). *(Courtesy of Thomas A. Weingeist, PhD, MD.)*

Uveal Trabecular Meshwork

The uveal meshwork is composed of cordlike trabeculae and has fewer elastic fibers than does the corneoscleral meshwork. The trabeculocytes usually contain pigment granules, and the trabecular apertures are less circular and larger than those of the corneoscleral meshwork.

Corneoscleral Meshwork

The corneoscleral meshwork consists of a series of thin, flat, perforated connective tissue sheets arranged in a laminar pattern. Each trabecular beam is covered by a monolayer of thin trabecular cells exhibiting multiple pinocytotic vesicles. The basal lamina of these cells forms the outer cortex of the trabecular beam; the inner core is composed of collagen and elastic fibers.

Aging changes to the trabecular meshwork include increased pigmentation, decreased number of trabecular cells, and thickening of the basement membrane beneath the trabecular cells. These changes can cause resistance to aqueous outflow or possibly glaucoma. This subject is covered in greater depth in BCSC Section 10, *Glaucoma*.

Pericanalicular Connective Tissue

Pericanalicular connective tissue invests the entire extent of the Schlemm canal. On its trabecular aspect, between the outermost layers of the corneoscleral meshwork and the endothelial lining of the Schlemm canal, lies the *endothelial meshwork,* a multilayered collection of cells forming a loose network. Between these cells are spaces up to 10 μm wide through which aqueous humor can percolate to reach the endothelial lining of the Schlemm canal. This region of the drainage system contributes the most to outflow resistance, partly because the pathway is narrow and tortuous and partly because of the resistance offered by extracellular proteoglycans and glycoproteins.

Schlemm Canal

The Schlemm canal is a circular tube that closely resembles a lymphatic vessel. It is formed by a continuous monolayer of nonfenestrated endothelium and a thin connective tissue wall. The basement membrane of the endothelium is poorly defined. The lateral walls of the endothelial cells are joined by tight junctions. Micropinocytotic vesicles are present at the apical and basal surfaces of the cells. Larger vesicles (so-called giant vacuoles) have been observed along the internal canal wall (Figs 2-11, 2-12). These vacuoles are lined

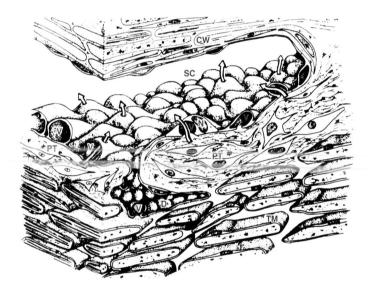

Figure 2-11 The walls of the Schlemm canal (SC) and adjacent trabecular meshwork (TM). The endothelial lining of the trabecular wall of the Schlemm canal is highly irregular; normally, the cells show luminal bulges corresponding to cell nuclei (N) and macrovacuolar configurations (V). The latter represent cellular invaginations from the basal aspect that eventually open on the apical aspect of the cell to form transcellular channels *(arrows)*, through which aqueous humor flows down a pressure gradient. A diverticulum (D)—its endothelial lining continuous with that of the canal—is shown on the inner wall of the Schlemm canal next to macrovacuolar configurations. Such blind, tortuous diverticula course for a variable distance into the trabecular meshwork but remain separated from the open spaces of the meshwork by their continuous endothelial lining. The endothelial lining of the trabecular wall is supported by interrupted, irregular basement membrane and a zone of pericanalicular connective tissue (PT) of variable thickness. The cellular element predominates in this zone, and the fibrous elements, especially elastic fibers, are irregularly arranged in a netlike fashion. Here, the open spaces are narrower than those of the trabecular meshwork. The corneoscleral trabecular sheets show frequent branching, and the endothelial covering may be shared between adjacent sheets. The corneoscleral wall (CW) of the Schlemm canal is more compact than the trabecular wall; a lamellar arrangement of collagen and elastic tissue predominates. *(Reproduced with permission from Tripathi RC, Tripathi BJ. Functional anatomy of the anterior chamber angle. In: Jakobiec FA, ed.* Ocular Anatomy, Embryology, and Teratology. *Philadelphia: Harper & Row; 1982.)*

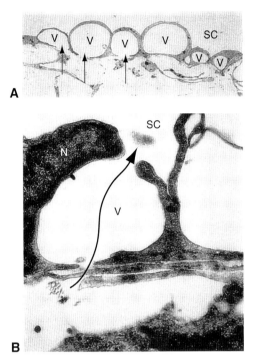

Figure 2-12 **A,** Low-magnification electron micrograph of the endothelial lining of the Schlemm canal (SC), showing that most of the vacuolar configurations (V) at this level have direct communication *(arrows)* with the subendothelial extracellular spaces, which contain aqueous humor (×3970). **B,** Electron micrograph of a vacuolar structure that shows both basal and apical openings, thus constituting a vacuolar transcellular channel *(arrow)*. Through this channel, the fluid-containing extracellular space on the basal aspect of the cell is temporarily connected with the lumen of the Schlemm canal, allowing bulk outflow of aqueous humor. N = indented nucleus of the cell (×23,825). *(Reproduced with permission from Tripathi RC. The functional morphology of the outflow systems of ocular and cerebospinal fluids. Exp Eye Res. 1977;25 Suppl:65–116.)*

by a single membrane, and their size and number are increased by a rise in intraocular pressure. They are thought to contribute to the pressure-dependent outflow of aqueous humor.

Collector Channels

Approximately 25–30 collector channels arise from the Schlemm canal (Fig 2-13) and drain into the deep and midscleral venous plexuses. Up to 8 of these channels drain directly into the episcleral venous plexus as aqueous veins (Fig 2-14), which are visible in the conjunctiva by biomicroscopy.

Aging causes a twofold to threefold thickening of trabecular sheets; the cortex thickens and the core thins. Endothelial cellularity is lost, connective tissue (eg, in the endothelial meshwork) increases, debris accumulates in the meshwork, and glycosaminoglycans accumulate in the extracellular space. Such changes are exaggerated in chronic open-angle glaucoma.

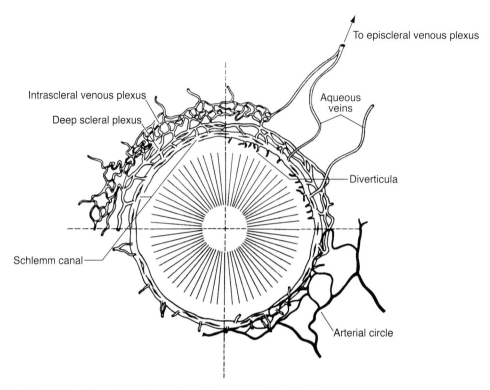

Figure 2-13   Schematic representation of the Schlemm canal and relationships of the arteriolar and venous vascular supply. For clarity, the various systems have been limited to only parts of the circumference of the canal. Small, tortuous, blind diverticula (so-called Sondermann channels) extend from the canal into the trabecular meshwork. Externally, the collector channels arising from the Schlemm canal anastomose to form the intrascleral and deep scleral venous plexuses. At irregular intervals around the circumference, aqueous veins arise from the intrascleral plexus and connect directly to the episcleral veins. The arteriolar supply closely approximates the canal, but no direct communication occurs between the two. *(Reproduced with permission from Tripathi RC, Tripathi BJ. Functional anatomy of the anterior chamber angle. In: Jakobiec FA, ed.* Ocular Anatomy, Embryology, and Teratology. *Philadelphia: Harper & Row; 1982:236.)*

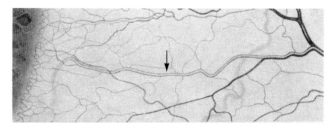

Figure 2-14   Aqueous vein *(arrow)*. Collector channels from the Schlemm canal drain into the episcleral venous plexus. With high magnification of the slit-lamp biomicroscope, they are visible near the limbus. Laminar flow and the mixing of aqueous and blood are visible. *(Reproduced with permission from Thiel R.* Atlas of Diseases of the Eye. *Amsterdam: Elsevier; 1963.)*

Uveal Tract

The uveal tract is the main vascular compartment of the eye. It consists of 3 parts:

1. iris
2. ciliary body (located in the anterior uvea)
3. choroid (located in the posterior uvea)

The uveal tract is firmly attached to the sclera at only 3 sites:

1. scleral spur
2. exit points of the vortex veins
3. optic nerve

These attachments account for the characteristic anterior balloons formed in choroidal detachment.

Iris

The iris is the most anterior extension of the uveal tract (Figs 2-15, 2-16). It is made of blood vessels and connective tissue, in addition to the melanocytes and pigment cells responsible for its distinctive color. The mobility of the iris allows the pupil to change size. During mydriasis, the iris is pulled into numerous ridges and folds; during miosis, its anterior surface appears relatively smooth. The iris diaphragm subdivides the anterior segment into the anterior and posterior chambers.

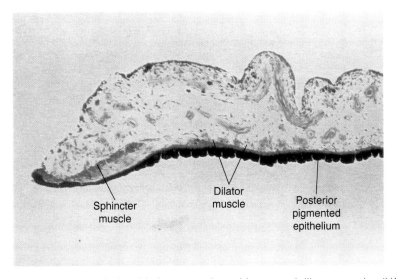

Figure 2-15 Iris. Note the relationship between the sphincter and dilator muscles (H&E ×20). *(Courtesy of Thomas A. Weingeist, PhD, MD.)*

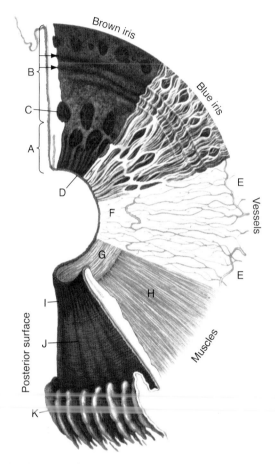

Figure 2-16 Composite drawing of the surfaces and layers of the iris, beginning at the upper left and proceeding clockwise. The iris cross section shows the pupillary (A) and ciliary (B) portions; the surface view shows a brown iris with its dense, matted anterior border layer. Circular contraction furrows are shown *(arrows)* in the ciliary portion of the iris. Fuchs crypts (C) are seen at either side of the collarette in the pupillary and ciliary portions and peripherally near the iris root. The pigment ruff is seen at the pupillary edge (D). The blue iris surface shows a less dense anterior border layer and more prominent trabeculae. The iris vessels are shown beginning at the major arterial circle in the ciliary body (E). Radial branches of the arteries and veins extend toward the pupillary region. The arteries form the incomplete minor arterial circle (F), from which branches extend toward the pupil, creating capillary arcades. The sector below demonstrates the circular arrangement of the sphincter muscle (G) and the radial processes of the dilator muscle (H). The posterior surface of the iris shows the radial contraction furrows (I) and the structural folds (J) of Schwalbe. Circular contraction folds are also present in the ciliary portion. The pars plicata of the ciliary body is shown at bottom (K). *(Reproduced with permission from Hogan MJ, Alvarado JA, and Weddell JE.* Histology of the Human Eye. *Philadelphia: WB Saunders; 1971.)*

Stroma

The iris stroma is composed of pigmented cells (melanocytes) and nonpigmented cells, collagen fibrils, and a matrix containing hyaluronic acid. The aqueous humor flows freely through the loose stroma along the anterior border of the iris, which contains multiple crypts and crevices that vary in size, shape, and depth. This surface is covered by an interrupted layer of connective tissue cells that merges with the ciliary body.

The overall structure of the iris stroma is similar in irides of all colors. Differences in color are related to the amount of pigmentation in the anterior border layer and the deep stroma. The stroma of blue irides is lightly pigmented, and brown irides have a densely pigmented stroma that absorbs light.

Vessels and Nerves

Blood vessels form the bulk of the iris stroma. Most follow a radial course, arising from the major arterial circle and passing to the center of the pupil. In the region of the *collarette* (the thickest portion of the iris), anastomoses occur between the arterial and venous arcades to form the minor vascular circle of the iris, which is often incomplete. The major arterial circle is located at the apex of the ciliary body, not the iris. In humans, the anterior border layer is normally avascular. The diameter of the capillaries is relatively large. Their endothelium is nonfenestrated and is surrounded by a basement membrane, associated pericytes, and a zone of collagenous filaments. The intima has no internal elastic lamina. Myelinated and nonmyelinated nerve fibers serve sensory, vasomotor, and muscular functions throughout the stroma.

Posterior Pigmented Layer

The posterior surface of the iris is densely pigmented and appears velvety smooth and uniform. It is continuous with the nonpigmented epithelium of the ciliary body and thence with the neurosensory portion of the retina. The polarity of its cells is maintained from embryogenesis. The basal surface of the pigmented layer borders the posterior chamber. The apical surface faces the stroma and adheres to the anterior pigmented layer, which gives rise to the dilator muscle (Fig 2-17).

The posterior pigmented layer of the iris curves around the pupillary margin and extends for a short distance onto the anterior border layer of the iris stroma as the pigment ruff. In rubeosis iridis, the pigmented layer extends farther onto the anterior surface of the iris, a condition called *ectropion*. The term *ectropion uveae,* which refers to an outfolding over the pupil of the iris pigment epithelium (IPE), is a misnomer because the IPE derived from neural ectoderm (not neural crest) and therefore is not considered part of the uvea.

Wright KW, Spiegel PH, eds. *Pediatric Ophthalmology and Strabismus.* New York: Springer; 2002.

Dilator Muscle

The dilator muscle is derived embryologically from the outer layer of the optic cup, which is neuroectoderm. It lies parallel and anterior to the posterior pigmented epithelium. The smooth muscle cells contain fine myofilaments and melanosomes. The myofibrils are confined mainly to the basal portion of the cells and extend anteriorly into the iris stroma. The melanosomes and the nucleus are in the apical region of each myoepithelial cell.

There is dual sympathetic and parasympathetic innervation. The dilator muscle contracts in response to sympathetic α_1-adrenergic stimulation; cholinergic parasympathetic stimulation may have an inhibitory role.

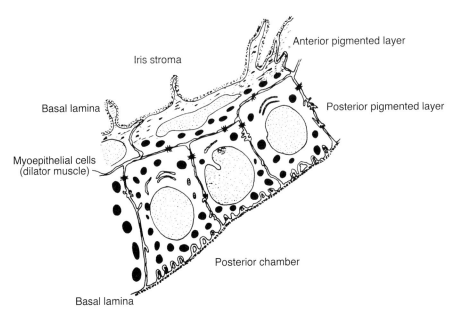

Figure 2-17 Posterior layer of the iris. *(Illustration by Thomas A. Weingeist, PhD, MD.)*

The *first-order neuron* of the sympathetic chain begins in the ipsilateral posterolateral hypothalamus and passes through the brainstem to synapse in the intermediolateral gray matter of the spinal cord, chiefly at thoracic level 1. The *second-order preganglionic neuron* exits the spinal cord, passes over the pulmonary apex and through the stellate ganglion without synapsing, and synapses in the superior cervical ganglion. The *third-order postganglionic neuron* originates here, joins the internal carotid plexus, enters the cavernous sinus, and travels with the ophthalmic division of cranial nerve (CN) V to the orbit and then to the dilator muscle. Interruption of the sympathetic nerve supply results in Horner syndrome, with miosis, in addition to ptosis and anhydrosis.

Sphincter Muscle

Like the dilator muscle, the sphincter muscle is derived from neuroectoderm. It is composed of a circular band of smooth muscle fibers and is located near the pupillary margin in the deep stroma, anterior to the pigment epithelium of the iris. Although dual innervation has been demonstrated morphologically, the sphincter muscle receives its primary innervation from parasympathetic nerve fibers that originate in the CN III nucleus, and it responds pharmacologically to muscarinic stimulation. The reciprocal sympathetic innervation to the sphincter appears to serve an inhibitory role, helping relax the sphincter in darkness.

The fibers subserving the sphincter muscle leave the Edinger-Westphal subnucleus and follow the inferior division of CN III after it bifurcates in the cavernous sinus. The fibers continue in the branch supplying the inferior oblique muscle, exit, and synapse with postganglionic fibers in the ciliary ganglion. The postganglionic fibers travel with the short ciliary nerves to the iris sphincter. They are unusual in that they are myelinated, presumably reflecting a need for fast conduction.

Ciliary Body

The ciliary body, which is triangular in cross section, bridges the anterior and posterior segments (see Fig 2-10). The apex of the ciliary body is directed posteriorly toward the ora serrata. The base of the ciliary body gives rise to the iris. The only attachment of the ciliary body to the sclera is at its base, via its longitudinal muscle fibers, where they insert into the scleral spur.

The ciliary body has 2 principal functions: (1) aqueous humor formation and (2) lens accommodation. It also plays a role in the trabecular and uveoscleral outflow of aqueous humor.

Ciliary Epithelium and Stroma

The ciliary body is 6–7 mm wide and consists of 2 parts: (1) the pars plana and (2) the pars plicata. The *pars plana* is a relatively avascular, smooth, pigmented zone; it is 4 mm wide and extends from the ora serrata to the ciliary processes. The safest posterior surgical approach to the vitreous cavity is through the pars plana, located 3–4 mm from the corneal limbus. The *pars plicata* is richly vascularized and consists of approximately 70 radial folds, or ciliary processes. The zonular fibers of the lens attach primarily in the valleys of the ciliary processes but also along the pars plana (see Fig 2-8).

The capillary plexus of each ciliary process is supplied by arterioles as they pass anteriorly and posteriorly from the major arterial circle; each plexus is drained by 1 or 2 large venules located at the crest of each process. Sphincter tone within the arteriolar smooth muscle affects the capillary hydrostatic pressure gradient. In addition, sphincter tone influences whether blood flows into the capillary plexus or directly to the draining choroidal vein, bypassing the plexus completely. Neuronal innervation of the vascular smooth muscle and humoral vasoactive substances may be important in determining regional blood flow, capillary surface area available for exchange of fluid, and hydrostatic capillary pressure. All of these factors affect the rate of aqueous humor formation.

The ciliary body is lined by a double layer of epithelial cells: the nonpigmented and the pigmented epithelium (Fig 2-18). The inner, nonpigmented epithelium is located between the aqueous humor of the posterior chamber and the outer, pigmented epithelium. The apices of the nonpigmented and pigmented cell layers are fused by a complex system of junctions and cellular interdigitations. Along the lateral intercellular spaces, near the apical border of the nonpigmented epithelium, are tight junctions (zonulae occludentes) that maintain the blood–aqueous barrier. The basal surface of the nonpigmented epithelium, which borders the posterior chamber, is covered by the basal lamina, which is multilaminar in the valleys of the processes. The basal lamina of the pigmented epithelium, which faces the iris stroma, is thick and more homogeneous than that of the nonpigmented epithelium.

The pigmented epithelium is relatively uniform throughout the ciliary body. Each of its cuboidal cells is characterized by multiple basal infoldings, a large nucleus, mitochondria, an extensive endoplasmic reticulum, and many melanosomes. The nonpigmented epithelium tends to be cuboidal in the pars plana but columnar in the pars plicata. It also has multiple basal infoldings, abundant mitochondria, and large nuclei. The endoplasmic reticulum and Golgi complexes in these cells are important for aqueous humor formation. Sometimes melanosomes are present, especially anteriorly, near the iris.

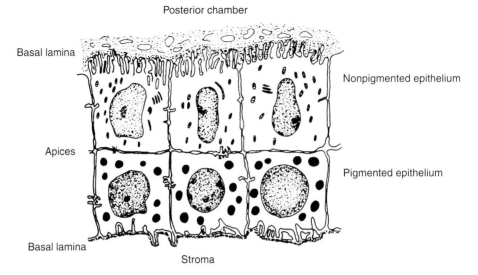

Figure 2-18 Ciliary epithelium. *(Illustration by Thomas A. Weingeist, PhD, MD.)*

The uveal portion of the ciliary body consists of comparatively large fenestrated capillaries, collagen fibrils, and fibroblasts. The main arterial supply to the ciliary body comes from the anterior and long posterior ciliary arteries, which join together to form a multilayered arterial plexus consisting of a superficial episcleral plexus; a deeper intramuscular plexus; and an incomplete major arterial circle often mistakenly attributed to the iris but actually located posterior to the anterior chamber angle recess, in the ciliary body. The major veins drain posteriorly through the vortex system, although some drainage also occurs through the intrascleral venous plexus and the episcleral veins into the limbal region.

Ciliary Muscle

The 3 layers of fibers in the ciliary muscle (Fig 2-19) are

1. longitudinal
2. radial
3. circular

Most of the ciliary muscle is made up of the outer layer of longitudinal fibers that attach to the scleral spur. The radial muscle fibers arise in the midportion of the ciliary body, and the circular fibers are located in the innermost portion. Clinically, the 3 groups of muscle fibers function as a unit. Presbyopia is associated with age-related changes in the lens (discussed in the section Lens, later in this chapter) rather than in the ciliary muscle. Even so, the muscle does change with age; the amount of connective tissue between the muscle bundles increases, and there is a loss of elastic recoil after contraction.

The ciliary muscles behave like other smooth, nonstriated muscle fibers. Ultrastructural studies reveal that they contain multiple myofibrils with characteristic electron-dense attachment bodies, mitochondria, glycogen particles, and a prominent nucleus. The smooth muscle cells are surrounded by a basal lamina separated from the cell membrane by a 300-Å space. Bundles of fibers are surrounded by a thin fibroblastic sheath rather

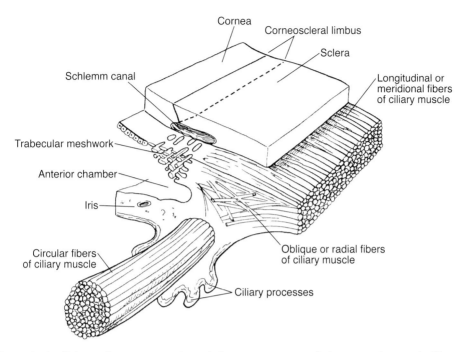

Figure 2-19 Schematic representation of the arrangement of the smooth muscle fibers in the ciliary body. Note the relationship of the ciliary body to the iris, the anterior chamber, the Schlemm canal, and the corneoscleral limbus. *(Reproduced with permission from Snell RS, Lemp MA.* Clinical Anatomy of the Eye. *Cambridge, MA: Blackwell Scientific Publications; 1989.)*

than by collagen. The muscle is rich in type VI collagen, which forms a sheath around the anterior elastic tendons. These tendons insert into the scleral spur and around the tips of the oblique and circular muscle fibers as they insert into the trabecular meshwork. Both myelinated and nonmyelinated nerve fibers are observed throughout the ciliary muscle. Innervation is derived mainly from parasympathetic fibers of CN III via the short ciliary nerves. Approximately 97% of these ciliary fibers are directed to the ciliary muscle, and about 3% are directed to the iris sphincter. Sympathetic fibers have also been observed and may play a role in relaxing the muscle. Cholinergic drugs contract the ciliary muscle. Because some of the muscle fibers form tendinous attachments to the scleral spur, their contraction increases aqueous flow by opening up the spaces of the trabecular meshwork.

Streeten BW. The ciliary body. In: Duane TD, Jaeger EA, eds. *Biomedical Foundations of Ophthalmology.* Philadelphia: Lippincott; 1995.

Choroid

The choroid, the posterior portion of the uveal tract, nourishes the outer portion of the retina (Fig 2-20). It averages 0.25 mm in thickness and consists of 3 layers of vessels:

1. the choriocapillaris, the innermost layer
2. a middle layer of small vessels
3. an outer layer of large vessels

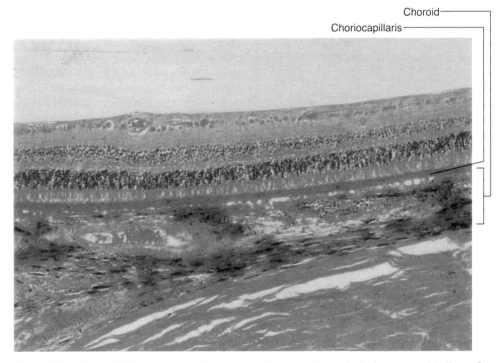

Choroid

Choriocapillaris

Figure 2-20 Choroid. The choriocapillaris lies just below the retinal pigment epithelium. Beneath are middle and outer vascular layers and multiple dendritic melanocytes (H&E ×32). *(Courtesy of Thomas A. Weingeist, PhD, MD.)*

Perfusion of the choroid comes both from the long and short posterior ciliary arteries and from the perforating anterior ciliary arteries. Venous blood drains through the vortex system. Blood flow through the choroid is high compared with that of other tissues. As a result, the oxygen content of choroidal venous blood is only 2%–3% lower than that of arterial blood.

Bruch Membrane

The Bruch membrane is a PAS-positive lamina resulting from the fusion of the basal laminae of the *retinal pigment epithelium (RPE)* and the choriocapillaris of the choroid (Fig 2-21). It extends from the margin of the optic disc to the ora serrata, and ultrastructurally it has 5 elements:

1. basal lamina of the RPE
2. inner collagenous zone
3. thicker, porous band of elastic fibers
4. outer collagenous zone
5. basal lamina of the choriocapillaris

The Bruch membrane, therefore, consists of a series of connective tissue sheets that are highly permeable to small molecules such as fluorescein. Defects in the Bruch membrane

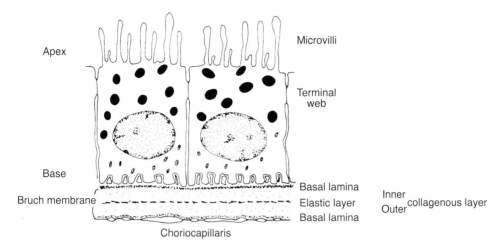

Figure 2-21 Retinal pigment epithelium and the Bruch membrane. *(Illustration by Thomas A. Weingeist, PhD, MD.)*

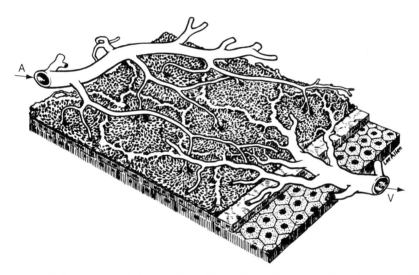

Figure 2-22 Lobular pattern of the choriocapillaris. Note that the retinal pigment epithelium is internal to the choriocapillaris. A = choroidal arteriole; V = choroidal venule. *(Reproduced with permission from Hayreh SS. The choriocapillaris. Albrecht Von Graefes Arch Klin Exp Ophthalmol. 1974;192(3):165–179.)*

develop spontaneously in myopia or pseudoxanthoma elasticum, or they result from trauma or inflammation.

Choriocapillaris

The choriocapillaris is a continuous layer of large capillaries (40–60 μm in diameter) lying in a single plane beneath the RPE (Fig 2-22). The vessel walls are extremely thin and contain multiple fenestrations, especially on the surface facing the retina (Fig 2-23). Pericytes are located along the outer wall.

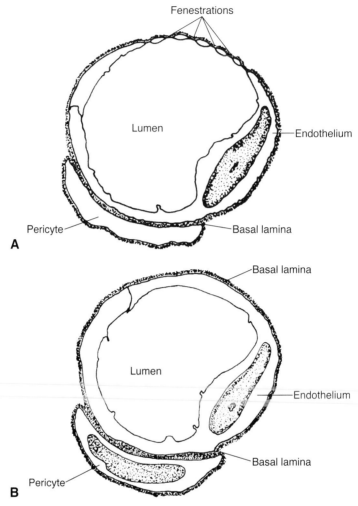

Figure 2-23 A, Fenestrated choroidal capillary. **B,** Nonfenestrated retinal capillary. *(Illustration by Thomas A. Weingeist, PhD, MD.)*

The middle and outer choroidal vessels are not fenestrated. The large vessels, typical of small arteries elsewhere, possess an internal elastic lamina and smooth muscle cells in the media. As a result, small molecules such as fluorescein, which diffuse across the endothelium of the choriocapillaris, do not leak through medium and large choroidal vessels. Abundant melanocytes, as well as occasional macrophages, lymphocytes, mast cells, and plasma cells, appear throughout the choroidal stroma. The intercellular space contains collagen fibers and nerve fibers. Melanosomes are absent from the RPE and choroid of albinos. In lightly pigmented eyes, pigmentation in the choroid is sparse compared with that of darkly pigmented eyes. The degree of pigmentation in the choroid must be considered by those performing photocoagulation, because it influences the absorption of laser energy.

Lens

The lens is a biconvex structure located directly behind the posterior chamber and pupil (Fig 2-24). The lens contributes 20.00 D of the 60.00 D of focusing power of the average adult eye (see Visual Acuity Conversion Chart on the inside front cover). The equatorial diameter is 6.5 mm at birth; it increases in the first 2–3 decades of life and remains approximately 9–10 mm in diameter in late life. The anteroposterior width of the lens is approximately 3 mm at birth and increases after the second decade of life to approximately 6 mm by age 80 years. This growth is accompanied by a shortening of the anterior radius of curvature of the lens, which would increase its optical power if not for a compensatory change in the refractive gradient across the lens substance.

In youth, accommodation for near vision is achieved by ciliary muscle contraction, which moves the ciliary muscle mass forward and inward. This contraction relaxes zonular tension and allows the lens to assume a globular shape, causing its anterior curvature to shorten. The increased lens thickness during accommodation is entirely due to a change in nuclear shape. With age, accommodative power is steadily lost. At age 8 years, the power is 14.00 D. By age 28 years, the accommodative power decreases to approximately 9.00 D, and it decreases further to 1.00 D by age 64 years. Causes of this power loss include the increased size of the lens, altered mechanical relationships, and the increased stiffness of the lens nucleus secondary to changes in the crystalline proteins of the fiber cytoplasm. Other factors, such as alterations in the geometry of zonular attachments with age and changes in lens capsule elasticity, may also play a role.

The lens has certain unusual features. It lacks innervation and is avascular. After regression of the hyaloid vasculature during embryogenesis, the lens depends solely on the aqueous and vitreous for its nourishment. From embryonic life on, it is entirely enclosed by a basal lamina, the lens capsule. BCSC Section 11, *Lens and Cataract*, discusses the lens in depth.

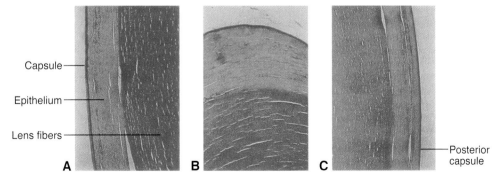

Figure 2-24 **A,** Lens: anterior capsule, epithelium, and lens fibers. **B,** Equator of the lens. Note the nuclei within the lens bow and the zonular fibers. **C,** Posterior lens capsule. Note the absence of lens epithelium (H&E ×32). *(Courtesy of Thomas A. Weingeist, PhD, MD.)*

Capsule

The lens is surrounded by a basal lamina, the lens capsule, which is a product of the lens epithelium (Fig 2-25). It is rich in type IV collagen and other matrix proteins. Synthesis of the anterior lens capsule (which overlies the epithelium) proceeds throughout life so that its thickness increases, whereas that of the posterior capsule remains relatively constant. Values of 15.5 µm for the thickness of the anterior capsule and 2.8 µm for the posterior capsule have been cited for the adult lens.

Morphologically, the lens capsule consists of fine filaments arranged in lamellae, parallel to the surface. The anterior lens capsule contains a fibrogranular material, identified as laminin, which is absent from the posterior capsule at the ultrastructural level. The thinness of the posterior capsule creates a potential for rupture during cataract surgery.

Epithelium

The lens epithelium lies beneath the anterior and equatorial capsule, but it is absent under the posterior capsule. The basal aspects of the cells abut the lens capsule without specialized attachment sites. The apices of the cells face the interior of the lens, and the lateral borders interdigitate, with practically no intercellular space. Each cell contains a prominent nucleus but relatively few cytoplasmic organelles.

Regional differences in the lens epithelium are important. The central zone represents a stable population of cells whose numbers slowly decline with age. An intermediate zone of smaller cells shows occasional mitoses. Peripherally, there are meridional rows of cuboidal preequatorial cells that form the germinative zone of the lens. Here, cells undergo mitotic division, elongate anteriorly and posteriorly, and form the differentiated fiber cells of the lens. In the human lens, cell division continues throughout life and is responsible for the continued growth of the lens. Germinative cells left behind after phacoemulsification can give rise to posterior capsular opacification as a result of aberrant proliferation and cell migration.

Fibers

The lens has an outer cortex and an inner nucleus. The nucleus is the part of the fiber mass that is formed at birth, and the cortex forms as new fibers are added postnatally. In optical section with the slit lamp, lamellar zones of discontinuity are visible; they differentiate the adult cortex into deep and superficial regions. The fiber cells are hexagonal in cross section, have a spindle shape, and possess numerous interlocking, fingerlike projections (Fig 2-26). Apart from the most superficial cortical fibers, the cytoplasm is homogeneous and contains few organelles. The high refractive index of the lens results from the high concentration of lens crystallins (α, β, and γ) in the fiber cytoplasm. The lens sutures are formed by the interdigitation of the anterior and posterior tips of the spindle-shaped fibers. In the fetal lens, this interdigitation forms the anterior Y-shaped suture and the posterior inverted Y–shaped suture. As the lens ages, further branches are added to the sutures; each new set of branch points corresponds to the appearance of a fresh optical zone of discontinuity.

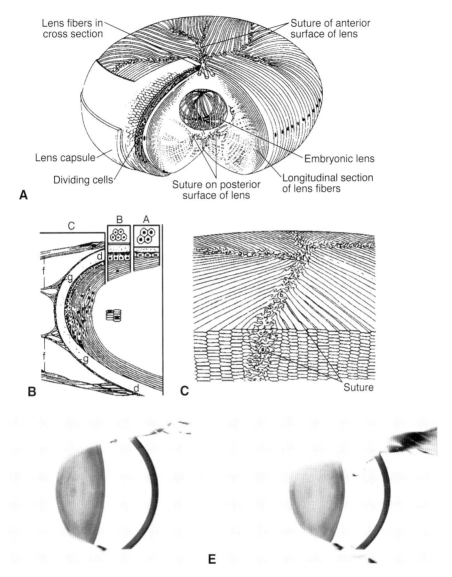

Figure 2-25 Organization of the lens. At areas where lens cells converge and meet, sutures are formed. **A,** Cutaway view of the adult lens showing an embryonic lens inside. The embryonal nucleus has a Y-shaped suture at both the anterior and posterior poles; in the adult lens cortex, the organization of the sutures is more complex. At the equator, the lens epithelium can divide, and the cells become highly elongated and ribbonlike, sending processes anteriorly and posteriorly. As new lens cells are formed, older cells come to lie in the deeper parts of the cortex. **B,** Cross section and corresponding surface view showing the difference in lens fibers at the anterior (A), intermediate (B), and equatorial (C) zones. The lens capsule, or basement membrane of the lens epithelium (d), is shown in relation to the zonular fibers (f) and their attachment to the lens (g). **C,** The diagram shows a closer view of lens sutures. **D** and **E,** Optical sections of the lens of a young adult human (25-year-old female) demonstrated by Scheimpflug photography. The cornea is to the right. **D,** Lens in the nonaccommodative state. **E,** Lens during accommodation. Note that the anterior radius of curvature is shortened in the latter case.
(Parts A–C reproduced with permission from Kessel RG, Kardon RH. Tissues and Organs: A Text-Atlas of Scanning Electron Microscopy. San Francisco: WH Freeman; 1979. Parts D and E courtesy of Jane Koretz.)

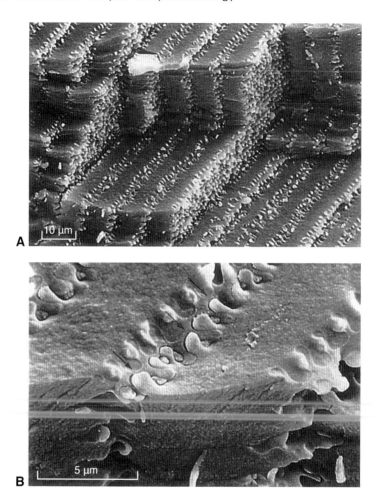

Figure 2-26 **A** and **B,** Scanning electron micrographs of the relationship between lens fiber packing and interdigitation *(arrows in B)*. *(Reproduced with permission from Kessel RG, Kardon RH. Tissues and Organs: A Text-Atlas of Scanning Electron Microscopy. San Francisco: WH Freeman; 1979.)*

Zonular Fibers (Suspensory Ligaments)

The lens is held in place by the system of zonular fibers that originate from the basal laminae of the nonpigmented epithelium of the pars plana and pars plicata of the ciliary body. These fibers attach chiefly to the lens capsule anterior and posterior to the equator. Each zonular fiber is made up of multiple filaments of fibrillin that merge with the equatorial lens capsule. In Marfan syndrome, mutations in the fibrillin gene lead to weakening of the zonule and subluxation of the lens.

When the eye is focused for distance, the zonule is under tension and the lens form is relatively flattened. During accommodation, contraction of the ciliary muscle moves the proximal attachment of the zonule forward and inward, so the lens becomes more globular and the eye adjusts for near vision (see Fig 2-25B).

Bourge JL, Robert AM, Robert L, Renard G. Zonular fibers, multimolecular composition as related to function (elasticity) and pathology. *Pathol Biol (Paris).* 2007;55(7):347–359. Epub 2007 Mar 12.

Streeten BW. Anatomy of the zonular apparatus. In: Duane TD, Jaeger EA, eds. *Biomedical Foundations of Ophthalmology.* Philadelphia: Harper & Row; 1992.

Retina

The *fundus oculi* is the part of the eye that is visible with ophthalmoscopy; it includes the retina, its vessels, and the *optic nerve head,* or *optic disc.* The *macula,* 5–6 mm in diameter, lies between the temporal vascular arcades. At the macula's center lies the *fovea,* which is rich in cones and responsible for color vision and the highest visual acuity. In the far periphery, the *ora serrata* (the junction between the retina and the pars plana) can be observed with gonioscopy or indirect ophthalmoscopy. The reddish color of the fundus is due to the transmission of light reflected from the posterior sclera through the capillary bed of the choroid.

The *retina* is a thin, transparent structure that develops from the inner and outer layers of the optic cup. In cross section, from outer to inner retina, the 10 layers of the neurosensory retina are

1. internal limiting membrane
2. nerve fiber layer
3. ganglion cell layer
4. inner plexiform layer
5. inner nuclear layer
6. middle limiting membrane
7. outer plexiform layer
8. outer nuclear layer
9. external limiting membrane
10. rod and cone inner and outer segments

The retina is also discussed in depth in BCSC Section 12, *Retina and Vitreous.*

Retinal Pigment Epithelium

The structure of the outer pigmented epithelial layer is relatively simple compared with that of the overlying inner, or neurosensory, retina. The RPE consists of a monolayer of hexagonal cells that extends anteriorly from the optic disc to the ora serrata, where it merges with the pigmented epithelium of the ciliary body. Its structure is deceptively simple considering its many functions:

- vitamin A metabolism
- maintenance of the outer blood–retina barrier
- phagocytosis of the photoreceptor outer segments
- absorption of light (reduction of scatter)

- heat exchange
- formation of the basal lamina of the Bruch membrane
- production of the mucopolysaccharide matrix surrounding the outer segments
- active transport of materials into and out of the RPE

Like other epithelial and endothelial cells, the RPE cells are polarized. The basal aspect is intricately folded and provides a large surface of attachment to the thin basal lamina that forms the inner layer of the Bruch membrane (see Fig 2-21). The apices have multiple villous processes that engage with the photoreceptor outer segments. Separation of the RPE from the neurosensory retina is called *retinal detachment.*

Contiguous RPE cells are firmly attached by a series of lateral, intercellular junctional complexes. The *zonulae occludentes* and *zonulae adherentes* not only provide structural stability but also play an important role in maintaining the outer blood–retina barrier. Zonulae occludentes consist of fused plasma membranes forming a circular band or belt between adjacent cells. A small intercellular space is present between zonulae adherentes.

The retina and RPE show important regional differences (Fig 2-27). The retina is thickest in the papillomacular bundle near the optic nerve (0.23 mm) and thinnest in the foveola (0.10 mm) and ora serrata (0.11 mm). RPE cells vary from 10 to 60 μm in diameter. Compared with RPE cells in the periphery, RPE cells in the fovea are taller and thinner, contain more melanosomes, and have larger melanosomes. These characteristics account in part for the decreased transmission of choroidal fluorescence observed during fundus fluorescein angiography. Cells in the periphery are shorter, broader, and less pigmented. The eye of a fetus or infant contains between 4 and 6 million RPE cells. Although the surface area of the eye increases appreciably with age, the increase in the number of RPE cells is relatively small. No mitotic figures are apparent within the RPE of the normal adult eye.

The cytoplasm of the RPE cells contains multiple round and ovoid pigment granules *(melanosomes).* These organelles develop in situ during formation of the optic cup and

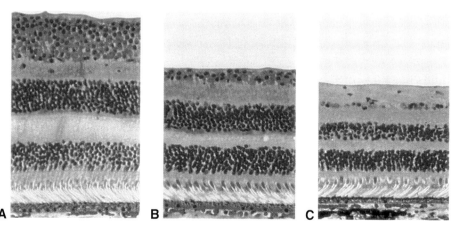

Figure 2-27 Regional differences in the retina. **A,** Papillomacular bundle. **B,** Macula. **C,** Peripheral retina. (H&E, all same magnification.) *(Courtesy of Thomas A. Weingeist, PhD, MD.)*

first appear as nonmelanized premelanosomes. Their development contrasts sharply with that of the pigment granules in uveal melanocytes, which are derived from the neural crest and later migrate into the uvea.

Lipofuscin granules probably arise from the discs of photoreceptor outer segments and represent residual bodies arising from phagosomal activity. This so-called wear-and-tear pigment is less electron dense than the melanosomes, and its concentration increases gradually with age. Clinically, these lipofuscin granules are responsible for the signal observed with fundus autofluorescence.

Phagosomes are membrane-enclosed packets of disc outer segments that have been engulfed by the RPE. Several stages of disintegration are evident at any given time. In some species, shedding and degradation of the membranes of rod and cone outer segments follow a diurnal rhythm synchronized with daily fluctuations of environmental light. The cytoplasm of the RPE also contains numerous mitochondria (which are involved in aerobic metabolism), rough-surfaced endoplasmic reticulum, a Golgi apparatus, and a large round nucleus.

Throughout life, incompletely digested residual bodies, lipofuscin pigment, phagosomes, and other material are excreted beneath the basal lamina of the RPE. These contribute to the formation of *drusen,* which are accumulations of this extracellular material. Drusen can vary in size and are commonly classified by their funduscopic appearance as either hard or soft. They are typically located between the basement membrane of the RPE cells and the inner collagenous zone of the Bruch membrane.

Neurosensory Retina

The neurosensory retina is composed of neuronal, glial, and vascular elements (Fig 2-28).

Neuronal elements

The photoreceptor layer of the neurosensory retina consists of highly specialized neuroepithelial cells called *rods* and *cones.* Each photoreceptor cell consists of an outer segment and an inner segment. The outer segments, surrounded by a mucopolysaccharide matrix, make contact with the apical processes of the RPE. Tight junctions or other intercellular connections do not exist between the photoreceptor cell outer segments and the RPE. The factors responsible for keeping these layers in apposition are poorly understood but probably involve active transport.

The rod photoreceptor consists of an outer segment that contains multiple laminated discs resembling a stack of coins and a central connecting cilium. The microtubules of the cilium have a 9-plus-0 cross-sectional configuration rather than the 9-plus-2 configuration found in motile cilia. The rod inner segment is subdivided into 2 additional elements: (1) an outer ellipsoid containing numerous mitochondria and (2) an inner myoid containing a large amount of glycogen; the myoid is continuous with the main cell body, where the nucleus is located (Fig 2-29). The inner portion of the cell contains the *synaptic body,* or *spherule,* of the rod, which is formed by a single invagination that accommodates 2 horizontal cell processes and 1 or more central bipolar dendrites (Fig 2-30). The outer segments of the cones have a different morphology depending on their location in the retina.

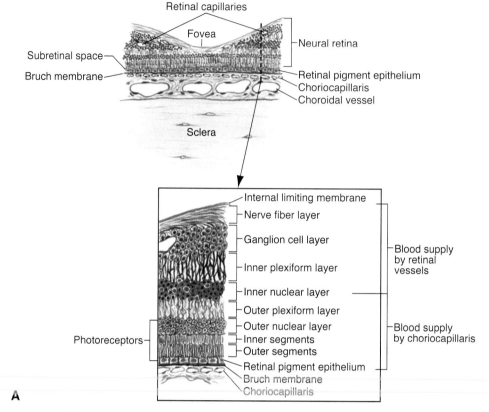

Figure 2-28   A, Cross section of retina illustrating the layers of retina and approximate location of blood supply to these layers.

The extrafoveal cone photoreceptors of the retina have conical ellipsoids and myoids, and their nuclei tend to be closer to the external limiting membrane than are the nuclei of the rods. Although the structure of the outer segments of the rods and cones is similar, at least 1 important difference exists. Rod discs are not attached to the cell membrane; they are discrete structures. Cone discs are attached to the cell membrane and are thought to be renewed by membranous replacement. The cone *synaptic body,* or *pedicle,* is more complex than the rod spherule. Cone pedicles synapse with other rods and cones as well as with horizontal and bipolar cell processes. Foveal cones have cylindrical inner segments similar to rods but otherwise are cytologically identical to extrafoveal cones. Horizontal cells make synaptic connections with many rod spherules and cone pedicles; they also extend cell processes horizontally throughout the outer plexiform layer. Bipolar cells are oriented vertically. Their dendrites synapse with either rod or cone synaptic bodies, and their axons make synaptic contact with ganglion cells and amacrine cells in the inner plexiform layer.

The axons of the ganglion cells bend to become parallel to the inner surface of the retina, where they form the nerve fiber layer and later the axons of the optic nerve. Each optic nerve has more than 1 million optic nerve fibers. The nerve fibers from

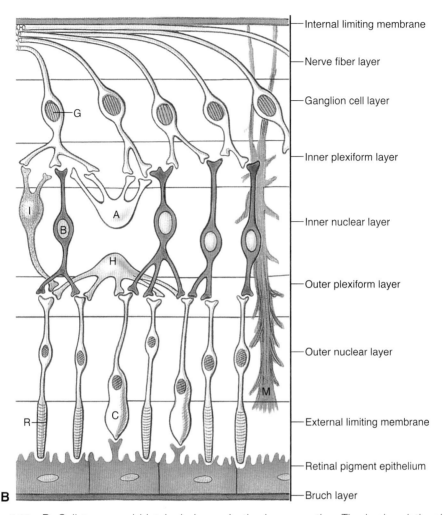

Internal limiting membrane

Nerve fiber layer

Ganglion cell layer

Inner plexiform layer

Inner nuclear layer

Outer plexiform layer

Outer nuclear layer

External limiting membrane

Retinal pigment epithelium

Bruch layer

Figure 2-28 **B,** Cell types and histologic layers in the human retina. The basic relationship between rod (R) and cone (C) photoreceptors as well as bipolar (B), horizontal (H), amacrine (A), inner plexiform cell (I), and ganglion (G) neurons is depicted. Note that the Müller cell (M) extends across almost the whole thickness of the retina; the apical processes of Müller cells form the external limiting membrane; the foot processes of Müller cells partially form the internal limiting membrane. *(Part A modified with permission from D'Amico DJ. Diseases of the retina. N Engl J Med. 1994;331:95–106. Part B illustration by Christine Gralapp.)*

the temporal retina follow an arcuate course around the macula to enter the superior and inferior poles of the optic disc. The papillomacular fibers travel straight to the optic nerve from the fovea. The nasal axons also pursue a radial course. The visibility of the nerve fibers is enhanced when they are viewed ophthalmoscopically using green (red-free) illumination.

The neuronal elements and their connections in the retina are highly complex. Many types of bipolar, amacrine, and ganglion cells exist. The neuronal elements of more than

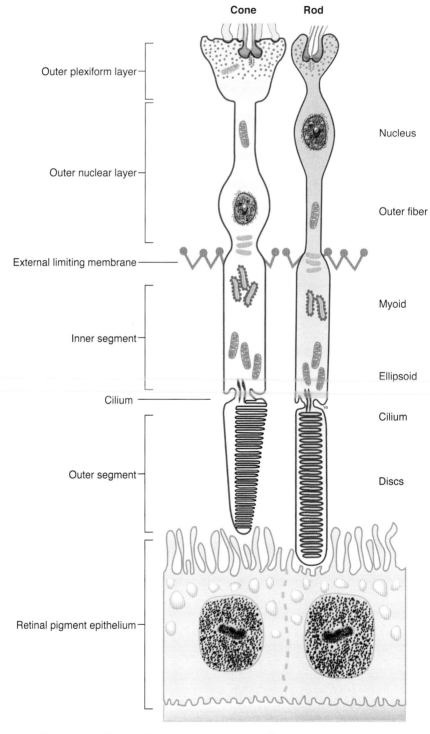

Figure 2-29 Rod and cone photoreceptor cells. *(Illustration by Sylvia Barker.)*

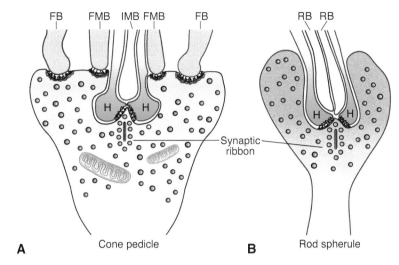

FB   FMB IMB FMB   FB

RB RB

Synaptic ribbon

A   Cone pedicle

B   Rod spherule

Figure 2-30   Synaptic bodies of photoreceptors. **A,** Cone pedicle with synapses to several types of bipolar cells. **B,** Rod spherule with synapses to bipolar cells. FB = flat bipolar; FMB = flat midget bipolar; H = horizontal cell processes; IMB = invaginating midget bipolar; RB = rod bipolar. *(Illustration by Sylvia Barker.)*

120 million rods and 6 million cones are interconnected, and signal processing within the neurosensory retina is significant.

Glial elements

Müller cells are glial cells that extend vertically from the external limiting membrane inward to the internal limiting membrane. Their nuclei are located in the inner nuclear layer. Müller cells, along with the other glial elements (the fibrous and protoplasmic astrocytes and microglia), provide structural support and nutrition to the retina and are crucial to normal physiology.

Vascular elements

The inner portion of the retina is perfused by branches of the central retinal artery. In addition, a cilioretinal artery can branch from the ciliary circulation to supply the macula; studies show this occurs in approximately 18%–32% of eyes.

The retinal blood vessels are analogous to the cerebral blood vessels and maintain the inner blood–retina barrier. This physiologic barrier is due to the single layer of nonfenestrated endothelial cells, whose tight junctions are impervious to tracer substances such as fluorescein and horseradish peroxidase. A basal lamina covers the outer surface of the endothelium. The basement membrane contains an interrupted layer of pericytes, or mural cells, surrounded by their own basement membrane material.

Müller cells and other glial elements are generally attached to the basal lamina of retinal blood vessels. Retinal blood vessels lack an internal elastic lamina and the continuous layer of smooth muscle cells found in other vessels in the body. Smooth muscle cells are occasionally present in vessels near the optic nerve head. They become a more discontinuous layer as the retinal arterioles pass farther out to the peripheral retina. The retinal blood vessels do not ordinarily extend deeper than the middle limiting membrane. Where venules and arterioles cross, they share a common basement membrane. Venous occlusive disorders are common at arteriovenous crossings.

Stratification of the neurosensory retina

The neurosensory retina can be subdivided into several layers (see Fig 2-28). The outermost layer, which is located next to the RPE, is the *external limiting membrane (ELM)*. It is not a true membrane and is formed by the attachment sites of adjacent photoreceptors and Müller cells. It is highly fenestrated.

The *outer plexiform layer (OPL)* is composed of the interconnections between the photoreceptor synaptic bodies and the horizontal and bipolar cells. In the macular region, the OPL is thicker and contains more fibers, because the axons of the rods and cones become longer and more oblique as they deviate from the fovea. In this region, the OPL is known as the *Henle fiber layer* (Fig 2-31). At the edge of the foveola, it lies almost parallel to the internal limiting membrane. The *inner nuclear layer (INL)* contains nuclei of bipolar, Müller, horizontal, and amacrine cells.

The next region is formed by a zone of desmosome-like attachments in the region of the synaptic bodies of the photoreceptor cells. The retinal blood vessels ordinarily do not extend beyond this point.

The *inner plexiform layer (IPL)* consists of axons of the bipolar and amacrine cells and dendrites of the ganglion cells and their synapses. The *ganglion cell layer (GCL)* is made up of the cell bodies of the ganglion cells that lie near the inner surface of the retina. The *nerve fiber layer (NFL)* is formed by axons of the ganglion cells. Normally, these axons

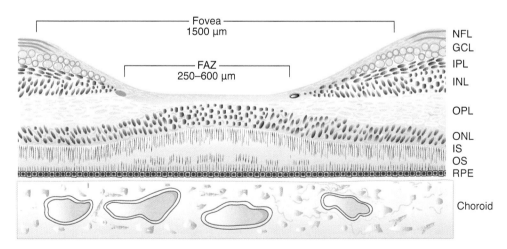

Figure 2-31 Schematic section through the fovea. FAZ = foveal avascular zone; GCL = ganglion cell layer; INL = inner nuclear layer; IPL = inner plexiform layer; IS = inner segment of the photoreceptor; NFL = nerve fiber layer; ONL = outer nuclear layer; OPL = outer plexiform layer (Henle fiber layer); OS = outer segment of the photoreceptors; RPE = retinal pigment epithelium. *(Illustration by Sylvia Barker.)*

do not become myelinated until after they pass through the lamina cribrosa of the optic nerve.

Similar to the ELM, the *internal limiting membrane (ILM)* is not a true membrane. It is formed by the footplates of the Müller cells and attachments to the basal lamina. The basal lamina of the retina is smooth on the vitreal side but appears undulating on the retinal side, where it follows the contour of the Müller cells. The thickness of the basal lamina varies. Overall, cells and their processes in the retina are oriented perpendicular to the plane of the RPE in the middle and outer layers but parallel to the retinal surface in the inner layers. For this reason, deposits of blood or exudates tend to form round blots in the outer layers (where small capillaries are found) and linear or flame-shaped patterns in the nerve fiber layer. At the fovea, the outer layers also tend to be parallel to the surface (Henle fiber layer). As a result, radial or star-shaped patterns may arise when these extracellular spaces are filled with serum and exudate.

Drexler W, Morgner U, Ghanta RK, Kärtner FX, Schuman JS, Fujimoto JG. Ultrahigh-resolution ophthalmic optical coherence tomography. *Nature Med.* 2001;7(4):502–507.

Macula

The terms *macula, macula lutea, posterior pole, area centralis, fovea,* and *foveola* have created confusion among anatomists and clinicians. Clinical retina specialists tend to regard the macula as the area within the temporal vascular arcades. Histologically, it is the region with more than 1 layer of ganglion cell nuclei (Figs 2-32, 2-33; also see Fig 2-28).

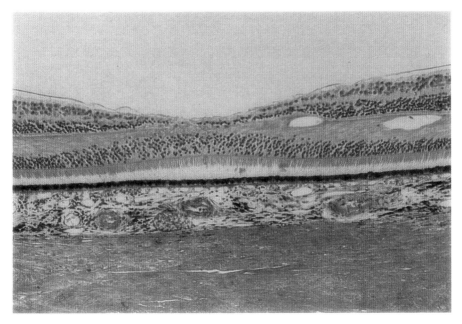

Figure 2-32 Light micrograph of the macula. Compare with Figure 2-31. *(Courtesy of Thomas A. Weingeist, PhD, MD.)*

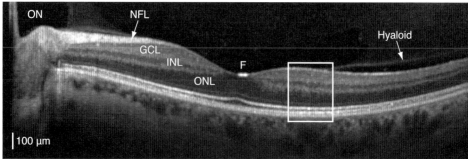

A Nasal   Temporal

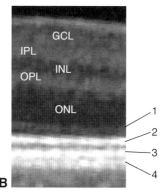

B

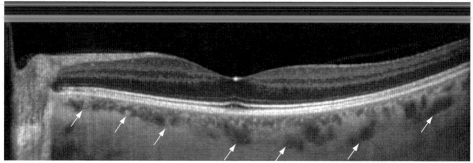

C Nasal   Temporal

Figure 2-33 **A,** Spectral-domain optical coherence tomography (SD-OCT) image of an 8.7-mm-long cross section along the horizontal meridian from the optic nerve (ON) through the foveal center (F) and extending into the temporal retina in a normal subject. The nuclear layers appear as darker bands and include the outer nuclear layer (ONL), the inner nuclear layer (INL), and the ganglion cell layer (GCL). Three layers of the inner retina appear hyperreflective (brighter): the outer plexiform layer (the band between the ONL and the INL), the inner plexiform layer (the band between the INL and the GCL), and the nerve fiber layer (NFL), the band of higher reflectivity that broadens nasally toward the optic nerve. The posterior hyaloid face of the vitreous is also visible as a thin reflective band that separates from the retinal surface. **B,** Magnification of the boxed portion of **A,** showing details that are deeper than or sclerad to the ONL. Four hyperreflective bands are grouped tightly: the external limiting membrane (1); the ellipsoid region of the photoreceptors in the transitional boundary region from the photoreceptor inner segment to the outer segment (2); the interdigitation between the tip of the outer segment and the retinal pigment epithelial (RPE) cell layer (3); and the RPE layer (4). The length of the photoreceptor outer segment spans the darker band between 2 and 3. **C,** An SD-OCT image of a cross section obtained with enhanced depth imaging, which allows for better visualization of deeper structures such as the choroid. *Arrows* indicate posterior margin of the choroid. *(Courtesy of Tomas S. Aleman, MD.)*

See BCSC Section 12, *Retina and Vitreous,* for further detail. The name *macula lutea* (which means *yellow spot*) derives from the yellow color of the central retina in dissected cadaver eyes. This color is due to the presence of carotenoid pigments, which are located chiefly in the Henle fiber layer. Two major pigments—zeaxanthin and lutein—have been identified whose proportions vary with their distance from the fovea. In the central area (0.25 mm from the fovea), the lutein-to-zeaxanthin ratio is 1:2.4, and in the periphery (2.2–8.7 mm from the fovea), the ratio is greater than 2:1. This variation in pigment ratio corresponds to the rod-to-cone ratio. Lutein is more concentrated in rod-dense areas of the retina; zeaxanthin is more concentrated in cone-dense areas. Lipofuscin, the yellow age pigment, has been observed in the cytoplasm of the perifoveal ganglion cells by electron microscopy.

The *fovea* is a concave central retinal depression approximately 1.5 mm in diameter; it is comparable in size to the optic nerve head (see Fig 2-31). Its margins are clinically inexact, but in younger subjects the fovea is evident ophthalmoscopically as an elliptical light reflex that arises from the slope of the thickened ILM of the retina. From this point inward, the basal lamina rapidly decreases in thickness as it dives down the slopes of the fovea toward the depths of the foveola, where it is barely visible, even by electron microscopy.

Around the fovea is the *parafovea,* 0.5 mm wide, where the GCL, the INL, and the OPL are thickest. Surrounding this zone is the most peripheral region of the macula, the *perifovea,* 1.5 mm wide. The masking of choroidal fluorescence observed in the macula during fundus fluorescein angiography is caused partly by xanthophyll pigment and partly by the higher melanin pigment content of the foveal RPE.

The *foveola* is a central depression within the fovea, located approximately 4.0 mm temporal and 0.8 mm inferior to the center of the optic disc. It is approximately 0.35 mm across and 0.10 mm thick at its center. The borders of the foveola merge imperceptibly with the fovea. The nuclei of the photoreceptor cells in the region of the foveola bow forward toward the ILM to form the fovea externa. Usually, only photoreceptors, Müller cells, and other glial cells are present in this area. Occasionally, light microscopy reveals ganglion cell nuclei just below the ILM.

The photoreceptor layer of the foveola is composed entirely of cones, whose close packing accounts for the high visual acuity for which this small area is responsible. The foveal cones are shaped like rods but possess all the cytologic characteristics of extramacular cones. The outer segments are oriented parallel to the visual axis and perpendicular to the plane of the RPE. In contrast, the peripheral photoreceptor cell outer segments are tilted toward the entrance pupil.

The *foveal avascular zone (FAZ),* or capillary-free zone (Fig 2-34; also see Fig 2-31), is an important clinical landmark in the treatment of subretinal neovascular membranes by laser photocoagulation. Its location is approximately the same as that of the foveola, and its appearance in fundus fluorescein angiograms varies greatly. The diameter of the FAZ varies from 250 to 600 μm or greater; often, a truly avascular, or capillary-free, zone cannot be identified.

Orth DH, Fine BS, Fagman W, Quirk TC. Clarification of foveomacular nomenclature and grid for quantitation of macular disorders. *Trans Sect Ophthalmol Am Acad Ophthalmol Otolaryngol.* 1977;83(3 Pt 1):OP506–514.

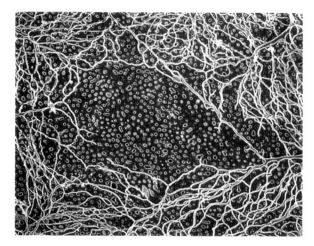

Figure 2-34 Scanning electron micrograph of a retinal vascular cast at the fovea, showing the foveal avascular zone and underlying choriocapillaris.

Ora Serrata

The ora serrata is the boundary between the retina and the pars plana. Its distance from the Schwalbe line is between 5.75 mm nasally and 6.50 mm temporally. In myopia, this distance is greater; in hyperopia, it is shorter. The Bruch membrane extends anteriorly, beyond the ora serrata, but is modified because there is no choriocapillaris in the ciliary body.

At the ora serrata, the diameter of the eye is 20 mm and the circumference is 63 mm; at the equator, the diameter is 24 mm and the circumference is 75 mm. Topographically, the ora serrata is relatively smooth temporally and serrated nasally. Retinal blood vessels end in loops before reaching the ora serrata.

The ora serrata is in a watershed zone between the anterior and posterior vascular systems, which may in part explain why peripheral retinal degeneration is relatively common. The peripheral retina in the region of the ora serrata is markedly attenuated. The photoreceptors are malformed, and the overlying retina frequently appears cystic in paraffin sections (Blessig-Iwanoff cysts) (Fig 2-35).

Vitreous

The vitreous cavity occupies four-fifths of the volume of the globe. The transparent vitreous humor is important to the metabolism of the intraocular tissues because it provides a route for metabolites used by the lens, ciliary body, and retina. Its volume is close to 4.0 mL. Although it has a gel-like structure, the vitreous is 99% water. Its viscosity is approximately twice that of water, mainly due to the presence of the mucopolysaccharide hyaluronic acid (Fig 2-36).

At the ultrastructural level, fine collagen fibrils (chiefly type II) and cells have been identified in the vitreous. The origin and function of these cells, termed *hyalocytes,* are unknown, but they probably represent modified histiocytes, glial cells, or fibroblasts. The

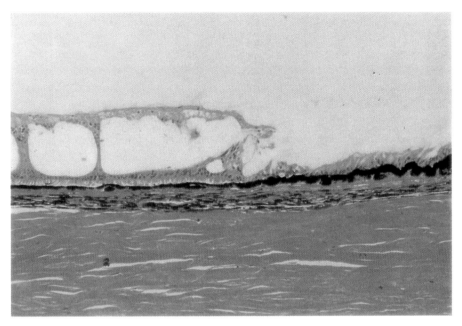

Figure 2-35 Ora serrata. Note the malformed appearance of the peripheral retina and the cystic changes at the junction between the pars plana and the retina (H&E ×32). *(Courtesy of Thomas A. Weingeist, PhD, MD.)*

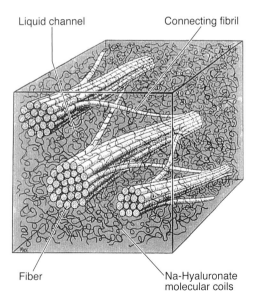

Liquid channel   Connecting fibril

Fiber   Na-Hyaluronate molecular coils

Figure 2-36 Three-dimensional representation of the molecular organization of the vitreous, showing the dissociation between hyaluronic acid molecules and collagen fibrils. The fibrils are packed into bundles, and the hyaluronic acid forms molecular "coils" that fill the intervening spaces to provide channels of liquid vitreous. *(Reproduced with permission from Sebag J, Balazs EA. Morphology and ultrastructure of human vitreous fibers.* Invest Ophthalmol Vis Sci. *1989;30(8):1867–1871.)*

fibrils at the vitreous base merge with the basal lamina of the nonpigmented epithelium of the pars plana and the ILM of the retina.

The vitreous adheres to the retina peripherally at the vitreous base, which extends from 2.0 mm anterior to the ora serrata to approximately 4.0 mm posterior to it. Additional attachments exist at the disc margin, at the perimacular region, along the retinal vessels, and at the periphery of the posterior lens capsule. The vitreous becomes more fluid with age and frequently separates from the inner retina (posterior vitreous detachment) (Fig 2-37). The associated peripheral retinal traction is a potential cause of rhegmatogenous retinal detachment (Figs 2-38 through 2-40). During embryonic development, regression of the hyaloid vasculature results in the formation of an S-shaped channel (the Cloquet canal), which passes sinuously from a point slightly nasal to the posterior pole of the lens (Mittendorf dot; Fig 2-41) to the margin of the optic nerve head. Remnants of this fetal vasculature may be observed clinically on the nerve head in the adult (vascular loops and Bergmeister papilla).

Lund-Andersen H, Sander B. The vitreous. In: Kaufman PL, Alm A, eds. *Adler's Physiology of the Eye*. 10th ed. St Louis: Mosby; 2003:293–316.

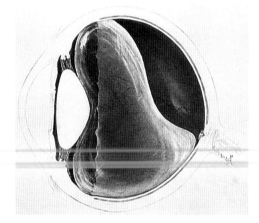

Figure 2-37 Typical posterior vitreous detachment. The cortical vitreous initially separates from the retina in the posterior pole and the superior quadrants. The detachment may then progress farther anteriorly until reaching the posterior margin of the vitreous base in the inferior quadrants. *(Reproduced with permission from Michels RG, Wilkinson CP, Rice TA, eds.* Retinal Detachment. *St Louis: Mosby; 1990.)*

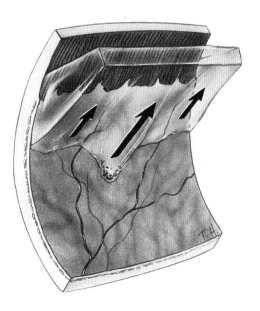

Figure 2-38 Localized posterior extension of the vitreous base with a firm underlying area of vitreoretinal attachment may result in greater traction in that area *(large arrow)* than along the adjacent vitreous base *(small arrows)*. *(Reproduced with permission from Michels RG, Wilkinson CP, Rice TA, eds.* Retinal Detachment. *St Louis: Mosby; 1990.)*

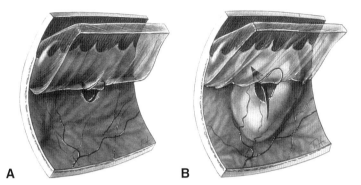

A **B**

Figure 2-39 **A,** Traction from the posterior vitreous surface on a site of firm vitreoretinal attachment is the usual mechanism causing a retinal break. **B,** Persistent traction on the flap of the retinal tear and fluid currents in the vitreous cavity contribute to retinal detachment. *(Reproduced with permission from Michels RG, Wilkinson CP, Rice TA, eds.* Retinal Detachment. *St Louis: Mosby; 1990.)*

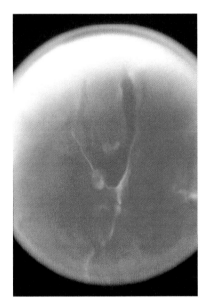

Figure 2-40 Fundus photograph of a flap retinal tear with associated retinal detachment. *(Courtesy of James Folk, MD.)*

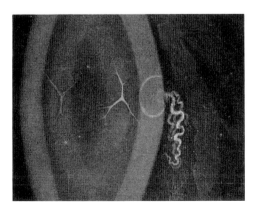

Figure 2-41 Mittendorf dot. In some individuals, a remnant of the hyaloid vasculature is visible on the posterior pole of the lens, as a normal variant. *(Reproduced with permission from Thiel R.* Atlas of Diseases of the Eye. *Amsterdam: Elsevier; 1963.)*

CHAPTER 3

Cranial Nerves: Central and Peripheral Connections

Cranial nerves (CN) I–VI are depicted in Figure 3-1 in relation to the bony canals and arteries at the base of the skull. The reader may find it useful to refer to this figure as each cranial nerve is discussed. CN VII is discussed later in this chapter. For further study, see BCSC Section 5, *Neuro-Ophthalmology,* which describes the cranial nerves and their functions and dysfunctions in detail.

Cranial Nerve I (Olfactory Nerve)

Cranial nerve I originates from small olfactory receptors in the mucous membrane of the nose. Unmyelinated CN I fibers pass from these receptors in the nasal cavity through the cribriform plate of the ethmoidal bone and enter the ventral surface of the olfactory bulb, where they form the nerve.

The olfactory tract runs posteriorly from the bulb beneath the frontal lobe of the brain in a groove (or sulcus) and lateral to the gyrus rectus (Fig 3-2). The gyrus rectus forms the anterolateral border of the suprasellar cistern. Meningiomas arising from the arachnoid cells in this area can cause important ophthalmic signs and symptoms associated with loss of olfaction.

Cranial Nerve II (Optic Nerve)

Cranial nerve II, the optic nerve, consists of more than 1 million axons that originate in the ganglion cell layer of the retina and extend toward the occipital cortex. The optic nerve may be divided into the following 4 topographic areas (Table 3-1):

1. intraocular region of the optic nerve: optic disc, or nerve head; prelaminar area; and laminar area
2. intraorbital region (located within the muscle cone)
3. intracanalicular region (located within the optic canal)
4. intracranial region (ending in the optic chiasm)

The organization of the optic nerve is similar to that of the white matter of the brain. Developmentally, the optic nerve is part of the brain, and its fibers are surrounded by glial

Figure 3-1 View from the right parietal bone looking downward into the skull base, showing the relationship between the bony canals **(A)**, nerves **(B)**, and arteries **(C)** at the base of the skull. The orbits are located to the right, out of the picture (the roof of the orbits is just visible). The floor of the right middle cranial fossa is in the lower part. **A,** AC = anterior clinoid; ACF = anterior cranial fossa; CC = carotid canal; FO = foramen ovale; FR = foramen rotundum; MCF = middle cranial fossa; OF = optic foramen; PC = posterior clinoid; SOF = superior orbital fissure; ST = sella turcica. **B,** I = olfactory nerve; II = optic nerve; III = oculomotor nerve; IV = trochlear nerve; V = trigeminal nerve, with ophthalmic V_1, maxillary V_2, and mandibular V_3 divisions; VI = abducens nerve; TG = trigeminal ganglion. **C,** ACoA (and *arrowhead*) = anterior communicating artery; BA = basilar artery; ICA = internal carotid artery; MCA = middle cerebral artery; OA = ophthalmic artery; PCA = posterior cerebral artery; PCoA = posterior communicating artery. *(Reproduced with permission from Zide BM, Jelks GW, eds.* Surgical Anatomy of the Orbit. *New York: Raven; 1985.)*

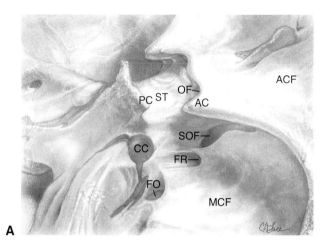

A

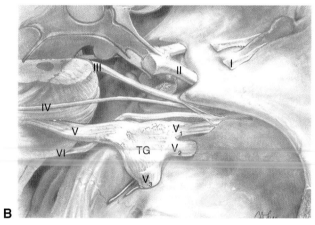

B

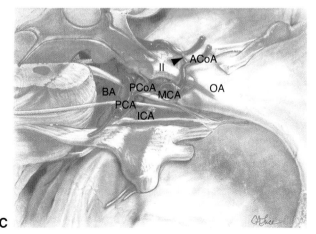

C

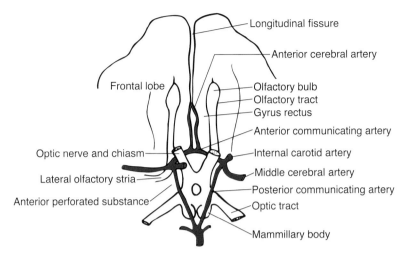

Figure 3-2 Inferior surface of the brain, depicting cranial nerve (CN) I, CN II, and surrounding structures. *(Illustration by Thomas A. Weingeist, PhD, MD.)*

Table 3-1 Regional Differences in the Optic Nerve

Segment	Length (mm)	Diameter (mm)	Blood Supply
Intraocular	1.0		Retinal arterioles
Optic disc		1.76 × 1.92	Branches of posterior ciliary arteries
Prelaminar area			
Laminar area			
Intraorbital	25	3–4	Intraneural branches of central retinal artery CRA; pial branches from CRA and choroid
Intracanalicular	4–10		Ophthalmic artery
Intracranial	10	4–7	Branches of internal carotid and ophthalmic arteries

(and not Schwann) cell sheaths. Part of the intraocular portion of the optic nerve is visible ophthalmoscopically as the *optic nerve head,* or optic disc. The intraorbital portion is approximately 25–30 mm long, which is greater than the distance between the back of the globe and the optic canal (18 mm). For this reason, when the eye is in the primary position, the optic nerve runs a sinuous course. Axial proptosis secondary to thyroid-related eye disease or a retrobulbar tumor can lead to stretching of the optic nerve, which may cause chronic nerve injury and optic neuropathy.

Cascone P, Rinna C, Reale G, Calvani F, Iannetti G. Compression and stretching in Graves orbitopathy: emergency orbital decompression techniques. *J Craniofac Surg.* 2012;23(5): 1430–1433.

Soni CR, Johnson LN. Visual neuropraxia and progressive vision loss from thyroid-associated stretch optic neuropathy. *Eur J Ophthalmol.* 2010;20(2):429–436.

Intraocular Region

The optic nerve head is the principal site of many congenital and acquired ocular diseases; therefore, detailed knowledge of its anatomy is important for the practicing ophthalmologist. Its anterior surface is visible ophthalmoscopically as the *optic disc,* an oval structure whose size reflects some ethnic and racial variance. The size of the optic disc varies widely, averaging 1.76 mm horizontally and 1.92 mm vertically. The cup-shaped depression, or *physiologic cup,* is located slightly temporal to the optic disc's geometric center and represents an axon-free region. The main branches of the central retinal artery (CRA) and the central retinal vein (CRV) pass through the center of the cup. The optic nerve head has 4 parts:

1. superficial nerve fiber layer
2. prelaminar area
3. laminar area
4. retrolaminar area

Jonas JB, Gusek GC, Naumann GO. Optic disc, cup and neuroretinal rim size, configuration and correlations in normal eyes. *Invest Ophthalmol Vis Sci.* 1988;29(7):1151–1158.

Superficial nerve fiber layer

As the nonmyelinated ganglion cell axons enter the nerve head, they retain their retinotopic organization, with fibers from the upper retina above and those from the lower retina below. Fibers from the temporal retina are lateral; those from the nasal side are medial. Macular fibers, which constitute approximately one-third of the nerve, are laterally placed. In the nerve head, foveal fibers are located peripherally, and peripapillary fibers are located centrally.

Prelaminar area

The ganglion cell axons that enter the nerve head are supported by a "wicker basket" of astrocytic glial cells and are segregated into bundles, or *fascicles,* that pass through the lamina cribrosa. These astrocytes invest the optic nerve and form continuous circular tubes that enclose groups of nerve fibers throughout their intraocular and intraorbital course, separating them from connective tissue elements at all sites. At the nerve head, the Müller cells that make up the internal limiting membrane (ILM) are replaced by astrocytes. Astrocytes constitute 10% of the nerve head volume and form an ILM that covers the surface of the nerve head and is continuous with the Müller cell–derived ILM of the retina. The pigment epithelium may be exposed at the temporal margin of the disc to form a narrow pigmented crescent. When the pigment epithelium and choroid fail to reach the temporal margin, crescents of partial or absent pigmentation may be observed. The relationship between the choroid and the prelaminar portion of the optic nerve partly accounts for the staining of the disc normally observed in late phases of fluorescein fundus angiography. The disc vessels do not leak, but the choroidal capillaries are freely permeable to fluorescein, which can therefore diffuse into the lamina.

When the optic nerve is damaged, axons and supporting glial elements can be lost, causing pathologic enlargement of the optic cup. This cupping may be the first objective sign of damage from glaucoma or other forms of optic neuropathy.

Laminar area

The *lamina cribrosa* comprises approximately 10 connective tissue plates, which are integrated with the sclera and whose pores transmit the axon bundles. The openings are wider above than below, which may imply less protection from the mechanical effects of pressure in glaucoma. The lamina contains type I and type III collagens, abundant elastin, laminin, and fibronectin. Astrocytes surround the axon bundles, and small blood vessels are present. The lamina cribrosa serves the following 3 functions: (1) scaffold for the optic nerve axons, (2) point of fixation for the CRA and CRV, and (3) reinforcement of the posterior segment of the globe. High-resolution optical coherence tomography is beginning to facilitate the systematic anatomical study of the lamina cribrosa in pathologic states such as glaucoma.

Retrolaminar area

Behind the lamina cribrosa, the diameter of the optic nerve increases to 3 mm as a result of myelination of the nerve fibers and the presence of oligodendroglia and the surrounding meningeal sheaths (pia, arachnoid, and dura) (Fig 3-3). The retrolaminar nerve continues proximally (as the intraorbital part of the optic nerve) to the apex of the orbit. The axoplasm of the neurons contains neurofilaments, microtubules, mitochondria, and smooth endoplasmic reticulum.

Intraorbital Region

Annulus of Zinn

The intraorbital part of the optic nerve lies within the muscle cone. Before passing into the optic canal, the nerve is surrounded by the annulus of Zinn, which is formed by the origins of the rectus muscles. The superior and medial rectus muscles partially share a connective tissue sheath with the optic nerve. This connection may partly explain why patients with retrobulbar neuritis report symptoms of pain on eye movement. At the optic canal, the dural sheath of the nerve fuses to the periosteum, completely immobilizing the nerve and rendering it susceptible to shearing forces from trauma transmitted to the orbital apex via the bony buttresses of the orbit.

Meningeal sheaths

The *pia mater* is the innermost layer of the optic nerve sheath. It is a vascular connective tissue coat, covered with meningothelial cells, that sends numerous septa into the optic nerve, dividing its axons into bundles. The septa continue throughout the intraorbital and intracanalicular regions of the nerve and end just before the chiasm. They contain collagen, elastic tissue, fibroblasts, nerves, and small arterioles and venules (Fig 3-4). They provide mechanical support for the nerve bundles and nutrition to the axons and glial cells. A mantle of astrocytic glial cells prevents the pia and septa from having direct contact with nerve axons.

The *arachnoid mater,* which is composed of collagenous tissue, small amounts of elastic tissue, and meningothelial cells, lines the dura mater and is connected to the pia across the subarachnoid space by vascular trabeculae. The subarachnoid space ends anteriorly at the level of the lamina cribrosa. Posteriorly, it is usually continuous with the

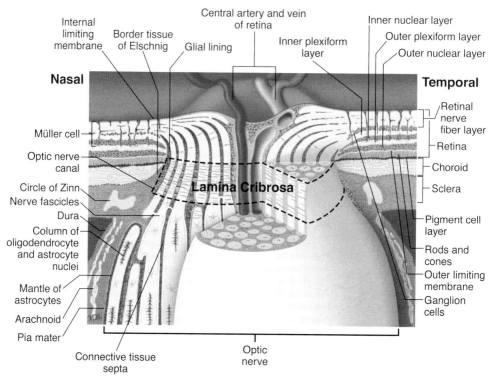

Figure 3-3 Schematic representation of the optic nerve head. The temporal retina has a thicker layer of ganglion cells, representing the increased ganglion cell concentration found in the macula. Müller glia traverse the neural retina to provide both structural and functional support. Where the retina terminates at the optic disc edge, the Müller cells are continuous with the astrocytes, forming the internal limiting membrane. The border tissue of Elschnig is the dense connective tissue that joins the sclera with the Bruch membrane, enclosing the choroid and forming the scleral ring that defines the margin of the optic disc. At the posterior termination of the choroid on the temporal side, the border tissue of Elschnig lies between the astrocytes surrounding the optic nerve canal and the stroma of the choroid. On the nasal side, the choroidal stroma is directly adjacent to the astrocytes surrounding the nerve. This collection of astrocytes surrounding the canal is known as the border tissue, which is continuous with a similar glial lining at the termination of the retina. The nerve fibers of the retina are segregated into approximately 1000 fascicles by astrocytes. On reaching the lamina cribrosa *(upper dashed line)*, the nerve fascicles and their surrounding astrocytes are separated from each other by connective tissue. The lamina cribrosa is an extension of scleral collagen and elastic fibers through the nerve. The external choroid also sends some connective tissue to the anterior part of the lamina. At the external part of the lamina cribrosa *(lower dashed line)*, the nerve fibers become myelinated, and columns of oligodendrocytes and a few astrocytes are present within the nerve fascicles. The bundles continue to be separated by connective tissue septa all the way to the chiasm. The septa are derived from the pia mater. This connective tissue is also derived from the pia mater and is known as septal tissue. A mantle of astrocytes, continuous anteriorly with the border tissue, surrounds the nerve along its orbital course. The dura, arachnoid, and pia mater are shown. The nerve fibers are myelinated. Within the bundles, the cell bodies of astrocytes and oligodendrocytes form a column of nuclei. The central retinal vessels are surrounded by a perivascular connective tissue throughout its course in the nerve. This connective tissue, known as the central supporting connective tissue strand, blends with the connective tissue of the lamina cribrosa. *(Illustration by Mark Miller.)*

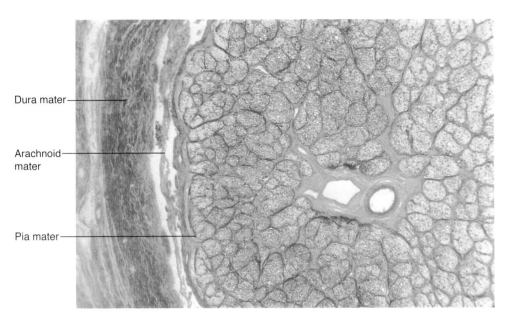

Figure 3-4 Meningeal sheaths. The dura mater, the outer layer, is composed of collagenous connective tissue. The arachnoid mater, the middle layer, is made up of fine collagenous fibers arranged in a loose meshwork lined by endothelial cells. The innermost layer, the pia mater, is made up of fine collagenous and elastic fibers and is highly vascularized. Elements from both the arachnoid and the pia are continuous with the optic nerve septa (Masson trichrome, ×64). *(Courtesy of Thomas A. Weingeist, PhD, MD.)*

subarachnoid space of the brain. Because the central retinal vessels cross this space, a rise in intracranial pressure can compress the retinal vein and raise the venous pressure within the retina above the intraocular pressure. This situation causes intraocular venous dilatation and the loss of spontaneous venous pulsation at the nerve head. Such an absence of pulsation may clinically indicate raised intracranial pressure.

The thick *dura mater* encases the brain and makes up the outer layer of the meningeal sheath of the optic nerve. It is 0.3–0.5 mm thick and consists of dense bundles of collagen and elastic tissue that fuse anteriorly with the outer layers of the sclera. The meninges of the optic nerve are supplied by sensory nerve fibers, which account in part for the pain experienced by patients with retrobulbar neuritis and other inflammatory optic nerve diseases.

Intracanalicular Region

Within the optic canal, the blood supply of the optic nerve is derived from pial vessels originating from the ophthalmic artery. The optic nerve and surrounding arachnoid are tethered to the periosteum of the bony canal within the intracanalicular region. Blunt trauma, particularly over the eyebrow, can transmit the force of injury to the intracanalicular region, causing shearing and interruption of the blood supply to the nerve in this area. Such nerve damage is called *indirect traumatic optic neuropathy*. In addition, optic nerve edema in this area can lead to a compartment syndrome, further compromising the function of the optic nerve within the confined space of the optic canal.

Intracranial Region

After passing through the optic canals, the 2 optic nerves lie above the ophthalmic arteries, above and medial to the *internal carotid arteries (ICAs)*. The anterior cerebral arteries cross over the optic nerves and are connected by the anterior communicating artery, which completes the anterior portion of the circle of Willis. The optic nerves then pass posteriorly over the cavernous sinus to join in the optic chiasm. The chiasm then divides into right and left optic tracts, which end in their respective lateral geniculate bodies. From these bodies arise the geniculocalcarine pathways (or optic radiations), which pass to each primary visual cortex. Lesions at different locations along the visual pathway produce characteristic visual field defects that help localize the site of damage (Fig 3-5).

Blood Supply of the Optic Nerve

The ophthalmic artery lies below the optic nerve. The CRA and, usually, 2 long posterior ciliary arteries branch off from the ophthalmic artery once it enters the muscle cone at the annulus of Zinn.

The blood supply of the optic nerve varies from one segment of the nerve to another. Although the blood supply can vary widely, a multitude of studies have revealed a basic pattern. The arterial supply of the optic nerve head is as follows: the retrolaminar nerve is supplied chiefly by pial vessels and short posterior ciliary vessels, with some help from

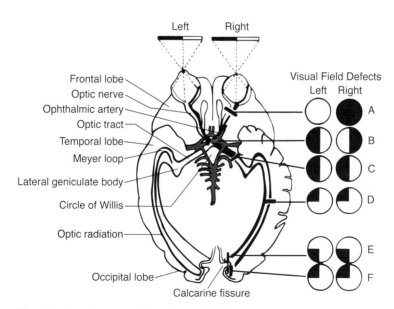

Figure 3-5 The visual pathway and the circle of Willis, showing lesions at different locations and their corresponding visual field defects. *(Illustration by Thomas A. Weingeist, PhD, MD.)*

the CRA and recurrent choroidal arteries. The lamina is supplied by short posterior ciliary arteries or by branches of the arterial circle of Haller and Zinn *(circle of Zinn-Haller)*. This circle arises from the paraoptic branches of the short posterior ciliary arteries and is usually embedded in the sclera around the nerve head. It is often incomplete and may be divided into superior and inferior halves. The CRA does not supply this region.

The prelaminar nerve is supplied by the short posterior ciliary arteries (cilioretinal arteries, if present) and recurrent choroidal arteries, although their relative contribution is debated. The nerve fiber layer is supplied by the CRA (Figs 3-6, 3-7). The posterior ciliary arteries are terminal arteries, and the area where the respective capillary beds from each artery meet is termed the *watershed zone*. When perfusion pressure drops, the tissue lying within this area is the most vulnerable to ischemia. Consequences can be significant when the entire optic nerve head or a part of it lies within the watershed zone.

The intraorbital region of the optic nerve is supplied proximally by the pial vascular network and by neighboring branches of the ophthalmic artery. Distally, it is also supplied by intraneural branches of the CRA. Most anteriorly, it is supplied by short posterior ciliary arteries and occasional peripapillary choroidal arteries.

The intracanalicular region of the optic nerve is supplied almost exclusively by the ophthalmic artery. The intracranial region of the optic nerve is supplied primarily by branches of both the ICA and the ophthalmic artery.

The lumen of the CRA is surrounded by nonfenestrated endothelial cells with typical zonulae occludentes that are similar to those in retinal vessels. The CRA, however, differs from retinal arterioles in that it contains a fenestrated internal elastic lamina and an outer layer of smooth muscle cells surrounded by a thin basement membrane. The retinal arterioles have no internal elastic lamina, and they lose their smooth muscle cells shortly after entering the retina. The CRV consists of endothelial cells, a thin basal lamina, and a thick collagenous adventitia.

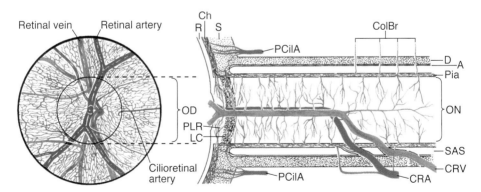

Figure 3-6 Schematic of the blood supply to the optic nerve head and intraorbital optic nerve. A = arachnoid; Ch = choroid; ColBr = collateral branches; CRA = central retinal artery; CRV = central retinal vein; D = dura; LC = lamina cribrosa; OD = optic disc; ON = optic nerve; PCilA = posterior ciliary arteries; PLR = prelaminar region; R = retina; S = sclera; SAS = subarachnoid space. *(Reproduced with permission from Hayreh SS. Anatomy and physiology of the optic nerve head. Trans Am Acad Ophthalmol Otolaryngol. 1974;78(2):OP240–254.)*

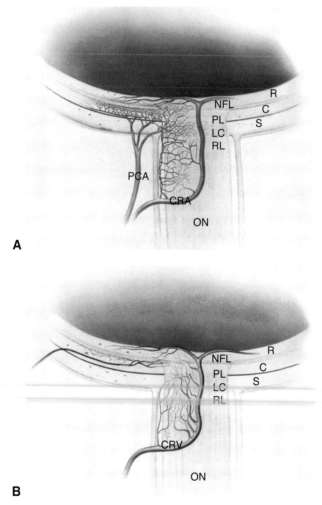

Figure 3-7 Anterior optic nerve vasculature. **A,** Arterial supply to the anterior optic nerve and peripapillary choroid (C). **B,** Venous drainage of the anterior optic nerve and peripapillary choroid (C). CRA = central retinal artery; CRV = central retinal vein; LC = lamina cribrosa; NFL = superficial nerve fiber layer; ON = optic nerve; PCA = posterior ciliary artery; PL = prelamina; R = retina; RL = retrolamina; S = sclera. *(Reproduced with permission from Wright KW, ed.* Textbook of Ophthalmology. *Baltimore: Williams & Wilkins; 1997:592, figs 44-2, 44-3. Originally from Ritch R, Shields MB, Krupin T, eds.* The Glaucomas. *2nd ed. St Louis: Mosby; 1996:178.)*

Chiasm

The optic chiasm makes up part of the anterior inferior floor of the third ventricle. It is surrounded by pia and arachnoid and is richly vascularized. The chiasm is approximately 12 mm wide, 8 mm long in the anteroposterior direction, and 4 mm thick. The extramacular fibers from the inferonasal retina cross anteriorly in the chiasm at the "Wilbrand knee" before passing into the optic tract. Extramacular superonasal fibers cross directly to the opposite tract. Extramacular temporal fibers remain uncrossed in the chiasm and optic tract. The macular projections are located centrally in the optic nerve and constitute

80%–90% of the total volume of the optic nerve and the chiasmal fibers. The temporal macular fibers pursue a direct course through the chiasm as a bundle of uncrossed fibers. Nasal macular fibers cross in the posterior part of the chiasm. Approximately 53% of the optic nerve fibers are crossed, and 47% are uncrossed.

Optic Tract

Each optic tract contains ipsilateral temporal and contralateral nasal fibers from the optic nerves. Fibers (both crossed and uncrossed) from the upper retinal projections travel medially in the optic tract; lower projections move laterally. The macular fibers adopt a dorsolateral orientation as they course toward the lateral geniculate body.

Lateral Geniculate Body

The lateral geniculate body, or nucleus, is the synaptic zone for the higher visual projections. It is an oval, caplike structure that receives approximately 70% of the optic tract fibers within its 6 alternating layers of gray and white matter. Layers 1, 4, and 6 of the lateral geniculate body contain axons from the contralateral optic nerve. Layers 2, 3, and 5 arise from the ipsilateral optic nerve. The 6 layers, numbered consecutively from below upward, give rise to the optic radiations.

Optic Radiations

The optic radiations connect the lateral geniculate body with the cortex of the occipital lobe. The fibers of the optic radiations leave the lateral geniculate body and wind around the temporal horn of the lateral ventricle, approaching the anterior tip of the temporal lobe, or *loop of Meyer*. They then sweep backward toward the visual area of the occipital lobe. Damage to the optic radiation in the anterior temporal lobe gives rise to a wedge-shaped, upper homonymous "pie in the sky" visual field defect.

Visual Cortex

The visual cortex, the thinnest area of the human cerebral cortex, has 6 cellular layers and occupies the superior and inferior lips of the calcarine fissure on the posterior and medial surfaces of the occipital lobes. Macular function is extremely well represented in the visual cortex and occupies the most posterior position at the tip of the occipital lobe. The most anterior portion of the calcarine fissure is occupied by contralateral nasal retinal fibers only. The posterior cerebral artery, a branch of the basilar artery, supplies the visual cortex almost exclusively. However, the blood supply to the occipital lobe does show anatomical variation; in some individuals, the middle cerebral artery contributes.

Trobe JD. *The Neurology of Vision.* New York: Oxford University Press; 2001:1–42.

Cranial Nerve III (Oculomotor Nerve)

Although CN III contains only 24,000 fibers, it supplies all the extraocular muscles except the superior oblique and the lateral rectus. It also carries cholinergic innervation to the pupillary sphincter and the ciliary muscle.

Cranial nerve III arises from a complex group of cells in the rostral midbrain, or *mes-encephalon,* at the level of the superior colliculus. This nuclear complex lies ventral to the periaqueductal gray matter, is immediately rostral to the CN IV nuclear complex, and is bounded inferolaterally by the medial longitudinal fasciculus.

The CN III nucleus consists of several distinct, large motor cell subnuclei, each of which subserves the extraocular muscle it innervates (Fig 3-8). Except for a single central caudal nucleus that serves both levator palpebrae superioris muscles, the cell groups are paired. Notably, the shared innervation of both levator muscles is responsible for Hering's law of equal innervation.

Fibers from the dorsal nucleus cross, or *decussate,* in the caudal aspect of the nucleus and therefore supply the contralateral superior rectus muscles. The Edinger-Westphal nucleus is cephalad and dorsomedial in location. It provides the parasympathetic pre-ganglionic efferent innervation to the ciliary muscle and pupillary sphincter. The most ventral subnuclei supply the medial rectus muscles. A subnucleus for ocular convergence has been described but is not consistently found in primates.

The fascicular portion of CN III travels ventrally from the nuclear complex, through the red nucleus, between the medial aspects of the cerebral peduncles, and through the cortico-spinal fibers. It exits in the interpeduncular space. In the subarachnoid space, CN III passes below the posterior cerebral artery and above the superior cerebellar artery, the 2 major branches of the basilar artery (Fig 3-9). The nerve travels forward in the interpeduncular cistern lateral to the posterior communicating artery and penetrates the arachnoid between the free and attached borders of the tentorium cerebelli. Aneurysms that affect CN III commonly occur at the junction of the posterior communicating artery and the ICA.

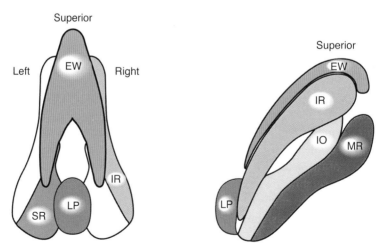

Figure 3-8 Diagram of the oculomotor nuclear complex, which is composed of different sub-nuclei that give rise to CN III. A central caudal nucleus supplies both levator muscles, and the nucleus for each superior rectus supplies the contralateral muscle. EW = Edinger-Westphal nucleus; IO = nucleus to the inferior oblique muscle; IR = nucleus to the inferior rectus muscle; LP = nucleus to the levator palpebrae muscle; MR = nucleus to the medial rectus muscle; SR = nucleus to the contralateral superior rectus muscle. *(Illustration by Sylvia Barker.)*

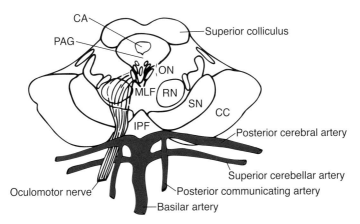

Figure 3-9 Schematic cross section through the midbrain at the level of the CN III nucleus. Note the relationship between CN III and the posterior cerebral, superior cerebellar, and posterior communicating arteries. CA = cerebral aqueduct; CC = crus cerebri (includes corticospinal tract); IPF = interpeduncular fossa; MLF = medial longitudinal fasciculus; ON = oculomotor nucleus; PAG = periaqueductal gray; RN = red nucleus; SN = substantia nigra.

The oculomotor nerve pierces the dura on the lateral side of the posterior clinoid process, initially traversing the roof of the cavernous sinus. It runs along the lateral wall of the cavernous sinus and above CN IV and enters the orbit through the superior orbital fissure.

Cranial nerve III usually separates into superior and inferior divisions after passing through the annulus of Zinn in the orbit. Alternatively, it may divide within the anterior cavernous sinus. The nerve maintains a topographic organization even in the midbrain, so lesions almost anywhere along its course may cause a divisional nerve palsy.

The superior division of CN III innervates the superior rectus and levator palpebrae muscles. The larger inferior division splits into 3 branches to supply the medial and inferior rectus muscles and the inferior oblique muscle.

The parasympathetic fibers wind around the periphery of the nerve, enter the inferior division, and course through the branch that supplies the inferior oblique muscle. They join the ciliary ganglion, where they synapse with the postganglionic fibers, which emerge as many short ciliary nerves. These nerves pierce the sclera and travel through the choroid to innervate the pupillary sphincter and the ciliary muscle. The superficial location of these fibers makes them more vulnerable to compression, such as from an aneurysm, than to ischemia. However, a pupil-sparing oculomotor nerve palsy, even in the context of systemic vascular disease, is not a perfect indicator of the absence of an enlarging aneurysm, and a growing number of neuro-ophthalmologists recommend emergent imaging (by computed tomography/computed tomography angiography or magnetic resonance imaging/magnetic resonance angiography) for anyone with new-onset CN III palsy with incomplete ptosis.

Trobe JD. Searching for brain aneurysm in third cranial nerve palsy. *J Neuro-Ophthalmol.* 2009;29(3):171–173.

Pathways for the Pupil Reflexes

Light reflex

The light reflex consists of a simultaneous and equal constriction of the pupils in response to illumination of one or the other eye. The afferent pupillary pathway coincides with that of the visual pathway and includes a decussation of nasal fibers in the chiasm. At the posterior part of the optic tract, the pupillary fibers leave the visual fibers and pass to the lateral side of the midbrain to reach the pretectal nuclei at the level of the superior colliculus. Here, efferent fibers arise and pass to the Edinger-Westphal nuclei, decussating partially (both ventral to the aqueduct and dorsally, in the posterior commissure). Preganglionic parasympathetic fibers leave each Edinger-Westphal nucleus and run in the oculomotor nerve as it leaves the brainstem. The fibers spiral downward to lie medially in the nerve at the level of the petroclinoid ligament and inferiorly in the inferior division of CN III as it enters the orbit. These fibers synapse in the ciliary ganglion and give rise to postganglionic myelinated short ciliary nerves, approximately 3%–5% of which are pupillomotor. The rest are designated for the ciliary muscle and are concerned with the near reflex.

Near reflex

The near reflex is a synkinesis that occurs when attention is changed from distance to near. This reflex includes accommodation, pupil constriction, and convergence. The reflex is initiated in the occipital association cortex, from which impulses descend along corticofugal pathways to relay in pretectal and possibly tegmental areas. From these relays, fibers pass to the Edinger-Westphal nuclei, the motor nuclei of the medial rectus muscles, and the nuclei of CN VI. Fibers for the near reflex approach the pretectal nucleus from the ventral aspect; thus, compressive dorsal lesions of the optic tectum spare the near pupil reflex relative to the light reflex (light–near dissociation). Efferent fibers for accommodation follow the same general pathway as do those for the light reflex, but their final distribution (via the short ciliary nerves) is to the ciliary muscle.

Cranial Nerve IV (Trochlear Nerve)

Cranial nerve IV contains the fewest nerve fibers (approximately 3400) of any cranial nerve, but it has the longest intracranial course (75 mm). The nerve nucleus is located in the caudal mesencephalon at the level of the inferior colliculus near the periaqueductal gray matter, ventral to the aqueduct of Sylvius. It is continuous with the caudal end of the CN III nucleus and differs histologically from that nucleus only in the smaller size of its cells. Like the CN III nucleus, it is bounded ventrolaterally by the medial longitudinal fasciculus.

The fascicles of CN IV curve dorsocaudally around the periaqueductal gray matter and decussate completely in the superior medullary velum. The nerves exit the brainstem just beneath the inferior colliculus. Thus, CN IV is the only cranial nerve that is completely decussated and the only motor nerve to exit dorsally from the nervous system. As it curves around the brainstem in the ambient cistern, CN IV runs beneath the free edge of the tentorium, passes between the posterior cerebral and superior cerebellar arteries, and then pierces the dura mater to enter the cavernous sinus.

Cranial nerve IV travels beneath CN III and above the ophthalmic division of CN V in the lateral wall of the cavernous sinus. It enters the orbit through the superior orbital fissure outside the annulus of Zinn and runs superiorly to innervate the superior oblique muscle. Because of its location outside the muscle cone, CN IV is usually not affected by injection of retrobulbar anesthetics.

Cranial Nerve V (Trigeminal Nerve)

Cranial nerve V, the largest cranial nerve, possesses both sensory and motor divisions. The sensory portion subserves the greater part of the scalp, forehead, face, eyelids, eyes, lacrimal glands, extraocular muscles, ears, dura mater, and tongue. The motor portion innervates the muscles of mastication through branches of the mandibular division.

The CN V nuclear complex extends from the midbrain to the upper cervical segments, often as caudal as C4. It consists of the following 4 nuclei, listed from above downward:

1. mesencephalic nucleus
2. main sensory nucleus
3. spinal nucleus and tract
4. motor nucleus located in the pons

Important interconnections exist between the different subdivisions of the CN V sensory nuclei and the reticular formation (Fig 3-10).

Mesencephalic Nucleus

The mesencephalic nucleus mediates proprioception and deep sensation from the masticatory, facial, and extraocular muscles. The nucleus extends inferiorly into the posterior pons as far as the main sensory nucleus.

Main Sensory Nucleus

The main sensory nucleus lies in the pons, lateral to the motor nucleus. It is continuous with the mesencephalic nucleus (above) and with the spinal nucleus (below). It receives its input from ascending branches of the sensory root, and it serves light touch from the skin and mucous membranes. The sensory root of CN V, upon entering the pons, divides into an ascending tract and a descending tract. The ascending tract terminates in the main sensory nucleus, and the descending tract ends in the spinal nucleus.

Spinal Nucleus and Tract

The spinal nucleus and tract extend through the medulla to C4. The nucleus receives pain and temperature afferents from the descending spinal tract, which also carries cutaneous components of CN VII, CN IX, and CN X that serve sensations from the ear and external auditory meatus. The sensory fibers from the ophthalmic division of

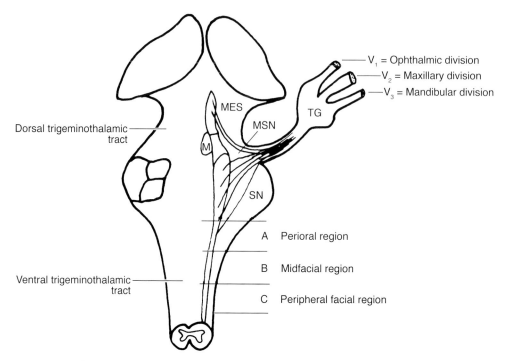

Figure 3-10 Cranial nerve V complex (dorsal view of brainstem). M = motor nucleus; MES = mesencephalic nucleus; MSN = main sensory nucleus; SN = spinal nucleus and tract; TG = trigeminal ganglion. A, B, and C represent portions of the caudal spinal nucleus that correspond to concentric areas of the face.

CN V (V_1) terminate in the most ventral portion of the spinal nucleus and tract. Fibers from the maxillary division (V_2) end in the midportion of the spinal nucleus (in a ventral–dorsal plane). The fibers from the mandibular division (V_3) end in the dorsal parts of the nucleus.

The cutaneous territory of each of the CN V divisions is represented in the spinal nucleus and tract in a rostral–caudal direction. Fibers from the perioral region are thought to terminate most rostrally in the nucleus; fibers from the peripheral face and scalp end in the caudal portion. The zone between them, the midfacial region, is projected onto the central portion of the nucleus. This "onionskin" pattern of cutaneous sensation has been revealed by clinical studies of patients with damage to the spinal nucleus and tract (Fig 3-11). Damage to the trigeminal sensory nucleus at the level of the brainstem causes bilateral sensory loss in concentric areas of the face, with the sensory area surrounding the mouth in the center. If a patient verifies this distribution of sensory loss, the lesion is in the brainstem. Conversely, sensory loss that follows the peripheral distribution of the trigeminal sensory divisions (ophthalmic, maxillary, and mandibular) indicates that the lesion lies in CN V after it exits the brainstem.

Axons from the main sensory, spinal, and portions of the mesencephalic nuclei relay sensory information to higher sensory areas of the brain. The axons cross the midline

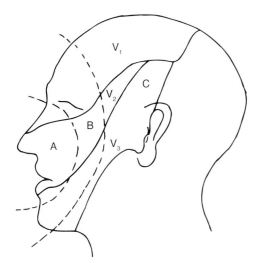

Figure 3-11 Cranial nerve V (trigeminal nerve): pattern of facial sensation. Lesions of the trigeminal sensory nucleus in the brainstem result in an "onionskin" distribution of altered sensation (regions A, B, and C) delineated by the *dashed lines;* lesions of the ophthalmic (V₁), maxillary (V₂), and mandibular (V₃) nerves result in the pattern of sensory loss delineated by the *solid lines.* *(Illustration by Thomas A. Weingeist, PhD, MD.)*

in the pons and ascend to the thalamus along the ventral and dorsal trigeminothalamic tracts. They terminate in the nerve cells of the ventral posteromedial nucleus of the thalamus. These cells, in turn, send axons through the internal capsule to the postcentral gyrus of the cerebral cortex.

The afferent limb of the oculocardiac reflex is mediated by the trigeminal nerve. Although the mechanism underlying the oculocardiac reflex is not known, the size and length of the trigeminal nucleus (see Fig 3-10) may suggest a physical etiology for the interaction between the trigeminal nerve and the vagus nerve (CN X).

Motor Nucleus

The motor nucleus is located medial to the main sensory nucleus in the pons. It receives fibers from both cerebral hemispheres, the reticular formation, the red nucleus, the tectum, the medial longitudinal fasciculus, and the mesencephalic nucleus. A monosynaptic reflex arc is formed by cells from the mesencephalic nucleus and the motor nucleus. The motor nucleus sends off axons that form the motor root, which eventually supplies the muscles of mastication (pterygoid, masseter, and temporalis), the tensor tympani muscle, tensor veli palatini muscle, mylohyoid muscle, and the anterior belly of the digastric muscle.

The intracranial portion of the fifth nerve emerges from the upper lateral portion of the ventral pons, passes over the petrous apex, forms the *trigeminal ganglion,* and then divides into 3 branches. The trigeminal ganglion, also called the *gasserian* or *semilunar ganglion,* contains the cells of origin of all the CN V sensory axons. The crescent-shaped ganglion occupies a recess in the dura mater posterolateral to the cavernous sinus. This recess, called the *Meckel cave,* is near the apex of the petrous part of the temporal bone in the middle cranial fossa. Medially, the trigeminal ganglion is close to the ICA and the posterior cavernous sinus.

Divisions of Cranial Nerve V

The 3 divisions of CN V are the ophthalmic (V_1), the maxillary (V_2), and the mandibular (V_3).

Ophthalmic division (CN V$_1$)

The ophthalmic division enters the cavernous sinus lateral to the ICA and courses beneath CN III and CN IV. Within the sinus, it gives off a tentorial–dural branch, which supplies sensation to the cerebral vessels, dura mater of the anterior fossa, cavernous sinus, sphenoid wing, petrous apex, Meckel cave, tentorium cerebelli, falx cerebri, and dural venous sinuses. CN V_1 passes into the orbit through the superior orbital fissure and divides into 3 branches: frontal, lacrimal, and nasociliary.

The frontal nerve divides into the supraorbital and supratrochlear nerves, which provide sensation to the medial portion of the upper eyelid and the conjunctiva, forehead, scalp, frontal sinuses, and side of the nose. According to common teaching, the supratrochlear nerve exits the orbit 17 mm from midline, whereas the supraorbital nerve exits at 27 mm from midline, through either a notch or a true foramen.

The lacrimal nerve innervates the lacrimal gland and the neighboring conjunctiva and skin. It was formerly suggested that postganglionic parasympathetic lacrimal secretory fibers, arising in the pterygopalatine ganglion, were carried to the lacrimal gland via a zygomaticotemporal connection with the lacrimal nerve. However, it is now thought more likely that the gland receives its parasympathetic supply directly from the retro-orbital plexus (discussed later, in the section Cranial Nerve VII). Occasionally, the lacrimal nerve exits the orbit via a lacrimal foramen to supply the lateral forehead. Otherwise, that area is supplied by branches of the supraorbital nerve (Fig 3-12).

The nasociliary nerve supplies sensation through nasal branches to the middle and inferior turbinates, septum, lateral nasal wall, and tip of the nose. The infratrochlear branch serves the lacrimal drainage system, the conjunctiva, and the skin of the medial canthal region. Long ciliary nerves carry sensory fibers from the ciliary body, the iris, and the cornea and provide sympathetic innervation to the dilator muscle of the iris. Sensation from the globe is carried by short ciliary nerves. The CN V fibers pass through the ciliary ganglion to join the nasociliary nerve. The ciliary nerves also contain postganglionic parasympathetic fibers from the ganglion to the pupillary sphincter and the ciliary muscle. The trigeminal nerve, like other sensory nerves, interacts with its innervated tissues. In the cornea, sensory innervation is important for corneal homeostasis, and loss of sensation leads to neurotrophic keratopathy.

Maxillary division (CN V$_2$)

The maxillary division leaves the trigeminal ganglion to exit the skull through the foramen rotundum, which lies below the superior orbital fissure. Cranial nerve V_2 courses through the pterygopalatine fossa into the inferior orbital fissure and then passes through the infraorbital canal as the infraorbital nerve. After exiting the infraorbital foramen, CN V_2 divides into an inferior palpebral branch supplying the lower eyelid, a nasal branch for the side of the nose, and a superior labial branch for the upper lip. The teeth, maxillary sinus, roof of the mouth, and soft palate are also innervated by branches of the maxillary division.

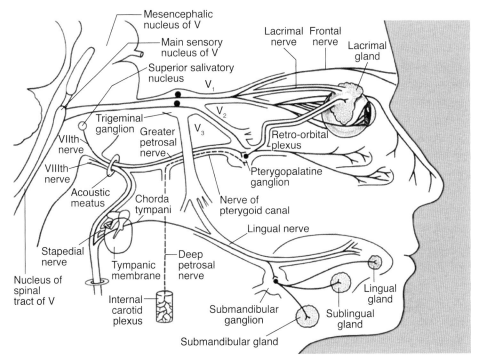

Figure 3-12 Lacrimal reflex arc (after Kurihashi). The afferent pathway is provided by the first and second divisions of CN V. The efferent path proceeds from the lacrimal nucleus (close to the superior salivary nucleus) via CN VII (nervus intermedius), through the geniculate ganglion, the greater superficial petrosal nerve, and the nerve of the pterygoid canal (where it is joined by sympathetic fibers from the deep petrosal nerve). The nerve then passes to the pterygo-palatine ganglion, where it synapses with postganglionic fibers. These fibers reach the lacrimal gland directly, via the retro-orbital plexus of nerves (particularly CN V1). The fibers carry cholin-ergic and vasoactive intestinal polypeptide (VIP)-ergic fibers to the gland. *(From Bron AJ, Tripathi RC, Tripathi BJ. Wolff's Anatomy of the Eye and Orbit. 8th ed. London: Chapman & Hall; 1997.)*

Mandibular division (CN V₃)

The mandibular division contains sensory and motor fibers. It exits the skull through the foramen ovale and provides motor input for the masticatory muscles. Sensation is supplied to the mucosa and skin of the mandible, lower lip, tongue, external ear, and tympanum.

> Standring S, ed. *Gray's Anatomy: The Anatomical Basis of Clinical Practice.* 39th ed. Edin-
> burgh, New York: Elsevier Churchill Livingstone; 2005.

Cranial Nerve VI (Abducens Nerve)

The nucleus of CN VI is situated in the floor of the fourth ventricle, beneath the facial col-liculus, in the caudal pons. Fibers of CN VII pass over or loop around the CN VI nucleus and exit in the cerebellopontine angle. The medial longitudinal fasciculus lies medial to

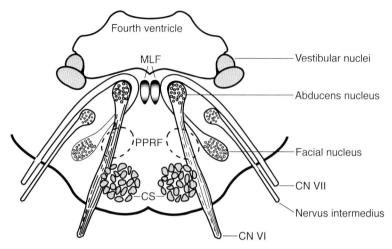

Figure 3-13 Cross section of the pons at the level of the CN VI (abducens nerve) nucleus. CS = corticospinal tract; MLF = medial longitudinal fasciculus; PPRF = pontine paramedian reticular formation. *(Illustration by Sylvia Barker.)*

the CN VI nucleus. The fascicular portion of the nerve runs ventrally through the paramedian pontine reticular formation and the pyramidal tract and leaves the brainstem in the pontomedullary junction (Fig 3-13).

Cranial nerve VI takes a vertical course along the ventral face of the pons and is crossed by the anterior inferior cerebellar artery. It continues through the subarachnoid space along the surface of the clivus, surrounded by the Batson venous plexus, to perforate the dura mater below the crest of the petrous portion of the temporal bone, approximately 2 cm below the posterior clinoid process. It then passes intradurally through or around the inferior petrosal sinus and beneath the petroclinoid (Gruber) ligament through the Dorello canal, where it enters the cavernous sinus. This long route, especially along the surface of the clivus and beneath the petroclinoid ligament, is responsible for this nerve's susceptibility to stretch injury leading to paresis in the context of increased intracranial pressure. In the cavernous sinus, CN VI runs below and lateral to the carotid artery and may transiently carry sympathetic fibers from the carotid plexus. It passes through the superior orbital fissure within the annulus of Zinn and innervates the lateral rectus muscle on its ocular surface.

Cranial Nerve VII (Facial Nerve)

Cranial nerve VII is developmentally derived from the second branchial arch. It is a complex mixed sensory and motor nerve. The motor root contains special visceral efferent fibers that innervate the muscles of facial expression.

The so-called sensory root of CN VII is the nervus intermedius, which contains special visceral afferent, general somatic afferent, and general visceral efferent fibers.

The special *visceral afferent fibers,* which convey the sense of taste from the anterior two-thirds of the tongue, terminate centrally in the nucleus of the tractus solitarius. The general *somatic afferent fibers* convey sensation from the external auditory meatus and the retroauricular skin; centrally, they enter the spinal nucleus of CN V. The general visceral efferent fibers provide preganglionic parasympathetic innervation by way of the spheno-palatine and submandibular ganglia to the lacrimal, submaxillary, and sublingual glands.

The motor nucleus of CN VII is a cigar-shaped column, 4 mm long, located in the caudal third of the pons. It is ventrolateral to the CN VI nucleus, ventromedial to the spinal nucleus of CN V, and dorsal to the superior olive. Four distinct subgroups within the nucleus innervate specific facial muscles; the ventral portion of the intermediate group probably supplies axons to the orbicularis oculi. The part of the nucleus supplying the upper half of the face receives corticobulbar input from both cerebral hemispheres. The lower half of the face is influenced by corticobulbar fibers from the opposite cerebral hemisphere.

Fibers from the motor nucleus course dorsomedially to approach the floor of the fourth ventricle and then ascend immediately dorsal to the CN VI nucleus. At the rostral end of the CN VI nucleus, the main facial motor fibers arch over its dorsal surface (forming the internal genu of CN VII) and then pass ventrolaterally between the spinal nucleus of CN V and the CN VII nucleus to exit the brainstem at the pontomedullary junction. The bulge formed by the CN VII genu in the floor of the fourth ventricle is the facial colliculus (see Fig 3-13).

The sensory nucleus of CN VII is the rostral portion of the tractus solitarius, some-times known as the *gustatory nucleus.* It lies lateral to the motor and parasympathetic nuclei in the caudal pons. Sensations of taste from the anterior two-thirds of the tongue are carried by special visceral afferent fibers to this nucleus. The impulses travel along the lingual nerve and chorda tympani; the cell bodies for these impulses are located in the geniculate ganglion. The impulses eventually reach the brain through the nervus intermedius.

Cranial nerve VII, the nervus intermedius, and CN VIII (the acoustic nerve) pass together through the lateral pontine cistern in the cerebellopontine angle and enter the internal auditory meatus in a common meningeal sheath. Cranial nerve VII and the intermedius nerve then enter the fallopian canal, the longest bony canal traversed by any cranial nerve (30 mm).

Cranial nerve VII can be divided into 3 segments in its course through this canal. After passing anterolaterally for a short distance known as the *labyrinthine segment,* the nerves bend sharply at the geniculate ganglion and are then directed dorsolaterally past the tympanic cavity. This 90° bend, known as the *tympanic segment,* is the external genu of CN VII. Two parasympathetic branches from the superior salivatory and lacrimal nuclei leave the nerve at the tympanic segment: the greater superficial petrosal nerve and a small filament that joins the inferior petrosal nerve. The third segment of the nerve, the *mastoid segment,* is directed straight down toward the base of the skull. The stapedius nerve leaves, and the chorda tympani joins CN VII in the mastoid segment. The CN VII trunk then exits the skull at the stylomastoid foramen and separates into a large temporofacial division and a small cervicofacial division between the superficial and deep lobes of the parotid gland. This area of branching is known as the *pes anserinus.*

The temporofacial division gives rise to the temporal, zygomatic, and buccal branches. The cervicofacial division is the origin of the marginal mandibular and colli branches. However, anastomoses and branching patterns are numerous. Commonly, the temporal branch supplies the upper half of the orbicularis oculi, and the zygomatic branch supplies the lower half. The frontalis, corrugator supercilii, and pyramidalis muscles are usually innervated by the temporal branch. The temporal (or frontal) branch of the facial nerve crosses the zygomatic arch as one or multiple "twigs" inside the deep layers of the temporoparietal fascia. The nerve is fairly superficial as it crosses the zygomatic arch at the junction of the anterior one-third and posterior two-thirds of the arch. It then enters the more superficial layer of the temporoparietal fascia while staying below the *superficial musculoaponeurotic system (SMAS).* A good approximation of the course of the nerve across the zygomatic arch follows the point at which a line between the tragus and the lateral eyelid commissure is bisected by a line that begins at the earlobe. The nerve can be injured in the context of perizygomatic or temple surgical approaches, such as Tenzel or Mustarde semicircular flap reconstruction of the eyelid, temporal artery biopsy, and cosmetic forehead and midface surgery.

The parasympathetic outflow originates in the superior salivatory nucleus and the lacrimal nucleus, both of which lie posterolateral to the motor nucleus and probably receive afferent fibers from the hypothalamus. The superior salivatory nucleus also receives input from the olfactory system. The hypothalamic fibers reaching the lacrimal nucleus may mediate emotional tearing, and there is supranuclear input from the cortex and the limbic system. Reflex lacrimation is controlled by afferents from the sensory nuclei of CN V. These preganglionic parasympathetic fibers pass peripherally as part of the nervus intermedius and divide into 2 groups near the external genu of CN VII. The lacrimal group of fibers passes to the pterygopalatine ganglion in the greater superficial petrosal nerve. The salivatory group of fibers projects through the chorda tympani nerve to the submandibular ganglion to innervate the submandibular and sublingual salivary glands.

The greater superficial petrosal nerve extends forward on the anterior surface of the petrous temporal bone to join the deep petrosal nerve (sympathetic fibers) and form the nerve of the pterygoid canal. This nerve enters the pterygopalatine fossa; joins the pterygopalatine ganglion; and gives rise to unmyelinated postganglionic fibers that innervate the globe, lacrimal gland, glands of the palate, and nose. Those parasympathetic fibers destined for the orbit enter it via the superior orbital fissure, along with branches of the ophthalmic nerve (CN V_1). Here, they are joined by sympathetic fibers from the carotid plexus and form a retro-orbital plexus of nerves, whose rami oculares supply orbital vessels or enter the globe to supply the choroid and anterior segment structures. Some of these fibers enter the globe directly; others enter via connections with the short ciliary nerves. The rami oculares also supply the lacrimal gland.

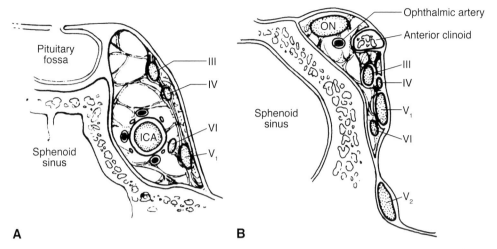

Figure 3-14 Cavernous sinus: coronal sections **(A)** at the level of the pituitary fossa and **(B)** at the level of the anterior clinoid process. ICA = internal carotid artery; ON = optic nerve. *(Reproduced with permission from Doxanas MT, Anderson RL. Clinical Orbital Anatomy. Baltimore: Williams & Wilkins; 1984.)*

Cavernous Sinus

The cavernous sinus is an interconnected series of venous channels located just posterior to the orbital apex and lateral to the sphenoidal air sinus and pituitary fossa (Fig 3-14). The following structures are located within the venous cavity:

- the ICA surrounded by the sympathetic carotid plexus
- CN III, CN IV, and CN VI
- the ophthalmic and maxillary divisions of CN V

Other Venous Sinuses

The cavernous sinus is only one part of an interconnecting series of venous channels that carry blood away from the brain and drain into the internal jugular veins. Other venous sinuses include the superior sagittal, transverse, straight, sigmoid, and petrosal sinuses. The various components of the venous system are depicted in Figure 3-15. Thrombosis in any portion of the venous sinuses can lead to increased venous pressure and may cause intracranial hypertension and papilledema.

Circle of Willis

The major arteries supplying the brain are the right and left ICAs (which distribute blood primarily to the rostral portion of the brain) and the right and left vertebral arteries (which join to form the basilar artery). The basilar artery distributes blood primarily to

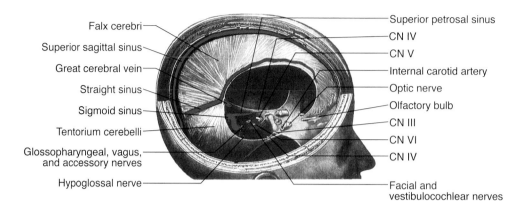

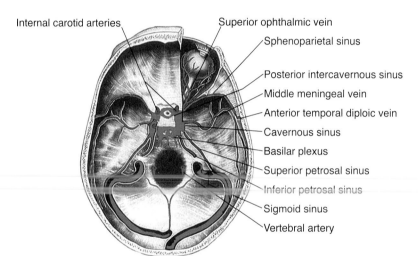

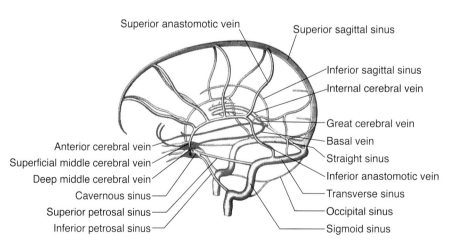

Figure 3-15 Drawings depicting the venous sinuses of the brain, their interconnections, and their relationships to the dura. *(Reproduced with permission from Williams PL, Warwick R. Gray's Anatomy. 38th ed. Edinburgh: Churchill Livingstone; 1995.)*

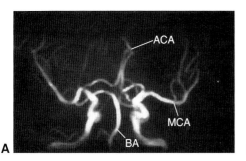 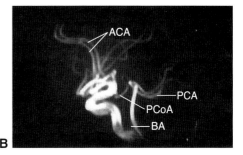

Figure 3-16 **A,** Magnetic resonance angiogram showing the circle of Willis in an anteroposterior view. **B,** An oblique view from the same patient. ACA = anterior cerebral artery; BA = basilar artery; MCA = middle cerebral artery; PCA = posterior cerebral artery; PCoA = posterior communicating artery. *(Courtesy of T. Talli, MD, and W. Yuh, MD.)*

the brainstem and the posterior portion of the brain. These arteries interconnect at the base of the brain at the circle of Willis (Fig 3-16; see also Figs 3-2, 3-5). These interconnections help distribute blood to all regions of the brain, even when a portion of the system becomes occluded.

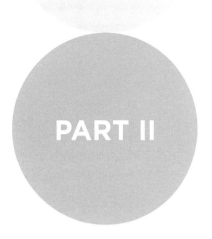

PART II

Embryology

CHAPTER 4

Ocular Development

General Principles

Embryogenesis can be thought of as a series of steps that build on one another; each step creates a ripple effect on all subsequent steps. These steps are regulated by genetic programs that are activated in specific cell types and in a specific order. These genetic programs consist of cascades of genes that are expressed in response to external cues. Often, the same genes participate in different cascades and play different roles in different contexts. For example, gene products that activate transcription in a particular program may repress transcription in the context of another program, depending on the position of the program within the overall developmental cascade. Regulating these cascades are diffusible ligands (growth factors and hormones) that create overlapping zones of concentration gradients that allow cells to triangulate their position within the developing embryo and decide which program to activate. Misactivation of genetic cascades, whether the result of gene mutations, oocyte abnormalities, or exposure to teratogens, causes embryologic abnormalities that, in the most severe cases, are embryonic lethal or, in less severe cases, give rise to congenital abnormalities.

During gastrulation, 3 germ layers form in all animal (metazoa) embryos: (1) ectoderm (superficial layer), (2) mesoderm (middle layer), and (3) endoderm (inner layer) (Fig 4-1). In addition, vertebrate embryos have an ectomesenchymal cell population that arises from neural ectoderm at the dorsal edge of the neural tube. These cells, known as neural crest cells, are transient migratory stem cells that can form tissues with ectodermal and mesodermal characteristics. The eye and orbital tissues develop from ectoderm, mesoderm, and neural crest cells, with the neural crest cells making a particularly large contribution (Figs 4-2, 4-3). In addition, neural crest cells make key contributions to facial, dental, and calvarial structures (Fig 4-4). For this reason, syndromes that arise from neural crest maldevelopment (eg, Goldenhar syndrome) often involve the eye as well as facial, dental, and calvarial abnormalities.

Following gastrulation, the ectoderm separates into surface and neural ectoderm. Each makes a key contribution to eye development (Table 4-1).

Billon N, Iannarelli P, Monteiro MC, et al. The generation of adipocytes by the neural crest. *Development.* 2007;134(12):2283–2292.

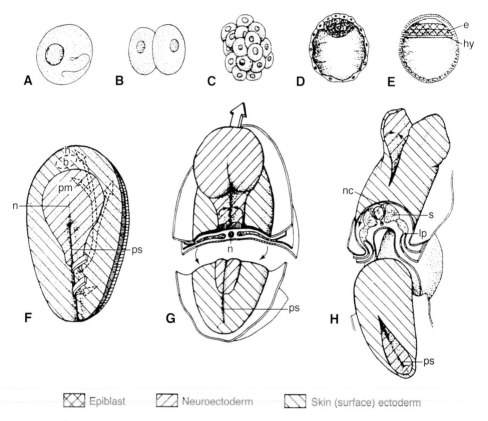

| Epiblast | Neuroectoderm | Skin (surface) ectoderm |

Figure 4-1 Early stages of human embryonic development. **A,** Fertilization. **B, C,** Earliest cell divisions to morula stage. **D,** Sectioned blastocyst. A fluid-filled cavity has formed, and the cells that will form the embryo (the darker area indicates the inner cell mass) are distinct from those that will develop into support tissues (eg, the placenta). **E,** Embryo-forming cells have now separated into 2 layers: the epiblast (e) and hypoblast (hy). **F,** Dorsal view of an embryo that is slightly more advanced than the sectioned embryo illustrated in **E.** Gastrulation movements *(arrows)* bring cells from the upper layer through the primitive streak (ps) into the potential space between the 2 layers to form the middle germ layer (mesoderm). Mesodermal cells fail to penetrate between the ectoderm and endoderm at the oral plate (b = buccopharyngeal membrane), which later forms the embryonic partition between the oral and pharyngeal cavities. At this stage, the heart primordium (h) lies anterior to the oral plate. The notochord (n) is formed from the anterior (cephalic) end of the primitive streak. The prochordal mesoderm (pm) is subjacent to the neural plate on the region between n and b. **G,** Early stages of neural tube folding and closure, and folding of the lateral body walls *(solid arrows).* The anterior neural plate has begun to "overgrow" *(open arrow)* the heart primordium and future oral region, including the buccopharyngeal membrane. **H,** Embryo folding is nearing completion. Migration of cranial neural crest cells (nc) in the hindbrain region has been initiated. In contrast to the trunk crest cells, most of those forming in the head region migrate laterally—under the surface ectoderm but superficial to the somites (s) and the lateral plate (lp) of the mesoderm. *(Reproduced with permission from Serafin D, Georgiade NG. Pediatric Plastic Surgery. St Louis: Mosby; 1984.)*

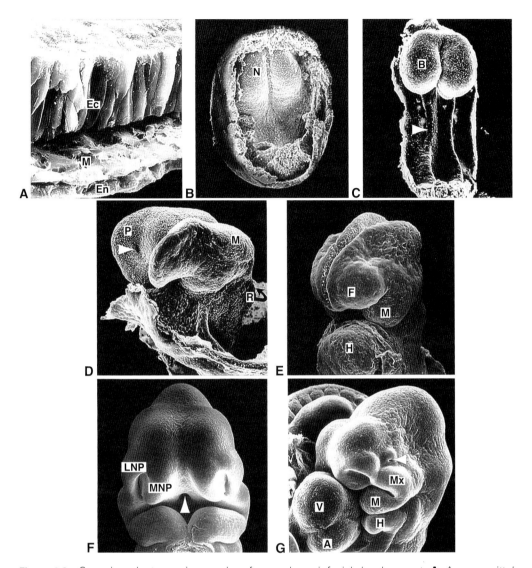

Figure 4-2 Scanning electron micrographs of normal craniofacial development. **A,** A parasagittal section through the cranial aspect of a gastrulation-stage mouse embryo. The cells of the 3 germ layers—ectoderm (Ec), mesoderm (M), and endoderm (En)—have distinct morphologies. **B,** The developing neural plate (N) is apparent in a dorsal view of this presomite mouse embryo. **C,** Neural folds *(arrowhead)* can be observed in the developing spinal cord region. The lateral aspects of the brain (B) region have not yet begun to elevate in this mouse embryo in the head-fold stage. **D,** Three regions of the brain can be distinguished at this 6-somite stage: prosencephalon (P), mesencephalon (M), and rhombencephalon (R, *curved arrow*). Optic sulci *(arrowhead)* are visible as evaginations from the prosencephalon. **E,** The neural tube has not yet fused in this 12-somite embryo. The stomodeum, or primitive oral cavity, is bordered by the frontonasal prominence (F), the first visceral arch (mandibular arch, M), and the developing heart (H). **F,** Medial and lateral nasal prominences (MNP, LNP) surround olfactory pits in this 36-somite mouse embryo. The Rathke pouch *(arrowhead)* can be distinguished in the roof of the stomodeum. **G,** In this lateral view of a 36-somite mouse embryo, the first and second (hyoid, H) visceral arches are apparent. The region of the first arch consists of maxillary (Mx) and mandibular (M) components. Note the presence of the eye with its invaginating lens *(arrowhead)*. Atrial (A) and ventricular (V) heart chambers can be distinguished.

(Reproduced with permission from Sulik KK, Johnston MC. Embryonic origin of holoprosencephaly: interrelationship of the developing brain and face. Scan Electron Microsc. 1982;(Pt 1):311.)

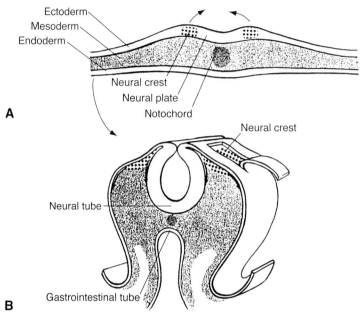

Figure 4-3 Cross sections through embryos before **(A)** and after **(B)** the onset of migration of crest cells *(diamond pattern)*. The ectoderm is peeled back in **B** to show the underlying neural crest cells. *(Reproduced with permission from Johnston MC, Sulik KK. Development of face and oral cavity. In: Bhaskar SN, ed. Orban's Oral Histology and Embryology. 11th ed. St Louis: Mosby; 1991.)*

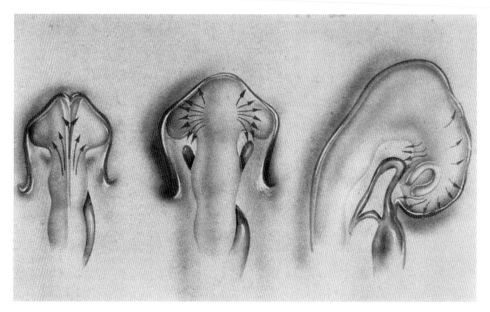

Figure 4-4 Migration of cranial neural crest cells from dorsal diencephalic and mesencephalic regions. *Left,* Cells begin migration anteriorly as tube closes. *Center,* Crest cells move in waves around the optic vesicle and lose continuity with the surface cells. *Right,* The neural tube flexes ventrally, carrying the optic cup and crest cells ventrally.

Table 4-1 **Derivatives of Embryonic Tissues**

Ectoderm

Neuroectoderm
  Neurosensory retina
  Optic nerve, axons, and glia
  Retinal pigment epithelium

Cranial neural crest
  Bones: midline and inferior orbital bones; parts of orbital roof and lateral rim
  Cartilage
  Choroidal stroma
  Ciliary ganglion
  Connective tissue of orbit
  Corneal stroma and endothelium
  Extraocular muscle sheaths and tendons
  Fat (also see Mesoderm)
  Iris pigment epithelium
  Melanocytes (uveal and epithelial)
  Meningeal sheaths of the optic nerve
  Optic nerve sheath
  Schwann cells of ciliary nerves
  Sclera (also see Mesoderm)
  Trabecular meshwork
  Vasculature: muscle and connective tissue sheaths of ocular and orbital vessels

Surface ectoderm
  Conjunctival epithelium
  Epithelium, glands, cilia of skin of eyelids, and caruncle
  Lacrimal drainage system
  Lacrimal gland (also from neural crest)
  Lens
  Vitreous (also see Mesoderm)

Mesoderm
  Extraocular muscle fibers
  Fat (also see Cranial neural crest)
  Iris sphincter and dilator muscles
  Iris stroma
  Sclera (also see Cranial neural crest)
  Vascular endothelium
  Vitreous (also see Surface ectoderm)

Eye Development

The earliest sign of eye development is the formation of the *lens placodes,* which are small surface ectoderm thickenings on both sides of the developing head (Table 4-2). At the same time, the neural ectoderm forms 2 optic pits that fill up to form pouches on either side of the midline; these pouches are termed the *optic vesicles.* The narrow neck of these vesicles directly connects the optic vesicle and the developing forebrain. Once the optic vesicle touches the inner aspect of the surface ectoderm, the vesicle invaginates to form a bilayered optic cup; the inner layer forms the neural retina, whereas the outer layer forms the retinal pigment epithelium (RPE; Fig 4-5). Although the physical space between layers eventually closes, it remains a potential space, given that retinal

Table 4-2 **Chronology of Embryonic and Fetal Development of the Eye**

22 days	Optic primordium appears in neural folds (1.5–3.0 mm).
25 days	Optic vesicle evaginates. Neural crest cells migrate to surround vesicle.
28 days	Vesicle induces lens placode.
Second month	Invagination of optic and lens vesicles.
	Hyaloid artery fills embryonic fissure.
	Closure of embryonic fissure begins.
	Pigment granules appear in retinal pigment epithelium.
	Primordia of lateral rectus and superior oblique muscles grow anteriorly.
	Eyelid folds appear.
	Retinal differentiation begins with nuclear and marginal zones.
	Migration of retinal cells begins.
	Neural crest cells of corneal endothelium migrate centrally. Corneal stroma follows.
	Cavity of lens vesicle is obliterated.
	Secondary vitreous surrounds hyaloid system.
	Choroidal vasculature develops.
	Axons from ganglion cells migrate to optic nerve.
	Glial laminal cribrosa forms.
	Bruch membrane appears.
Third month	Precursors of rods and cones differentiate.
	Anterior rim of optic vesicle grows forward, and ciliary body starts to develop.
	Sclera condenses.
	Vortex veins pierce sclera.
	Eyelid folds meet and fuse.
Fourth month	Retinal vessels grow into nerve fiber layer near optic disc.
	Folds of ciliary processes appear.
	Iris sphincter develops.
	Descemet membrane forms.
	Schlemm canal appears.
	Hyaloid system starts to regress.
	Glands and cilia develop.
Fifth month	Photoreceptors develop inner segments.
	Choroidal vessels form layers.
	Iris stroma is vascularized.
	Eyelids begin to separate.
Sixth month	Ganglion cells thicken in macula.
	Recurrent arterial branches join the choroidal vessels.
	Dilator muscle of iris forms.
Seventh month	Outer segments of photoreceptors differentiate.
	Central fovea starts to thin.
	Fibrous lamina cribrosa forms.
	Choroidal melanocytes produce pigment.
	Circular muscle forms in ciliary body.
Eighth month	Chamber angle completes formation.
	Hyaloid system disappears.
Ninth month	Retinal vessels reach the periphery.
	Myelination of fibers of optic nerve is complete to lamina cribrosa.
	Pupillary membrane disappears.

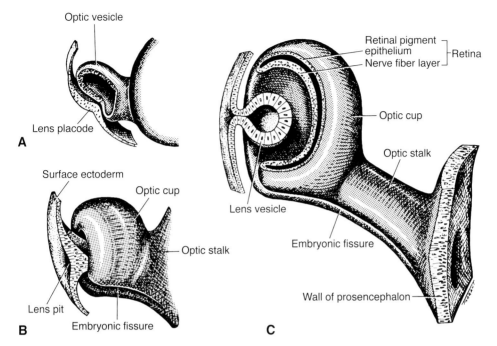

Figure 4-5 Development of the human optic cup. The optic vesicle and cup are partly cut away in **A** and **C**, and the lens vesicle is sectioned for clarity. **A,** A 4.5-mm embryo (27 days). **B,** A 5.5-mm embryo. **C,** A 7.5-mm embryo (28 days). *(Reproduced from Tripathi RC. Comparative aspects of aqueous outflow. In: Davson H, ed. The Eye. Vol 1a. 3rd ed. Orlando: Academic Press; 1984.)*

detachments are commonly observed. As the optic cup forms, 2 processes take place. First, the surface ectoderm begins to invaginate to form the lens. Second, the area between the cup and the surface ectoderm fills with a combination of mesodermal and neural crest–derived cells—the ectomesenchyme that will form much of the anterior segment of the eye.

The invagination of the optic cup occurs asymmetrically (Figs 4-6, 4-7, 4-8), with a ventral fissure that facilitates entry of mesodermal and neural crest cells (Fig 4-9). The fissure closes at its center first and then "zips" both anteriorly and posteriorly. Failure of fissure closure leads to a coloboma. Anterior colobomas are the most common (they cause iris and occasionally anterior scleral defects); central colobomas are the least common; and posterior colobomas occur with a frequency somewhere in between (they give rise to optic nerve head defects). The location of fissure closure correlates with the inferonasal quadrant, which is where colobomas are clinically found.

Lens and Anterior Segment Formation

Lens formation begins with proliferation of surface ectoderm cells to form a lens plate, followed by inward invagination of the plate to form a lens pit. As the pit deepens, it closes

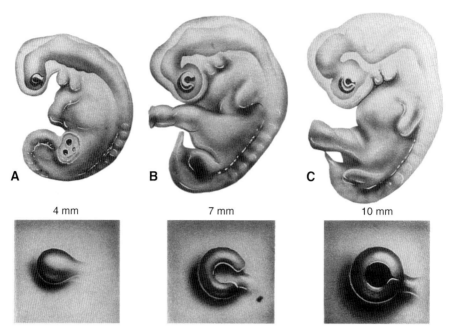

Figure 4-6 Ocular and somatic development. **A,** Flexion of the neural tube and ballooning of the optic vesicle. **B,** Upper-limb buds appear as the optic cup and embryonic fissure emerge. **C,** Completion of the optic cup with closure of the fissure. Convolutions appear in the brain, and leg buds appear. Measurements show the size of the fetus. *Bottom,* Optic vesicle; optic cup with open embryonic fissure; cup with fissure closing.

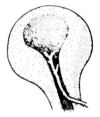

Figure 4-7 Optic cup and stalk with open embryonic fissure below. The hyaloid artery from the dorsal ophthalmic artery enters the cavity through the posterior aspect of the embryonic fissure. The rim of the optic cup is above. The lens is not shown.

anteriorly and detaches from the surface to form the lens vesicle (Fig 4-10). The remaining cells at the surface form the corneal epithelium. Invading ectomesenchymal cells form the corneal stroma and endothelium, along with other anterior segment structures.

The lens vesicle is a single-layered structure composed of cuboidal cells surrounding a large lumen, and it sits within the optic cup. The anterior cells remain cuboidal and single layered throughout life, but the rest of the lens epithelium cells become elongated, and their proliferation fills the optic vesicle. These cells form the primary lens fibers that eventually form the embryonal nucleus. The remaining outer cells form a true basement membrane known as the *lens capsule.* The lens is a unique structure in that its basement membrane surrounds its cellular component. The lens capsule is transparent,

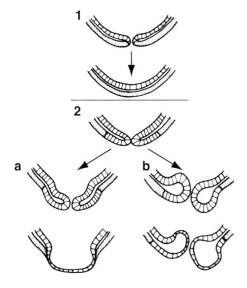

Figure 4-8 Closure of lips of the embryonic fissure. **1,** Normal closure. Inner layers (neurosensory retina) and outer layers (retinal pigment epithelium, or RPE) *(dotted area)* meet and merge. Basement membrane forms on both surfaces. **2,** Coloboma formation. Ectropion of the inner retina at the lips of the fissure results in imperfect fusion; pigment epithelium is displaced laterally by cells of the neurosensory retina. **a,** A simple coloboma results in a defective retina and RPE. The uvea and sclera (not shown) are thin and dysgenic. **b,** In a cystic coloboma, the primary vesicular cavity enlarges adjacent to the point of defective closure.

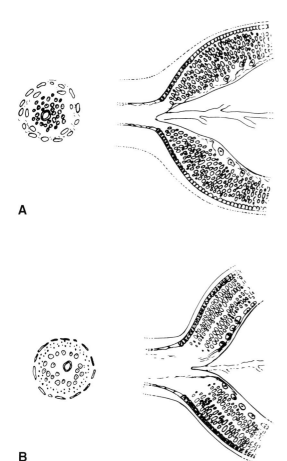

Figure 4-9 Development of the retina and optic nerve. **A,** *Right,* The fetal neurosensory retina develops from neuroectoderm as ganglion cells migrate from the outer primitive zone of closely packed nuclei to the inner marginal zone of fibrils. A few axons from ganglion cells grow toward the optic nerve. The RPE begins melanization in the posterior pole. *Left,* A cross section shows the fetal optic nerve with a center of vacuolating primitive cells through which axons from the ganglion cells will grow toward the brain. Neural crest cells as mesenchyme loosely ring the nerve. The hyaloid artery enters the vitreous (fifth week). **B,** *Right,* The migration of nuclei results in 3 nuclear and plexiform layers. *Left,* A cross section of the optic nerve shows axons of ganglion cells *(black dots)* migrating through vacuolating cells, first in the periphery of the nerve. Neural crest cells condense to meningeal sheaths of optic nerve (seventh week).

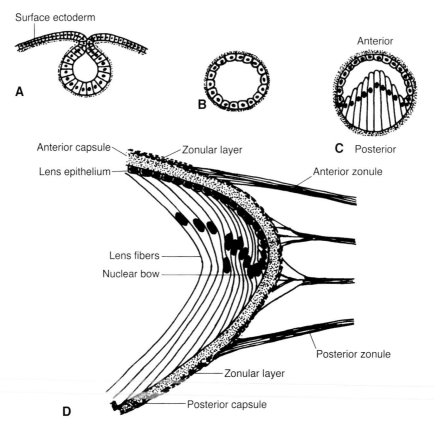

Figure 4-10 Stages in the development of the lens and its capsule. **A,** Formation of the lens vesicle from invagination of surface ectoderm together with its basal lamina in an embryo corresponding to 32 days of gestation. **B,** Separation of the vesicle from the surface ectoderm and its surrounding basal lamina. **C,** Obliteration of the lens vesicle cavity by elongation of posterior cells at approximately 35 days of gestation. **D,** Equatorial region of the fully formed lens. Attachment of zonular fibers to the anterior, posterior, and equatorial regions of the lens periphery becomes apparent at approximately 5½ weeks of gestation. Note the change in polarity of cells from anterior to posterior regions of the lens. *(Modified from Tripathi RC. Anatomy of the human eye, orbit, and adnexa. In: Davson H, Graham LT Jr, eds.* The Eye. *Vol 5. Orlando: Academic Press; 1974.)*

thickest at its equator, and thinnest posteriorly. It is composed of type IV collagen and glycosaminoglycans (GAGs). The elasticity of the lens capsule is key to facilitating changes in lens shape to achieve accommodation. The anterior lens (cuboidal) epithelium continues to form new lens fibers throughout life, leading to the lenticular thickening observed with age. The zonules of the lens form as part of the vitreous and ciliary body, with mostly ectomesenchymal contributions.

The cornea develops from both surface ectoderm (corneal epithelium) and neural crest–derived ectomesenchymal cells (stroma and endothelium) (Figs 4-11, 4-12). The Bowman membrane is a condensed layer of collagen that serves as the basement membrane for the corneal epithelial cells; it is evident mostly in primates. The corneal stroma consists of collagen fibers that are arranged in an optically optimal lattice formation. The Descemet membrane is the basement membrane of the corneal endothelial cells, which

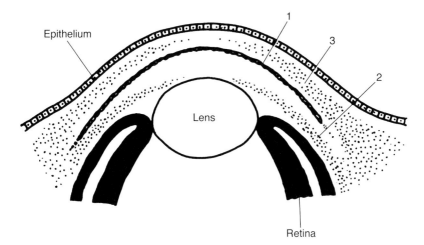

Figure 4-11 Three successive waves of ingrowth of neural crest cells associated with differentiation of the anterior chambers. **1,** First wave forms the corneal endothelium. **2,** Second wave forms the iris and part of the pupillary membrane. **3,** Third wave forms keratocytes. *(Reproduced with permission from Tripathi RC. Comparative aspects of aqueous outflow. In: Davson H, Graham LT Jr, eds. The Eye. Vol 5. Orlando: Academic Press; 1974.)*

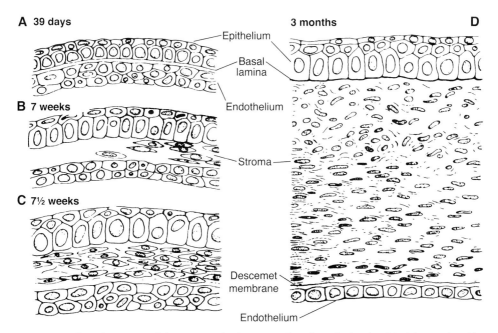

Figure 4-12 Development of the cornea in the central region. **A,** At day 39, 2-layered epithelium rests on the basal lamina and is separated from the endothelium (2–3 layers) by a narrow acellular space. **B,** At week 7, mesenchymal cells from the periphery migrate into the space between the epithelium and the endothelium. **C,** Mesenchymal cells (future keratocytes) are arranged in 4–5 incomplete layers by 7½ weeks; a few collagen fibrils are present among the cells. **D,** By 3 months, the epithelium has 2–3 layers of cells, and the stroma has approximately 25–30 layers of keratocytes that are arranged more regularly in the posterior half. Thin, uneven Descemet membrane lies between the most posterior keratocytes and the now-single layer of endothelium. *(Reproduced from Cook CS, Ozanics B, Jakobiec FA. Prenatal development of the eye and its adnexa. In: Tasman W, Jaegaer EA, eds. Duane's Foundations of Clinical Ophthalmology. Vol 1. Philadelphia: Lippincott; 1987.)*

form a monolayer of cuboidal cells on the inner surface of the cornea. These endothelial cells appear to be derived from neural crest cells, but after development, they do not regenerate. Instead, they stretch to fill in regions left empty by cell death. The endothelium is very rich in mitochondria and expends significant energy moving water out of the cornea to maintain corneal transparency.

Uvea

The uvea, including the choroid, ciliary body, and iris, develops from a combination of neural ectoderm, mesoderm, and neural crest cells. The neural crest contributes the pigmented and epithelial components of the uvea, whereas the muscles of the sphincter and iris dilator are likely of mesodermal origin. The mesoderm also contributes the nonpigmented parts of the uvea, namely, the iris stroma and the ciliary muscle.

Retina and Posterior Segment

The retina forms as 2 overlapping layers: (1) the neural retina forms from the inner surface of the optic cup, whereas (2) the RPE forms from the outer surface. The vitreous is likely formed by both mesodermal and ectodermal components: neural ectoderm cells of the inner optic cup probably contribute the primary vitreous connective fibers, and the mesoderm forms the hyaloid vasculature (Fig 4-13). The primary vitreous forms a central conical structure that contains the hyaloid vasculature and is surrounded by secondary vitreous, which eventually replaces the primary vitreous by the sixth fetal month. The zonular fibers of the lens also develop at this time; they are distinct from the primary and secondary vitreous.

Neural (inner) retinal development is driven by overlapping cascades of genetic programs; several "master" switches help determine lineages and drive cell fate, such as Nrl (neural retinal leucine zipper), a transcription factor of the Maf subfamily that serves as an intrinsic regulator of rod photoreceptor development. Retinal development occurs concentrically, beginning in the center of the optic cup and extending peripherally. Lamination of the neural retina occurs at approximately 8–12 weeks of gestation. Ganglion cells appear to be the first to differentiate; they proliferate rapidly early in the second trimester. The internal and external limiting membranes form when cells cease to proliferate and begin to differentiate. Retinal vasculature follows the same concentric pattern of development.

The RPE forms from proliferating pseudostratified columnar epithelial cells that create tight junctions and deposit a basement membrane. The Bruch membrane is composed of 5 layers:

1. basement membrane of the RPE
2. inner collagenous zone
3. elastic fibers
4. outer collagenous zone
5. basement membrane of the choriocapillaris

35 days

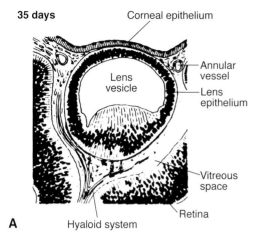

A

2 months

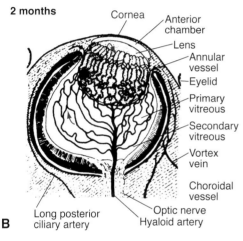

B

3–4 months

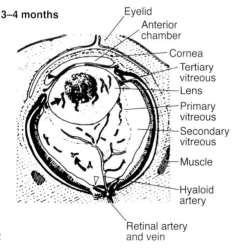

C

Figure 4-13 Vitreous development and the regression of the hyaloid system, as illustrated in sagittal sections. **A,** At 35 days, hyaloid vessels and their branches, the vasa hyaloidea propria, occupy the space between the lens and the neural ectoderm. A capillary net joins the capsula perilenticularis fibrosa, which is composed of ectodermal fibrils associated with vasoformative mesenchyme from the periphery. The ground substance of the primary vitreous is finely fibrillar. **B,** By the second month, the vascular primary vitreous reaches its greatest extent. Arborization of the vasa hyaloidea propria *(curved arrow)* fills the retrolental area and is embedded in collagen fibrils. An avascular secondary vitreous of more finely fibrillar composition forms a narrow zone between the peripheral (outer) branches of the vasa hyaloidea propria and the retina. The *bent arrow (at top)* points to the vessel of the pupillary membrane. The drawing is a composite of embryos at 15–30 mm. **C,** During the fourth month, hyaloid vessels and the vasa hyaloidea propria, together with the tunica vasculosa lentis, atrophy progressively; the smaller peripheral channels regress first. The *curved arrow* points to remnants of involuted vessels of the superficial portion of the vasa hyaloidea propria in the secondary vitreous. The *black arrowhead (upper left)* indicates the pupillary membrane. The *straight arrow* points to the remnants of the atrophied capsulopupillary vessels. Zonular fibers (tertiary vitreous) begin to stretch from the growing ciliary region toward the lens capsule. Vessels through the center of the optic nerve connect with the hyaloid artery and vein and send small loops into the retina *(open arrowhead)*. The drawing is a composite of fetuses at 75–110 mm. *(Reproduced with permission from Cook CS, Ozanics V, Jakobiec FA. Prenatal development of the eye and its adnexa. In: Tasman W, Jaeger EA, eds.* Duane's Foundations of Clinical Ophthalmology. *Philadelphia: Lippincott; 1991.)*

The RPE is the only pigmented tissue in the body that is not derived from neural crest cells, although these cells are located at the anterior-most edge of the neural crest, suggesting shared evolutionary origins.

The optic nerve develops from the optic stalk, which is the narrow stalk that connects the optic vesicle with the forebrain. The optic stalk is highly active in regulating cell migration into and around the developing eye, mostly through release of ligands and expression of growth factor receptors. The stalk initially forms from neuroectodermal cells surrounded by neural crest cells. In the sixth week of gestation, neuroectodermal cells begin to vacuolate and degenerate, providing space for axons from the ganglion cells of the inner retina. The surrounding neural crest cells form meninges, whereas neuroectodermal cells form surrounding oligodendrocytes (to make myelin sheaths). Peripheral nerves, including most cranial nerves, are surrounded by myelin supplied by Schwann cells. The exception is the optic nerve, which is surrounded by oligodendrocytes. This difference is an important reason the optic nerve is susceptible to optic neuritis.

Sclera

The sclera is formed from mesodermal and neural crest–derived ectomesenchyme elements. The sclera joins the developing cornea near the equator of the developing eye, but the sclera continues to develop and expand to surround the developing optic cup. The sclera spur and Tenon capsule form later, at the time of extraocular muscle (EOM) insertion.

Orbit and Extraocular Muscles

Orbital development involves key contributions from ectodermal, mesodermal, and neural crest–derived elements. The EOMs form from paraxial and prechordal mesoderm, following cues from the developing eye as well as from surrounding neural crest mesenchyme. Indeed, the interactions among the optic cup, mesoderm, and neural crest cells are crucial to the proper development and organization of the EOMs. If the optic cup fails to form and the eye vesicle turns into a cyst, the EOMs often develop anomalously, an outcome that is likely because signals from the optic cup are necessary for proper migration of neural crest cells into the eye and surrounding tissues, and subsequent signals from these neural crest–derived cells are required for proper development and organization of the EOMs. Interestingly, eyeless blind cave fish still develop embryonic eyes, likely because the developing eyes serve as important organizers of facial and head development (possibly through the morphogenic actions of retinoic acid).

Congenital cranial dysinnervation disorders involving the EOMs include Duane retraction syndrome, Marcus Gunn jaw-winking syndrome, and congenital fibrosis of the extraocular muscles (CFEOM; see BCSC Section 6, *Pediatric Ophthalmology and Strabismus*). Genetic studies have identified mutations in genes for neuron biology and axon guidance (eg, *KIF21A, PHOX2A*) that cause these EOM syndromes. By extrapolation, congenital ptosis and other congenital EOM disorders probably result from delays in muscle innervation. Current models suggest that as the muscle mesenchyme and associated nerve jointly develop, a delay in the innervation of the muscle mesenchyme can cause premature differentiation of that mesenchyme into connective tissue (ie, fibrosis). The extent of delay may correlate with the severity of fibrosis (eg, severity of the congenital ptosis and levator muscle dysfunction). Furthermore, the delay in, or absence of, innervation may provide a window for inappropriate innervation by another cranial nerve, such as trigeminal innervation of the levator muscle (Marcus Gunn jaw-winking syndrome) or oculomotor innervation of the lateral rectus muscle (Duane syndrome).

By the fourth week of gestation, the frontonasal and maxillary processes of neural crest cells occupy the space that surrounds the optic cups. The bones, cartilage, fat, and connective tissues of the orbit develop from these cells. All bones of the orbit are membranous except the sphenoid, which is initially cartilaginous. Ossification begins during the third month of gestation, and fusion occurs between the sixth and seventh months.

The upper eyelid first develops at 4–5 weeks of gestation as a proliferation of surface ectoderm in the region of the future outer canthus. During the second month, both the upper and lower eyelids become discernible as undifferentiated skinfolds that surround mesenchyme of neural crest origin (Fig 4-14). Later, mesodermal mesenchyme infiltrates the eyelids and differentiates into the palpebral musculature. The eyelid folds grow toward each other as well as laterally. Starting near the inner canthus, the margins of the folds fuse at approximately 10 weeks of gestation. As the folds adhere to each other, evolution of cilia and glands continues. The orbicularis muscle condenses in the fold in week 12. The eyelid adhesions gradually break down late in the fifth month, coincident with the secretion of sebum from the sebaceous glands and cornification of the surface epithelium.

The lacrimal gland begins to develop between the sixth and seventh weeks of gestation. Solid cords of epithelial cells proliferate from the basal cell layer of the conjunctiva in the temporal region of the fornix. Neural crest–derived mesenchymal cells aggregate

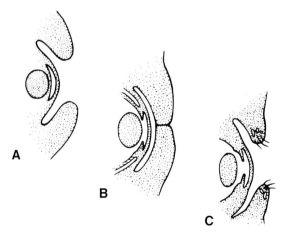

Figure 4-14 Development of the eyelids. **A,** During the seventh week, the upper and lower eyelid folds grow over the eye. **B,** Eyelids fuse during the eighth week; fusion starts along the nasal margin. **C,** From the fifth to seventh months, as cilia and glandular structures develop, eyelids gradually open.

at the tips of the cords and differentiate into acini. At approximately 3 months, ducts of the gland form by vacuolation of the cord cells and the development of lumina. Lacrimal gland (reflex) tear production does not begin until 20 or more days after birth. Therefore, newborn infants cry without tears. Between the third and sixth months of gestation, eyelid appendages and pilosebaceous units develop from invaginations of epithelial cells into the underlying mesenchyme.

Engle EC. Human genetic disorders of axon guidance. *Cold Spring Harb Perspect Biol.* 2010; 2(3):a001784.

Genetic Cascades and Morphogenic Gradients

The embryonic genome is not transcribed until the stage of midblastula transition, which takes place several hours after fertilization. Instead, maternal messenger RNA (mRNA) is found in the oocyte, providing the initial genetic instruction set to the fertilized egg. Once embryonic transcription begins, it follows a set of predefined genetic programs.

Homeobox Gene Program

The blueprint for the embryonic program involves the homeobox (Hox) genes. These genes are so named because they contain a distinctive and highly conserved segment of DNA, approximately 180 base pairs long, that encodes a conserved 60–amino acid sequence constituting the homeodomain. The homeodomain provides a protein with specific DNA-binding capabilities. The term *homeo* originates from Edward B. Lewis's discovery of Hox genes in the fruit fly *Drosophila melanogaster.* In these experiments, conducted in the 1940s and 1950s, Lewis discovered that incorrect expression of Hox genes transforms one body segment into another. This transformation is a homeotic transformation because the new segment mimics a segment elsewhere in the body. Later research by Christiane Nüsslein-Volhard and Eric F. Wieschaus involved performance of genetic screens in *D melanogaster* to identify genes that serve as master regulators of embryonic development. Importantly, they determined that Hox genes have this role, and they further characterized chromosomal regions that contained sequential series of Hox genes, revealing a spatiotemporal pattern of expression that drives sequential steps in embryogenesis. For their pioneering work on embryonic development, Drs. Lewis, Nüsslein-Volhard, and Wieschaus shared the Nobel Prize in Physiology or Medicine in 1995.

The function of Hox genes as master regulators arises from the ability of these genes to regulate expression of downstream genes through homeodomain binding to DNA promoter sequences, wherein they act as switches of gene transcription. Each set of switches drives a particular cell fate, and transcriptional cascades of these switches lead to the development of different tissues and organs.

As expected, specific Hox genes are crucial for the development of the eye. The *PAX6* (PAired homeoboX 6) gene in particular appears to be a master switch for eye development. It is expressed very early in the primordial eye field, and ectopic expression of *PAX6* can lead to ectopic eyes. Other Hox genes that play key roles in eye development include *PAX2, RX,* and *PitX2.*

Growth Factors, Diffusible Ligands, and Morphogens

Gene-expression cascades are clearly crucial for eye development, just as they are for development of most organs. However, to respond to cues in real time, cells in the developing eye require additional signals. These signals take the form of diffusible extracellular factors (termed *morphogens*) that are active in the earliest stages of embryonic development. The most important of these factors include retinoic acid (RA), Wnt, fibroblast growth factors (FGFs), and the hedgehog family members Shh and Ihh. These factors fall into 2 broad groups: Group 1 ligands interact with intracellular receptors that directly regulate gene expression (eg, RA). Group 2 ligands interact with cell-surface receptors that initiate an intracellular signaling cascade (eg, Wnt, FGF), often involving protein phosphorylation cascades, to eventually affect gene expression and intracellular remodeling (eg, cytoskeleton), cell motility, protein trafficking, and other processes. Cells respond differently to ligands depending on ligand concentration in the context of a concentration gradient (also termed *morphogenic gradient*). In many cases, cells and tissues that have multiple potential fates utilize these diffusible ligands to activate a particular fate. For example, FGF signaling in the optic vesicle regulates expression of the basic helix-loop-helix transcription factor MITF (microphthalmia transcription factor) in the optic cup, which in turn regulates the balance between development of neural retina and pigment epithelium. The interested reader is referred to several excellent reviews on the topic of eye development and diffusible ligands in embryogenesis.

Kish PE, Bohnsack BL, Gallina D, Kasprick DS, Kahana A. The eye as an organizer of craniofacial development. *Genesis*. 2011;49(4):222–230.

Rogers KW, Schier AF. Morphogen gradients: from generation to interpretation. *Annu Rev Cell Dev Biol*. 2011;27:377–407.

Tabata T. Genetics of morphogen gradients. *Nat Rev Genet*. 2001;2:620–630.

Future Directions

The embryologic study of how a single cell (zygote) gives rise to a multitude of cell and tissue types has led to the fledgling field of stem cell biology. Stem cells range from totipotent to pluripotent to multipotent as they become more limited in their potential to form the entire range of cell and tissue types. The strict definition of stem cells refers to cells that have the ability to self-renew via asymmetric cell division; the more colloquial and common definition refers to multipotent but lineage-restricted progenitor cells (eg, limbal stem cells). Although stem cell research has generally depended on the study of embryonic stem cells, the advent of induced pluripotent stem cells (iPSCs) has provided a more easily accessible and less politically charged model for the study of pluripotency. Stem cell models have been extremely useful in the study of organogenesis, tissue differentiation, and associated genetic cascades, but future therapies employing regenerative approaches are more likely to utilize lineage-restricted progenitor cells so as to increase the likelihood of proper regeneration of function while reducing the risk of cancer.

Bohnsack BL, Gallina D, Thompson H, et al. Development of extraocular muscles requires early signals from periocular neural crest and the developing eye. *Arch Ophthalmol*. 2011; 129(8):1030–1041.

Eiraku M, Takata N, Ishibashi H, et al. Self-organizing optic-cup morphogenesis in three-dimensional culture. *Nature.* 2011;472(7341):51–56.

Gage PJ, Zacharias AL. Signaling "cross-talk" is integrated by transcription factors in the development of the anterior segment in the eye. *Dev Dyn.* 2009;238(9):2149–2162.

Graw J. The genetic and molecular basis of congenital eye defects. *Nat Rev Genet.* 2003;4(11): 876–888.

Kish PE, Bohnsack BL, Gallina D, Kasprick DS, Kahana A. The eye as an organizer of craniofacial development. *Genesis.* 2011;49(4):222–230.

Shaham O, Menuchin Y, Farhy C, Ashery-Padan R. Pax6: a multi-level regulator of ocular development. *Prog Retin Eye Res.* 2012;31(5):351–376.

Swaroop A, Kim D, Forrest D. Transcriptional regulation of photoreceptor development and homeostasis in the mammalian retina. *Nat Rev Neurosci.* 2010;11(8):563–576.

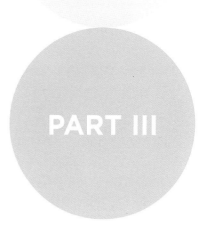

PART III

Genetics

Introduction

Genetics is the study of heredity and the variations in inherited characteristics and diseases. Although genetics is a relatively new science compared with such disciplines as anatomy and physiology, its significance in the overall understanding of human life cannot be overstated. Genetic knowledge can enhance our understanding of the processes of cellular function, embryology, and development, as well as our concepts of disease. Many researchers think that as much as 90% of medical disease either has a major genetic component or involves genetic factors that may significantly influence the disease.

The discovery of previously unknown genes has opened new areas of understanding of physiology at the cellular or tissue level, an important example of which is the discovery of *homeobox genes* (eg, the *HOX* and *PAX* gene families) that regulate, guide, and coordinate early embryologic development and differentiation. (These genes, also called *homeotic selector genes,* are also discussed in Part II.) Another example is the identification of the genes that appear to be transcribed as initiating events in the process of *apoptosis,* or programmed cell death, which itself appears crucial for normal embryogenesis as well as for degenerative diseases.

Genetic disorders affect approximately 5% of live-born infants in the United States. Approximately 50% of childhood blindness has a genetic cause. Some 20,000–25,000 human genes involving about 180,000 exons are known. In approximately 10%–15% of known genetic diseases, clinical findings are limited to the eye; a similar percentage includes systemic disorders with ocular manifestations.

Terminology

Not knowing the vocabulary of genetics and molecular biology is one of the greatest impediments to understanding these fields. Modern online resources allow readers to easily look up unfamiliar terms. The following glossary includes many key genetics terms.

Glossary

Allele Alternative form of a gene or DNA sequence that may occupy a given locus on a pair of chromosomes. Clinical traits, gene products, and disorders are said to be *allelic* if they are determined to be at the same locus and *nonallelic* if they are determined to reside at different loci.

Allelic association See *Linkage disequilibrium.*

Allelic heterogeneity When different alleles at the same locus are capable of producing an abnormal phenotype.

Aneuploidy An abnormal number of chromosomes.

Anticipation The occurrence of a dominantly inherited disease at an earlier age (often with greater severity) in subsequent generations. Now known to occur with expansion of a trinucleotide repeat sequence. Observed, for example, in fragile X syndrome, myotonic dystrophy, and Huntington disease.

Antisense strand of DNA That strand of double-stranded DNA that serves as a template for RNA transcription. Also called the *noncoding,* or *transcribed,* strand.

Apoptosis The process by which internal or external messages trigger expression of specific genes and their products, resulting in the initiation of a series of cellular events that involve fragmentation of the cell nucleus, dissolution of cellular structure, and orderly cell death. Unlike traumatic cell death, apoptosis results in the death of individual cells rather than clusters of cells and does not lead to the release of inflammatory intracellular products. Also called *programmed cell death (PCD).*

Assortative mating Mating between individuals with a preference for or against a specific phenotype or genotype; that is, nonrandom mating.

Autosome Any chromosome other than the sex (X and Y) chromosomes. The normal human has 22 pairs of autosomes.

Barr body Inactive X chromosome found in the nucleus of some female somatic cells.

Base pair (bp) Two complementary nitrogen bases that are paired in double-stranded DNA. Used as a unit of physical distance or length of a sequence of nucleotides.

Carrier An individual who has a pair of genes consisting of 1 normal and 1 abnormal, or *mutant,* gene. Usually, such individuals are by definition phenotypically "normal," although in certain disorders biochemical evidence of a deficient or defective gene product may be present. Occasionally, carriers of an X-linked disorder may show partial expression of a genetic trait.

Centimorgan (cM) A measure of the crossover frequency between linked genes. One centimorgan equals 1% recombination and represents a physical distance of approximately 1 million bp.

Centromere The constricted region of the chromosome. It is associated with spindle fibers during mitosis and meiosis and is important in the movement of chromosomes to the poles of the dividing cell.

Chorionic villus sampling (CVS) Transcervical procedure in which chorionic villi are retrieved with a flexible suction catheter and used in studies to establish a prenatal diagnosis.

Chromatid One of the duplicate arms (also called *sister chromatids*) of chromosomes that are created after DNA replication during mitosis or the first division of meiosis.

Chromatin The complex of DNA and proteins that is present in chromosomes. Chromatin is found in 2 varieties: euchromatin and heterochromatin. Euchromatin is a lightly packed form of chromatin that is often under active transcription. Heterochromatin consists primarily of genetically inactive satellite sequences such as centromeres, telomeres, and the Barr body.

CLIA (Clinical Laboratory Improvement Amendments) A federal program that sets standards for clinical laboratory testing in the United States. Clinicians are advised to use a CLIA-certified laboratory to provide feedback to patients.

Clinical heterogeneity Different mutations at the same locus producing different phenotypes. Examples include macular dystrophy and retinitis pigmentosa from differing mutations of peripherin/*RDS* and Crouzon, Pfeiffer, and Apert syndromes from differing mutations of *FGFR2*.

Codominance Simultaneous expression of both alleles of a heterozygous locus (eg, ABO blood groups).

Codon A sequence of 3 adjacent nucleotides that forms the basic unit of the genetic code. The DNA molecule is a chain of nucleotide bases read in units of 3 bases *(triplets),* each of which will translate (through messenger RNA) into an amino acid. Thus, each triplet codon specifies a single amino acid.

Complementary DNA (cDNA) DNA created by the action of reverse transcriptase from messenger RNA. In contrast to genomic DNA, cDNA does not have introns.

Complex genetic disorder (multigene disorder) A trait or medical disorder that does not follow Mendelian patterns of inheritance. Close relatives have a higher risk of the disorder, suggesting that the state is determined by genes at multiple loci (and that environmental factors are possibly involved).

Compound heterozygote Individual with a gene locus having different, abnormal alleles on each homologous chromosome.

Congenital Present at birth. The term has no implications about the origin of the congenital feature, which could be genetic or environmental.

Consanguinity The genetic relationship of individuals who are the descendants of a sexual union between blood relatives; in other words, individuals who share a recent common ancestor (eg, offspring of a marriage between cousins).

Conservation When a similar genetic sequence or nucleotide position is present among different species at 1 gene or related genes of similar sequence. In such cases, the sequence or position is said to be conserved or to show conservation.

Copy number variation A structural variation in the genome resulting from deleted or inserted nucleotides, exons, or genes (also referred to as *indels*). Indels have been used as

DNA markers to locate genes but may also cause disease by adding amino acids (eg, in triplet-repeat disorders) or may affect gene expression (eg, the expression of color opsins on the X chromosome).

Crossing over A process in which matching segments of homologous chromosomes (chromatids) break, are exchanged to the other chromosome, and are reconnected to the other chromosome by repair of the breaks. Crossing over is a regular event in meiosis but occurs only rarely in mitosis. Also termed *recombination.*

Database of Genotypes and Phenotypes (dbGaP) Funded by the US National Institutes of Health, a catalog of genetic information (genotypes) linked to clinical information (phenotypes) from results of genome-wide association studies (GWAS).

Degeneracy of genetic code The redundancy of the genetic code stemming from the fact that most of the 20 amino acids are coded for by more than 1 of the 64 possible triplet codons. The genetic code is termed *degenerate.*

Digenic inheritance Simultaneous inheritance of 2 nonallelic mutant genes, giving rise to a genetic disorder in which inheritance of only 1 of the 2 is insufficient to cause disease. Digenic inheritance is the simplest form of polygenic inheritance. An example is retinitis pigmentosa caused by simultaneous inheritance in the heterozygous state of otherwise tolerable mutations of both the *ROM1* and peripherin/*RDS* genes.

Diploid The number of chromosomes in most somatic cells, which in humans is 46. The diploid number is twice the haploid number (the number of chromosomes in gametes).

Direct-to-consumer genetic testing Genetic tests marketed directly to consumers. An individual orders a test kit directly from a genetic testing laboratory and mails a tissue sample (saliva or blood) back to the laboratory, which runs a series of DNA tests, usually single-nucleotide polymorphisms (SNPs) or in some cases sequencing. These DNA tests may be specific to certain genes or diseases or may involve a large panel of genes and diseases. Lack of counseling, quality control, and appropriate scientific interpretation of data are major challenges to direct-to-consumer testing.

DNA code The sequences of DNA trinucleotides corresponding to the amino acids.

Dominant An allele that is expressed in the phenotype when inherited along with a normal allele. See *Recessive.*

Dominant medical disorder A distinctive disease state that occurs in an individual with a genotype that is heterozygous for a dominant disease-producing allele. Homozygotes for dominant disease-producing alleles are rare and are usually more severely affected than heterozygotes. By definition, normal dominant traits give the same phenotype in both the heterozygous and the homozygous states.

Dominant negative An autosomal dominant mutation that disrupts the function of the normal or wild-type allele in the heterozygous state, giving a phenotype approaching that of the homozygous mutant.

ENCODE (ENCyclopedia Of DNA Elements) A catalog of functional elements in the human genome (see http://genome.gov/encode).

Endonuclease A phosphodiester-cleaving enzyme, usually derived from bacteria, that cuts nucleic acids at internal positions. Restriction endonucleases cut at specific recognition sites determined by the occurrence of a specific recognition sequence of 4, 5, or 6 bp. Endonuclease specificity may also be confined to substrate conformation, nucleic acid species (DNA, RNA), and the presence of modified nucleotides.

Enhancer Any sequence of DNA upstream or downstream of the coding region that acts in *cis* (ie, on the same chromosome) to increase (or, as a negative enhancer, to decrease) the rate of transcription of a nearby gene. Enhancers may display tissue specificity and act over considerable distances.

Epigenetics/epigenomics The study of modifications of the expression of the genetic code by factors that may themselves be genetically or environmentally influenced; examples of such factors include cytosine methylation and histone formation.

Eukaryote Organisms with their DNA located within a nucleus (includes all multicellular and higher unicellular organisms).

Exome sequencing A strategy to selectively sequence the coding regions of the genome as a less expensive alternative to whole-genome sequencing. Approximately 180,000 exons constitute 1% of the human genome, or about 30 megabases (Mb).

Exon A coding sequence of DNA is represented in the mature mRNA product. See *Intron*.

Expressed-sequence tag (EST) A partial sequence of a gene that uniquely identifies the gene's message. These tags are useful, in reverse transcriptase polymerase chain reaction (RT-PCR) detection, for determining the expression levels of large numbers of genes in parallel reactions.

Expressivity The variation in clinical manifestation among individuals with a particular genotype, usually a dominant medical disorder. The variability may be a difference in either age of onset (manifestation) or severity. See *Penetrance*.

Fragile sites Reproducible sites of secondary constrictions, gaps, or breaks in chromatids. Fragile sites are transmitted as Mendelian codominant traits and are not usually associated with abnormal phenotype. The most notable exceptions are the association of fragile X chromosomes with X-linked mental retardation and postpubertal macro-orchidism (fragile X syndrome). See *Trinucleotide repeat expansion*.

Frameshift mutation (framing error, frameshift) Any mutation, usually a deletion or insertion of a nucleotide or a number of nucleotides not divisible by 3, that results in a loss of the normal sequences of triplets, causing the new sequence to code for entirely different amino acids from the original. The mutation usually leads to the eventual chance formation of a *stop codon*.

Gene The segment of DNA and its associated regulatory elements coding for a single trait, usually a single polypeptide or mRNA. The definition was expanded to include any expressed sequence of nucleotides that has functional significance, including DNA sequences that govern the transcription of a gene (promoter sequences immediately upstream of the gene or enhancer sequences that may be more distantly located).

Gene-tailored drug therapy See *Pharmacogenetics/pharmacogenomics.*

Genetic Information Nondiscrimination Act (GINA) A law enacted by the US Congress in 2008 to prohibit the improper use of genetic information by health insurance providers and employers.

Genome The sum total of the genetic material of a cell or an organism.

Genome-wide association studies (GWAS) Research studies that examine the associations between single-nucleotide polymorphisms (SNPs) and traits or diseases by comparing the DNA of a group of people with a particular disease (cases) and another, similar group without that disease (controls). Hundreds of thousands of SNPs are read on arrays in studies designed to find common ancestral mutations that contribute risk for disease.

Genomics The study of the genome. Names for the fields of *transcriptomics, proteomics,* and *metabolomics* were coined in a similar fashion.

Genotype The genetic constitution of an organism. Also, the specific set of 2 alleles inherited at a locus.

Germinal mosaicism The occurrence of 2 populations of gametes in an individual, 1 population with a normal allele and the other with a disease-producing mutant gene. Of new cases of some autosomal-dominant diseases (eg, osteogenesis imperfecta), 5%–10% are thought to result from germinal mosaicism; offspring of the affected parent are at significant risk for the same disease.

Haploid Half the number of chromosomes in most somatic cells; equal to the number of chromosomes in gametes. In humans, the haploid number is 23. Also used to denote the state in which only 1 of a pair or set of chromosomes is present. See *Diploid.*

Haploid insufficiency (haploinsufficiency) The condition of dominant genetic disease caused by reduction in gene product to levels that are insufficient to produce the desired function of the protein. For example, aniridia and Waardenburg syndrome result from insufficiency of the single functional copy of the *PAX6* and *PAX3* genes, respectively, to activate transcription of the genes that they normally control.

Haplotype A series of contiguous alleles along the length of a single chromosome that may be inherited as a block. Also referred to as a *haploblock.*

HapMap The haplotype map of the human genome describing the common patterns of human genetic variation. A key resource in finding variants affecting health and disease.

Hemizygous (hemizygote) Having only 1 allele at a locus; usually refers to X-linked loci in males, who normally have only 1 set of X-linked genes. An individual who is missing an entire chromosome or a segment of 1 chromosome is considered hemizygous for the genes on the homologous chromosome.

Hereditary Genetically transmitted or capable of being genetically transmitted from parent to offspring. Not quite synonymous with *heritable,* which implies the ability to be transmitted to the next generation but does not intrinsically connote inheritance from the prior generation.

Heterogeneity (genetic heterogeneity) The production of a phenotype (or apparently similar phenotypes) by different genetic entities. Refers to genetic disorders that are found to be 2 or more fundamentally distinct entities. See *Clinical heterogeneity.*

Heteroplasmy The presence of 2 or more different populations of mitochondria within a cell, each population carrying a different allele (or the presence or absence of a mutation) at a given locus.

Heterozygous (heterozygote) Having 2 unlike alleles at a particular locus. See *Hemizygous, Homozygous.*

Homeobox A conserved 180-bp sequence of DNA, first detected within homeobox genes (also known as *homeotic selector genes*), that helps determine the cell's fate.

Homeobox genes Transcription factor genes that regulate the activity or expression of other genes, eventually guiding the embryonic development of cells into body segments, body parts, and specialized organ systems. Examples are the *HOX* and *PAX* families of developmental genes. Whereas *HOX* genes are involved in early body plan organization, *PAX* genes are involved in somewhat later organ and body part development. See the discussion of homeobox genes in Chapter 4, Ocular Development.

Homologous chromosomes The 2 members of a matched pair of (sister) chromosomes, 1 derived from each parent, that have the same gene loci, but not necessarily the same alleles, in the same order.

Homoplasmy The presence of a single population of mitochondria within a cell, each carrying the same allele (or the same presence or absence of a mutation) at a given locus.

Homozygous (homozygote) Having 2 like or identical alleles at a particular locus in the diploid genome. The term is sometimes misused to refer to *compound heterozygote* (see earlier entry).

Human Genome Project (HGP) The international scientific research project that identified and mapped the approximately 20,000–25,000 human genes. A working draft of the genome was announced in 2000, and the genome was completed in 2003.

Hybridization The bonding (by Watson-Crick base pairing) of single-stranded DNA or RNA into double-stranded DNA or RNA. The ability of stretches of DNA or RNA to hybridize with each other is highly dependent on complementarity of the base-pair sequence.

Imprinting The reversible marking or inactivation of an allele by inheritance (through either the maternal or the paternal lineage), which may significantly alter gene expression. The imprinting is reversed if the gene is passed through the opposite parental line in subsequent generations. This phenomenon occurs in Prader-Willi and Angelman syndromes; it may also occur with mutations of the Wilms tumor gene. One mechanism of imprinting is thought to involve methylation of 5′ elements of the gene.

Intron A segment of DNA that is transcribed into heterogeneous RNA but is ultimately removed from the transcript by splicing together the sequences on either side of it (exons) when mature mRNA is produced.

Karyotype An image of an individual's chromosome set arranged in a standard pattern in pairs by size, shape, band pattern, and other identifiable physical features.

Kilobase (kb) 1000 bp of DNA or 1000 bases of single-stranded RNA.

Library A complete set of clones presumably including all genetic material of interest from an organism, tissue, or specific cell type at a specified stage of development. A *genomic library* contains cloned DNA fragments from the entire genome; a *cDNA library* contains fragments of cloned DNA generated by reverse transcription from mRNA. Genomic libraries are useful sources to search for genes, whereas cDNA libraries give information about expression within the source cell or tissue.

Linkage A concept that refers to loci rather than to the alleles that reside on those loci. Exists when the loci of 2 genes or DNA sequences are physically close enough to each other on the same chromosome that alleles at the 2 loci do not assort independently at meiosis but tend to be inherited together.

Linkage disequilibrium The state in which alleles that reside at loci close together in the genome remain inherited together through many generations because the close physical distance makes crossover between the loci extremely unlikely. Thus, alleles that are in linkage disequilibrium are present in subpopulations of individuals (eg, those with a given disease) in greater-than-expected frequencies. Also called *allelic association.*

Locus The physical site on a chromosome occupied by a particular gene. The term is often colloquially used interchangeably with *gene.*

Locus heterogeneity The term for when a similar phenotype is produced by mutations at different loci, for example, X-linked retinitis pigmentosa resulting from *RP2* at Xp11 and *RP3* at Xp21.

LOD score (*l*ogarithm of *od*ds, or logarithm of the likelihood ratio) A statistical method that tests whether a set of linkage data indicates that 2 loci are linked or unlinked. The LOD score is the logarithm to the base 10 of the odds favoring linkage. By convention, an

LOD score greater than 3 (1000:1 odds in favor of linkage) is generally accepted as proof of linkage.

Lyonization Inactivation of genes on either the maternally or the paternally derived X chromosome in somatic cells. The timing of inactivation is variable but may occur about the time of implantation. First proposed by Mary Lyon.

Manhattan plot A type of plot used in genome-wide association studies (GWAS). Genomic coordinates are displayed along the x-axis, with the negative logarithm of the association *P* value for each single-nucleotide polymorphism (SNP) displayed on the y-axis. The strongest associations appear as peaks, calling to mind the profile of skyscrapers towering above lower buildings.

Meiosis The special form of cell division that occurs in germ cells by which gametes of haploid chromosomal number are created. Each of the chromatids, which are clearly visible by prophase, contains a long double helix of DNA associated with histones and other chromosomal proteins. At anaphase, the chromatids separate at the centromere and migrate to each half of the dividing cell; thus, each daughter cell receives an identical set of chromatids (which become the chromosomes for that cell). During the first, or *reduction,* division of meiosis, the chromatids of homologous chromosomes undergo crossover (during the diplotene phase), and the number of chromosomes is reduced to the haploid number by the separation of homologous chromosomes (with duplicate chromatids) to each daughter cell. During the second division of meiosis, the sister chromatids separate to form the haploid set of chromosomes of each gamete.

Mendelian disorder (single-gene disorder) A trait or medical disorder that follows patterns of inheritance suggesting the state is determined by a gene at a single locus (eg, autosomal dominant, autosomal recessive, or X-linked recessive inheritance).

Methylation The attachment of methyl groups to DNA at CpG (cytosine-phosphate-guanine) sites. CpG islands are associated with the promoters of many genes, and there is an inverse relationship between CpG methylation and transcriptional activity.

MicroRNA (miRNA) Small single-stranded RNA fragment (of approximately 22 nucleotides) that directly interacts with target mRNA through complementary base pairing and inhibits translation of the target genes. miRNA modifies gene expression at transcriptional and posttranscriptional levels.

Microsatellite (eg, dinucleotide or trinucleotide repeats) Tandemly repeated segments scattered throughout the genome of varying numbers of 2–4 nucleotides in a row, for example, a stretch of consecutive CA combinations of bases (NNNCACACACACACACACACA-CANN or $[CA]_{10}$, where N is any base) in a DNA strand. The repeats are inherently unstable and can undergo mutation at a rate of up to 10%. Defects of some microsatellites are associated with cancer and insulin-dependent diabetes mellitus, although most have no known biological significance. Other terms used are *variable number of tandem repeats (VNTR)* and *variable tandem repeats (VTR).* The highly variable nature of the number of repeats provides information useful as markers for establishing linkage to disease loci.

Missense mutation A mutation, often the change of a single nucleotide, that results in the substitution of 1 amino acid for another in the final gene product.

Mitosis The ordinary form of cell division, which results in daughter cells identical in chromosomal number to the parent cell.

Mosaic An individual or tissue with at least 2 cell lines of different genotype or distinctive chromosomal constitution that develop after the formation of the zygote.

Multifactorial inheritance The combined operation of several unspecified genetic and environmental factors in the inheritance of a particular trait or disease. See *Polygenic inheritance.*

Mutation Any alteration of a gene or genetic material from its "natural" state, regardless of whether the change has a positive, neutral, or negative effect.

Next-generation sequencing (massively parallel DNA sequencing) Sequencing technology that speeds the process, producing thousands or millions of DNA sequences at once. This technology has allowed for rapid, large-scale DNA sequencing at much lower cost.

Nondisjunction Failure of 2 chromosomes to separate during meiosis or mitosis.

Nonsense mutation Any mutation that either results directly in the formation of a stop codon or creates a stop codon in the downstream sequence after a frameshift mutation.

Nucleoside The combination of a nitrogen-containing base and a 5-carbon sugar. The 5 nucleosides are adenosine (A), guanosine (G), cytidine (C), uridine (U), and thymidine (T). Note that the abbreviations are the same as those for the nitrogen bases that characterize the nucleoside.

Nucleosome The primary unit of chromatin, consisting of a 146-bp sequence of DNA wrapped twice around a core composed of 8 histone molecules.

Nucleotide The combination of a nucleoside and 1 or more phosphate groups. *Purine nucleotides* have a nitrogen-containing base of adenine (A) and guanine (G) in DNA or RNA. *Pyrimidine nucleotides* have a nitrogen-containing base of thymine (T) and cytosine (C) in DNA and uracil (U) in RNA.

OMIM (Online Mendelian Inheritance in Man) An online database of genes and genetic disorders (see www.ncbi.nlm.nih.gov/omim).

Oncogene A gene that, when dysregulated, is capable of transforming cells to a neoplastic phenotype characterized by loss of growth control and/or tumorigenesis in a suitable host or site. In many cases, cancer is caused by the growth-stimulating effects of increased expression, protein activation, or aberrant regulation of transcription factors required for normal growth. Certain oncogenes are produced by chromosomal translocations of normal transcription factor genes to regions adjacent to more abundantly expressed genes, causing inappropriate excessive expression. See *Tumor-suppressor genes.*

Open reading frame (ORF) Any part of the genome that could be translated into a protein sequence because of the absence of stop codons. An exon is an example of an ORF. See *Exon.*

p arm The short arm of a chromosome in relation to the centromere. From *petit.*

Penetrance The proportion of individuals of a given genotype who show any evidence of an associated phenotype. Usually refers to the proportion of individuals heterozygous for a dominant disease who show any evidence of the disease. Nonpenetrance is the lack of phenotypic evidence of the genotype. See *Expressivity.*

Personalized genetics The use of personal genomic data to determine patient care, including drug treatment, for an individual patient.

Pharmacogenetics/pharmacogenomics The fields of biochemical genetics concerned with genetically controlled variations in drug responses.

Phenocopy The occurrence of a particular clinical phenotype as a result of either a non-mutagenic environmental factor (eg, exposure to a drug or virus) or an atypical genetic defect, when the more usually associated genetic defect is absent.

Phenotype An observable feature of an individual, resulting from interaction of the genotype with the environment (in medicine, often a disease phenotype).

Pleiotropism Multiple end effects (in different organ systems) arising from a single, mutant gene or gene pair.

Polygenic inheritance Determined by the operation of 2 or more genes. See *Multifactorial inheritance.*

Polymerase chain reaction (PCR) A technique by which segments of DNA or RNA can be amplified by use of flanking oligonucleotides called *primers* and repeated cycles of amplification with DNA polymerase. The steps involve

- heating to separate the molecules into single-stranded DNA
- repeated annealing to the complementary target DNA sequences or primers specifically designed to delimit the beginning and ending of the target segment
- extension of the primer sequences with the enzyme DNA polymerase, creating double-stranded DNA
- separation of the products into single-stranded DNA

In effect, the amount of DNA is doubled with each cycle. Often, 30 or more cycles are used to obtain sufficient amplification for further testing.

Real-time PCR, or *quantitative PCR (qPCR),* is used to simultaneously amplify and quantify a targeted DNA molecule. *Digital PCR (dPCR)* is a refinement used to directly quantify and clonally amplify nucleic acids. dPCR is a more precise method than qPCR because it allows for more reliable collection and more sensitive measurement of nucleic acid amounts. Quantitative PCR has been demonstrated as useful for studying variations in gene sequences (eg, copy number variants and point mutations) and is routinely used to amplify samples for *next-generation sequencing.*

Polymorphism A genetic variation in which the frequency of the minor allele in a given population is greater than 1%.

Posttranslational modification Biochemical changes to or modifications of gene products after translation, including removal of amino acids from the end of the peptide, addition or removal of sugars, and addition of lipid side chains or phosphate groups to specific sites in the protein. Often, such changes are essential for proper protein localization or function.

Proband The affected person whose disorder, or concern about a disorder, brings a family or pedigree to be genetically evaluated. Also called the *propositus* (male), *proposita* (female), or *index case.*

Promoter That sequence of nucleotides upstream (5′) from the coding sequence of a gene that determines the site of binding of RNA polymerase and, hence, initiation of transcription. Different promoters for the same gene may exist and can result in alternately spliced gene products and tissue-specific expression. The promoter may contain the consensus DNA sequence (the so-called TATA box) approximately 25–30 bp (5′) upstream from the transcription start site.

Pseudodominance The appearance of vertical transmission of a recessive genetic disorder from one generation to the next due to an unusually high carrier frequency of a recessive allele and the resultant mating of an affected homozygote with an unaffected heterozygote, which produces affected offspring. Pseudodominance implies recessive disease that has the appearance of dominant inheritance.

Pseudogene A defective copy of a gene that often lacks introns and is rarely, if ever, expressed. Some pseudogenes are thought to arise by reverse transcription of mRNA that has had the introns spliced out. Others, such as globin pseudogenes, arise from silencing of a tandem duplicate. Because they are released from conservation (the maintenance of essential DNA sequences necessary for function) through selection, pseudogenes often contain numerous base-pair changes and other mutational events (compared with the original functional gene).

q arm The long arm of a chromosome. See *p arm.*

Recessive Classically, a gene that results in a phenotype only in the homozygous or compound heterozygous state. See *Dominant.*

Recessive medical disorder A disease state whose occurrence requires a homozygous (or compound heterozygous) genotype—that is, a double "dose" of the mutant allele. Heterozygotes are essentially clinically normal.

Recombinant An individual with a combination of genes on a single chromosome unlike that in either parent. Usually applied to linkage analysis, in which *recombinant* refers to a haplotype (a set of alleles on a specific chromosome) that is not present in either parent because of a recombination crossover.

Recombinant DNA DNA that has been cut out of a single organism, reinserted into the DNA of a vector (plasmid or phage), and then reimplanted into a host cell. Also, any DNA that has been altered for further use.

Recombination The formation of a new set of alleles on a single chromosome unlike that in either parent; due to crossover during meiosis.

Reference genomes DNA sequences from control subjects in selected populations including the International HapMap and 1000 Genomes Projects.

Relatives, first-degree Individuals who share on average half of their genetic material with the proband: parents, siblings, offspring.

Relatives, second-degree Individuals who share on average one-fourth of their genetic material with the proband: grandparents, aunts and uncles, nieces and nephews, grandchildren.

Replication Creation of a new linear DNA copy by the enzyme DNA polymerase, proceeding from the 5′ side of bound primer to the 3′ end of the DNA sequence. Replication of DNA occurs during chromosomal duplication.

Replication slippage An error of DNA replication or copying. Because of the similarity of repeated base-pair sequences, 1 or more repeats may be skipped over and not represented in the copied DNA sequence.

Replicative segregation The process by which, through partitioning of copies of mtDNA to each daughter cell during division, some cells receive a preponderance of normal or mutant copies. Replicative segregation tends to result in conversion of heteroplasmy to homoplasmy with associated development of disease within the affected tissue, if the tissue becomes homoplasmic for the mutant mtDNA. This phenomenon explains the development of new organ-system involvement in multisystem mitochondrial diseases.

Reverse transcription The process, performed by the enzyme reverse transcriptase, in which mRNA is converted back to DNA. If the introns have already been spliced out of the precursor mRNA, the product of this process is cDNA.

Sanger sequencing The chain-termination method of sequencing DNA based on incorporating dideoxynucleotide molecules.

Segregation The separation of pairs of alleles at meiosis.

Sex linked Genes on the X or Y (sex) chromosome. The term is often used improperly to mean X-linked.

Short interfering RNA (siRNA) A double-stranded RNA molecule (of 20–25 nucleotides) that plays a role in the RNA interference pathway, where it interferes with the expression of genes with complementary nucleotide sequences. Also known as *small interference RNA.*

Simplex A term denoting that only a single individual within a given family is affected and implying no inheritance type. Thus, a single male or female with a genetic disease is called a *simplex case.* The term *isolated* is also sometimes used.

Single-nucleotide polymorphism (SNP) Variation in a single base pair in a nucleotide sequence in the genome. SNPs are rarely mutations that cause disease, are occasionally linked to disease-causing mutations, and most often are of unknown significance.

Splice junction site The DNA region that demarcates the boundaries between exons and introns. The specific sequence determines whether the site acts as a 5′ donor or a 3′ acceptor site during splicing. Single base-pair changes or mutations that involve splice junction sites may result in skipping of the following exon or incorporation of part of the adjacent intron into the mature mRNA.

Splicing Process by which the introns are removed from the precursor mRNA and the exons are joined together as mature mRNA prior to translation. Takes place within *spliceosomes.*

Sporadic A trait that occurs in a single member of a kindred with no other family members affected. The term has been used by some geneticists to imply that the trait is nongenetic.

Stop codon (termination codon) The DNA triplet that causes translation to end when the translation is coded into mRNA. The DNA stop codons are TAG, TAA, and TGA. Expressed as mRNA, these are UAG, UAA, and UGA.

Telomeric DNA A type of highly repetitive satellite DNA that forms the tips of chromosomes and prevents them from fraying or joining. It decreases in size as a consequence of the normal mechanisms of DNA replication in mitosis and may be important in cellular senescence. Defects in the maintenance of telomeres may play a role in cancer formation.

1000 Genomes Project An international collaboration, launched in 2008, to compile the most detailed public catalog of human genetic variation.

Threshold In polygenic or multifactorial inheritance, a relatively sharp qualitative difference beyond which individuals are considered affected. The threshold is presumed to have been reached by the cumulative effects of the polygenic and multifactorial influences.

Transcription The synthesis as catalyzed by a DNA-dependent RNA polymerase of a single-stranded RNA molecule from the antisense strand of a double-stranded DNA template in the cell nucleus.

Translation The process by which a polypeptide is synthesized from a sequence of specific mRNA.

Translocation The transfer of a part of 1 chromosome to a nonhomologous chromosome.

Trinucleotide repeat expansion/contraction The process by which long sequences of multiple triplet codons (see *Microsatellite*) are lengthened or shortened in the course of gene replication. The process of expansion of trinucleotide repeats over consecutive generations results in the genetic phenomenon of *anticipation*. The underlying mechanisms for expansion (or contraction) appear to be replication slippage and unequal crossing over in the region of the repeats. Most disorders involving trinucleotide repeats are dominant in inheritance (eg, fragile X syndrome, myotonic dystrophy, Huntington disease, and Kennedy disease), but one is autosomal recessive (Friedreich ataxia).

Tumor-suppressor genes Genes that must be present in 1 fully functional copy in order to keep cells from uncontrolled proliferation. Two "hits" (inactivations) of the gene, one for each allele, must occur in a given cell for tumor formation to occur. Examples include the genes for retinoblastoma, Wilms tumor, tuberous sclerosis, p53, ataxia-telangiectasia, and von Hippel–Lindau disease. Also called *antioncogenes*. See *Oncogene*.

Unequal crossing over An error in the events of chromosomal duplication and cell division occurring during meiosis and, rarely, during mitosis. Probably because of similar sequences or repeated segments, chromosomal exchange occurs between nonhomologous regions of the chromosome, resulting in duplication and deletion of genetic material in the daughter cells.

Uniparental disomy The conveyance to an offspring of 2 copies of an abnormal gene or chromosome by only 1 parent (the other parent makes no contribution). The child can be affected with autosomal recessive disease even if only 1 of the parents is a carrier of the abnormal gene. This occurrence has been reported in Stargardt disease, cystic fibrosis, Prader-Willi syndrome, and Angelman syndrome.

Untranslated region (UTR) The regions upstream (5′ UTR) and downstream (3′ UTR) of the open reading frame of a gene. The 5′ UTR contains the promoter and part or all of the regulatory regions of the gene. The 3′ UTR presumably also serves important functions in regulation and mRNA stability.

Vector A viral, bacteriophage, or plasmid DNA molecule into which a stretch of genomic DNA or cDNA or a specific gene can be inserted. The λ-bacteriophage can accept segments of DNA up to 25 kb long. Cosmid vectors can accommodate a segment 40 kb long. BAC (bacterial artificial chromosome) and YAC (yeast artificial chromosome) vectors can accept much larger fragments of DNA. Viral vectors such as adeno-associated viruses (AAV) have been used in gene therapy trials.

Western blot A technique to detect and analyze specific proteins in a blood or tissue sample. Based on their mass, proteins are separated from one another using polyacrylamide gel electrophoresis (PAGE). After PAGE, the separated proteins are transferred from the gel to a membrane (blot) and visualized using antibodies to specific targets.

Wild type A normal phenotype of an organism. Also, a normal allele as compared with a mutant allele.

X-linked Term that refers to genes on the X chromosome.

Y-linked Term that refers to genes on the Y chromosome.

CHAPTER 5

Molecular Genetics

This chapter provides a review of molecular genetics (with emphasis on clinical applications in ophthalmology), an overview of the techniques for manipulating DNA in the laboratory, and an appreciation of the power and implications of molecular investigations for the study of inherited diseases.

Gene Structure

Composed of DNA, *genes* are the molecular units of heredity and are located primarily in the cell nucleus, where they are assembled into *chromosomes* of varying sizes. Paired chromosomes are numbered from largest (1) to smallest (22), and there are 2 additional sex chromosomes (XY or XX). The 4 bases present in DNA—adenine (A), cytosine (C), guanine (G), and thymine (T)—are combined into a double-helix structure that allows replication, transcription, and translation. The genetic structure (Fig 5-1) can be likened to the sections of an encyclopedia, with genes the chapters, *exons* the sentences, *trinucleotides* the words, and *nucleotides* the letters.

 Mitochondria are the power plants of the cell, where oxidative phosphorylation occurs. The mitochondria are a vestige of a symbiotic relationship between 2 primitive unicellular organisms that merged to form eukaryotic organisms (most animals and plants). The fact that mitochondria still contain their own DNA is a reminder of their independent origin. Each mitochondrion contains 2–10 copies of a very short, circular segment containing 13 protein-coding genes involved in oxidative phosphorylation. Because mitochondria contain several segments of DNA and each cell contains several mitochondria, there may be variation of the mitochondrial DNA (mtDNA) within a cell and between cells of the same person, a state known as *heteroplasmy*. Humans acquire mitochondria from the ovum, and thus mtDNA follows maternal line inheritance.

 Chromosomal DNA replication and RNA synthesis (transcription) occur within the nucleus. Messenger RNA (mRNA) is transported to ribosomes in the cytoplasm, where translation to the amino acid sequences of proteins occurs. Following the mRNA molecule's initiation codon (start sequence) is the structural *open reading frame (ORF),* which is composed of *exons* (sequences that code for amino acids that will be present in the final protein) and *introns* (sequences that are spliced out during the processing of mRNA). Following the last exon is the *3′ untranslated region (3′ UTR).* The function of this region is partly regulatory.

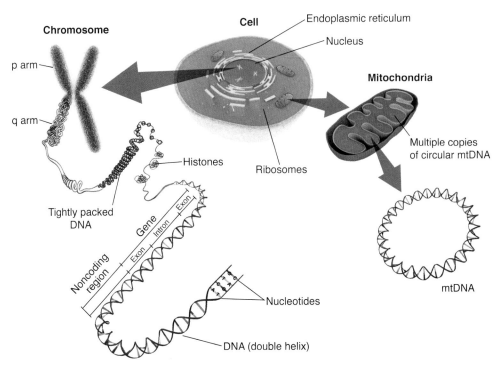

Figure 5-1 Structures of the cell showing the location of DNA within chromosomes and mitochondria. The basic double helix of nucleotides is divided into noncoding regions, introns, and exons to form genes.

The development of introns in higher organisms may have had evolutionary benefits. The compartmentalization of coding segments into exons may have allowed for more rapid evolution of proteins by allowing for alternative processing of precursor RNA (alternative splicing) and for rearrangements of exons during gene duplication (exon shuffling). Some introns contain complete, separate genes, and some of these may cause disease or influence the expression of other genes. Expansion of unstable repeats within introns can cause abnormal splicing and result in genetic disease. Small insertions and deletions are very common and referred to as *indels*.

The Cell Cycle

The cell cycle is the series of events that take place in a cell leading to its division and duplication (Fig 5-2). The 4 distinct phases are G_1 (growth), S (synthesis), G_2 (growth), and M (mitosis). The M phase consists of 2 processes: *mitosis,* in which the cell's chromosomes are divided between the 2 sister cells, followed by *cytokinesis,* in which the cell's cytoplasm divides in half and forms distinct cells. Cells that have temporarily stopped dividing are said to have entered a state of quiescence called the G_0 phase. The M phase can be subdivided into several distinct, sequential phases: *prophase* (chromatin is condensed

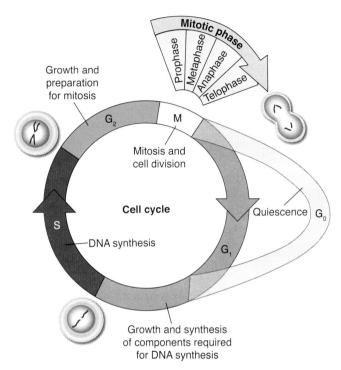

Figure 5-2   In the cell cycle, the progression from DNA synthesis (S) to mitosis (M) includes phases before (G$_1$) and after (G$_2$) the replication of DNA. On receiving signals to differentiate, cells leave the cycle and enter the final stage of cell differentiation, or terminal differentiation. Under certain circumstances, cells may enter the pathway to programmed cell death (apoptosis). G$_0$ = quiescence.

into chromosomes), *metaphase* (chromosomes align in the middle of the cell), *anaphase* (chromosomes split and migrate to opposite poles of the cell), and *telophase* (2 daughter nuclei form in the cell).

Meiosis is a specialized type of cell division necessary for sexual reproduction in eukaryotes because the cells produced by meiosis are ova and sperm. Unlike in mitosis, in meiosis the chromosomes undergo a recombination that shuffles the genes from each parent, producing a different genetic combination in each gamete. The outcome of meiosis is 4 genetically unique haploid cells, whereas the outcome of mitosis is 2 genetically identical diploid cells.

Interphase consists of the G$_1$ and S phases (there is no G$_2$ phase in meiosis) and is followed by meiosis I and then meiosis II. Meiosis I and II are each divided into prophase, metaphase, anaphase, and telophase stages, as in the mitotic cell cycle. The G$_1$ phase occurs when each of the chromosomes consists of a single (very long) molecule of DNA. At this stage in humans, the cells contain 46 chromosomes, the same number as in somatic cells. The S phase takes place when the chromosomes duplicate, so that each of the 46 chromosomes becomes a complex of 2 identical sister chromatids.

Meiosis I consists of the separation of each pair of homologous chromosomes into 2 cells. The entire haploid content of each chromosome is contained in each of the resulting daughter cells; the first meiotic division therefore reduces the ploidy of the original cell by half.

During meiosis II, each chromosome's sister strands (the chromatids) are decoupled, and the individual chromatids are segregated into haploid daughter cells. The 2 cells resulting from meiosis I divide during meiosis II, creating 4 haploid daughter cells.

Chromosomal *crossing over* is the exchange of genetic material between homologous chromosomes (1 from each parent) that results in recombinant chromosomes. It occurs during prophase I of meiosis, usually when matching regions on matching chromosomes break and then reconnect to the other chromosome. Although the same genes appear in the same order, the alleles are different. It is theoretically possible to have any combination of parental alleles in an offspring. This theory of *independent assortment* of alleles is fundamental to genetic inheritance. However, the chances of recombination are greater the farther apart 2 genes are from each other. The genetic distance is described in centimorgans (cM; named for Thomas Hunt Morgan, who described crossing over), and a distance of 1cM between genes represents a 1% chance of their crossing over in 1 meiosis.

Genetic *linkage* describes the tendency of genes to be inherited together as a result of their nearby location on the same chromosome. *Linkage disequilibrium* occurs when combinations of genes or genetic markers are present more or less frequently in a population than would be expected based on their distances apart from each other. This concept is applied in searches for a gene that may cause a particular disease.

Although crossovers typically occur between homologous regions of matching chromosomes, a mismatch or unbalanced recombination may occur. This rare event can be a local duplication or deletion of genes on 1 chromosome, a translocation of part of 1 chromosome onto a different one, or an inversion of a part of the chromosome.

Noncoding DNA

Approximately 95% of the base sequences in human DNA do not code for proteins or RNA or have any other known function. The roles for this previously named *junk DNA* will emerge when the structures and functions of the genome, chromosomes, nucleus, and nuclear proteins are fully understood. It has been suggested that RNA transcribed from noncoding DNA may directly influence the transcription of other sequences and participate in normal genome repair and regulation. Some of the repetitive sequences of nontranscribed DNA form *telomeric DNA,* which is essential for the correct formation and maintenance of chromosomes. Loss of telomeric DNA correlates with cell senescence and carcinogenesis. Therefore, sequences within noncoding DNA may influence the transcription or otherwise regulate the expression of numerous other genes.

Noncoding DNA is composed of highly repetitive sequences, some of which include *satellites, microsatellites, short interspersed elements (SINEs),* and *long interspersed elements (LINEs).* The 300-base-pair (bp) *Alu* sequence, named after the restriction enzyme used to identify it, is the repetitive DNA that appears most frequently.

Gene Transcription and Translation:
The Central Dogma of Genetics

The central dogma of gene transcription and translation is that the DNA code is tran-scribed as messenger RNA (mRNA) code and then translated as amino acid code of the resulting protein (Fig 5-3). The trinucleotides that correspond with amino acids have some redundancy in the system, so that a nucleotide change may not necessarily result in a change in amino acid. The coding region of DNA is composed of exons, several of which are spliced together to make the full coding sequence of RNA. The noncoding portion of DNA, which accounts for the majority of DNA, comprises introns, promoters, and other regions and is involved in regulating gene expression and exon splicing. Although the central dogma specifies that DNA determines RNA sequence and that RNA determines amino acid sequence, there are feedback and regulatory mechanisms of gene expression that are both genetically and environmentally determined. These mechanisms, such as methylation and histone formation, can silence gene expression. In addition, small seg-ments of RNA can block mRNA. The influence of these regulatory mechanisms in gene and disease expression is known as *epigenetics.*

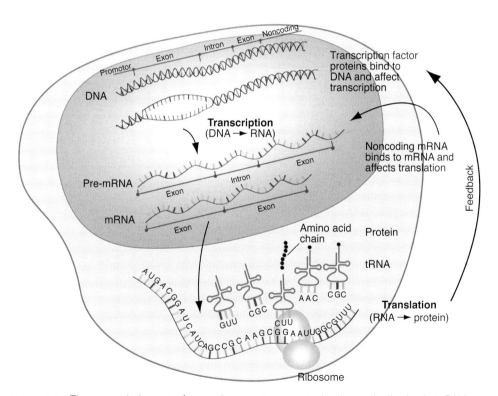

Figure 5-3 The central dogma of genetics, as represented schematically, is that DNA se-quence codes are transcribed to the mRNA sequence, and then the mRNA transcription is translated into the amino acid sequence of the coded protein. However, proteins in the form of transcription factors and complementary short RNA sequences can modify translation and transcription. These proteins are being investigated as potential forms of genetic therapy.

s control cellular activity through 2 processes:

1. transcription *(expression),* in which DNA molecules give rise to RNA molecules, followed by translation in most cases
2. *translation,* in which RNA directs the synthesis of proteins. Translation occurs in ribosomes, where mRNA induces transfer RNA (tRNA)–mediated recruitment of amino acids to "build" a protein. A more in-depth description of translation is beyond the scope of this chapter.

Transcription factors are proteins that bind to specific DNA sequences and thus control the flow (or transcription) of genetic information from DNA to mRNA. Transcription factors perform this function by promoting or repressing the recruitment of RNA polymerase to specific genes.

Approximately 10% of genes in the human genome code for transcription factors. They contain one or more DNA-binding domains, which attach to specific sequences of DNA adjacent to the genes that they regulate. There are numerous families of these genes, including the homeobox and paired box genes. *PAX6* acts as a master control gene for the development of the eye and is an example of the importance of transcription factors in embryogenesis.

Many ophthalmic diseases result from transcription-factor mutations. *PAX2* mutations cause colobomas of the optic nerve and renal hypoplasia. *PAX3* mutations cause Waardenburg syndrome with dystopia canthorum (types WS1 and WS3). *PAX6* mutations are the basis of virtually all cases of aniridia, occasional cases of Peters anomaly, and several other rarer phenotypes, specifically autosomal dominant keratitis and dominant foveal hypoplasia.

Fitzpatrick DR, van Heyningen V. Developmental eye disorders. *Curr Opin Genet Dev.* 2005; 15(3):348–353.

Intron Excision

Messenger RNA undergoes excision of the introns by a highly organized process called *splicing,* which leaves the mRNA composed of only exons, or coding segments. The exons can then undergo translation in the ribosomes. Splicing takes place in specialized structures called *spliceosomes,* which are composed of RNA and proteins. Errors of splicing can lead to genetic disease. Approximately 15% of point mutations that cause human disease do so by the generation of splicing errors that result in aberrations such as exon skipping, intron retention, or use of a cryptic splice site. For example, mutations in proteins important in splicing can cause retinitis pigmentosa (RP).

Alternative Splicing and Isoforms

Alternative splicing is the creation of multiple pre-mRNA sequences from the same gene by the action of different promoters. These promoters cause certain exons to be skipped during transcription of the gene. The protein products of alternative splicing are often called *isoforms.* The promoters are usually tissue specific, so different tissues express different isoforms. The gene for dystrophin is an example of alternative splicing: full-length dystrophin is the major isoform expressed in muscle; shorter isoforms predominate in the retina, peripheral nerve, and central nervous system. Another example of alternative splicing's relevance underlies the basis of the cornea's avascularity. Vascular endothelial growth factor (VEGF) receptor 1 is a key blood vessel receptor that binds and transduces a signal from the primary mediator of angiogenesis, VEGF. In the cornea, high levels of an alternatively spliced isoform, soluble VEGF receptor 1 (sVEGFR-1), are expressed. As this isoform is soluble, it is present in the extracellular matrix and serves as an endogenous VEGF trap or decoy receptor. Without it, the cornea becomes vulnerable to vascular invasion.

> Ambati BK, Nozaki M, Singh N, et al. Corneal avascularity is due to soluble VEGF receptor-1. *Nature.* 2006;443(7114):993–997.

Methylation

Regions of DNA that are undergoing transcription lack 5-methyl cytosine residues, which normally account for 1%–5% of total DNA. Evidence suggests a close correlation between methylation and gene inactivation. Regulation of DNA methylation may be responsible for imprinting control. Methylation may account for variation in phenotypic expression of some diseases.

> Hjelmeland LM. Dark matters in AMD genetics: epigenetics and stochasticity. *Invest Ophthalmol Vis Sci.* 2011;52(3):1622–1631.

X-Inactivation

The random inactivation of 1 of the 2 X chromosomes in the female, resulting in the lack of expression of the majority of genes on that chromosome, is a significant event during early development of the human embryo. The time of X-inactivation is not precisely known but is thought to vary over a period of several cell divisions during the blastocyst–gastrula transition. X-inactivation is also known as *lyonization,* after its discoverer, Mary Lyon. Lyonization affects the severity of the phenotype of several X-linked retinal conditions, such as RP and incontinentia pigmenti.

Imprinting

Genetic imprinting, also called *allele-specific marking,* is a heritable yet reversible process by which a gene is modified, depending on which parent provides it. The mechanism is unclear but appears to operate at the chromatin organization level and involves heterochromatization and methylation of CpG (cytosine-phosphate-guanine) sites. Examples of genes that can be imprinted include the Wilms tumor–suppressor gene and the human *SNRPN* (small nuclear ribonucleoprotein polypeptide N) gene.

Prader-Willi and Angelman syndromes are examples of diseases resulting from abnormalities of imprinting. Approximately 70%–80% of patients with Prader-Willi syndrome harbor a deletion of the paternally derived chromosome 15q11–q13, resulting in the loss of this region's normal contribution from the paternal line. About 70%–80% of patients with Angelman syndrome also have a deletion of 15q11–q13, but from the maternally derived chromosome, resulting in loss of the maternal contribution. Uniparental disomy, wherein both 15 chromosomes are inherited from the same parent, can also cause each syndrome. Again, the 2 chromosome 15s in uniparental disomy are maternal in Prader-Willi syndrome and paternal in Angelman syndrome. The *SNRPN* gene maps to 15q11–q13 but appears to be expressed only from the paternally inherited allele.

DNA Damage and Repair

DNA is constantly sustaining damage from mutagens such as ultraviolet light, chemicals, and spontaneous deamination. Each cell loses 10,000 bases per day from spontaneous DNA breakdown related to normal body temperature alone. In the absence of repair, these mutations would accumulate and result in tumor formation. Damaged DNA is estimated to cause approximately 80%–90% of cancers in humans.

Repair

Damaged DNA sites are repaired chiefly by 2 mechanisms: *excision repair* and *mismatch repair*. The processes of replication, transcription, mismatch repair, excision repair, and gene expression are closely coordinated by cross-acting systems. Enzymes that cut or patch segments of DNA during crossing over at meiosis are also involved in DNA repair. Molecules that unwind double-stranded DNA (called *helicases*) are involved in replication, transcription, and DNA excision repair.

The *antioncogene p53* appears to play an extremely important role as the "guardian of the genome" by preventing cells from proliferating if their DNA is irreparably damaged. Levels of p53 increase after ultraviolet or ionizing radiation. p53 inhibits DNA replication directly and binds with 1 of the RNA polymerase transcription factors, TFIIH. If the degree of damage is slight, increased production of p53 induces reversible cell arrest until DNA repair can take place. If DNA damage is too great or irreversible, p53 production is massively increased and apoptosis occurs, probably through stimulation of the expression of the *BAX* gene, whose product promotes apoptosis. Loss of p53 causes cells to fail to arrest in response to DNA damage, and these cells do not enter apoptosis. Thus, mutations of p53 predispose to tumorigenesis.

The gene mutated in ataxia-telangiectasia (Louis-Bar syndrome), a protein kinase called *ATM,* also appears to be integrally involved in DNA repair, possibly by informing the cell of radiation damage. The *ATM* gene product associates with synaptonemal complexes, promotes chromosomal synapsis, and is required for meiosis. People with ataxia-telangiectasia have a threefold greater risk of cancer.

Xeroderma pigmentosa is a severe condition in which DNA-repair enzyme functions are crippled. Patients with this condition typically have diffuse pigmented anomalies on their sun-exposed skin surfaces and are at high risk for squamous cell carcinoma of the ocular surface.

Apoptosis

Apoptosis is a Greek word to describe the dropping off of leaves from trees. (*Ptosis,* drooping of the upper eyelid, comes from the same root.) Apoptosis is the process of programmed cell death that occurs in multicellular organisms, in contrast to necrosis, a form of traumatic cell death that results from acute cellular injury. Biochemical events in apoptosis result in characteristic cell changes and cell death. Morphological changes include cell shrinkage, nuclear fragmentation, chromatin condensation, and chromosomal DNA fragmentation. Several key events in apoptosis focus on the mitochondria, including the release of caspase activators, changes in electron transport, loss of mitochondrial transmembrane potential, altered cellular reduction-oxidation (redox) reactions, and activation of pro- and antiapoptotic Bcl-2 family proteins. Apoptosis is important in the developing human embryo; scaffolding cells such as those involved in eyelid opening are removed by epidermal apoptosis. In later life, excessive apoptosis causes atrophy, such as occurs in RP or glaucoma, whereas insufficient apoptosis results in uncontrolled cell proliferation, such as occurs in cancers including retinoblastoma.

Mutations and Disease

Mutations Versus Polymorphisms

Mutations are changes in DNA that lead to disease, whereas polymorphisms are variations in DNA that were previously thought to rarely cause disease. The difference is not always easy to determine. In general, mutations change amino acid sequence or, more dramatically, lead to a shortening or nonproduction of the protein encoded by the gene. Polymorphisms tend not to cause a change in the amino acid sequence (because of the built-in redundancy in the DNA code) or a change from one amino acid to a similar amino acid. However, some synonymous changes, although not changes in amino acid sequence, could affect splicing. Many of the disease-associated single-nucleotide polymorphisms (SNPs) identified in genome-wide association studies (GWAS) are found in the noncoding regions of the genome.

Mutations

Mutations can involve a change in a single base pair; simple deletion or insertion of DNA material; or more complex rearrangements such as inversions, duplications, or translocations. Deletion, insertion, or duplication of any number of base pairs in other than groups of 3 creates a frameshift in the entire DNA sequence downstream, resulting in the eventual formation of a stop codon and truncation of the message.

Mutations that result in no active gene product being produced are called *null mutations.* Null mutations include missense or nonsense mutations that (1) produce either a stop mutation directly or a frameshift with creation of a premature stop codon downstream or (2) cause the loss or gain of a donor or acceptor splice junction site, resulting in the loss of exons or inappropriate incorporation of introns into the spliced mRNA.

Mutations can also lead to a gain of function that may be beneficial (leading to evolution) or detrimental (leading to disease). An example of a beneficial gain in function is the emergence, among bacteria, of antibiotic resistance. An example of a detrimental gain of function is a receptor protein that binds too tightly with its target protein, creating loss of normal physiologic function. Most autosomal dominant disorders are of this type.

Single base-pair mutations may code for the same amino acid or a tolerable change in the amino acid sequence, leading to harmless polymorphisms or DNA variations that are in turn inherited. These are called *conserved base-pair mutations.*

Polymorphisms

A polymorphism is any variation in DNA sequence that occurs, by convention, at a frequency of 1% or greater in the normal population. Key polymorphisms associated with disease include those in the region of the *CFH* gene in age-related macular degeneration and the *LOXL1* gene in exfoliation syndrome. Many polymorphisms are silent and just linked to the disease mutation, but some may influence disease.

Cancer Genes

Cancer can result from any of a number of genetic mechanisms, including the activation of oncogenes and the loss of tumor-suppressor genes. The product of proto-oncogenes is often involved in signal transduction of external messages to the intracellular machinery that governs normal cell growth and differentiation. As such, the DNA sequences of proto-oncogenes are highly conserved in nature between such different organisms as humans and yeast. Proto-oncogenes can be activated to oncogenes by loss or disruption of normal regulation.

Oncogenes

Oncogenes were first detected in retroviruses, which had acquired them from their host in order to take control of cell growth. Such oncogenes are often identified by names that refer to the viral source, an example being *ras* (*rat* sarcoma virus). They are found to be activated not only in virus-induced malignancies but in common nonviral cancers in humans. Oncogenes behave the same way that autosomal dominant traits behave, and only 1 mutant allele is needed for tumor formation, presumably by a dominant negative effect on regulation of signal transduction.

Tumor-suppressor genes

Tumor-suppressor genes, also called *antioncogenes,* are genes that must be present in 1 functional copy to prevent uncontrolled cell proliferation. Although some may represent genes whose products participate in checkpoints for the cell cycle, a characteristic of tumor-suppressor genes is the diversity of their normal functions. Some examples of tumor-suppressor genes include the genes for retinoblastoma, Wilms tumor, neurofibromatosis types 1 and 2, tuberous sclerosis, ataxia-telangiectasia, and von Hippel–Lindau disease. All of these examples (except ataxia-telangiectasia) behave as autosomal dominant traits, but the mechanism of tumor formation for tumor-suppressor genes is very different from that for oncogenes. If 1 allele is already defective because of a hereditary mutation, the other allele must also be lost for tumor formation to occur (also known as the *2-hit hypothesis*). This loss of the second allele is termed *loss of heterozygosity*, and it can occur from a second mutation, gene deletion, chromosomal loss, or mitotic recombination.

Mitochondrial Disease

A significant number of disorders associated with the eye or visual system involve mitochondrial deletions and mutations. Mitochondrial diseases should be considered whenever the inheritance pattern of a trait suggests maternal transmission. Although the inheritance pattern might superficially resemble that of an X-linked trait, maternal transmission differs in that all of the offspring of affected females—both daughters and sons—can inherit the trait, but only the daughters can pass it on.

The phenotype and severity of mitochondrial disease appear to depend on the nature of the mutation, the presence or degree of heteroplasmy (coexistence of more than 1 species of mitochondrial DNA [mtDNA]—ie, wild type and mutant), and the oxidative needs of the tissues involved. Spontaneous deletions and mutations of mtDNA accumulate with age, and the effect of this accumulation is to decrease the efficiency and function of the electron transport system, reducing the availability of adenosine triphosphate (ATP). When energy production becomes insufficient to maintain the function of cells or tissue, disease occurs. There appears to be an important interaction between age and tissue threshold of oxidative phosphorylation and the expression of inherited mutations of mtDNA.

With each cell division, the number of mutant mtDNA copies that are partitioned to a given daughter cell is random, unlike in Mendelian inheritance. After a number of cell divisions, some cells, purely by chance, receive more normal or more mutant copies of mtDNA, resulting in a drift toward homoplasmy in subsequent cell lines. This process is called *replicative segregation*. With mtDNA deletions, preferential replication of the smaller deleted molecules causes an increase of deleted copy over time. The trend toward homoplasmy helps explain why disease worsens with age and why organ systems not previously involved in multisystem mitochondrial disease become involved.

Mitochondrial diseases can be subdivided into these categories:

- disorders resulting from large rearrangements of mtDNA (deletions and insertions), such as chronic progressive external ophthalmoplegia (CPEO), Kearns-Sayre syndrome, and Pearson marrow-pancreas syndrome
- mutations of mtDNA-encoded ribosomal RNA (rRNA), such as occur in maternally inherited sensorineural deafness and aminoglycoside-induced deafness
- mutations of mtDNA-encoded tRNA, such as occur in the syndromes of mitochondrial encephalomyopathy, lactic acidosis, and strokelike episodes (MELAS); myoclonic epilepsy with ragged red fibers (MERRF); type 2 diabetes mellitus and deafness; and (in about 30% of cases) CPEO
- missense and nonsense mutations, such as are present in Leber hereditary optic neuropathy (LHON) and neuropathy, ataxia, and retinitis pigmentosa (NARP)

Chronic Progressive External Ophthalmoplegia

CPEO is a disorder involving progressive ptosis and paralysis of eye muscles associated with a ragged red myopathy, usually as a result of deletion of a portion of the mitochondrial genome. Patients with CPEO commonly have pigmentary retinopathy that does not create significant visual disability. Infrequently, they may have more marked retinal or other system involvement, the so-called *CPEO-plus syndromes.* In Kearns-Sayre syndrome, CPEO is associated with heart block and severe RP with marked visual impairment. Pearson marrow-pancreas syndrome results from a large deletion of mtDNA and presents in younger patients with an entirely different phenotype involving sideroblastic anemia and pancreatic exocrine dysfunction. However, in patients afflicted during their later years, Pearson marrow-pancreas syndrome can present with a phenotype resembling Kearns-Sayre syndrome.

Although roughly 50% of patients with CPEO have demonstrable mtDNA deletions, virtually all patients with Kearns-Sayre syndrome have large deletions. As many as 30% of patients with CPEO who do not harbor demonstrable mtDNA deletions may have a point mutation at nucleotide position 3243, the same mutation in the tRNA for leucine that in other people is associated with MELAS syndrome. For all of the syndromes associated with deletions, such as Kearns-Sayre and CPEO, detection of the deletion usually requires study of the muscle tissue.

Leber Hereditary Optic Neuropathy

The most important ophthalmic disease of mitochondria is Leber hereditary optic neuropathy (LHON), which is more prevalent in males than in females but does not fit a classic X-linked pattern of transmission. The trait is not transmitted to the offspring of affected males, but virtually every daughter and son of a female patient with LHON inherits the trait. In approximately 50% of cases, LHON development is correlated with a single base change (G to A at nucleotide position 11778 in the *ND-4* gene) in human mtDNA involved in the synthesis of NADH dehydrogenase. In addition to optic atrophy, patients can exhibit peripapillary microangiopathy. LHON can also occur from other so-called primary mutations at nucleotide positions 3460 of *ND-1* and 14484 of *ND-6*, as well as several other rare mutations. At least 12 secondary mutations have been associated with LHON, often when multiple mutations are present in an individual's mitochondria. Some authors think that these secondary mutations cause disease by additive detrimental effects on the electron transport system of oxidative phosphorylation. Most of these secondary mutations appear in the general population, and debate persists on whether each mutation alone is truly pathogenic.

The likelihood of improvement with time in the recovery of visual acuity appears to differ among patients with the separate mutations associated with LHON. Mutation at nucleotide position 11778 is associated with the least likelihood of recovery, and mutation at nucleotide position 14484 is associated with the greatest likelihood.

Neuropathy, Ataxia, and Retinitis Pigmentosa

NARP is associated with a single base-pair mutation at nucleotide position 8993 in the *ATPase-6* gene. The NARP phenotype occurs when the percentage of mutant mtDNA is less than 80%, whereas the same mutation present at much higher proportions (greater than 95%) can cause Leigh syndrome, a severe neurodegenerative disease of infancy and early childhood. The 8993 mutation is demonstrable in fibroblasts and lymphoblasts.

MELAS and MIDD

Two different disorders—mitochondrial encephalomyopathy, lactic acidosis, and stroke-like episodes (MELAS) and maternally inherited diabetes and deafness (MIDD)—are associated with an A to G 3243 mtDNA point mutation, which affects an mt transfer RNA. Macular retinal pigment epithelial atrophy has been described with this mutation.

> Yu-Wai-Man P, Griffiths PG, Hudson G, Chinnery PF. Inherited mitochondrial optic neuropathies. *J Med Genet.* 2009;46(3):145–158.

The Search for Genes in Specific Diseases

A variety of methods have been used to assign individual genes to specific chromosomes, to link individual genes to one another, and to link diseases to specific genes.

Genetic Markers

Occasionally in cytogenetic studies, a genetic marker such as a large deletion or translocation (eg, 11p13 in aniridia) may be visible. Other markers used to identify the location of genes include blood groups (eg, as in Duffy blood group and Coppock cataract); restriction fragment length polymorphisms (RFLPs; eg, as in RP); microsatellites of variable number of tandem repeats (VNTRs); and most recently SNPs, as used in many GWAS. Cytogenetic tests are conducted on white blood cells, whereas the other genetic markers test DNA that is extracted most commonly from peripheral blood or saliva.

If a specific chromosomal structure is abnormal or even normally variant, its transmission through a family with a hereditary disease, as mapped by a pedigree, may support the assumption that the mutant gene and the variant chromosome are comigrating. Thus, the mutant gene is likely to be physically located on the variant chromosome—that is, the gene is a cytogenetic marker for the disease.

Gene Dosage

If a portion of a chromosome containing a specific gene is deleted, the amount of the gene product will be determined only by the remaining homologue. For example, people with an interstitial deletion of part of the long arm of chromosome 13 may have serum levels of esterase D that are 50% of normal. When several such individuals were also found to have retinoblastoma, it was suggested that both the esterase and the retinoblastoma genes are located in the missing segment. In contrast to the reduced activity caused by a deletion, a duplication may produce 150% of normal activity of a given gene product, as a result of either a chromosomal trisomy or a triplication of a specific chromosomal segment. Gene dosage appears to be a mechanism of disease in anterior segment dysgenesis (ASD), caused by duplication or deletion of the *FOXC1* gene; both 50% and 150% of the transcription factor lead to ASD.

Linkage and Disease Association

Even if no information is known about the nature or function of a gene for a disease, linkage studies may be able to localize the gene to a given chromosome or a specific marker. In 1937, Bell and Haldane recognized the first linkage between 2 diseases on a human chromosome: congenital color vision deficiency and hemophilia on the X chromosome. Subsequent investigations have led to the chromosomal mapping of a large number of different human ocular diseases.

Gene assignments

Every chromosome has numerous defined genes. The Human Genome Project (HGP) has identified and mapped approximately 20,000–25,000 genes. In addition, the database OMIM (Online Mendelian Inheritance in Man; see www.ncbi.nlm.nih.gov /omim) lists information on all known mendelian disorders. Human gene mapping has 2 major applications. The first is identification of the gene for a specific genetic disease by its linkage to a known marker. For example, suppose gene A causes a hereditary disease and gene B is a known enzyme or polymorphic marker closely linked to A. Even though no biochemical test exists for A, a tight linkage to B would allow a reasonable probability of identifying the disease for prenatal diagnosis and sometimes for carrier detection. The second impact of linkage is as an aid to understanding the cause of the phenotypic malformations in specific chromosomal diseases. For example, the phenotype of Down syndrome may result from triplication of only the distal long arm of chromosome 21 through a chromosome rearrangement rather than trisomy of the entire chromosome.

It is possible to detect linkage by observing the frequency with which a polymorphic marker is inherited with a disease trait. The physical distance represented by 1 cM corresponds to approximately 1 million bp (1000 kb) and to a 1% chance that recombination will result from a single meiosis (a 0.01 recombination fraction). When a genetic marker is sufficiently close to a disease gene, both are rarely separated by meiotic recombination. The frequency of this separation by chromosomal exchange at meiosis is termed the *recombination frequency.* To be linked, markers should be no more than approximately 20 cM apart. For perspective, the average chromosome contains about 150 cM, and there are approximately 3300 cM in the entire human genome, which corresponds to 3×10^9 bp.

When determining linkage between a gene and a marker, geneticists compare different models by calculating likelihood ratios. When the likelihood ratio is 1000:1 that the odds of one model are greater than those of another, the first is accepted over the second. The base 10 logarithm of the likelihood ratio (*LOD score;* logarithm of *odds* score) is usually reported. An LOD score of 1–2 is of potential interest in terms of linkage; 2–3 is suggestive; and greater than 3 is generally considered proof of linkage. Although an LOD score of 3 gives a probability ratio of 1000:1 in favor of linkage versus independent assortment, this score does not indicate a type I error as low as 0.001 but, in fact, indicates an error that is close to 0.05, the standard significance level used in statistics. (BCSC Section 1, *Update on General Medicine,* explains these concepts in depth.)

Candidate Gene Approaches

Candidate gene screening

The process of candidate gene screening involves screening for mutations of genes that are abundantly expressed within a tissue and are either important for function or specifically expressed only in that tissue. Sometimes, the candidate gene is one that recapitulates the human disease in transgenic animals. Examples of candidate gene screening discoveries include the findings of mutations of peripherin/*RDS* in autosomal dominant RP and macular dystrophies and the finding of mutations of the rod cyclic guanosine monophosphate (cGMP) β-subunit of rod phosphodiesterase and the cGMP–gated cation channel in autosomal recessive RP.

Positional candidate gene screening

Whenever linkage studies localize a gene to a given chromosomal region, genes already known to reside in the same region become candidate genes for that disease. Following are some examples of disease localization that resulted from linkage to a given region, which in turn led to finding the disease-causing gene by screening for mutations of genes in the region: autosomal dominant RP from rhodopsin mutations (3q); Sorsby fundus dystrophy from *TIMP3* mutations (22q); and Oguchi disease from point deletions within the arrestin gene (2q).

Mutation Screening

Direct Sequencing

One of the most important advances in molecular genetics has been the development of techniques for rapid sequencing of DNA. Currently, it costs far less to sequence a stretch of DNA than to sequence and characterize the amino acid peptide that the DNA produces.

Although other mutation screening techniques exist, sequencing of DNA is the surest and most direct. Sequencing of complementary DNA (cDNA) derived from mRNA provides a quick look at the reading frames (exons) of the gene, whereas sequencing of genomic DNA is more time-consuming because of the presence of introns between the exons. The intron–exon boundaries must be known and multiple PCR assays set up in order to screen not only the exons and their splice junction sites but also upstream and downstream regions that may be important for gene activation and regulation.

DNA sequencing techniques currently in use include the enzymatic (or Sanger sequencing) method, which can be automated (Fig 5-4 illustrates this procedure), and next-generation sequencing (NGS), also known as *massively parallel sequencing*. NGS offers the ability to sequence the entire genome of an individual. Some NGS methods use as probes allele-specific oligonucleotides that are constructed to use hybridization to recognize a specific DNA sequence in order to detect a specific point mutation (Figs 5-5 through 5-8).

Sanger Dideoxy Sequencing

1. Four DNA synthesis reactions incorporating chain-terminating dideoxy nucleotides lead to ending of the sequence at each A, T, C, or G, each labeled with a separate nucleotide.

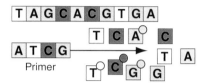

2. Each reaction thus generates fragments of increasing size, ending at the base specified by the reaction, ie, each A, T, C, or G.

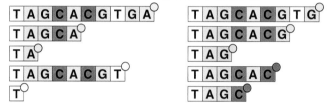

3. Fragments are resolved on a gel or automated sequencing machine.

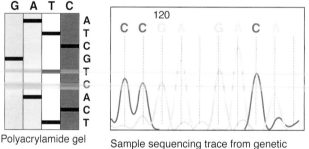

Polyacrylamide gel

Sample sequencing trace from genetic analyzer, which separates the DNA fragments by size and reads the fluorescence at the end of each fragment (which comes from the chain-terminating nucleotide).

Figure 5-4 Schematic representation of the original Sanger dideoxy chain-termination se-quencing method. The results produced are shown in step 3: DNA fragments resolved on a polyacrylamide gel and a sequencing trace from a modern automated sequencing machine. *(Redrawn with permission by Mark Miller from What's so special about next generation sequencing? Oxbridge Biotech Roundtable. www.oxbridgebiotech.com/review/research/whats-so-special-about-next-generation-sequencing. Published August 19, 2012. Accessed October 3, 2013.)*

Early methods of mutation detection included Sanger sequencing using radioactive and later fluorescent probes; the single-stranded conformational polymorphism (SSCP) technique; denaturing gradient gel electrophoresis (DGGE); and the use of restriction fragment length polymorphisms (RFLPs).

Complete exome sequencing will identify many potential mutations; however, consid-erable bioinformatic information is required to identify true disease-causing mutations.

Zhang J, Chiodini R, Badr A, Zhang G. The impact of next-generation sequencing on geno-mics. *J Genet Genomics.* 2011;38(3):95–109.

Whole-Genome Shotgun Sequencing

1. Genomic DNA randomly sheared and cloned in *E coli*

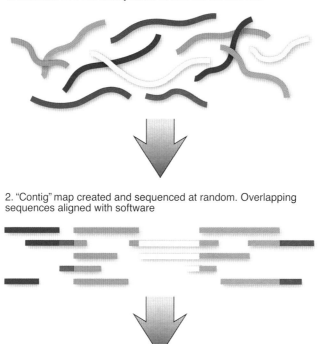

2. "Contig" map created and sequenced at random. Overlapping sequences aligned with software

3. Final sequence generated

Figure 5-5 Schematic summary of the whole-genome shotgun sequencing method of next-generation sequencing (NGS). At a basic level, all NGS technologies use the same principle: fragment the DNA, add primers/adapters, amplify, and sequence. In whole-genome shotgun sequencing, a DNA sample is randomly broken into numerous small fragments that are then sequenced using the chain-termination method. Multiple overlapping DNA fragments produced from numerous repetitions of this process are then assembled into a single continuous sequence on a computer program. *(Redrawn by Mark Miller with permission from What's so special about next generation sequencing? Oxbridge Biotech Roundtable. Available at www.oxbridgebiotech.com/review/research/whats-so-special-about-next-generation-sequencing. Published August 19, 2012. Accessed October 3, 2013.)*

Genome-Wide Association Studies

Although karyotyping and linkage analysis can still be used to identify disease-associated genes, most research is now centered on GWAS and NGS. Following the creation of the human gene map, the next project (called the International HapMap Project) compared the DNA sequence of 1184 reference individuals from 11 global populations (creating a catalog called the *HapMap*) to identify regions of variation between individuals and racial groups. By using the HapMap to study individuals from a similar population, genetics researchers find that many people will share a series of SNPs or a haplotype. Thus, it is possible to test only one or a few SNPs but to infer a large number of adjacent SNPs

454 Method

1. DNA broken into smaller fragments

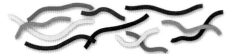

2. Adapters attached to the DNA fragments to allow amplification of the sequences

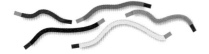

3. Beads added that contain small sequences matching parts of the adapters. DNA binds to the beads, aiming for one DNA fragment per bead

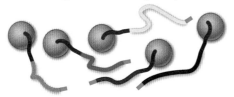

4. DNA strands amplified on bead, and DNA strands denatured to make single-stranded fragments

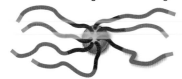

5. Single beads transferred into the wells of a 96-well plate with polymerase enzyme beads

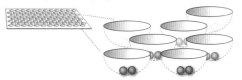

6. Nucleotides fed in waves, ie, only A, then T, then C, then G. Incorporation of the nucleotides measured by the release of light when a nucleotide is incorporated

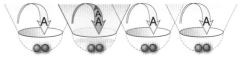

7. Release of light for each nucleotide plotted for each fragment, allowing determination of the sequence

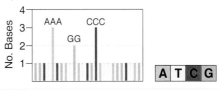

Figure 5-6   Schematic representation of the 454 NGS method, which uses the sequencing-by-synthesis principle. This method uses light generated after a base is incorporated to measure the signals (hence it is also called *pyrosequencing*). *(Redrawn by Mark Miller with permission from What's so special about next generation sequencing? Oxbridge Biotech Roundtable. Available at www.oxbridgebiotech .com/review/research/whats-so-special-about-next-generation-sequencing. Published August 19, 2012. Accessed October 3, 2013.)*

by imputation. Chip or bead platforms enable the investigation of 100,000 to millions of SNPs across the genome, forming the basis of a GWAS.

Results of a GWAS are usually presented in a Manhattan plot, so named because it brings to mind the New York City skyline. In a Manhattan plot, the chromosomes are arranged in order along the x-axis, and the P value of the association of the disease or trait with the particular SNP at that chromosomal location is given on the y-axis. Figure 5-9 shows a Manhattan plot for glaucoma. A significant gene association (threshold ~5×10^{-8}) will often have multiple adjacent SNPs at high levels of significance, and thus a column of points will rise on the plot. It is rare that the SNPs themselves are the disease-causing mutations. Usually they are linked in the haploblock to the mutation, which is why researchers will then use fine-mapping of the region by looking at a large number of SNPs in the nearby region.

Solexa Technology

1. Double-stranded DNAs are sheared into shorter fragments.

2. Adapters (short DNA sequences) are bound to the fragments.

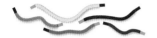

3. Fragments are placed on a hollow slide with a lawn of primers.

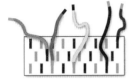

4. DNA fragments bend over and bind to a complementary primer on the slide surface.

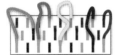

5. DNA fragments are amplified, forming dense DNA clusters on each channel of the slide.

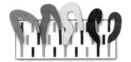

6. One type of the strand is discarded to make sequencing more efficient. DNA polymerase and labeled nucleotides are added.

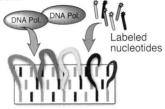

7. As bases are incorporated, a laser is used to activate fluorescence.

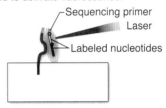

8. Each DNA cluster is monitored by a computer and the color of each cluster noted as each base is incorporated.

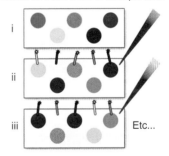

Figure 5-7 Illustration depicting the concept of the Solexa technology method of NGS, which uses the sequencing-by-synthesis principle as in the 454 method but measures signals through the use of fluorescent dye. *(Redrawn by Mark Miller with permission from What's so special about next generation sequencing? Oxbridge Biotech Roundtable. Available at www.oxbridgebiotech.com/review/research/whats-so -special-about-next-generation-sequencing. Published August 19, 2012. Accessed October 3, 2013.)*

Combining numerous studies, usually of multiple ethnic groups, in meta-analyses allows for identification of additional associated gene regions. Figure 5-10 shows how GWAS meta-analyses combine data from individual GWAS. Figure 5-11 shows the meta-analysis of GWAS for age-related macular degeneration (AMD), with 19 loci now identified. The effect size for all of these genes is usually small, but cumulatively they account for approximately 40% of AMD heritability.

Comparison of GWAS from different ethnic groups can help clarify whether the SNP itself is disease causing or just linked to the true disease-causing mutation(s). An example

Nanopore Sequencing Technology

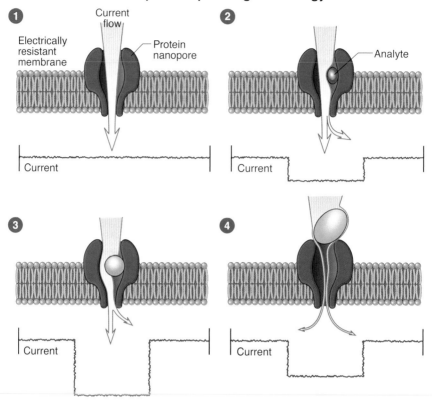

Figure 5-8 In the nanopore sequencing technology method of NGS, an ionic current is passed through protein nanopores that are set in an electrically resistant membrane bilayer. Different analytes to be sequenced are depicted by the *red* and *blue dots* and the *green oval*. A characteristic current disruption occurs when an analyte passes through the pore or near its aperture, and the analyte can be identified in this manner. In one application, a sample DNA strand can be fed through the nanopore by an enzyme, and the 4 standard DNA bases can be identified in sequence as the strand passes through. *(Redrawn by Mark Miller with permission from Introduction to nanopore sensing. Oxford Nanopore Technologies Ltd website. Available at https://www.nanoporetech.com/technology/introduction-to -nanopore-sensing/. Accessed October 3, 2013.)*

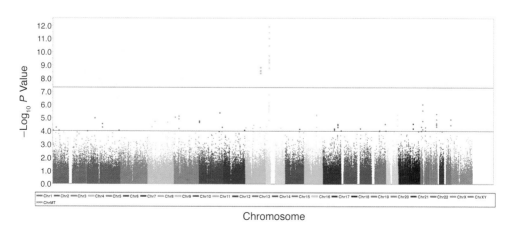

Figure 5-9 Manhattan plot for glaucoma, identifying the *CDKN2BAS* region at 9p21 and the *SIX1/SIX6* region at 14q23. *(Reproduced with permission from Wiggs JL, Yaspan BL, Hauser MA, et al. Common variants at 9p21 and 8q22 are associated with increased susceptibility to optic nerve degeneration in glaucoma. PLoS Genet. 2012;8(4):e1002654.)*

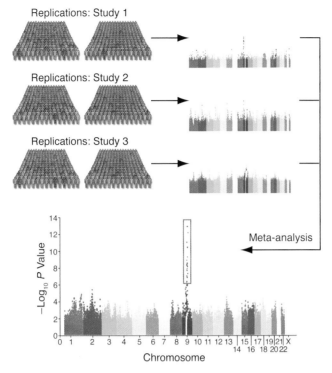

Figure 5-10 Meta-analysis of Manhattan plots. *(Reproduced with permission from Manolio TA. Genome-wide association studies and assessment of the risk of disease. N Engl J Med. 2010;363(2):166–176.)*

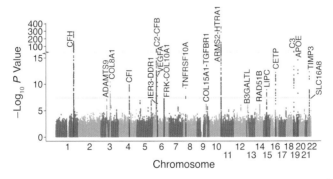

Figure 5-11 Manhattan plot for age-related macular degeneration meta-analysis identifying numerous associated genes. *(Reproduced with permission from Fritsche LG, Chen W, Schu M, et al. Seven new loci associated with age-related macular degeneration. Nat Genet. 2013;45(4):433-439.)*

is the *LOXL1* gene associated with exfoliation syndrome. One SNP was associated with disease in the Caucasian population, but disease was associated with the opposite SNP in the Japanese population (Fig 5-12A). Thus, it is unlikely that this SNP is actually disease causing but more likely that different SNPs are associated with the true disease-causing mutation in East Asian and white, or Caucasian-derived, populations. In contrast, another SNP had equivalent association in both populations (Fig 5-12B).

For a catalog of GWAS including ophthalmic studies, see www.genome.gov/GWA Studies.

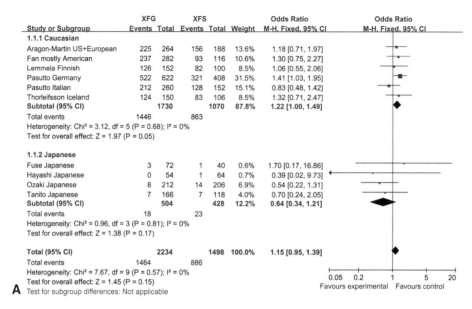

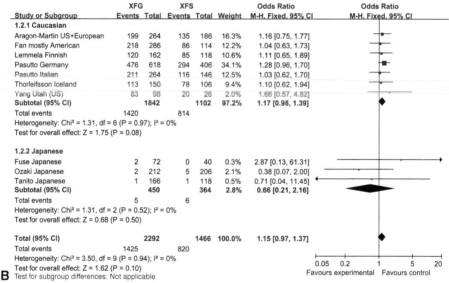

Figure 5-12 Forest plots *(at right)* of meta-analyses for single-nucleotide polymorphisms (SNPs) near *LOX1* in exfoliation syndrome (XFS) and exfoliation glaucoma (XFG). A forest plot is a graphical display designed to illustrate the relative strength of effects found in different quantitative scientific studies that address the same question; essentially, it graphically represents a meta-analysis of the results. **A,** Meta-analysis of the association of SNP rs1048661 with a combined group of XFS and XFG cases. Subgroup meta-analysis indicated that the odds ratios (ORs) of SNP rs1048661 G allele are reversed in Caucasian and Japanese populations. **B,** Meta-analysis of the association of SNP rs3825942 with a combined group of XFS and XFG cases. Subgroup meta-analysis indicated that the ORs of SNP rs3825942 G allele are consistent in Caucasian and Japanese populations. Square = study-specific OR, with the size of the square proportional to the weight of the study; horizontal line = 95% confidence interval (CI); diamond = summary OR with its corresponding 95% CI. *(Reproduced with permission from Chen H, Chen LJ, Zhang M, et al. Ethnicity-based subgroup meta-analysis of the association of LOXL1 polymorphisms with glaucoma. Ml Vis. 2010;16:167–177.)*

Gene Therapy

Gene therapy holds much promise, but the field remains in its infancy. The potential for cure is not matched by either technology or understanding. No clinical ophthalmic applications yet exist. Key challenges remain in characterizing linkages of genes to major diseases (especially chronic diseases that, although common, are likely multifactorial), understanding the pathogenic relevance of identified linked genes, and developing proper delivery systems for curative gene constructs (the main long-term gene therapy vehicle—viruses—is currently limited by inflammatory effects and the risk of oncogenesis).

Replacement of Absent Gene Product in X-Linked and Recessive Disease

For genetic diseases in which the mutant allele produces either no message or an ineffective gene product (called a *null allele*), correction of the disorder may be possible by simple replacement of the gene in the deficient cells or tissues. It is theoretically possible to transfer normal genes into human cells that harbor either null or mutant genes not producing a stable, translated product. Vectors used to carry the genetic material into the cells include adenoviruses, retroviruses (especially adeno-associated viruses [AAVs]), and plasmid–liposome complexes. AAV vector gene therapy has been successful in curing many disorders in animal models, such as the *RPE65* gene mutation that causes RP in the Briard dog.

Human gene therapy trials with *RPE65* are under way, with preliminary studies suggesting no major early adverse effects and possibly even some improvement in visual function in adults. Studies of younger subjects are also under way, and several other retinal dystrophy genes are being investigated for human gene therapy trials.

> Carvalho LS, Vandenberghe LH. Promising and delivering gene therapies for vision loss. *Vision Res.* 2015;111(Pt B):124–133.

Strategies for Dominant Diseases

Dominant diseases are caused by production of a gene product that is either insufficient *(haploid insufficiency)* or conducive to disease *(dominant-negative effect).* Theoretically, haploid insufficiency should be treatable by gene replacement therapy as outlined in the previous section for X-linked and recessive diseases. For dominant disorders produced by defective developmental genes, this correction would have to occur in early uterine development.

Disorders resulting from a dominant-negative effect require a different approach. Thus, strategies for treatment of dominant disease differ, depending on whether a functional gene product is produced. Some genes code for RNA molecules that can bind to mRNA from another gene and block the other molecule's ability to be translated. Greater understanding of these genes may allow for creation of either drugs or new gene-encoded RNA molecules that can block the translation of mRNA for defective alleles, thus allowing only the normal allele to be expressed.

Another approach is the use of oligonucleotides that are designed to bind with mRNA from mutant alleles, stopping the mRNA from being translated by ribosomes (Fig 5-13). Although many problems need to be worked out for such therapy to be effective, this

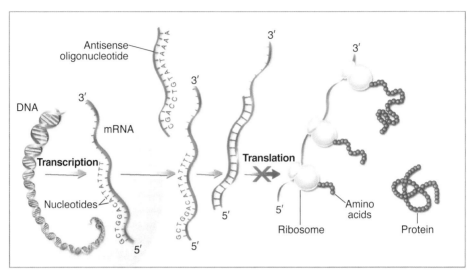

Figure 5-13 Blockade of translation by antisense oligonucleotides. Normal gene transcription of DNA into mRNA is followed by translation of mRNA into protein. Antisense oligonucleotides complementary to a portion of mRNA bind mRNA, preventing translation—either by the steric effect of the binding process itself or (possibly) by inducing degradation of the mRNA by RNase. *(Reproduced with permission from Askari FK, McDonnell WM. Antisense-oligonucleotide therapy. N Engl J Med. 1996;334(5):316–318.)*

approach holds promise for autosomal dominant disorders in which disease is caused by expression of the mutant gene product.

One approach to the treatment of autosomal dominant diseases is to target the translated strand of the mutant allele by antisense DNA, a sequence of DNA designed to anneal to and block the processing or translation of the abnormal mRNA. The use of ribozymes, RNA molecules that have the ability to cleave certain RNA molecules, provides another approach. A third method utilizes *short interfering RNA (siRNA)*, also known as *small interference RNA*, to bind to mRNA and lead to the eventual degradation of specific mRNA molecules. The use of siRNA molecules as potential therapeutic agents has become increasingly popular in the past few years, and this approach has proven to be a powerful means by which to study the function of novel gene products. However, therapy with siRNA faces difficulty in achieving intracellular delivery and from cell-surface TLR3 receptor stimulation, which can induce immune or antiangiogenic processes as a generic class property. A new form of genome editing known as CRISPR–Cas (clustered, regularly interspaced, short palindromic repeats–CRISPR-associated) has been used to correct point mutations in the DNA sequence of cells.

CHAPTER 6

Clinical Genetics

The most valuable tool in clinical genetics is the phrase, "Does anyone else in the family have . . . ?"

A positive family history currently carries greater specificity and sensitivity than most laboratory genetic tests. Even with all the DNA mutations currently known for diseases, the vast majority of mutations remain to be identified, and the full hand of genetic cards dealt to each person is not known. Genetics is important in every ophthalmic consultation, from those involving rare inborn errors of metabolism or congenital malformations to common eye diseases, such as myopia, glaucoma, cataract, and age-related macular degeneration (AMD). Even susceptibility to infection and trauma can be genetic. An understanding of the genetic basis of a disease may be particularly useful for arriving at a correct diagnosis when another family member has a similar disease. In addition, it is important for clinicians to recognize that a patient presenting with a particular eye problem may be at increased risk for an unrelated disease such as glaucoma because of an affected parent.

The ophthalmologist has an important obligation to patients with genetic eye diseases either to provide genetic counseling or to arrange for referral to a geneticist or genetic counselor. Clinicians now have patients presenting with DNA test results for themselves or their families. The results may range from the identification of high-risk retinoblastoma gene mutations (which will significantly influence the management of at-risk children within the family) to genetic associations that are of no more value than iridology (genes have been associated with iris crypts and furrows). It is important to understand the clinical settings in which a genetic test is crucial, useful, or irrelevant to patient management. These distinctions will change in the future as new clinical trials define treatments based on genetic background. When a patient presents with a DNA result for a disease for which no effective treatment based on such results is currently available and asks, "What should we do about this?" the best answer is, "Participate in, or help fund, research so we can find out what the best treatments are." The US National Institutes of Health (NIH) website www.clinicaltrials.gov is a good place to refer these patients.

The key recommendations of the American Academy of Ophthalmology (AAO) Task Force on Genetic Testing policy are given at the end of this chapter. When faced with the option of ordering genetic tests, clinicians should ask the same question they ask before ordering any tests, "How will this change management?" The best utilization of genetic testing comes from knowledge of the family history. An accurate family history might help an ophthalmologist save not only a patient's sight but, in cases of retinoblastoma or Marfan syndrome, even the patient's life.

Pedigree Analysis

Establishing a pedigree or drawing a family tree is the key to clinical genetics. The most useful strategy is to start with open questions such as, "Are there any eye diseases in the family?" and proceed further to more targeted questions such as—in the case of potential Leber hereditary optic neuropathy (LHON)—"Did any men on the maternal side of your family lose vision as a young adult?" For patients with a family history, it is best to convert the information into a pedigree diagram (this can be a challenge in some electronic medical records). An initial, rough outline can be drawn on paper and the information entered into a simple or more sophisticated pedigree-drawing software program. The standard protocol for pedigree symbols is outlined in Figure 6-1.

Drawing one's own extended family tree is a useful exercise for the clinician. A male is represented by a square and a female by a circle. The index case, or *proband,* is the patient who brings attention to the pedigree, and he or she is usually marked with an arrow. A basic pedigree should include parents, siblings, and children, and it should note those affected and unaffected by the disorder of interest. Often, specific inquiry of grandparents, uncles, aunts, and cousins can help clarify the inheritance pattern.

The interviewer should always ascertain whether brothers and sisters are half siblings or full siblings. This procedure may not only limit the possible patterns of inheritance but also identify other individuals at risk for the disorder under consideration. Information about parentage must be pursued aggressively (but always privately and confidentially). Both incest and nonpaternity are sensitive issues, but clearly neither is rare in our society. In considering rare autosomal recessive diseases, the interviewer must ask specifically about consanguinity. Are the parents cousins? Are there common last names in the families of both parents? Were the parents born in the same area or do they belong to known ethnic or religious isolates?

Age at death may be useful in specific situations and can be recorded near the appropriate symbols. In the case of a child with ectopia lentis and no family history of similar ocular disease, a clinician may find the identification of a relative who died from a

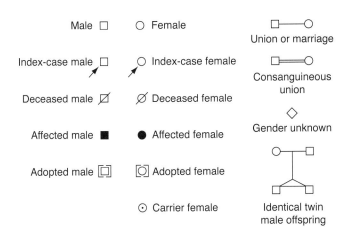

Figure 6-1 Symbols commonly used for pedigree analysis. *(Courtesy of David A. Mackey, MD.)*

dissecting thoracic aorta in his fourth decade of life very informative, leading to a tentative consideration of Marfan syndrome in the differential diagnosis. In another example, the clinician's casual observation of multiple patches of congenital hypertrophy of the retinal pigment epithelium (RPE) in each eye in a young adult may trigger remembrance that a parent had died at age 50 years from metastatic adenocarcinoma of the colon and a sibling from a brain tumor at age 10 years. Taken together, this information may lead to a diagnosis of Gardner syndrome and referral to a gastroenterologist for further diagnostic evaluation.

Taking a family history does not end with the first consultation because it may be the first time a patient has heard of the disease. On discussing the new diagnosis with the family, the patient (particularly a male) may discover additional family history. Clinicians should encourage patients to talk to their families and then have them update the family history on subsequent consultations. For more complicated genetic diseases, a genetic counselor will be able to assist patients with an extensive pedigree.

Bennett RL, Steinhaus KA, Uhrich SB, et al. Recommendations for standardized human pedigree nomenclature. Pedigree Standardization Task Force of the National Society of Genetic Counselors. *Am J Hum Genet.* 1995;56(3):745–752.

Patterns of Inheritance

Many of the terms used in this section are defined in the Introduction to Part III of this volume, which includes a glossary. See also the section, later in this chapter, Terminology: Hereditary, Genetic, Familial, Congenital.

Dominant Versus Recessive

The terms *dominant* and *recessive* were first used by Gregor Mendel. In classical genetics, a dominant gene is always expressed with similar phenotype, whether the mutant gene is present in a homozygous or heterozygous state. Stated simply, a dominant gene is expressed when present in only a single copy. A gene is called *recessive* if its expression is masked by a normal allele or, more precisely, if it is expressed only in the homozygote (or compound heterozygote) state when both alleles at a specific locus are mutant.

A *trait* is the consequence of the gene's action. In actuality, it is the trait, or phenotypic expression of the gene at a clinical level, rather than the gene itself that is dominant or recessive. A trait is recessive if its expression is suppressed by the presence of a normal gene (as in galactosemia) and dominant if it is apparently unaffected by a single copy of the normal allele (as in Marfan syndrome). If the alleles are different and yet are both manifested in the phenotype, they are said to be *codominant*. Examples of phenotypes with codominant inheritance patterns include the ABO blood types, HLA types, and hemoglobin variants (as involved in sickle cell disease).

As a result of epigenetic factors, a gene may have a greater or lesser effect on the individual or an organ, and therefore the trait may be more or less apparent. Thus, the designation of a trait as either dominant or recessive depends on the testing method used. Although classically a dominant gene has the same phenotype when the mutant allele is present in either the heterozygous or the homozygous state, most dominant medical diseases act more like codominant diseases, in which individuals who are homozygous for a mutant allele or who harbor 2 mutant alleles will have more severe expression than will those with only 1 mutant allele.

In experiments, the biochemical mechanisms of dominant hereditary diseases appear different from those of recessive disorders. Recessive traits usually result from enzyme deficiencies caused by mutations of the gene specifying the affected enzyme. The altered enzyme often can be shown to be structurally abnormal or unstable. Heterozygotes usually have approximately 50% of normal enzyme activity but are clinically unaffected, implying that half of the normal enzyme activity is compatible with near-normal function. If adequate biochemical testing can be performed and the specific enzyme isolated, the reduced enzyme activity can be quantified and the heterozygous genetic state inferred. Thus, clinically unaffected heterozygotes can be detected for such disorders as homocystinuria (decrease in cystathionine β-synthase), galactokinase deficiency (low blood galactokinase activity), classic galactosemia (galactose-1-phosphate uridyltransferase deficiency), gyrate atrophy of the choroid and retina (decreased ornithine-δ-aminotransferase), and Tay-Sachs disease (decreased hexosaminidase A). Table 6-1 outlines many disorders with ocular manifestations for which an enzyme defect is known.

Rajappa M, Goyal A, Kaur J. Inherited metabolic disorders involving the eye: a clinico-biochemical perspective. *Eye.* 2010;24(4):507–518.

Autosomal Recessive Inheritance

An autosomal recessive disease is expressed fully only in the presence of a mutant gene at the same locus on both homologous chromosomes (ie, homozygosity for a mutant gene) or of 2 different mutant alleles at the same locus (compound heterozygosity). A single mutant allele is sufficient to cause a recessive disorder if the normal allele on the homologous chromosome is deleted. A recessive trait can remain latent through several generations until the chance mating of 2 heterozygotes for a mutant allele gives rise to an affected individual. The frequency of heterozygotes for a given disorder will always be considerably greater than that of homozygotes. It is estimated that all human beings inherit numerous mutations for different recessive disorders for which they are heterozygotes.

Enzymatic defects

Autosomal recessive diseases often result from defects in enzymatic proteins. Most of the so-called inborn errors of metabolism that result from enzymatic defects are autosomal recessive traits, although a few are X-linked recessive disorders (eg, Lesch-Nyhan syndrome).

In some other disorders with genetic blocks in metabolism, the phenotypic consequences are related to the lack of a normal product distal to the block. An example is *albinism,* in which the metabolic block involves a step between the amino acid tyrosine and the formation of melanin. In still other inborn errors of metabolism, the phenotypic expression results from excessive production of a product through a normally alternative and minor metabolic pathway.

Table 6-1 Known Enzyme Disorders and Corresponding Ocular Signs

Disorder	Defective Enzyme	Ocular Sign
Storage diseases		
Fabry disease	Ceramide trihexosidase (α-galactosidase)	Corneal epithelial verticillate changes; aneurysmal dilation and tortuosity of retinal and conjunctival vessels
GM$_1$ gangliosidosis, type I (generalized gangliosidosis)	β-Galactosidase	Macular cherry-red spot; optic atrophy; corneal clouding (mild)
GM$_2$ gangliosidosis, type I (Tay-Sachs disease)	Hexosaminidase A	Macular cherry-red spot; optic atrophy
GM$_2$ gangliosidosis, type II (Sandhoff disease)	Hexosidase A and B	Macular cherry-red spot
Krabbe leukodystrophy	Cerebroside α-galactosidase	Macular cherry-red spot; optic atrophy
Mannosidosis	α-Mannosidase	Lenticular opacities
Metachromatic leukodystrophy	Arylsulfatase A	Retinal discoloration, degeneration
Mucopolysaccharidosis I H (Hurler syndrome)	α-L-Iduronidase	Corneal opacity; pigmentary retinal degeneration
Mucopolysaccharidosis I S (Scheie syndrome)	α-L-Iduronidase	Corneal opacity; pigmentary retinal degeneration
Mucopolysaccharidosis II (Hunter syndrome)	Sulfoiduronate sulfatase	Corneal opacity (mild type); older-age patients
Mucopolysaccharidosis III (Sanfilippo syndrome)	Heparan sulfate sulfatase	Pigmentary retinal degeneration; optic atrophy
Metabolic disorders		
Albinism	Tyrosinase	Foveal hypoplasia; nystagmus; iris transillumination
Alkaptonuria	Homogentisic acid oxidase	Dark sclera
Crigler-Najjar syndrome	Glucuronide transferase	Extraocular movement
Ehlers-Danlos syndrome VI	Lysyl hydroxylase	Microcornea; retinal detachment; ectopia lentis; blue scleras
Familial dysautonomia	Dopamine-β-hydroxylase	Alacrima; corneal hypoesthesia; exodeviation; methacholine-induced miosis
Galactokinase deficiency	Galactokinase	Cataracts
Galactosemia	Galactose-1-phosphate uridyltransferase	Cataracts
Gyrate atrophy of the choroid and retina	Ornithine aminotransferase	Degeneration of the choroid and retina; cataracts; myopia
Homocystinuria	Cystathionine synthase	Dislocated lens
Hyperglycinemia	Glycine cell transport	Optic atrophy
Intermittent ataxia	Pyruvate dicarboxylase	Nystagmus
Leigh necrotizing encephalopathy	Pyruvate carboxylase	Optic atrophy
Maple syrup urine disease	Branch chain decarboxylase	Ophthalmoplegia; nystagmus
Niemann-Pick disease	Sphingomyelinase	Macular cherry-red spot
Refsum syndrome	Phytanic acid oxidase	Retinal degeneration
Sulfite oxidase deficiency	Sulfite oxidase	Ectopia lentis
Tyrosinemia	Tyrosine aminotransferase	Lens opacity
Tyrosinosis	Tyrosine aminotransferase	Corneal dystrophy

Carrier heterozygotes

The heterozygous carrier of a mutant gene may show minimal evidence of the gene defect, particularly at a biochemical level. Thus, carrier heterozygotes have been detected by a variety of methods:

- identification of abnormal metabolites by electrophoresis (eg, galactokinase deficiency)
- hair bulb assay (eg, oculocutaneous albinism and Fabry disease)
- monitoring of enzyme activity in leukocytes (eg, galactose-1-phosphate uridyl-transferase in galactosemia)
- skin culture for analysis of enzyme activity in fibroblasts (eg, ornithine-δ-aminotransferase deficiency in gyrate atrophy of the retina and choroid)
- assay of serum and tears (eg, hexosaminidase A in Tay-Sachs disease)

In contrast to the transmission of dominant traits, most reproduction resulting in transmission of recessive disorders involves phenotypically normal heterozygous parents. Out of 4 offspring produced by parents carrying the same gene for an autosomal recessive disease, on average, 1 will be affected (homozygote), 2 will be carriers (heterozygotes), and 1 will be genetically and phenotypically normal. Thus, clinically normal heterozygous parents will produce offspring with a ratio of 1 clinically affected to 3 clinically normal. There is no predilection for either sex. In 2-child families, the patient with a recessive disease is frequently the only affected family member. For instance, approximately 40%–50% of patients with retinitis pigmentosa (RP) have no family history of the disorder. However, their age of onset, rate of progression, and other phenotypic characteristics are similar to those with defined recessive inheritance patterns.

Once 1 child is born with a recessive disorder, the genetic risk for each subsequent child of the same parents is 25%. This concept has specific implications for genetic counseling. All offspring of an affected individual will be carriers; they are unlikely to be affected with the disorder unless their clinically unaffected parent is also by chance a carrier of the gene. The normal-appearing sibling of a child with a recessive disorder has a statistical risk of 2 chances in 3 of being a genetic carrier. As the genes for recessive diseases are identified, these individuals and their offspring will benefit from predictive DNA testing.

Consanguinity

The mating of close relatives can increase the probability that their children will inherit a homozygous genotype for recessive traits, particularly for relatively rare ones. For example, the probability that the same allele is present in first cousins is 1 in 8. In the offspring of a first-cousin sexual union, 1 of every 16 of the genes is commonly present in a homozygous state. It follows that each offspring from a first-cousin union has a 1 in 16 chance of manifesting an autosomal recessive trait within a given family. Approximately 1% of all sexual unions may be consanguineous. A vigorous search for consanguinity between the parents should be made in any case of a rare recessive disease.

In contrast, the expression of common recessive genes is less influenced by inbreeding because most homozygous offspring are the progeny of unrelated parents. This pattern is usually the case with such frequent disorders as sickle cell disease and cystic fibrosis. The characteristics of autosomal recessive inheritance are summarized in Table 6-2.

Table 6-2 Characteristics of Autosomal Recessive Inheritance

The mutant gene usually does not cause clinical disease (recessive) in the heterozygote.

Individuals inheriting both the genes (homozygotes) of the defective type express the disorder.

Typically, the trait appears only in siblings, not in their parents or offspring or in other relatives.

The ratio of normal to affected in a sibship is 3:1. The larger the sibship, the more often will more than one child be affected.

The sexes are affected in equal proportions.

Parents of the affected person may be genetically related (consanguinity); the rarer the trait, the more likely.

Affected individuals have children who, although phenotypically normal, are carriers (heterozygotes) of the gene.

Pseudodominance

Occasionally, an affected homozygote mates with a heterozygote. Of their offspring, 50% will be carriers and 50% will be affected homozygotes. Because this segregation pattern mimics that of dominant inheritance, it is called *pseudodominance*. Fortunately, such matings are usually rare and are unlikely to affect more than two vertical generations.

Autosomal Dominant Inheritance

When an autosomal allele leads to a regular, clearly definable abnormality in the heterozygote, the trait is termed *dominant*. Autosomal dominant traits often represent defects in structural nonenzymatic proteins, such as in fibrillin in Marfan syndrome or collagen in Stickler syndrome. In addition, a dominant mode of inheritance has been observed for some malignant neoplastic syndromes, such as retinoblastoma, von Hippel–Lindau disease, tuberous sclerosis, and Gardner syndrome. Although the neoplasias in these diseases are inherited as autosomal dominant traits, the tumors themselves result from loss of function of both alleles of autosomal recessive tumor-suppressor genes.

Almost all bearers of dominant disorders in the human population are heterozygotes. In dominant inheritance, the heterozygote is clinically affected, and a single dose of the mutant gene interferes with normal function. Occasionally, depending on the frequency of the abnormal gene in the population and the phenotype, 2 carriers of the same abnormality produce children. Any offspring of 2 heterozygous parents has a 25% risk of being an affected homozygote.

It has been suggested that dominant diseases are caused by mutations affecting structural proteins, such as cell receptor growth factors (eg, *FGFR2* in Crouzon disease), or by functional deficits generated by abnormal polypeptide subunits (eg, unstable hemoglobins). The dominant disorders aniridia and Waardenburg syndrome result from loss of 1 of the 2 alleles for the developmental transcription factors *PAX6* and *PAX3*, respectively.

In some instances, dominantly inherited traits are not clinically expressed. In other instances—such as in some families with autosomal dominant RP—pedigree analysis infrequently shows a defective gene in individuals who do not manifest any discernible clinical or functional impairment. This situation is called *incomplete penetrance* or *skipped generation*.

Conclusive evidence of autosomal dominant inheritance requires demonstration of the disease in at least 3 successive generations. Transmission of the disorder from male to male offspring, with both sexes showing the typical disease, must also occur. The characteristics of autosomal dominant inheritance with complete (100%) penetrance are summarized in Table 6-3. In the usual clinical situation, any offspring of an affected heterozygote with a dominant disorder, regardless of sex, has a 1 in 2 chance of inheriting the mutant gene and thereby demonstrating some effect. The degree of variability in the expression of certain traits is usually more pronounced in autosomal dominantly inherited disorders than in other types of genetic disorders. Moreover, when a clinical disorder is inherited in more than one mendelian pattern, the dominantly inherited disorder is, in general, clinically less severe than the recessively inherited one.

Counseling for recurrence risk of autosomal dominant traits must involve thorough examination of not only the affected person (who may have the full syndrome) but also the parents. If 1 parent is even mildly affected, the risk of additional genetically affected siblings rises to 50%. It is unacceptable to miss variable expressivity when parents and other family members can be examined. In some ocular disorders, family members can inherit a gene for a dominant trait and not show clinically apparent manifestations. In these cases, electrophysiologic testing or genetic testing can be used to detect the impairment. For example, a relatively inexpensive genetic test can show which clinically normal family members carry the mutation for Best vitelliform macular dystrophy.

X-Linked Inheritance

A trait determined by genes on either of the sex chromosomes is properly termed *sex-linked*. This genetic pattern became widely known with the occurrence of hemophilia in European and Russian royal families.

The rules governing all modes of sex-linked inheritance can be derived logically by considering the chromosomal basis. Females have 2 X chromosomes, 1 of which will go to each ovum. Males have both an X and a Y chromosome. The male parent contributes his only X chromosome to all his daughters and his only Y chromosome to all his sons. Traits

---

Table 6-3 Characteristics of Autosomal Dominant Inheritance With Complete Penetrance

The trait appears in multiple generations (vertical transmission).

Affected males and females are equally likely to transmit the trait to male and female offspring. Thus, male-to-male transmission occurs.

Each affected individual has an affected parent, unless the condition arose by new mutation in the given individual.

Males and females are affected in equal proportions.

Unaffected persons do not transmit the trait to their children.

The trait is expressed in the heterozygote but is more severe in the homozygote.

The age of fathers of isolated (new mutation) cases is usually advanced.

The more severely the trait interferes with survival and reproduction, the greater the proportion of isolated (new mutation) cases.

Variability in expression of the trait from generation to generation and between individuals in the same generation is expected.

Affected persons transmit the trait on average to 50% of their offspring.

---

determined by genes carried on the Y chromosome are transmitted from a father to 100% of his sons. Among these Y chromosomal genes is the *testis-determining factor* (*TDF*—also called *sex-determining region Y, or SRY*). Genes controlling tooth size, stature, spermatogenesis, and hairy pinnae are also on the Y chromosome. All other sex-linked traits or diseases are thought to result from genes on the X chromosome and are properly termed *X-linked.* Some X-linked conditions have considerable frequencies in human populations; the various protan and deutan color vision defects were also among the first human traits assigned to a specific chromosome.

The distinctive feature of X-linked inheritance, both dominant and recessive, is the absence of father-to-son transmission. Because the male X chromosome passes only to daughters, all daughters of an affected male will inherit the mutant gene.

X-linked recessive inheritance

A male has only 1 copy of any X-linked gene and therefore is said to be *hemizygous* for the gene, rather than homozygous or heterozygous. Because there is no normal gene to balance a mutant X-linked gene in the male, its resulting phenotype, whether dominant or recessive, will always be expressed. A female may be heterozygous or homozygous for a mutant X-linked gene. X-linked traits are commonly called *recessive* if they are caused by genes located on the X chromosome, as these genes express themselves fully only in the absence of the normal allele. Thus, males (with their single X chromosome) are predominantly affected. All their phenotypically healthy but heterozygous daughters are carriers. By contrast, each son of a heterozygous woman has an equal chance of being normal or hemizygously affected.

A female will be affected with an X-linked recessive trait under a limited number of circumstances:

- She is homozygous for the mutant gene by inheritance (ie, from an affected father and a heterozygous mother).
- Her mother is heterozygous and her father contributes a new mutation.
- She has Turner syndrome, with only 1 X chromosome, or a partial deletion of 1 X chromosome and therefore is effectively hemizygous.
- She has a highly unusual skewing of inactivation of her normal X chromosome, as explained by the Lyon hypothesis (discussed in the section Lyonization later in this chapter).
- Her disorder is actually an autosomal genocopy of the X-linked condition.

Table 6-4 summarizes the characteristics of X-linked recessive inheritance, which should be considered if all affected individuals in a family are males, especially if they are related through historically unaffected women (eg, uncle and nephew, or multiple affected half brothers with different fathers). Many X-linked RP pedigrees have been mislabeled as autosomal dominant because of manifesting female carriers. The key feature of an X-linked pedigree is no male-to-male transmission.

X-linked dominant inheritance

X-linked dominant traits are caused by mutant genes expressed in a single dose and carried on the X chromosome. Thus, both heterozygous women and hemizygous men are clinically affected. Females are affected nearly twice as frequently as males. All daughters

Table 6-4 Characteristics of X-Linked Recessive Inheritance

Usually only males are affected.

An affected male transmits the gene to all of his daughters (obligate carriers) and none of his sons.

All daughters of affected males, even those phenotypically normal, are carriers.

Affected males in a family either are brothers or are related to one another through carrier females (eg, maternal uncles).

If an affected male has children with a carrier female, on average 50% of their daughters will be homozygous and affected and 50% will be heterozygous and carriers.

Heterozygous females may rarely be affected (manifesting heterozygotes) because of lyonization.

Female carriers transmit the gene on average to 50% of their sons, who are affected, and to 50% of their daughters, who will be carriers.

of males with the disease are affected. However, all sons of affected males are free of the trait unless their mothers are also affected. Because only children of affected males provide information in discriminating X-linked dominant from autosomal dominant disease, it may be impossible to distinguish these modes on genetic grounds when the pedigree is small or the available data are scarce. Some X-linked dominant disorders, such as incontinentia pigmenti (Bloch-Sulzberger syndrome), may prove lethal to the hemizygous male. The characteristics of X-linked dominant inheritance are summarized in Table 6-5.

X-linked disorders

Females with X-linked diseases have milder symptoms than males. Occasionally, males may be affected severely enough that they die before the reproductive period, thus preventing transmission of the gene. Such is the case with Duchenne muscular dystrophy, in which most affected males die before their midteens. In other disorders, males are so severely affected that they die before birth, and only females survive. Families with such disorders would include only affected daughters, unaffected daughters, and normal sons at a ratio of 1:1:1. Incontinentia pigmenti is one such lethal genetic disorder. Perinatally, affected females develop an erythematous, vesicular skin eruption, which progresses to marbled, curvilinear pigmentation. The syndrome includes dental abnormalities, congenital or secondary cataracts, proliferative retinopathy and pseudogliomas, and tractional retinal detachment.

Among the most severe X-linked dominant disorders with lethality for the hemizygous males is Aicardi syndrome. No verified birth of a male with this entity has ever been reported. Females have profound cognitive disabilities and delays; muscular hypotonia; blindness associated with a characteristic lacunar juxtapapillary chorioretinal dysplasia and optic disc anomalies; and central nervous system abnormalities, the most common characteristic of which is agenesis of the corpus callosum. No recurrences have been reported among siblings, and parents can be reassured that the risk in subsequent children is minimal. All instances of the disease appear to arise from a new X-dominant lethal mutation, and females do not survive long enough to reproduce. The crucial area appears to be on the distal end of the short arm of the X chromosome, because some

Table 6-5 Characteristics of X-Linked Dominant Inheritance

Both males and females are affected, but the incidence of the trait is approximately twice as high in females as in males (or exclusively in females if the trait is lethal in the male).
An affected male transmits the trait to all of his daughters and to none of his sons.
Heterozygous affected females transmit the trait to both sexes with equal frequency.
The heterozygous female tends to be less severely affected than the hemizygous male.

patients with a deletion in this region have also been shown to have features of Aicardi syndrome.

Maternal Inheritance

When nearly all offspring of an affected woman appear to be at risk for inheriting and expressing a trait, and the daughters are at risk for passing the trait on to the next generation, the pattern of inheritance is called *maternal inheritance*. The disease stops with all-male offspring, whether affected or not. This form of inheritance is highly suggestive of a mitochondrial disorder. The structure and molecular aspects of the mitochondrial genome and a general discussion of mitochondrial disease are covered in Chapter 5, Molecular Genetics.

Terminology: Hereditary, Genetic, Familial, Congenital

Hereditary indicates that a disease or trait under consideration results directly from an individual's particular genetic composition (or *genome*) and that it can be passed from one generation to another. *Genetic* denotes that the disorder is caused by a defect of genes, whether acquired or inherited. In some instances, such as mutations in genes related to ocular melanoma, the disease is clearly genetic, but it is not passed to subsequent generations and is therefore not hereditary. Thus, the terms *hereditary* and *genetic* are not exactly synonymous but are sometimes used to convey similar concepts. Both hereditary and genetic disorders may be congenital or develop later in life.

A condition is *familial* if it occurs in more than one member of a family. It may, of course, be hereditary but need not be. A familial disorder can be caused by common exposure to infectious agents (eg, adenoviral conjunctivitis), excess food intake (eg, obesity), or environmental agents such as cigarette smoke. Genetic factors, however, may contribute to the effects of exposure to these environmental factors and cloud the picture.

The term *congenital* refers to characteristics present at birth. These characteristics may be hereditary or familial, or they may occur as an isolated event, often as the result of an infection (eg, rubella, toxoplasmosis, or cytomegalovirus) or a toxic agent (eg, thalidomide embryopathy or fetal alcohol syndrome). The presence of such characteristics *at birth* or shortly after (in the first weeks) is the defining factor. Pediatric ophthalmology literature refers to congenital nystagmus, congenital esotropia, congenital glaucoma, and congenital cataract, but in many cases these disorders are not present at birth and should be referred to as *infantile*.

Heritability refers to the proportion of phenotypic variation in a population that is attributable to genetic variation among individuals. Estimation of heritability aims to answer the "nature versus nurture" debate and to allow researchers to pursue genetic and/or environmental determinants of disease, although most cases involve a combination of the 2 determinants. Heritability studies compare the phenotypic similarity of close genetically related individuals with that of less closely related individuals. The best example of this type of study is a comparison of the correlation of identical twins (monozygotic twins sharing 100% of their DNA sequence) with that of nonidentical twins (dizygotic twins sharing 50% of their DNA sequence). With both twins sharing the same age and similar intrauterine and early childhood environments, most of the variation is thought to be due to genetic factors. An example of a twin study concerning the highly heritable trait of central corneal thickness is shown in Figure 6-2.

A condition known to be genetic and hereditary (eg, RP) may appear in only 1 individual of a family. Such an individual is said to have a *simplex,* or *isolated,* form of a genetic disease. A genetically determined trait may be isolated in the pedigree for several reasons:

- The pedigree is small.
- The full expression of the disease has not been sought or has not manifested in other relatives.
- The disorder represents a new genetic mutation or chromosomal change.
- The disorder is recessive, and the investigation to determine whether the parents are carriers has been inadequate.
- There is nonpaternity.

Clinically similar disorders may be inherited in several different ways—for example, RP can occur from an autosomal dominant, autosomal recessive, X-linked recessive, or

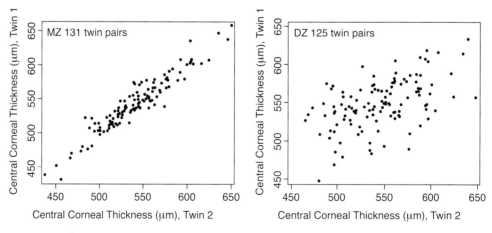

Figure 6-2 Comparison of correlation level for central corneal thickness in a set of monozygotic (MZ) twins with that of a set of dizygotic (DZ) twins. *Left,* Comparison for the MZ twins (correlation, 0.95). *Right,* Comparison for the DZ twins (correlation, 0.52). The difference in the correlation levels of the 2 sets of twins allows for calculation of the heritability of central corneal thickness, which in this example is 95%. *(Courtesy of David A. Mackey, MD.)*

mitochondrial mutation. These various genetic forms represent distinct gene defects with different alterations in gene structure and different biochemical pathogeneses, each of which has similar clinical phenotypic expressions. Clarification of genetic heterogeneity is important, because only with the proper diagnosis and correct identification of the inheritance pattern can appropriate genetic counseling and prognosis be offered.

Some genetic disorders originally thought to be a single and unique entity are found, on close scrutiny, to be two or more fundamentally distinct entities. Further clarification of the inheritance pattern or biochemical analysis permits separation of initially similar disorders. Such has been the case for Marfan syndrome and homocystinuria. Although both disorders cause unusual body habitus and ectopia lentis, the presence of dominant inheritance, aortic aneurysms, and valvular heart disease in Marfan syndrome distinguishes it from the recessive pattern and thromboembolic disease of homocystinuria.

Genetic heterogeneity is a general term that applies to the phenotypic similarity that may be produced by two or more fundamentally distinct genetic entities; this term implies that the genes are nonallelic. Leber congenital amaurosis, which has more than 14 causative genes, is a good example (Fig 6-3). Once the location on a chromosome is determined for a particular disease gene and once the gene's molecular structure is identified, most examples of genetic heterogeneity cease to be a problem for diagnosis or classification. However, clinical, allelic, and locus heterogeneity can remain perplexing issues. For example, mutations of the Norrie disease gene, *NDP,* usually result in the typical phenotype of pseudoglioma from exudative retinal detachments, but some mutations of *NDP* have been associated with X-linked exudative vitreoretinopathy without any systemic associations.

Sanfilippo PG, Hewitt AW, Hammond CJ, Mackey DA. The heritability of ocular traits. *Surv Ophthalmol.* 2010;55(6):561–583.

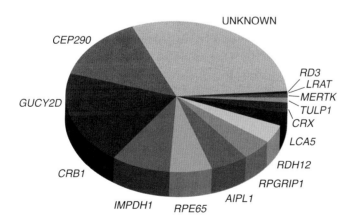

Figure 6-3 Prevalence of the 14 causative genes known in 2008 for cases of Leber congenital amaurosis (led by *CEP290* in approximately 15% of cases). Mutations for approximately 30% of cases remain to be identified. *(Reproduced with permission from den Hollander AI, Roepman R, Koenekoop RK, Cremers FP. Leber congenital amaurosis: genes, proteins and disease mechanisms. Prog Retin Eye Res. 2008;27(4):391–419.)*

Genes and Chromosomes

In 1909, the Danish biologist Wilhelm Johannsen coined the word *genes,* from the Greek for "giving birth to," as a term for individual units of hereditary information. Genes are the basic units of inheritance, and they include the sequence of nucleotides that codes for a single trait or a single polypeptide chain and its associated regulatory regions. Human genes vary substantially in size, from approximately 500 base pairs (bp) to more than 2 million bp. However, more than 98% range in size from less than 10 kilobase pairs (kb; 1 kb = 1000 bp) to 500 kb. Many are considerably larger than 50 kb. Whereas a single human cell contains enough DNA for 6 million genes, approximately 20,000–25,000 genes are found among the 23 pairs of known chromosomes. The function of the remaining 95% of the genetic material is likely to be involved in regulation of gene expression but is largely unknown.

The relative sequence of the genes, which are arranged linearly along the chromosome, is called the *genetic map.* The physical position or region on the chromosome occupied by a single gene is known as a *locus.* The physical contiguity of various gene loci becomes the vehicle for close association of genes with one another *(linkage)* and their clustering in groups that characteristically move together or separately *(segregation)* from one generation to the next.

Each normal human somatic cell has 46 chromosomes composed of 23 homologous pairs. Each member of a homologous pair carries matched, although not necessarily identical, genes in the same sequence. One member of each chromosome pair is inherited from the father, the other from the mother. Each normal sperm or ovum contains 23 chromosomes, 1 representative from each pair; thus, each parent transmits half of his or her genetic information to each child. Of the 46 chromosomes, 44 are called autosomes because they provide information on somatic characteristics; the remaining 2 chromosomes are X and Y. See the earlier section in this chapter, X-Linked Inheritance.

Alleles

The alternative forms of a particular gene at the same locus on each of an identical pair of chromosomes are called *alleles* (Greek for "reciprocals"). If both members of a pair of alleles for a given autosomal locus are identical (ie, the DNA sequence is the same), the individual is *homozygous* (a *homozygote*); if the allelic genes are distinct from each other (ie, the DNA sequence differs), the individual is *heterozygous* (a *heterozygote*). Different gene defects can cause dramatically different phenotypes and still be allelic. For example, sickle cell disease (SS hemoglobinopathy) caused by homozygosity of 1 mutant gene is substantially different from the phenotypic expression of SC hemoglobinopathy, yet the *Hb S* gene and the *Hb C* gene are allelic.

The term *polyallelism* refers to the many possible variants or mutations of a single gene. Mutant proteins that correspond to mutant alleles frequently have been shown to possess slightly different biochemical properties. Among the mucopolysaccharidoses, for example, the enzyme alpha-L-iduronidase is defective in both Hurler and Scheie syndromes. Because these disorders stem from mutations of the same gene, they are abnormalities of the same enzyme and thus allelic. However, the clinical severity of these 2 disorders (age of onset; age of detection; and severity of affliction of skeleton, liver, spleen, and cornea) is entirely different, presumably because the function of the mutant enzyme is less altered by the Scheie syndrome mutation. Because the enzyme is a protein composed of hundreds of amino acids, a mutation resulting in a base substitution within a certain codon might cause a change in one or more amino acids in a portion of the enzyme remote from its active site, thus reducing its effect on the enzyme's function. However, the substitution of 1 amino acid at a crucial location in the enzyme's active site might abolish most or all of its enzymatic activity. Several examples of allelic disorders appear among the mucopolysaccharidoses.

The phenotype of the usual heterozygote is determined by 1 mutant allele and 1 "normal" allele. However, the genotype of a compound heterozygote comprises 2 different mutant alleles, each at the same locus. The genetic Hurler-Scheie compound heterozygote is biochemically proven and clinically manifests features intermediate between the homozygotes of the 2 alleles. Whenever detailed biochemical analysis is performed, the products of the 2 alleles manifest slightly different properties (such as rates of enzyme activity or electrophoretic migration).

In contrast, and as noted earlier, some genetic disorders originally thought to be single and unique may, on close scrutiny, reveal two or more fundamentally distinct entities. Occasionally, this genetic heterogeneity is observed with diseases that are inherited in the same manner, such as tyrosinase-negative and tyrosinase-positive oculocutaneous albinism. Because these 2 conditions are phenotypically similar and each is inherited as an autosomal recessive trait, it was assumed for some time that they were allelic. When a tyrosinase-negative person with albinism bears children with a tyrosinase-positive person with albinism, the offspring appear clinically normal. This observation excludes the possibility that these 2 conditions are allelic: each condition occurs only when an offspring is heterozygous for the gene causing the condition. Defects in separate gene loci (the tyrosinase gene and the *P* gene) are now known to cause oculocutaneous albinism. The offspring of matings of individuals with phenotypically similar but genotypically different disorders are called *double heterozygotes* because they are heterozygous for each of the 2 loci.

Ashworth JL, Biswas S, Wraith E, Lloyd IC. Mucopolysaccharidoses and the eye. *Surv Ophthalmol.* 2006;51(1):1–17.

Mitosis

A cell may undergo 2 types of cell division: mitosis and meiosis. Mitosis gives rise to the multiple generations of genetically identical cells needed for the growth and maintenance of the organism. When mitosis is about to begin, the cell accurately duplicates all of its chromosomes. The replicated chromosomes then separate into 2 identical groups that migrate apart and eventually reach opposite sides of the cell. The cell and its contents then divide, forming 2 genetically identical daughter cells, each with the same diploid chromosome number and genetic information as the parent cell.

Meiosis

In contrast to mitosis, meiosis leads to the production of cells that have only 1 member of each chromosome pair (Fig 6-4). The specialized cells that arise from meiosis and participate in sexual reproduction are called *gametes.* The male gamete is a sperm, and the female gamete, an ovum. During meiosis, a modified sequence of divisions systematically reduces the number of chromosomes in each cell by one-half to the *haploid* number. Consequently, each gamete contains 23 chromosomes, 1 representative of each pair. This assortment occurs randomly, except that 1 representative of each pair of chromosomes is incorporated into each sperm or egg.

At conception, a sperm and an ovum unite, forming a *zygote,* a single cell that contains 46 chromosomes. Because both parents contribute equally to the genetic makeup of their offspring, new and often advantageous gene combinations may emerge.

Segregation

Two allelic genes, which occupy the same gene locus on 2 homologous chromosomes, separate with the division of the 2 chromosomes during meiosis, and each goes to a

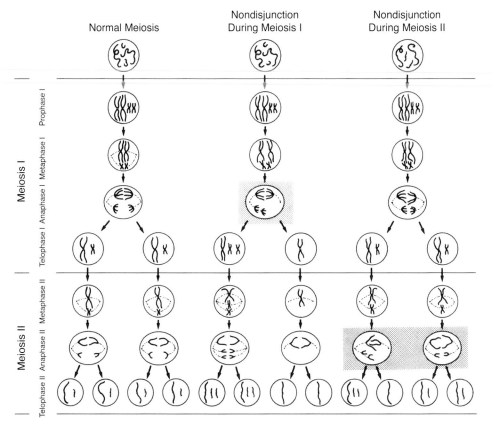

Figure 6-4 Normal meiosis and chromosomal nondisjunction occurring at different phases of meiosis.

different gamete. Thus, the genes are said to *segregate,* a property limited to allelic genes, which cannot occur together in a single offspring of the bearer. For example, if a parent is a compound heterozygote for both hemoglobin S and hemoglobin C, which occupy the same genetic locus on homologous chromosomes, none of the offspring will inherit both hemoglobins from that parent; each will inherit either one or the other.

Independent Assortment

Genes on different *(nonhomologous)* chromosomes may or may not separate together during meiotic cell division. This random process, called *independent assortment,* states that nonallelic genes assort independently of one another. Because *crossing over* (exchange of chromosomal material between the members of a pair of homologous chromosomes) can occur in meiosis, 2 nonallelic genes originally on opposite members of the chromosomal pair may end up together on either of the 2 or remain separated, depending on their original positions and on the sites of genetic interchange. Thus, the gametes of an individual with 2 nonallelic dominant traits, or *syntenic traits,* located on the same chromosome could produce 4 possible offspring. A child may inherit:

- both traits if the separate alleles remain on the same chromosome and the child inherits this chromosome
- neither trait if the genes remain on 1 chromosome but the child inherits the opposite chromosome with neither allele
- only 1 of the 2 alleles if crossing over occurred between the loci, and the child receives the chromosome with that particular allele

This scheme for nonallelic traits depends on the independent assortment of chromosomes in the first division of meiosis. Approximately 50 crossovers (1–3 per chromosome) occur during an average meiotic division.

Linkage

Linkage is the major exception or modification to the law of independent assortment. Nonallelic genes located reasonably close together on the same chromosome tend to be transmitted together, from generation to generation, more frequently than chance alone would allow for; thus, they are said to be linked. The closer together the 2 loci are, the less likely they are to be affected by crossovers. Linear physical proximity along a chromosome cannot be considered an automatic guarantor of linkage, however. In fact, certain sites on each chromosome may be more vulnerable to homologous crossing over than others.

Chromosomal Analysis

Cytogenetics is the branch of genetics concerned with the study of chromosomes and their properties. Chromosomal defects are changes in the chromosome number or structure that damage sensitive genetic functions and lead to developmental or reproductive disorders. These defects usually result from (1) a disruption of the mechanisms controlling chromosome movement during cell division or (2) alterations of chromosome structure that lead to changes in the number or arrangement of genes or to abnormal chromosomal behavior.

Chromosomal abnormalities occur in approximately 1 of 200 term pregnancies and in 1%–2% of all pregnancies involving parents over the age of 35 years. About 7% of perinatal deaths and some 40%–50% of retrievable spontaneous abortuses have significant chromosomal aberrations. Virtually any change in chromosome number during early development profoundly affects the formation of tissues and organs and the viability of the entire organism. Most major chromosomal disorders are characterized by both developmental delay and cognitive disability, as well as a variety of somatic abnormalities.

Indications for Chromosome Analysis

Ophthalmologists should be aware of the value of learning the constitutional and tumor karyotypes for infants with retinoblastoma, especially if the tumor represents a new genetic mutation. Chromosome analysis is also suggested in patients with isolated (nonfamilial) aniridia (which is often associated with Wilms tumor) and other systemic malformations.

A chromosomally abnormal state in a previous child warrants consideration of amniocentesis or chorionic villus sampling for prenatal diagnosis in subsequent pregnancies to avoid the risk of recurrence. An alternative is the use of preimplantation genetic diagnosis (PGD).

Karyotype

The systematic display of chromosomes from a single somatic cell is called a *karyotype*. Chromosome preparations are most commonly obtained from peripheral venous blood, although bone marrow, skin fibroblasts, and cells from amniotic fluid or chorionic villi are useful under specific circumstances. Chromosome analysis can be obtained directly from neoplastic tissues, as in retinoblastoma and Wilms tumor, for example.

Fluorescence in situ hybridization and chromosome arm painting

With the fluorescence in situ hybridization (FISH) technique, DNA fragments from genes of interest are first tagged with a fluorescent compound and then annealed or hybridized to chromosomes. In the process of chromosome arm painting, the regions of interest are stained to determine whether duplication, deletion, or rearrangement has occurred. Such fluorescent molecular probes can be used to detect and often quantify the presence of specific DNA sequences on a chromosome and can identify microscopic abnormalities that would be indiscernible by conventional cytogenetic methods.

Using microdissections of chromosomal regions and FISH, probes have been developed that label entire arms of chromosomes and each of the individual chromosomes (multicolor spectral karyotyping and combinatorial multifluor FISH). With 2-color FISH, both arms of each chromosome can be labeled simultaneously (Fig 6-5). These probes are valuable for detecting and understanding the mechanisms of complex chromosomal rearrangement.

Speicher MR, Gwyn Ballard S, Ward DC. Karyotyping human chromosomes by combinatorial multi-fluor FISH. *Nat Genet.* 1996;12(4):368–375.

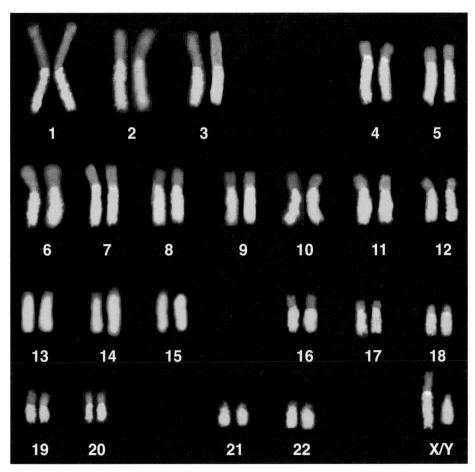

Figure 6-5 Composite karyotype of all human chromosomes hybridized with chromosome arm painting. Metaphase chromosomes were hybridized simultaneously with corresponding short-arm *(red)* and long-arm *(green)* painting probes, and a composite karyotype was generated. *(Reproduced with permission from Guan XY, Zhang H, Bittner M, Jiang Y, Meltzer P, Trent J. Chromosome arm painting probes. Nat Genet. 1996;12(1):10–11.)*

Aneuploidy of Autosomes

Aneuploidy denotes an abnormal number of chromosomes in cells. The presence of 3 homologous chromosomes in a cell rather than the normal pair is termed *trisomy*. *Monosomy* is the presence of only 1 member of any pair of autosomes or only 1 sex chromosome. The absence of a single autosome is almost always lethal to the embryo; an extra autosome is often catastrophic to surviving embryos. Aneuploidy of sex chromosomes (such as X, XXX, XXY, and XYY) is less disastrous. Monosomies and trisomies are generally caused by mechanical accidents that increase or decrease the number of chromosomes in the gametes. The most common type of accident, meiotic *nondisjunction,* results from a disruption of chromosome movement during meiosis (see Fig 6-4).

Trisomy 21 syndrome, or Down syndrome, is the most common chromosomal syndrome in humans; it has an overall incidence of 1:800 live births. Clinical features of this syndrome have been well known since the British physician John Langdon Down originally described them in 1866.

The most important risk factor for having a child with Down syndrome is maternal age. The frequency of Down syndrome increases from approximately 1:1400 live births for mothers aged 20–24 years to approximately 1:40 live births for mothers aged 44 years. However, the frequency of Down syndrome is greater (1:1250) for mothers between 15 and 19 years of age than it is in the next-higher age range. Above age 50 years, the frequency is 1:11 live births. The eponym *Down syndrome* summarizes a clinical description of certain distinctive, if variable, phenotypic features, whereas the karyotype describes the chromosomal constitution of the cells and tissues studied.

In more than 80% of cases of Down syndrome, the genetic error occurs in the first meiosis, and in more than 95%, the error occurs in maternal rather than paternal meiosis. Approximately 5% of patients with Down syndrome have a *translocation* resulting from attachment of the long arm of chromosome 21 to the long arm of another acrocentric chromosome, usually 14 or 22. These translocations cause pairing problems during meiosis, and the translocated fragment of chromosome 21 appears in one of the daughter cells along with a normal chromosome 21. As in nondisjunction, the fragment becomes trisomic on fertilization. Trisomy of only the distal one-third of chromosome 21q is sufficient to cause the disorder. Genes that lie within the q22 band of chromosome 21 appear to be specifically responsible for the pathogenesis of Down syndrome.

Patients with Down syndrome may exhibit the following features:

- cognitive disabilities
- characteristic facies: oblique eye fissure, epicanthus, flat nasal bridge, and protruding tongue
- short, broad hands and wide space between first and second toes; characteristic dermatoglyphics
- hypotonia
- congenital heart disease
- immunologic, hematologic anomalies
- gastrointestinal anomalies
- atlantoaxial instability
- epilepsy
- Alzheimer disease
- short stature
- infertility
- dental hypoplasia

Ophthalmic features of Down syndrome are presented in Table 6-6.

Leonard S, Bower C, Petterson B, Leonard H. Medical aspects of school-aged children with Down syndrome. *Dev Med Child Neurol.* 1999;41(10):683–688.

Mosaicism

Occasionally, an individual or a tissue contains two or more cell lines with distinctly different chromosomal constitutions. Such individuals or tissues are termed *mosaics.*

Table 6-6 Ocular Findings in Down Syndrome (Trisomy 21)

Almond-shaped palpebral fissures
Upslanting (mongoloid) palpebral fissures
Prominent epicanthal folds
Blepharitis, usually chronic, with cicatricial ectropion
Nasolacrimal duct obstruction
Strabismus, usually esotropic
Nystagmus (typically horizontal)
Aberrant retinal vessels (at disc)
Iris stromal hypoplasia
Brushfield spots
Keratoconus
Cataract
Myopia
Optic atrophy

Sometimes the peripheral blood, which is the usual source for chromosomal analysis, contains populations of cells with completely different chromosomal constitutions. One population of cells may be so infrequent that a second tissue, such as skin fibroblasts, must be analyzed to demonstrate the mosaicism.

The clinical effects of mosaicism are difficult to predict because the distribution of abnormal cells in the embryo is determined by the timing of the error and other variables. If mitotic nondisjunction immediately follows conception, the zygote divides into 2 abnormal cells: 1 trisomic and 1 monosomic. The monosomic cells rarely survive and may decrease in number or even disappear entirely over time. Mitotic nondisjunction may occur when the embryo is composed of a small population of cells. Thus, 3 populations of cells are established—1 normal and 2 abnormal—although some abnormal cell lines may be "discarded" or lost during development. If mitotic nondisjunction occurs at a more advanced stage of development, resulting abnormal populations constitute a minority of the embryo's cells, and mosaicism may have little or no measurable effect on development.

A small population of aneuploid mosaic cells may not have a direct effect on development. However, when cells of this type occur in the reproductive tissues of otherwise normal people, some of the gametes may carry extra chromosomes or be missing some entirely. Consequently, mosaic parents tend to be at high risk for having chromosomally abnormal children.

The most common example of autosomal mosaicism is *trisomy 21 mosaicism*. Some patients with trisomy 21 mosaicism have the typical features of Down syndrome; others show no abnormalities in appearance or intelligence. The crucial variables seem to be the frequency and the embryologic distribution of the trisomic cells during early development, which do not necessarily correlate with the percentage of trisomic cells in any one tissue, such as peripheral blood.

Several types of sex chromosome mosaicism may occur. Again, the physical effects tend to vary, probably reflecting the quantity and distribution of the abnormal cells during development. For example, the cell population that lacks 1 of the X chromosomes can arise in a female embryo, leading to 45,X/46,XX mosaicism. In some cases, these patients develop normally; in other cases, some or all of the features of Turner syndrome appear.

Similarly, the Y chromosome may be lost in some cells of a developing male embryo. This produces 45,X/46,XY mosaicism. X/XY mosaics may develop as normal males, as females with the features of Turner syndrome, or as individuals with physical characteristics intermediate between the sexes (*intersexes,* or *pseudohermaphrodites*).

Ophthalmically Important Chromosomal Aberrations

Long arm 13 deletion (13q14) syndrome: retinoblastoma

Retinoblastoma is one of several heritable childhood malignancies. Ocular tumors, which are usually noted before the age of 4 years, affect between 1 in 15,000 and 1 in 34,000 live births in the United States. The disease exhibits both hereditary occurrence (approximately 30%–40%), in which tumors tend to be bilateral and multicentric, and sporadic occurrence, in which unilateral and solitary tumors are the rule. Only about 10% of patients with hereditary retinoblastoma have a family history of the disease; the remaining 90% have a new mutation in their germ cells.

Retinoblastoma does not develop in approximately 10% of all obligate carriers of a germline mutation (ie, incomplete penetrance). In addition, a karyotypically visible deletion of part of the long arm of chromosome 13 occurs in 3%–7% of all cases of retinoblastoma. The larger this deletion is, the more severe is the phenotypic syndrome, which includes cognitive disabilities and developmental delays, microcephaly, hand and foot anomalies, and ambiguous genitalia.

Although the hereditary pattern in familial retinoblastoma is that of an autosomal dominant mutation, the defect is recessive at the cellular level. The predisposition to retinoblastoma is caused by hemizygosity of the Rb locus within human chromosome band 13q14. The Rb locus is a member of a class of genes called *recessive tumor-suppressor genes*. The alleles normally present at these loci help prevent tumor formation. At least one active normal allele is needed to prevent the cell from losing control of proliferation. Patients who inherit a defective allele from 1 parent are at greater risk for losing the other allele through a number of mechanisms. Thus, tumor formation in retinoblastoma is caused by the loss of function of both normal alleles. Homozygous deletions within the 13q14 region have been noted in retinoblastomas derived from enucleated eyes.

The first step in tumorigenesis is a recessive mutation of 1 of the homologous alleles at the retinoblastoma locus by inheritance, germinal mutation, or somatic mutation. Hereditary retinoblastomas arise from a single additional somatic event in a cell that carries an inherited mutation, whereas sporadic cases require 2 somatic events. In approximately 50% of tumors, homozygosity for such a recessive mutation results from the mitotic loss of a portion of chromosome 13, including the 13q14 band. The resulting homozygosity for recessive mutant alleles at this locus allows the genesis of the tumor. Retinoblastoma, therefore, seemingly represents a malignancy caused by defective gene regulation rather than by the presence of a dominant mutant oncogene. Those who inherit a mutant allele at this locus have a high incidence of nonocular second tumors thought to be caused by the same mutation. Almost half of these tumors are osteosarcomas.

Short arm 11 deletion (11p13) syndrome: aniridia

Aniridia occurs from a defect in a gene that encodes a transcription factor needed for development of the eye. This developmental gene, *PAX6*, is located at 11p13. Aniridia is a panophthalmic disorder characterized by the following features:

- subnormal visual acuity
- congenital nystagmus
- strabismus
- keratitis due to limbal stem cell failure
- cataracts (usually anterior polar)
- ectopia lentis
- glaucoma
- optic nerve hypoplasia
- foveal or macular hypoplasia
- iris absence or severe hypoplasia

When working with a new patient with aniridia, the ophthalmologist should, if possible, conduct a careful examination of the patient's parents for the variable expression of autosomal dominant aniridia. Although almost all cases of aniridia result from *PAX6* mutations, a rare autosomal recessive disorder called *Gillespie syndrome* (phenotype OMIM number 206700) also produces partial aniridia, cerebellar ataxia, mental deficiency, and congenital cataracts.

Aniridia (often with cataract and glaucoma) can also occur sporadically in association with Wilms tumor, other genitourinary anomalies, and mental retardation, the so-called *WAGR syndrome.* This complex of findings is called a *contiguous gene-deletion syndrome* because it results from a deletion involving nearby genes. Most affected patients have a karyotypically visible interstitial deletion of a segment of chromosome 11p13. Patients with aniridia that is not clearly part of an autosomal dominant trait and those with coincident systemic malformations should undergo chromosomal analysis and observation for possible Wilms tumor.

The *PAX6* gene product is a transcription factor required for normal development of the eye. Mutations of *PAX6* have also been reported in Peters anomaly, autosomal dominant keratitis, and dominant foveal hypoplasia. The mechanism for disruption of normal embryology and the degenerative disease in aniridia and other *PAX6* disorders appears to be *haploinsufficiency,* which, in this case, is the inability of a single active allele to activate transduction of the developmental genes regulated by the *PAX6* gene product. In this way, aniridia is different from retinoblastoma and Wilms tumor, which result from an absence of both functional alleles at each of the homologous gene loci.

Mutations

Change in the structure or sequence of a gene is called a *mutation.* A mutation can occur more or less randomly anywhere along the DNA sequence of a gene and may result when one nucleotide is substituted for another (sometimes called a *point mutation*). A mutation that occurs in a noncoding portion of the gene may or may not be of clinical consequence. Similarly, a mutation may structurally alter a protein but in a manner that does not notably compromise its function. A new mutation that compromises function may appear in a given gene as the gene is transmitted from parent to offspring.

More gross mutations may involve deletion, translocation, insertion, or internal duplication of a portion of the DNA. Some mutations cause either destruction of the offspring or sterility. Others are less harmful or are potentially beneficial and become established in subsequent generations. Mutations can occur spontaneously for reasons that are not understood. They may also be induced by exposure to a variety of environmental agents called *mutagens*, such as radiation, viruses, and certain chemicals.

Mutations may arise in somatic as well as germinal cells, but these are not transmitted to subsequent generations. Somatic mutations in humans are difficult to identify, but some account for the inception of certain forms of neoplasia (eg, retinoblastoma).

Polymorphisms

Many mutations have either little or no deleterious effect on the organism. A *polymorphism* is defined as the occurrence of two or more alleles at a specific locus with a frequency greater than 1% each. Single-nucleotide polymorphisms are important for gene mapping in genome-wide association studies (GWAS).

Genome, Genotype, Phenotype

The genome is the sum total of the genetic material within a cell or an organism—thus, the total genetic endowment. By contrast, the genotype defines the genetic constitution, and thus biological capacity, with regard to a specific locus (eg, individual blood groups or a specific single enzyme). Phenotype indicates the total observable or manifest physical, physiologic, biochemical, or molecular characteristics of an individual, which are determined by the genotype but can be modified by the environment.

A clinical picture produced entirely by environmental factors that nevertheless closely resembles, or is even identical to, a phenotype is known as a *phenocopy*. Thus, for example, the pigmentary retinopathy of congenital rubella has occasionally been confused with a hereditary dystrophic disorder of the RPE. Similarly, amiodarone-induced changes in the corneal epithelium resemble those observed as cornea verticillata in the X-linked dystrophic disorder Fabry disease.

Single-Gene Disorders

Approximately 4500 different diseases are known to be caused by a defect in a single gene. As a group, these disorders are called *monogenic,* or *mendelian,* diseases. They most often show 1 of 3 patterns of inheritance: autosomal dominant, autosomal recessive, or X-linked. Disorders of mitochondrial DNA are inherited in a fourth manner, termed *maternal inheritance.*

Anticipation

Variability is an intrinsic property of human genetic disease that reflects the quantitative and qualitative differences in phenotype among individuals with the "same" mutant allele. Even within a single family with a genetic disease, each affected individual may manifest the disease to a different degree, with different features, or at a different age. Steinert myotonic dystrophy, for example, presents its features of motor myotonia, characteristic cataracts, gonadal atrophy, and presenile baldness with a wide variation in severity and age of detection. Even within a single family, the cataracts may begin to affect vision any time from the second to the seventh decade of life.

Such variability of clinical manifestation led to the concept of *anticipation,* the phenomenon of apparently earlier and more severe onset of a disease in successive generations within a family. Before 1990, most geneticists thought that anticipation was not a biological phenomenon but an artifact of ascertainment. With the relatively recent discovery of triplet or trinucleotide tandem-repeat expansion diseases, anticipation has been shown to reflect the increased length of trinucleotide tandem repeats from one generation to the next. Myotonic dystrophy, fragile X syndrome, Huntington disease, and Kennedy disease (a form of spinobulbar muscular atrophy) are some of the diseases whose discovery contributed to the rejuvenation of the concept of anticipation.

Some human variability may result from the intrinsic differences in genetic background of every human being. Other recognizable or presumptive influences on the variable intra- or interfamilial phenotype of the same gene include the following factors:

- sex influences or limitations
- maternal factors such as intrauterine environment and even cytoplasmic (eg, mitochondrial) inheritance factors
- modifying loci
- genetic heterogeneity, including both isoalleles and genocopies
- gene alterations induced either by position effects with other genes or by somatic mutations
- epigenetic factors, methylation, and histone formation

Obviously, nongenetic factors such as diet, temperature, and drugs may affect gene expression, either as phenocopies or through ecologic parameters.

Penetrance

The presence or absence of any effect of a gene is called *penetrance.* If a gene generates any evidence of phenotypic features, no matter how minimal, it is termed *penetrant;* if it is not expressed at any level of detection, it is termed *nonpenetrant.* Thus, penetrance is an all-or-nothing concept, statistically representing the fraction of individuals carrying a given gene that manifests any evidence of the specific trait. In families with an autosomal dominant mutant gene that has 100% penetrance of the phenotype, an average of 50% of the offspring will inherit the gene and show evidence of the disease.

Even though penetrance has an exact statistical definition, its clinical ascertainment is affected by diagnostic awareness and the methods of physical examination. For example, many mild cases of Marfan syndrome would be missed without careful biomicroscopy of the fully dilated pupil and echocardiography of the heart valves and great vessels. Similarly, if the criteria for identification of the retinoblastoma gene include indirect ophthalmoscopy and scleral depression, some "nonpenetrant" parents or siblings in families with "dominantly inherited" retinoblastoma may be found to have a spontaneously involuted tumor, which clearly identifies them as bearers of the gene. In another example, some family members who have a gene for Best macular dystrophy will be identified not by clinical ophthalmoscopic examination but only by electro-oculographic testing. Therefore, in examining a potential bearer of a gene, the examiner must carefully search for any manifestations of the gene's effects in all susceptible tissues before dismissing someone as from a "skipped generation."

Expressivity

The presence of a defective gene does not necessarily imply a complete expression of every potential manifestation. The variety of ways and levels of severity in which a particular genetic trait manifests its presence among different affected individuals is called *expressivity*. In von Recklinghausen disease, for example, an affected child may have only café-au-lait spots. The affected parent may have Lisch nodules of the iris, extensive punctiform and pedunculated neurofibromas of the skin, a huge plexiform neurofibroma of 1 lower extremity, and a glioma of the anterior visual pathway. It is extremely rare that all affected members in the same family have uniform textbook presentations of the disorder.

Differences in the age of onset of manifestation are one way that expressivity commonly varies in dominant disorders. In von Recklinghausen disease, the affected child at first may have only café-au-lait spots at birth, then develop iris Lisch nodules that gradually increase in number and size at about age 5–10 years, develop punctiform neurofibromas of the skin in early adolescence, experience subareolar neurofibromas postpuberty (in females), and experience visual impairment from the effect of an optic glioma in the late teens. Although all of these features are phenotypic components of the mutant gene, each feature has a characteristic age of onset and a natural history of growth and effect within the umbrella of the total disease.

Pleiotropism

Alteration within a single mutant gene may have consequences in various tissues in a given individual. The presentation of multiple phenotypic abnormalities produced by a single mutant gene is termed *pleiotropism*. For example, in Marfan syndrome, ectopia lentis is coupled with arachnodactyly, aortic aneurysms, and long extremities. Optic atrophy is found in association with juvenile diabetes mellitus, diabetes insipidus, and moderate perceptive hearing impairment in an autosomal recessive syndrome known as the *DIDMOAD (diabetes insipidus, diabetes mellitus, optic atrophy, and neural deafness) syndrome.* Neurosensory hearing loss can also be associated with hereditary hematuric nephritis, lenticular changes (anterior lenticonus, spherophakia, cataracts), arcus juvenilis, and whitish yellow retinal lesions in the dominantly inherited Alport syndrome. Similarly, the Bardet-Biedl syndrome comprises pigmentary retinopathy, obesity, genital hypoplasia, mental debility, and polydactyly. In each of these disorders, a single mutant gene is responsible for dysfunction in multiple systems.

Racial and Ethnic Concentration of Genetic Disorders

Most genetic diseases occur without regard to the affected individual's racial or ethnic background. Some, however, are concentrated in certain population groups.

Tay-Sachs disease (GM$_2$ gangliosidosis, type I), with its characteristic macular cherry-red spot, occurs predominantly in persons of Eastern European Jewish (Ashkenazi) ancestry. An estimated rate of 1 in 30 for carriers of this disorder in the Jewish population of New York City compares with an estimated carrier rate of 1 in 300 in non-Jewish Americans. In addition, familial dysautonomia *(Riley-Day syndrome)* with hypolacrima, corneal hypoesthesia, exodeviation, and methacholine-induced miosis also occurs more frequently in persons of Ashkenazi ancestry, as do *MAK-associated retinitis pigmentosa, Gaucher disease,* and *Niemann-Pick disease.*

A variety of *achromatopsia* (complete color blindness) with *myopia* is common on the South Pacific island of Pingelap, affecting 5% of the Pingelapese population in the Caroline Islands of Micronesia. *Oguchi disease* is observed primarily, although not exclusively, in Japanese people. Similarly, *sickle cell hemoglobinopathies* are inherited largely among African Americans.

The prevalence of *oculocutaneous albinism* is high among the Kuna Indians in Panama. *Hermansky-Pudlak syndrome (HPS)* occurs with a higher frequency in persons of Puerto Rican ancestry. HPS is an autosomal recessively inherited oculocutaneous albinism; its findings include a history of easy bruisability and bleeding tendency, associated with a prolonged bleeding time and abnormal platelet aggregation.

Lyonization

In classical human genetics, females with a gene for a recessive disease or trait on only 1 X chromosome should have no manifestations of the defect. However, ophthalmic examples of structural and functional abnormalities in females heterozygous for supposedly recessive X-linked traits abound. Such *carrier states,* usually mild but occasionally severe, have been described in carriers of choroideremia, X-linked Nettleship-Falls ocular albinism, X-linked RP, X-linked sutural cataracts, Lowe syndrome, Fabry disease, and color vision defects of the protan and deutan types, among others (Fig 6-6; Table 6-7).

Detection of these carrier states of the X-linked traits has become clinically relevant, especially for sisters and maternal aunts of affected males. In 1961, Mary Lyon (a British geneticist) advanced an explanation for the unanticipated or partial expression of a trait by a heterozygous female. Briefly, lyonization (X-chromosome inactivation) stated that in every somatic cell of a female, only 1 X chromosome is actively functioning. The second X chromosome is inactive and forms a densely staining marginal nuclear structure demonstrated as a Barr body in a buccal smear or in "drumsticks," pedunculated lobules of the nucleus identified in about 5% of the leukocytes of the normal female. X-chromosome inactivation occurs randomly to 1 X chromosome in early embryogenesis. The same X chromosome will be irreversibly inactive in every daughter of each of these "committed" primordial cells. The active gene is dominant at a cellular level. Thus, a heterozygous female for an X-linked disease will have 2 clonal cell populations (mosaic phenotype), 1 with normal activity for the gene in question and the other with mutant activity.

The proportion of mutant to normal X chromosomes inactivated usually follows a normal distribution, because presumably the inactivations in various cells are random events. Thus, an average of 50% of paternal X chromosomes and 50% of maternal

Figure 6-6 **A,** Yellow, "gold-dust" tapetal-like reflex in the left retina of a carrier for X-linked retinitis pigmentosa. **B,** Nasal midperipheral retina in the left eye of a carrier for X-linked retinitis pigmentosa, showing patchy bone spicule–like pigment clumping. **C,** Peripheral retina from the left eye of a carrier of choroideremia, showing a "moth-eaten" fundus appearance from areas of hypopigmentation and hyperpigmentation. **D,** Characteristic iris transillumination from a carrier of X-linked ocular albinism. **E,** Midperipheral retina from the left eye of a carrier for ocular albinism, showing a chocolate-brown pigmentation from areas of apparently enhanced pigmentation and clusters of hypopigmentation.

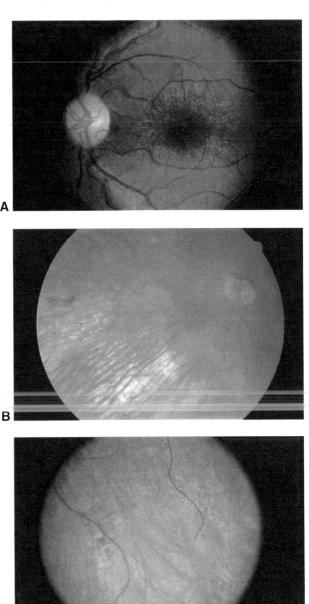

X chromosomes are inactivated. It is conceivable, however, that in some cases the mutant X is active in almost all cells; in other cases, the mutant X is inactivated in nearly all cells. By this mechanism, a female may express an X-linked disorder, and rare cases are known of women who have a classic color deficiency or X-linked ocular albinism, X-linked RP, or choroideremia.

Carriers of the X-linked variety of Nettleship-Falls ocular albinism may have a mottled mosaic fundus: in the pigmented retinal epithelial cells, the normal X chromosome

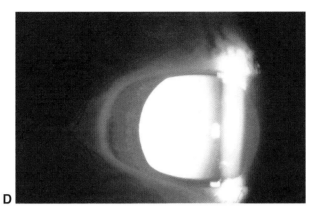

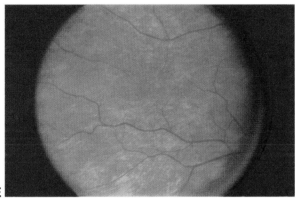

Table 6-7 Ocular Findings in Carriers of X-Linked Disorders

Disorder	Ocular Findings
Blue-cone monochromatism	Abnormalities in cone function on ERG, psychophysical thresholds, and color vision testing
Choroideremia	"Moth-eaten" fundus pigmentary changes, with areas of hypopigmentation, mottling, and pigment clumping in a striated pattern near the equator
Congenital stationary night blindness with myopia	Reductions in ERG oscillatory potentials
Fabry disease	Fingerprint or whorl-like (verticillata) changes within the corneal epithelium
Lowe syndrome	Scattered punctate lens opacities on slit-lamp examination
Ocular albinism	Chocolate brown clusters of pigment prominent in the midperipheral retina; mottling of macular pigment; iris transillumination
Red-green color vision deficiencies (protan and deutan)	Abnormally wide or displaced color match on a Nagel anomaloscope; decrease in sensitivity to red light in protan carriers (Schmidt sign)
X-linked retinitis pigmentosa	Regional fundus pigmentary changes, "gold-dust" tapetal-like reflex; ERG amplitude and implicit time abnormalities

is active; in the nonpigmented cells, the mutant X is active. However, these distinguishing features of the carrier state are not always present. The possibility that the patient is a carrier cannot be entirely eliminated if a given sign is not present, because a female might have undergone chance inactivation of the mutant X chromosome in most of her primordial cells, which evolved into the specific tissue observed and may appear phenotypically normal. This subtlety is even more important in evaluating family members with X-linked disease if the phenotypic carrier state is age dependent; thus, even in obligate carrier females for Lowe syndrome, lenticular cortical opacities are not necessarily present before the third decade of life.

Complex Genetic Disease: Polygenic and Multifactorial Inheritance

In chromosomal and mendelian (single-gene) disorders, genetic analysis of phenotypic, biochemical, or molecular parameters is imperative. However, a simple mode of inheritance cannot be assigned and a recurrence risk cannot be predicted for many common normal characteristics or disorders for which genetic variability clearly exists. Such traits as stature, refractive error, intraocular pressure (IOP), central corneal thickness, and iris color are usually distributed as a continuous variation over a wide range without sharp distinction between normal and abnormal phenotypes. This normal distribution contrasts with the bimodal curve (or trimodal curve in codominant models) noted for conditions transmitted by a single gene. Such conditions are often termed *polygenic,* implying that they result from the operation of multiple collaborating genes, each with rather minor additive effects. Many of these common genes with small effect have been identified through GWAS. With the exception of AMD, the discovered genes account for only a small percentage of the genetic effect for the traits and diseases investigated.

The term *multifactorial* denotes a combination of genetic and environmental factors in the etiology of disease without specifying the nature of the genetic influence. Examples of disorders involving these factors in humans include refractive error, glaucoma, and AMD.

Counseling for recurrence may be difficult in this type of inheritance. Ideally, empirical data are summarized from exhaustive analyses of similarly affected families in the population. In general, the risk is intermediate between population risk and mendelian risk. For example, the population risk for primary open-angle glaucoma (POAG) is 2%–3%, whereas the risk for glaucoma in families with severe myocilin mutations is near 50%. The risk for first-degree relatives of POAG patients is approximately 20%. The more severe the abnormality in the index case, the higher the risk of recurrence of the trait in relatives, presumably because either a greater number of deleterious genes are at work or a fixed population of more harmful genes exists. The risk of recurrence in future children is increased when more than one member of a family is affected, which is not true for mendelian disorders. Such observations have been offered for various forms of strabismus, glaucoma, and significant refractive errors.

Finally, if the malformation or disorder has occurred in both paternal and maternal relatives, the recurrence risk is distinctly higher because of the sharing of multiple unspecifiable but potentially harmful genes in their offspring.

Pharmacogenetics

The study of heritable factors that determine how drugs are chemically metabolized in the body is called *pharmacogenetics.* This field addresses genetic differences among population segments that are responsible for variations in both the therapeutic and adverse effects of drugs. Investigations in pharmacogenetics are important not only because they may lead to more rational approaches to therapy but also because they facilitate a deeper understanding of drug pharmacology. For more detail, see Part V, Ocular Pharmacology.

The drug isoniazid provides an example of how pharmacogenetics works. This antituberculosis drug is normally inactivated by the liver enzyme acetyltransferase. A large segment of the population, which varies by geographic distribution, has a reduced amount of this enzyme; these individuals are termed *slow inactivators.* When they take isoniazid, the drug reaches higher-than-normal concentrations, causing a greater incidence of adverse effects. Family studies have shown that a reduced level of acetyltransferase is inherited as an autosomal recessive trait.

Several other well-documented examples demonstrate how pharmacogenetics works. One example involves 10% of the male African-American population, a high percentage of male Sephardic Jews, and males from a number of other ethnic groups. An X-linked recessive trait causes a deficiency in glucose-6-phosphate dehydrogenase enzyme in the erythrocytes of affected males. As a consequence, a number of drugs (including sulfacetamide, vitamin K, acetylsalicylic acid, quinine, chloroquine, dapsone, and probenecid) may produce acute hemolytic anemia in these individuals. Pharmacogenetic causes have also been ascribed to variations in response to ophthalmic drugs, such as the increased IOP noted in a segment of the population after prolonged use of topical corticosteroids.

Several drugs have been shown to cause greater reaction in children with Down syndrome than in children without the syndrome. As a result of hypersensitivity, some children with Down syndrome have died after systemic administration of atropine. In some of the children, this hypersensitivity is also found with topical use of atropine. In these patients, atropine exerts a greater-than-normal effect on pupillary dilation. In several children with Down syndrome being treated for strabismus, hyperactivity occurred several hours after local instillation of echothiophate iodide, 0.125%.

One of the earliest examples of an inherited deficit in drug metabolism involved succinylcholine, a strong muscle relaxant that interferes with acetylcholinesterase, the enzyme that catabolizes acetylcholine at neuromuscular junctions. Normally, succinylcholine is rapidly destroyed by plasma cholinesterase (sometimes called *pseudocholinesterase*) so that its effect is short-lived—usually no more than a few minutes. Some people are homozygous for a recessive gene that codes for a form of cholinesterase with a considerably lower substrate affinity. Consequently, at therapeutic doses of succinylcholine, almost no destruction occurs, and the drug continues to exert its inhibitory effect on acetylcholinesterase, resulting in prolonged periods of apnea.

Clinical Management of Genetic Disease

Genetic disease may not be curable, but in most cases the patient benefits considerably from the physician's appropriate medical management. Such care should include all of the following steps.

Accurate Diagnosis

Unfortunately, because health care practitioners may not be as knowledgeable about genetic diagnoses as they are about other areas of medicine, many cases are not precisely diagnosed or, worse yet, are diagnosed incorrectly. A case of deafness and pigmentary retinopathy may be labeled rubella syndrome when the patient really has Usher syndrome. This latter syndrome, associated with RP, may not be recognized in patients with RP. For example, patients with RP and congenital polydactyly (surgically corrected in infancy) may not be recognized as having Bardet-Biedl syndrome. The correct diagnosis in such cases is important to ensure that the patient's educational and lifetime support needs are truly met.

Complete Explanation of the Disease

Patients are often very anxious when they do not understand the nature of their disease. A careful explanation of the disorder, as currently understood, will often dispel myths patients may have about their disease and their symptoms.

Virtually all genetic disorders confer burdens that may interfere with certain activities later in life. The appropriate time to discuss these burdens with patients and family members is often when they first ask about the consequences of a disease. Such explanations need to be tempered with empathy and with an understanding of the possible emotional and psychological effects of this information.

Treatment of the Disease Process

Definitive cures—that is, reversing or correcting underlying genetic defects—are yet to emerge for the majority of heritable disorders. However, some conditions in which metabolic defects have been identified can often be managed through 5 fundamental approaches:

1. dietary control
2. chelation of excessive metabolites
3. enzyme or gene-product replacements
4. vitamin and cofactor therapy
5. drug therapy to reduce accumulation of harmful products

Some genetic disorders affecting the eye that arise from an inborn error of metabolism can be managed effectively through dietary therapy. These conditions include homocystinuria, Refsum disease, gyrate atrophy galactokinase deficiency, and galactosemia. Implementing a galactose-free diet can reverse some of the main clinical signs of galactosemia, such as hepatosplenomegaly, jaundice, and weight loss. Progression of cortical cataracts can be avoided, and less extensive lens opacities may even regress with a galactose-free diet. With time, galactosemic patients are able to metabolize galactose through alternative pathways, obviating the need for lifelong dietary restriction.

Disorders that result from enzyme or transport protein deficiencies may lead to the accumulation of a metabolite or metal that harms various tissues. For example, in Wilson disease, decreased levels of serum ceruloplasmin result in poor transport of free copper (Cu^{2+}) ions and in storage of copper in tissues such as the brain, liver, and cornea. Resultant clinical signs can be reversed, at least partially, after the administration of D-penicillamine, a chelator of Cu^{2+} ions. Other copper chelators, such as British antilewisite (BAL), can be used, along with a copper-deficient diet, to reverse the clinical signs of Wilson disease (hepatolenticular degeneration).

Enzyme replacement therapy via plasma infusions in patients with Fabry disease has succeeded in temporarily decreasing plasma levels of the accumulated substrate ceramide trihexoside. The drugs are expensive, approximately $150,000 yearly (as of 2014), presenting a barrier to successful treatment for many patients around the world. Enzyme replacement therapy is not a cure, but it improves metabolism, curbs disease progression, and potentially reverses some symptoms.

Organ transplantation can be considered a form of regionalized enzyme replacement. In patients with cystinosis, cystine crystals accumulate in the kidneys. When a normal kidney, with its rich source of enzymes, is transplanted into a patient with cystinosis, cystine does not accumulate in the cells of the renal tubules and renal function tends to remain normal. In a complementary approach, stem cell transplantation is being investigated to treat various diseases, including those of the eye.

Vitamin therapy appears to be of benefit in 2 autosomal recessive disorders. In at least some patients with homocystinuria, vitamin B_6 (pyridoxine) administration has been shown to decrease homocystine accumulation in plasma and to reduce the severity of the disorder. Vitamin A and vitamin E therapy have been noted to benefit some patients with neurologic impairment due to abetalipoproteinemia; such therapy is also likely to slow or lessen the development and progression of retinal degeneration. More long-term therapeutic trials are necessary to better define the efficacy of vitamin therapy for these and perhaps other metabolic disorders.

Various genetically determined disorders can be managed by use of an appropriate drug. For example, excess accumulation of uric acid in primary gout can be prevented or reduced by (1) blocking the activity of the enzyme xanthine oxidase with the drug allopurinol or (2) increasing excretion of uric acid by the kidneys with the use of probenecid. In addition, the elevated serum cholesterol levels in familial hypercholesterolemia can often be reduced through the use of various cholesterol-lowering drugs or substances that bind bile acids in the gastrointestinal tract.

Appropriate management of sequelae and complications

Some of the sequelae of genetic diseases, such as glaucoma in Rieger syndrome or cataracts in RP, can be managed successfully to preserve or partially restore vision. However, patients need to understand how treatment of the sequelae or complications may differ according to their individual situations.

Gene therapy

Although only a few clinical trials for a limited number of genes are under way, viral-mediated gene replacement for inherited retinal diseases is available. The ophthalmologist is obliged either (1) to carefully search the Internet and the published literature for treatment trials that the patient may qualify for or (2) to refer the patient to another professional who will conduct such a search for treatment trials for which the patient may qualify. (For a database of clinical studies, see www.clinicaltrials.gov.)

Genetic Counseling

The ophthalmologist who understands the principles of human genetics has a foundation for counseling patients about their diseases. Genetic counseling imparts knowledge of human disease, including a genetic diagnosis and its ocular and systemic implications. The genetic counseling process helps individuals, couples, and families understand the risk of occurrence or recurrence of the disorder within the family. It provides information about appropriate use and implications of available genetic testing along with results interpretation, reproductive options, and facts about therapies, research, and resources. Psychosocial issues are also an integral part of the discussion. Genetic counseling is nondirective and addresses ethical issues as well as ethnic and cultural diversity with sensitivity. All genetic counseling is predicated on the following essential requirements:

- *Accurate diagnosis:* The physician must be sufficiently aware of the range of human ocular pathology to derive an accurate and specific diagnosis. It is impossible to counsel or refer patients on the basis of "congenital nystagmus" or "color blindness" or "macular degeneration"; these are signs, not diagnoses.
- *Complete family history:* A family history will narrow the choices of possible inheritance patterns, but it may not necessarily exclude new mutational events, isolated occurrences of recessive diseases, and chromosomal rearrangements in individual circumstances. The ophthalmologist must examine (or arrange to have examined) the parents, siblings, and other family members for mild manifestations of dominant diseases or characteristic carrier states in X-linked disorders. Only an ophthalmologist will be cognizant of, and attentive to, the atypical findings of hereditary ocular disorders. For example, identification of 1 young adult with the findings of Usher syndrome—prelingual deafness; night blindness; visual field constriction; and, ultimately, deterioration of central vision—obligates the ophthalmologist to evaluate a younger sibling who is congenitally deaf but "historically" has no eye problems. The probability is overwhelming that the sibling has the same disease.

- *Understanding the genetic and clinical aspects of the disorder:* The ophthalmologist should appreciate, perhaps more intimately than any other physician, how some clinically similar diseases inherited in the same pattern may be the result of different and even nonallelic defects. For example, the visual implications of, and prognoses for, tyrosinase-positive and tyrosinase-negative oculocutaneous albinism are considerably different. Some entities that are clinically similar may be inherited differently and thus have a different impact on other family members. In another example, pseudoxanthoma elasticum in both its autosomal dominant and recessive modes is often a late-onset disease that has serious implications for cardiovascular disease, stroke, and gastrointestinal bleeding. Informed counseling falls short if the ophthalmologist advises affected patients only about visual disability associated with angioid streaks without attention to the complete disease and the risks to other family members.

Issues in Genetic Counseling

The ophthalmologist must remember the possibility that an individual affected by a heritable condition may have a homozygous recessive trait. Thus, the ophthalmologist should search for parental consanguinity or ambiguous parentage (nonpaternity, incest, and even occult adoption) or for a new mutation and should inquire about advanced paternal (or maternal grandparental) age. Heterogeneity may complicate the diagnosis. Somatic mutations also occur, as with segmental neurofibromatosis or unilateral unifocal retinoblastoma. Nonpenetrance or mild expressivity in other family members should be excluded through diligent examination. Chromosomal abnormalities and phenocopies caused by infections or drugs may account for the isolated affected person. Nonetheless, the ophthalmologist's obligation to explain the disorder begins with an accurate diagnosis and establishment of the mode of heritability.

The genetic counseling process is nondirective; the genetic counselor informs rather than advises. It is inappropriate, perhaps even unethical, for a counselor to tell the patient what to do (for instance, not to have any children). Counselors recognize the ability of individuals and families to make appropriate decisions for themselves about their own health and reproductive choices in accordance with their personal beliefs and opinions, and they support them in the decision-making process.

In some instances, genetic testing for ocular disorders may provide individuals with information about their specific genetic mutation. While such testing can assist in the diagnosis and potentially give patients options to participate in clinical trials of new treatments, it may also identify carrier status and mutations in asymptomatic individuals who have known familial mutations, facilitating early diagnosis and subsequent intervention when available. The implications of these results require careful consideration and counseling because the information can affect not just the individuals who underwent testing but other family members as well. Genetic testing requests have to be carefully evaluated for compliance with existing guidelines and position statements covering the related ethical issues. For example, genetic testing for an adult-onset condition in a child, on the parents' request when there is no immediate medical benefit for the child, is not recommended.

Reproductive Issues

With a genetic diagnosis, the counseling ophthalmologist should outline the options available for family planning. Some people may accept a high statistical risk and choose to have children. This decision is based on how they perceive the social and psychological burdens of the disorder. Attitude toward reproduction may be considerably different, for instance, for a female carrier of protanopia than for a female carrier of X-linked RP or choroideremia, even though the statistical risk for an affected son is the same for each carrier. Some may elect to delay childbearing in the hope of future medical advances. For a variety of personal and ethical considerations, others may opt for contraception, termination of pregnancy, sterilization, and/or adoption.

Artificial insemination by a donor is a useful option in family planning if the father has a dominant disease or if both parents are carriers of a biochemically detectable recessive disorder. However, it is clearly not applicable if the mother is the carrier of an X-linked or mitochondrial disorder or if the mother is the individual affected by an autosomal dominant mutation. Finally, although its acceptance and legal implications may lag behind, donor eggs and embryos and surrogate motherhood may be useful alternatives for some families.

In some circumstances, an individual or couple may use the results of genetic testing and consider prenatal testing or in vitro fertilization (IVF) technology with preimplantation genetic diagnosis (PGD) to avoid recurrence in their children. Knowledge of these options and of the potential ethical, social, and cultural issues they raise is important for clinicians.

Prenatal diagnosis (PND) with amniocentesis or chorionic villus sampling (CVS) for biochemically identifiable disorders (eg, Tay-Sachs disease, many mucopolysaccharidoses, and more than 100 other diseases) is also useful in the proper genetic scenarios. However, because most genes are expressed in a tissue-specific manner, biochemical diagnostic techniques are limited to diseases for which the gene products are expressed in amniocytes.

Other possible indications for PND include advanced maternal age or positive results from prenatal screening, both of which carry an increased risk of chromosomal abnormalities; elevated maternal serum α-fetoprotein, suggesting a neural tube defect; the presence of soft markers or fetal abnormalities that could suggest a chromosomal abnormality or a genetic disease; and the presence of a familial disease detectable by DNA analysis.

Amniocentesis is usually performed at 15–16 weeks of gestation, when enough fluid and cells can be obtained for culture and the maternal risk of abortion is relatively low. The risk of spontaneous abortion or fetal morbidity from the procedure is approximately 0.5%. Earlier prenatal diagnosis of chromosomal abnormalities, at about 10 weeks of gestation, is available through the use of CVS. In this procedure, tissue from the placenta is obtained under ultrasound visualization. It is then cultured and karyotyped in a manner similar to that used for amniocentesis. As a first-trimester procedure, CVS allows for an earlier diagnosis and a safer means of pregnancy termination. The rate of spontaneous abortion associated with this procedure is estimated at 1%–2%. Because the yield of DNA is greater than that from the 20 mL of amniotic fluid withdrawn in amniocentesis, direct DNA analysis of cells can often be done without prior cell culture. Thus, information can be obtained considerably sooner than with amniocentesis.

Couples who elect PND in the form of either CVS or amniocentesis may face considerable anxiety about complications such as pregnancy loss, waiting time to obtain the genetic results, and potentially, the difficult decision of whether to terminate an affected pregnancy—a dilemma that couples are aware they may face repeatedly with each consecutive pregnancy.

PGD has the advantage of selecting unaffected embryos through testing prior to implantation. Embryos are created using *intracytoplasmic sperm injection (ICSI),* in which a single sperm is injected into each egg in an attempt to achieve fertilization. On day 3, when each embryo consists of 6–8 cells, 1 cell (blastomere) is removed per embryo. DNA is extracted from these cells and amplified using fluorescent polymerase chain reaction (F-PCR) to make millions of copies of the relevant region of DNA. This region is then sequenced to provide a reliable diagnosis of the status of the genetic mutation in each embryo. Unaffected embryos are transferred to the uterus on day 4 or 5. Usually no more than 1 or 2 embryos can be transferred, to avoid the possibility of multiple births.

PGD is acceptable to many couples, and for some, it represents a valuable alternative to PND. For some couples with a moral or religious objection to pregnancy termination and who are at risk of having a child with a genetic condition, this technique may provide the opportunity to have an unaffected child. However, PGD may be associated with stress and anxiety for couples similar to that discussed earlier. Other concerns include the high cost of IVF and genetic testing and the low IVF pregnancy rates. PGD has raised ethical issues about embryo destruction and sex selection. Furthermore, the issue of eugenics (selection for perceived favorable nonmedical traits) has also been debated. Just as diseases differ among individuals, so do the concerns and beliefs of different parents; thus the acceptability of different reproductive technologies should be discussed individually with each couple.

Referral to Providers of Support for Persons With Disabilities

Individuals and families often receive considerable benefit from referral to local, regional, or national agencies, support groups, or foundations that provide services for those with a particular disease. These organizations include local and state agencies for the blind or visually impaired, special school education programs, and appropriate consumer groups. Particularly when a disability is chronic and progressive, these agencies or support groups can greatly aid the individual or family in adjusting to changing visual disabilities. They also allow individuals or families with a particular genetic disorder to meet others with the same condition, providing them with support and possible advice.

National Human Genome Research Institute website. Genetic counseling, support and advocacy groups online. Available at www.genome.gov/11510370. Accessed October 23, 2013.

Online Mendelian Inheritance in Man website. Available at www.ncbi.nlm.nih.gov/omim. Accessed October 23, 2013.

Recommendations for Genetic Testing of Inherited Eye Disease

The AAO Task Force on Genetic Testing has stated that when properly performed, interpreted, and acted upon, genetic tests can improve the accuracy of diagnosis, prognosis, and genetic counseling; lead to reduced risk of disease recurrence in families at risk; and facilitate delivery of personalized care. Like other forms of medical intervention, genetic testing carries specific risks that vary from patient to patient and from family to family.

The results of a genetic test may affect plans to have children, create guilt or anxiety, and complicate family relationships. For these reasons, skilled counseling should be provided to all individuals who undergo genetic testing to maximize benefits and minimize risks.

The task force's 7 recommendations are as follows:

1. Offer genetic testing to patients who have clinical findings suggestive of a mendelian disorder for which causative gene or genes have been identified. If unfamiliar with such testing, refer the patient to a physician or counselor with such experience. In all cases, ensure that the patient receives counseling from a physician with expertise in inherited disease or a certified genetic counselor.

2. Use Clinical Laboratories Improvement Amendments (CLIA)–approved laboratories for all clinical testing. When possible, use laboratories that include in their reports estimates of the pathogenicity of observed genetic variants that are based on a review of the medical literature and databases of disease-causing and non–disease-causing variants.

3. Provide a copy of each genetic test report to the patient so that she or he will be able independently to seek mechanism-specific information, such as the availability of gene-specific clinical trials, should the patient wish to do so.

4. Avoid use of direct-to-consumer genetic testing and discourage patients from obtaining such tests themselves. Encourage the involvement of a trained physician, genetic counselor, or both for all genetic tests so that appropriate interpretation and counseling can be provided.

5. Avoid unnecessary parallel testing; order the most specific test(s) available given the patient's clinical findings. Restrict the use of massively parallel strategies like whole-exome sequencing and whole-genome sequencing to research studies conducted at tertiary care facilities.

6. Avoid routine genetic testing for genetically complex disorders like age-related macular degeneration and late-onset primary open-angle glaucoma until specific treatment or surveillance strategies have been shown in one or more published clinical trials to be of benefit to individuals with specific disease-associated genotypes. In the meantime, confine the genotyping of such patients to research studies.

7. Avoid testing asymptomatic minors for untreatable disorders except in extraordinary circumstances. For the few cases in which such testing is believed to be warranted, the following steps should be taken before the test is performed: (1) the parents and child should undergo formal genetic counseling, (2) the certified counselor or physician performing the counseling should state his or her opinion in writing that the test is in the family's best interest, and (3) all parents with custodial responsibility for the child should agree in writing with the decision to perform the test.

GTR: Genetic Testing Registry website. www.ncbi.nlm.nih.gov/gtr/. Accessed October 8, 2013.

Stone EM, Aldave AJ, Drack AV, et al. Recommendations for genetic testing of inherited eye diseases. Report of the American Academy of Ophthalmology Task Force on Genetic Testing. *Ophthalmology.* 2012;119(11):2408–2410.

Traboulsi EI, ed. *Genetic Diseases of the Eye.* 2nd ed. Oxford University Press; 2012.

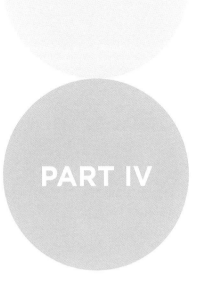

PART IV

Biochemistry and Metabolism

Introduction

Considerable progress has been made in understanding the biochemistry of vision over the past 15 to 20 years, as witnessed by the numerous reviews, research articles, and books that have been published during this time. Part IV, Biochemistry and Metabolism, was written for practitioners and residents in ophthalmology, as well as for students and researchers seeking a concise picture of the current state of knowledge in the biochemistry of the eye. With the recent growth in new information about vision biochemistry has come increasing specialization among ophthalmic researchers. These chapters cover most areas of research in ocular biochemistry, including tear film, cornea, iris and ciliary body, aqueous humor, lens, vitreous, retina, retinal pigment epithelium, and free radicals and antioxidants. The text attempts to relate basic science to clinical problems that may be faced during residency training and in subsequent practice.

CHAPTER **7**

Tear Film

The primary functions of the tear film are to

- provide a smooth optical surface at the air–cornea interface
- serve as a medium for removal of debris
- protect the ocular surface

The tear film carries tear constituents and debris to the puncta. In addition, it contains a vast number of antimicrobial agents, lubricates the cornea–eyelid interface, and prevents desiccation of the ocular surface.

Human tears are distributed among the marginal tear strip (or *tear meniscus*), the preocular film covering the exposed bulbar conjunctiva and cornea (precorneal tear film), and the conjunctival sac (between the eyelids and bulbar conjunctiva).

The *precorneal tear film* is a trilaminar structure consisting conceptually of an outer lipid layer, a middle aqueous layer, and an inner mucin layer. Measurements of tear-film thickness have differed widely. Original measurements of the precorneal tear film gave an average thickness of approximately 8–9 μm, with the aqueous layer constituting nearly all the thickness (Fig 7-1). More recent, and presumably more accurate, studies using optical coherence tomography (OCT) and reflectometry have found the tear film to be only

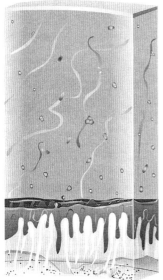

Outer lipid layer

Middle aqueous layer

Inner mucin layer

Microvilli of epithelium
extend into and stabilize
mucin layer

Figure 7-1 Schematic drawing of the structure of the tear film showing the outer lipid layer; middle, aqueous layer; inner mucin layer; and microvilli on the apical cells of the ocular surface epithelium. *(From Marshall D. Tear layer mechanics. In: Bennett ES, Weissman BA, eds.* Clinical Contact Lens Practice. *Philadelphia: JB Lippincott; 1991:2.)*

Table 7-1 Approximate Properties of Human Tear Film

Composition	Water	98.2%
	Solid	1.8%
Thickness	Total	3.4 μm
	Lipid layer	0.1–0.2 μm
Volume	Unanesthetized	7.4 μL
	Anesthetized	2.6 μL
Secretory rate	Unanesthetized	
	Schirmer	3.8 μL/min
	Fluorophotometry	0.9 μL/min
	Anesthetized	
	Schirmer	1.8 μL/min
	Fluorophotometry	0.3 μL/min
Turnover rate	Normal	12%–16%/min
	Stimulated	300%/min
Evaporation rate		0.06 μL/cm^2/min
Osmolarity		296–308 mOsm/L
pH		6.5–7.6
Electrolytes (mmol/L)	Na$^+$	134–170
	K$^+$	26–42
	Ca^{2+}	0.5
	Mg^{2+}	0.3–0.6
	Cl$^-$	120–135
	HCO$_3^-$	26

approximately 3.4 μm thick. The separation between the mucin and aqueous layers may not be distinct because mucins absorb electrolytes and water. The steady-state volume of tears is 7.4 μL for the unanesthetized eye and 2.6 μL for the anesthetized eye; this volume decreases with age. Some properties of the normal human tear film are given in Table 7-1.

Lipid Layer

The lipid layer has the following functions:

- retard evaporation
- contribute to the optical properties of the tear film because of its position at the air–tear film interface
- maintain a hydrophobic barrier *(lipid strip)* that prevents tear overflow by increasing surface tension
- prevent damage to eyelid margin skin by tears

The anterior layer of the tear film (approximately 100 molecules thick) contains polar and nonpolar lipids secreted primarily by the *meibomian (tarsal) glands* (Fig 7-2). These glands are located in the tarsal plate of the upper and lower eyelids and are supplied by parasympathetic nerves that are cholinesterase-positive and contain vasoactive intestinal polypeptide (VIP). Sympathetic and sensory nerves are present but sparsely distributed. Neuropeptide Y (NPY)–positive nerves are also abundant. There are approximately

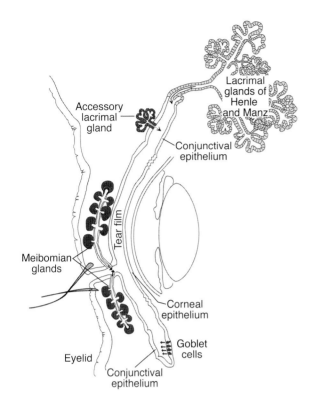

Figure 7-2 Schematic drawing of the major tear glands and ocular surface epithelia that contribute to the tear film. Shown are the meibomian glands (secrete oily layer); accessory lacrimal glands and lacrimal glands of Henle and Manz (secrete aqueous layer); conjunctival epithelium; corneal epithelium; and conjunctival goblet cells (secrete mucus layer). *(From Dartt DA, Sullivan DA. Wetting of the ocular surface. In: Albert DM, Jakobiec FA, eds. Principles and Practice of Ophthalmology. Philadelphia: Saunders; 1994:967.)*

30–40 meibomian glands in the upper eyelid and 20–30 meibomian glands in the lower eyelid. Each gland orifice opens onto the skin of the eyelid margin, between the tarsal *gray line* and the mucocutaneous junction. The sebaceous glands of Zeis, located at the eyelid margin close to the eyelash roots, also secrete lipid, which is incorporated into the tear film.

Because the polar lipids are charged compounds *(phospholipids)*, they are located at the aqueous–lipid interface. The fatty acids of the phospholipids interact with the other hydrophobic lipids (cholesterol and wax esters, which make up the bulk of the lipid layer) through noncovalent, noncharged bonds. Tear lipids are not susceptible to lipid peroxidation because they contain extremely low levels of polyunsaturated fatty acids.

Aqueous Layer

The aqueous layer has the following functions:

- supply oxygen to the avascular corneal epithelium
- maintain a constant electrolyte composition over the ocular surface epithelium
- provide an antibacterial and antiviral defense
- smooth minute irregularities of the anterior corneal surface
- wash away debris
- modulate corneal and conjunctival epithelial cell function

The middle, aqueous layer is secreted by the main and accessory lacrimal glands (see Fig 7-2). It consists of electrolytes, water, and proteins. The main lacrimal gland is divided into 2 anatomical parts, the *orbital* and the *palpebral* portions, by the *levator aponeurosis.* The *glands of Krause,* which constitute two-thirds of the accessory lacrimal glands, are located in the lateral part of the upper fornix. A number of Krause glands are also present in the lower fornix. The *glands of Wolfring* are variably located along the proximal margin of each tarsus. The accessory lacrimal glands are structurally like the main lacrimal gland.

The main lacrimal gland is richly innervated by parasympathetic nerves containing the neurotransmitters acetylcholine and VIP. The sympathetic innervation is less dense than the parasympathetic and contains norepinephrine and NPY as neurotransmitters. The sensory nerves are sparsely supplied with the neurotransmitters substance P and calcitonin gene–related peptide (CGRP). The accessory lacrimal glands are densely innervated, but the majority of nerves are unidentified. Some of this innervation consists of nerves containing VIP, substance P, and CGRP. Corneal innervation is predominantly sensory, but there is also sympathetic and (to a lesser extent) parasympathetic innervation. The conjunctival epithelium is innervated by parasympathetic, sympathetic, and sensory nerves.

The aqueous layer of tears consists of electrolytes, water, protein, and a variety of other solutes secreted by the main and accessory lacrimal glands, as well as by the corneal and conjunctival epithelia. In addition, with conjunctival inflammation and in response to drugs such as histamine, the blood vessels of the conjunctiva can leak a plasmalike fluid into the aqueous layer of tears.

Electrolytes and small molecules regulate the osmotic flow of fluids between the corneal epithelial cells and the tear film, buffer tear pH, and serve as enzyme cofactors in controlling membrane permeability. The Na^+ concentration of tears parallels that of serum; the concentration of K^+ is 5–7 times greater than that in serum. Na^+, K^+, and Cl^- regulate the osmotic flow of fluids from the cornea to the tear film. Bicarbonate regulates tear pH. Other tear electrolytes (Fe^{2+}, Cu^{2+}, Mg^{2+}, Ca^{2+}, PO_4^{3-}) are enzyme cofactors.

Tear-film solutes include urea, glucose, lactate, citrate, ascorbate, and amino acids. All enter the tear film via the systemic circulation, and their concentrations parallel those of serum levels. Fasting tear glucose levels are 3.6–4.1 mg/mL in those with and without diabetes mellitus. However, after a 100-mg oral glucose load, tear glucose levels exceed 11 mg/mL in 96% of diabetic persons tested.

Proteins in the tear film include immunoglobulin A (IgA) and secretory IgA (sIgA). IgA is formed by plasma cells in interstitial tissues of the main and accessory lacrimal glands and by the substantia propria of the conjunctiva. The secretory component is produced within lacrimal gland acini, and sIgA is secreted into the lumen of the main and accessory lacrimal glands. IgA plays a role in local host-defense mechanisms of the external eye, as shown by increased levels of IgA and IgG in human tears associated with ocular inflammation. Other immunoglobulins in tears are IgM, IgD, and IgE. Vernal conjunctivitis causes elevated tear and serum levels of IgE, increased IgE-producing plasma cells in the giant papillae of the superior tarsal conjunctiva, and elevated histamine levels. Increased levels of tear histamine support the concept of conjunctival mast-cell degranulation triggered by IgE–antigen interaction.

Lysozyme, lactoferrin, group II phospholipase A_2, lipocalins, and defensins are important tear antimicrobial constituents. Also present in tears is interferon, which inhibits viral replication and may be efficacious in limiting the severity of ulcerative herpetic keratitis. In addition, tears contain a wide array of cytokines and growth factors, including transforming growth factor βs, epidermal growth factor, β fibroblast growth factor, interleukin 1α and 1β, and tumor necrosis factor α. These constituents may play a role in the proliferation, migration, and differentiation of corneal and conjunctival epithelial cells. They may also regulate wound healing of the ocular surface.

Mucin Layer

The mucin layer of the tear film coats the microplicae of the superficial corneal epithelial cells and forms a fine network over the conjunctival surface. It contains mucins, proteins, electrolytes, and water. Functions of the mucin layer include the following:

- convert the corneal epithelium from a hydrophobic to a hydrophilic layer, which is essential for the even and spontaneous distribution of the tear film
- interact with the tear lipid layer to lower surface tension, thereby stabilizing the tear film
- trap exfoliated surface cells, foreign particles, and bacteria (by the loose mucin network covering the bulbar conjunctiva)
- lubricate the eyelids as they pass over the globe

Tear mucins are secreted principally by the conjunctival goblet cells and the stratified squamous cells of the conjunctival and corneal epithelia and minimally by lacrimal glands of Henle and Manz (see Fig 7-2). Goblet-cell mucin production is 2–3 μL/day, which contrasts with the 2–3 mL/day of aqueous tear production. Both conjunctival and tear mucins are negatively charged, high-molecular-weight glycoproteins. Tear dysfunction may result when tear mucins are deficient in number (eg, in avitaminosis A and conjunctival destruction), excessive in number (eg, in hyperthyroidism; foreign-body stimulation; and allergic, vernal, and giant papillary conjunctivitis), or biochemically altered (eg, in keratoconjunctivitis).

Tear Secretion

The lacrimal secretory system was once thought to have 2 components: *basic secretors* and *reflex secretors*. Basic secretion was ascribed to the accessory lacrimal glands of Krause and Wolfring; and reflex secretion, to the main lacrimal gland. However, it is now thought that all lacrimal glands respond as a unit. In addition, the cornea and conjunctiva can respond by secreting electrolytes, water, and mucins. Although the meibomian glands are innervated, it is not known whether nerves mediate lipid secretion from these glands. Reflex tear secretion is neurally mediated and induced in response to physical irritation (ie, superficial corneal and conjunctival sensory stimulation by mechanical, thermal, or chemical means), psychogenic factors, and bright light via the optic nerve. Induction of sensory nerves by a local neural reflex activates the parasympathetic and sympathetic nerves that innervate the tear glands and epithelia, causing secretion.

Parasympathetic and sympathetic nerves release their neurotransmitters, which interact with specific G-protein–linked receptors in the lacrimal glands, cornea, and conjunctiva; these receptors then activate their respective signaling pathways. There are 2 main signaling pathways: a Ca^{2+}/protein kinase C–dependent pathway and a cyclic adenosine monophosphate (cAMP)–dependent pathway (Figs 7-3, 7-4). In most tissues, the Ca^{2+}/protein kinase C–dependent pathway is activated by acetylcholine and, except in the main lacrimal gland, by norepinephrine. Acetylcholine, released from parasympathetic nerves, activates muscarinic receptors; norepinephrine, released from sympathetic nerves, activates α_1-adrenergic receptors. Stimulation of muscarinic and α_1-adrenergic receptors activates a guanine nucleotide–binding protein (G protein) of the $G\alpha_{q/11}$ subtype, which then turns on phospholipase C. Phospholipase C breaks down a membrane lipid— phosphatidylinositol 4,5,-bisphosphate—into inositol 1,4,5-trisphosphate (IP_3) and diacylglycerol. IP_3 releases intracellular Ca^{2+}. The depletion of Ca^{2+} from intracellular stores causes the influx of extracellular Ca^{2+} to refill these stores. Ca^{2+} (either by itself or by activating Ca^{2+}-calmodulin–dependent protein kinases) stimulates protein and/or electrolyte and water secretion. The increase in diacylglycerol activates protein kinase C, a family of 11 isozymes that stimulate protein and/or electrolyte and water secretion.

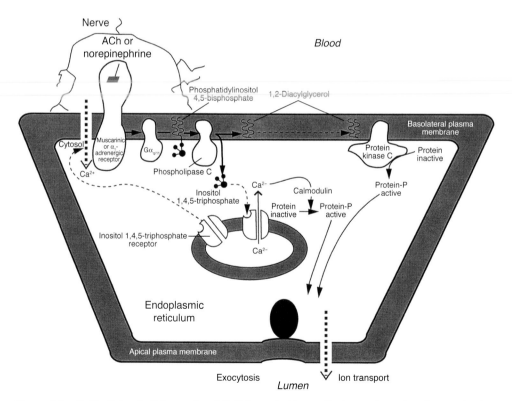

Figure 7-3 Epithelial cell. Schematic of Ca^{2+}/protein kinase C–dependent signal transduction pathway activated by cholinergic and α_1-adrenergic agonists in epithelial cells to stimulate mucin, protein, or electrolyte and water secretion. ACh = acetylcholine; $G\alpha_{q/11}$ = q/11 subtype of guanine nucleotide–binding protein; Protein-P = phosphorylated (activated) protein. *(Modified from Dartt DA. Regulation of tear secretion.* Adv Exp Med Biol. *1994;350:4.)*

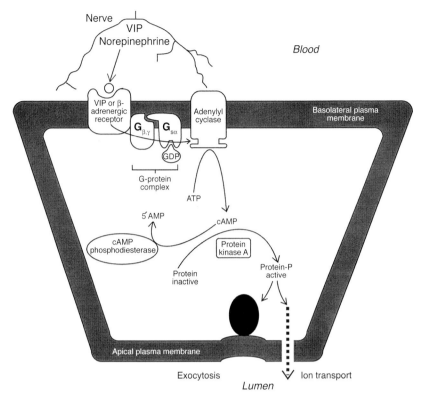

Figure 7-4 Epithelial cell. Schematic of 3′,5′-cyclic adenosine monophosphate (cAMP)–dependent signaling pathway activated by vasoactive intestinal polypeptide (VIP) or norepinephrine to stimulate mucin, protein, or electrolyte and water secretion in epithelial cells. 5′ AMP = adenosine 5′-monophosphate; ATP = adenosine 5′-triphosphate; $G_{\beta,\gamma}$ = β- and γ-subunits of guanine nucleotide–binding protein; $G_{s\alpha}$ = stimulatory α-subunit of guanine nucleotide–binding protein; GDP = guanosine 5′-diphosphate; Protein-P = phosphorylated (activated) protein. *(Modified from Dartt DA. Regulation of tear secretion.* Adv Exp Med Biol. *1994;350:5.)*

The cAMP-dependent pathway is activated by VIP and norepinephrine. VIP, released from parasympathetic nerves, interacts with VIP receptors; norepinephrine, released from sympathetic nerves, activates β-adrenergic receptors. Stimulation of VIP or β-adrenergic receptors activates G protein $G_{s\alpha}$ subtypes, which in turn stimulate adenylyl cyclase. Activation of adenylyl cyclase produces cAMP from ATP. cAMP activates cAMP-dependent protein kinases to stimulate protein and/or electrolyte and water secretion. The action of cAMP is terminated when it is broken down by cAMP-dependent phosphodiesterases.

Another mechanism for stimulating tear secretion (in addition to nerves) is peptide and steroid hormones. Peptide hormones, including α-melanocyte-stimulating hormone and adrenocorticotropic hormone (ACTH), stimulate protein secretion from the main lacrimal gland. These hormones activate the cAMP-dependent pathway described for VIP and β-adrenergic receptors. The steroid hormones, specifically the androgens, stimulate secretion of sIgA from the main lacrimal gland and lipid secretion from the meibomian glands. Androgens diffuse into the nucleus and bind to receptors, which are members of the steroid/thyroid hormone/retinoic acid family of transcription factors. The monomeric-activated androgen-receptor complex then associates with the response elements in the regulating region of the target gene (eg, for sIgA secretion, the target is the secretory component gene). This association promotes dimerization of 2 androgen-receptor complexes, a process that then activates gene transcription and eventually protein synthesis.

Eyelid movement is important in tear-film renewal, distribution, turnover, and drainage. As the eyelids close in a complete blink, the superior and inferior fornices are compressed by the force of the preseptal muscles, and the eyelids move toward each other, with the upper eyelid moving over the longer distance and exerting force on the globe. This force clears the anterior surface of debris and any insoluble mucin and expresses secretions from meibomian glands. The lower eyelid moves horizontally in a nasal direction and pushes tear fluid and debris toward the superior and inferior puncta. When the eyelids are opened, the tear film is redistributed. The upper eyelid pulls the aqueous phase of the tear film by capillary action. The lipid layer spreads as fast as the eyelids move, so that no area of the tear film is left uncovered by lipid. The lipid layer increases tear-film thickness and stabilizes the tear film. Polar lipids, present in the meibomian secretions, concentrate at the lipid–water interface and enhance the stability of the lipid layer.

Tear Dysfunction

A qualitative or quantitative abnormality of the tear film may occur as a result of

- change in the amount of tear-film constituents
- change in the composition of tear film
- uneven dispersion of the tear film because of corneal surface irregularities
- ineffective distribution of the tear film caused by eyelid–globe incongruity

The amount or composition of the tear film can change because of aqueous deficiency, mucin deficiency or excess (with or without associated aqueous deficiency), lipid abnormality (meibomian gland dysfunction), and/or ocular surface exposure. For example, increases in tear-film osmolarity have been observed in patients with keratoconjunctivitis sicca (KCS, or dry eye syndrome) or blepharitis and in those who use contact lenses. The preocular tear film is dispersed unevenly with an irregular corneal or limbal surface (inflammation, scarring, dystrophic changes) or poor contact lens fit. Eyelid–globe incongruity results from congenital, traumatic, or neurogenic eyelid dysfunction or absent or dysfunctional blink mechanism. With age, the quality and quantity of the tear film diminish. Diagnostic tests for tear dysfunction include tear breakup time, fluorescein staining, lissamine green staining, rose bengal staining, osmolarity test, and Schirmer test.

The tear-constituent imbalance can be corrected by decreasing the evaporation of tears (through reduced room temperature or increased humidity) and exchanging contact lenses for glasses. Tear-film instability (secondary to aqueous and/or mucin deficiency) can be reduced by the use of topical tear substitutes. Reduction of tear drainage by punctal occlusion prolongs the effect of artificial tears and preserves the natural tears. Thus, tear dysfunction is managed by creating a more regular corneal or conjunctival contour or by facilitating eyelid–globe congruity. Unfortunately, all these treatments are palliative (and not curative) in nature.

There is increasing evidence that KCS is associated with ocular surface inflammation. In various studies, adhesion molecule expression by conjunctiva epithelial cells, T-cell infiltration of the conjunctiva, and increases in soluble mediators (cytokines and proteases) in the tear film have been found in patients with KCS (Fig 7-5). Preliminary clinical studies have shown that using tear substitutes to treat patients with KCS may reduce tear osmolarity and improve ocular symptoms. Moreover, therapy with a multitude of anti-inflammatory drugs (including corticosteroids, cyclosporine, matrix metalloproteinases, and doxycycline) has been observed to improve the clinical symptoms of patients with KCS (Fig 7-6). Topical cyclosporine A emulsion is approved by the FDA for treating the inflammatory component of dry eye syndrome. This fungal-derived peptide emulsion has been shown effective in stimulating aqueous tear production in patients with

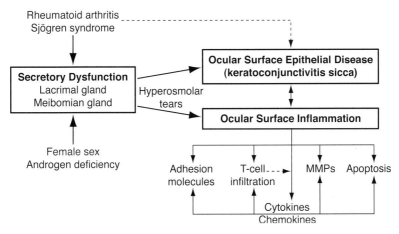

Figure 7-5 Inflammatory mediators in keratoconjunctivitis sicca. MMPs = matrix metalloproteinases. *(Reproduced with permission from Pflugfelder SC. Antiinflammatory therapy for dry eye. Am J Ophthalmol. 2004;137(2):338.)*

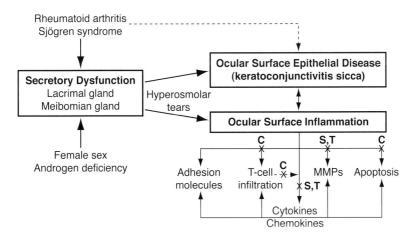

Figure 7-6 Targets of anti-inflammatory therapies for keratoconjunctivitis sicca. C = cyclosporin A; MMPs = matrix metalloproteinases; S = corticosteroids; T = tetracycline. *(Reproduced with permission from Pflugfelder SC. Antiinflammatory therapy for dry eye. Am J Ophthalmol. 2004;137(2):340.)*

KCS. No significant adverse systemic or ocular events (except for burning symptoms) were observed.

BCSC Section 7, *Orbit, Eyelids, and Lacrimal System,* discusses the lacrimal system in depth, with numerous illustrations. See also BCSC Section 8, *External Disease and Cornea,* which discusses keratoconjunctivitis sicca in greater detail.

Pflugfelder SC. Antiinflammatory therapy for dry eye. *Am J Ophthalmol.* 2004;137(2):337–342.

Tiffany JM. Tears and conjunctiva. In: Harding JJ, ed. *Biochemistry of the Eye.* London: Chapman & Hall Medical; 1997:1–15.

Tsubota K. Tear dynamics and dry eye. *Prog Retin Eye Res.* 1998;17(4):565–596.

CHAPTER **8**

Cornea

The cornea is a remarkable structure; it has a high degree of transparency and excellent self-protective and reparative properties. The cornea consists of the following histologic layers (Fig 8-1):

- epithelium with basement membrane
- Bowman layer
- stroma (or *substantia propria*)
- Descemet membrane
- endothelium

The human cornea has a rich afferent innervation. The long posterior ciliary nerves (branches of V_1, the ophthalmic division of cranial nerve V) penetrate the cornea in 3 planes: scleral, episcleral, and conjunctival. Peripherally, approximately 70–80 branches of the long posterior ciliary nerves enter the cornea and lose their myelin sheath 1–2 mm

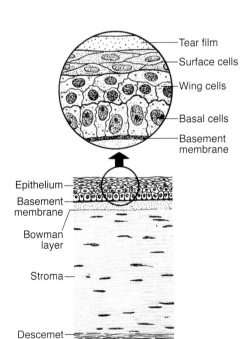

Figure 8-1 Diagram of different layers of the cornea. *(Reproduced with permission from Kanski JJ. Clinical Ophthalmology: A Systematic Approach. 3rd ed. Oxford: Butterworth-Heinemann; 1994:100.)*

from the limbus. A plexus posterior to the Bowman layer sends branches anteriorly into the epithelium.

Oxygen to the cornea is provided by the preocular tear film, eyelid vasculature, and aqueous humor. The primary metabolic substrate for the epithelial cells, stromal keratocytes, and endothelium is glucose. The stroma receives glucose primarily from the aqueous humor by carrier-mediated transport through the endothelium; the epithelium receives glucose by passive diffusion through the stroma. The preocular tear film and limbal vessels supply approximately 10% of the glucose used by the cornea. Glucose is metabolized in the cornea by all 3 metabolic pathways:

1. tricarboxylic acid (TCA) cycle
2. anaerobic glycolysis
3. hexose monophosphate (HMP) shunt

In the epithelium and endothelium, the HMP pathway breaks down 35%–65% of the glucose, but the keratocytes of the stroma metabolize very little glucose via this pathway. The keratocytes appear to lack 6-phosphogluconate dehydrogenase, an important enzyme in the HMP pathway. The TCA cycle is much more active in the endothelium than in the epithelium. Pyruvic acid, the end product of glycolysis, is converted either to carbon dioxide and water (via the TCA cycle under aerobic conditions) or to lactic acid (under anaerobic conditions). Production of lactic acid increases in conditions of oxygen deprivation, as in the case of tight-fitting contact lenses of low oxygen permeability. Accumulation of lactic acid in the cornea has detrimental consequences to vision, such as edema (due to an increase in an osmotic solute load) or stromal acidosis, which can change endothelial morphology and function.

Human corneas possess a remarkably high level of aldehyde dehydrogenase and transketolase. Together, these 2 proteins constitute 40%–50% of the soluble proteins in corneal stroma. Like enzyme crystallins of the lens, both aldehyde dehydrogenase and transketolase are thought to contribute to the optical properties of the cornea. Both proteins are also thought to protect corneal cells against free radicals and oxidative damage by absorbing UVB irradiation.

Epithelium

The epithelium is typically approximately 50 μm thick and constitutes 5%–10% of total corneal thickness. It is composed of 4–6 layers, which include 1–2 layers of superficial squamous cells, 2–3 layers of broad wing cells, and the innermost layer of the columnar basal cells. Surface projections (microvilli and microplicae) are present on the apical surface of the most superficial cell layer of epithelium. These projections are coated with filamentous material known as *glycocalyx*. Mucin glycoproteins, the major constituents of glycocalyx, are thought to promote both stability of the tear film and wettability of the corneal surface. Plasma membrane proteins and the lipids of corneal epithelial cells, like those of other cell types, are heavily glycosylated and play an important role in cell–cell adhesion as well as in adhesion of the basal cells of the corneal epithelium to the underlying basement membrane. The sugar residues of the plasma membrane glycoproteins and the glycolipids of corneal epithelium also play a role in wound-healing mechanisms; they do so by mediating corneal epithelial sheet migration over the wound surface following ocular injury. They also have a role in pathogenesis of corneal infection by serving as attachment sites for microbes.

Hydrophilic molecules penetrate the epithelium poorly, but they may pass through intercellular tight junctions if the polar molecule is less than 500 daltons in apparent molecular mass. Knowing the ionic dissociation constant of a molecule is important for determining its permeability across the cornea. To diffuse across the epithelium, organic molecules should exist in an uncharged state. However, a charged molecule more readily penetrates the stroma. Therefore, to penetrate the cornea and enter the anterior chamber, an organic molecule should be able to dissociate at physiologic pH and temperature (ie, within the stroma).

Bowman Layer

The Bowman layer, or Bowman membrane, is immediately posterior to the epithelial basal lamina. This layer is 8–12 μm thick and is composed of randomly packed type I and type V collagen fibers that are 30 nm in diameter. The fibers are enmeshed in a matrix consisting of proteoglycans and glycoproteins. The Bowman layer is secreted during embryogenesis by the anterior stromal keratocytes and epithelium. It is acellular, and it does not regenerate when damaged. It is thought that this layer, by virtue of its acellularity and packing distribution, serves to prevent exposure of stromal corneal keratocytes to growth factors secreted by epithelial cells, such as transforming growth factor βs (TGF-βs). This effect is notable because, during excimer laser surgery (photorefractive keratectomy [PRK] or laser subepithelial keratomileusis [LASEK]), the Bowman layer along with anterior corneal stromal tissue is removed. In these procedures, corneal haze is a potentially significant postoperative visual complication, presumably because stromal keratocytes are exposed to regenerating epithelial growth factors and take on fibroblastic behaviors. On the other hand, in laser in situ keratomileusis (LASIK), the Bowman layer is transected but still retained, and thus central corneal haze is extremely rare.

Stroma

The stroma makes up 90% of the corneal thickness. Stromal cells are known as *keratocytes*. There is loss of keratocyte density with age; therefore, depending on age, keratocytes constitute 10%–40% of corneal volume. Usually, these cells reside between the collagen lamellae. The stroma is made up of roughly 200 layers of lamellae, which are 1.5–2.5 μm thick and composed of collagen fibrils enmeshed in a matrix consisting of proteoglycans, proteins, and glycoproteins. The stromal fibrils within each lamella are narrow and uniform in diameter. In humans, the average fibril diameter is 30 nm.

Collagen fibrils within each lamella run parallel to each other from limbus to limbus. Adjacent lamellae are positioned at roughly right angles to each other: less than 90° in the anterior stroma but almost 90° in the posterior stroma. That is, alternate arrays of fibrils are nearly perpendicular, and they are observed tangentially in electron micrographs of cross sections of corneal stroma. Also, collagen fibrils in each lamella are regularly spaced, with a center-to-center distance of 55–60 nm. The narrow and uniform diameter of collagen fibrils and their regular arrangement are characteristic of collagen of the corneal stroma and are necessary for the transparency of this tissue. It has been hypothesized that the posterior-most 15 micrometers of stroma represent a distinct, tough acellular layer (Dua's layer). Type I is the major collagen component of the corneal stroma; it constitutes approximately 70% of the total stromal dry weight. Immunohistochemical and biochemical studies have demonstrated that normal adult corneal stroma also contains collagen types V, VI, VII, XII, and XIV. Type III collagen production is associated uniquely with stromal wound healing.

After collagen, proteoglycans are the second most abundant biological constituents of the cornea; they constitute approximately 10% of the dry weight of the cornea. It is the proteoglycans that confer hydrophilic properties to the stroma. Proteoglycans are glycosylated proteins with at least 1 glycosaminoglycan (GAG) chain covalently bound to the protein core. GAGs are composed of repeating disaccharides. The GAGs found in corneal stroma include

- keratan sulfate
- chondroitin sulfate
- dermatan sulfate

Two major proteoglycan populations have been identified in corneal stroma, one containing keratan sulfate chains and the other containing both dermatan sulfate and chondroitin sulfate chains. Regulation of spacing between the stromal collagen fibrils is thought to result from highly specific interactions between the proteoglycans and the collagen fibrils. When these interactions are disturbed, the ability of the cornea to remain transparent is profoundly affected.

Matrix metalloproteinases (MMPs) are a family of Zn^{2+}-dependent enzymes responsible for degradation of the components of the extracellular matrix (including proteoglycans and various types of collagens) during normal development as well as in disease processes. Of more than a dozen known metalloproteinases, only MMP-2 proenzyme has been found in the normal healthy cornea. However, after corneal injury, additional MMPs (including MMP-1, MMP-3, and MMP-9) are synthesized. The proteinase inhibitors of the cornea play a key role in corneal protection by restricting damage during corneal inflammation, ulceration, and wound healing. The following proteinase inhibitors have thus far been identified in the cornea:

- α_1-proteinase inhibitor
- α_1-antichymotrypsin
- α_2-macroglobulin
- plasminogen activator inhibitors 1 and 2
- tissue inhibitors of metalloproteinases

Many of these inhibitors are synthesized by resident cells of the cornea; some are derived from tears, aqueous humor, and limbal blood vessels.

Descemet Membrane and Endothelium

The Descemet membrane is a specialized basement membrane, 10–12 μm thick, present between the endothelium and the posterior stroma. It is secreted by endothelium and comprises an anterior banded portion and a posterior nonbanded portion. Type IV is the most abundant collagen in the Descemet membrane.

The corneal endothelium is a single layer posterior to the Descemet membrane and is composed of polygonal cells 20 μm in diameter. In young adults, the normal endothelial cell count is approximately 3000/mm². The number of endothelial cells decreases with age, and there is a concomitant spreading and thinning of the remaining cells. A group of tight junctions forms the apical junctional complex between cells that occludes the lateral extracellular spaces from the aqueous humor. Approximately 20–30 short microvilli per cell extend from the apical plasma membrane into the aqueous humor. The endothelium functions as a permeability barrier between the aqueous humor and the corneal stroma and as a pump to maintain the cornea in a dehydrated state by generating the negative hydrostatic pressure that also serves to hold free corneal flaps (eg, LASIK flaps) in place. In vivo, the endothelium derives sufficient oxygen from the aqueous humor to maintain normal pump function.

If the endothelium is injured, healing occurs mainly via cell migration, rearrangement, and enlargement of the residual cells. Substantial cell loss or damage results in irreversible edema because human corneal endothelial cells have a limited ability to divide after birth. Infiltration of polymorphonuclear leukocytes in response to severe corneal injury induces endothelial cells to become fibroblastic and to synthesize *retrocorneal fibrous membrane (RCFM)*. RCFM forms between the Descemet membrane and the corneal endothelium and causes a significant decrease in visual acuity. Unlike normal corneal endothelial cells, which accumulate little type I collagen protein, the fibroblastic cells isolated from the RCFM predominantly express type I collagen.

Panjwani N. Cornea and sclera. In: Harding JJ, ed. *Biochemistry of the Eye*. London: Chapman & Hall Medical; 1997:16–51.

CHAPTER 9

Aqueous Humor, Iris, and Ciliary Body

Introduction to the Aqueous Humor

In the physiology of the mammalian eye, the aqueous humor has several important functions:

- It provides nutrients (eg, glucose and amino acids) to support the function of tissues of the anterior segment, such as the avascular lens, cornea, and trabecular meshwork.
- It removes metabolic waste products (eg, lactic acid, pyruvic acid) from these tissues.
- It helps maintain appropriate intraocular pressure (IOP).

These functions are essential to maintaining the eye's structural integrity. In addition, because the aqueous humor is devoid of blood cells and of more than 99% of the plasma proteins, it provides an optically clear medium for the transmission of light along the visual path.

Dynamics of the Aqueous Humor

The aqueous humor *(aqueous)*, the transparent fluid that fills the anterior and posterior chambers, is secreted by the nonpigmented ciliary epithelium (NPE) from a substrate of blood plasma. Aqueous is the major nutrient source for the avascular lens and cornea and provides a route for the removal of waste products. Aqueous humor is essentially protein-free, which allows for optical clarity. The total protein level in human aqueous, approximately half of which is albumin, is very low—only about one five-hundredth that in plasma. Other components include growth factors and several enzymes; these constituents include carbonic anhydrase, lysozyme, diamine oxidase, plasminogen activator, dopamine-β-hydroxylase, phospholipase A_2 (PLA_2) and prostaglandins (PGs), cyclic adenosine monophosphate (cAMP), catecholamines, steroid hormones, and hyaluronic acid.

Ocular fluids are separated from blood by barriers formed by tight junctions between epithelial and endothelial cells. These barriers are called either *blood–aqueous* or *blood–retina*, depending on their location in the eye. Because of these barriers, the composition and amounts of all materials entering and leaving the eye, except for materials that exit through the Schlemm canal, can be carefully controlled. Perturbations of these *blood–ocular barriers* cause blood constituents to mix with ocular fluids; this mixing may be the cause of plasmoid aqueous, retinal exudates, or retinal edema.

Aqueous enters the posterior chamber from the ciliary processes by means of active and passive physiologic mechanisms:

- *active:* energy-dependent secretion, including carbonic anhydrase II (CA II) activity
- *passive:* diffusion and ultrafiltration

Diffusion involves the movement of ions such as sodium across a membrane toward the side with the most negative potential. Ultrafiltration is the nonenzymatic component of aqueous formation that depends on IOP, blood pressure, and the blood osmotic pressure in the ciliary body. In humans, CA II is present in both pigmented epithelium (PE) and NPE. Its inhibitors reduce the rate of entry of sodium and bicarbonate into the aqueous, causing a reduction in aqueous flow. The formation of aqueous is largely a product of active secretion by the inner NPE and involves membrane-associated Na^+,K^+-ATPase.

The aqueous humor is secreted by the ciliary epithelium at a flow rate of 2–3 µL/min. The ciliary epithelium is a bilayer of polarized epithelial cells lining the surface of the ciliary body; the 2 cell layers are the NPE, which faces the aqueous humor through the cells' basal plasma membrane, and the PE, which faces the stroma, also through the cells' basal plasma membrane. Therefore, the apical plasma membranes of NPE and PE cells appose each other, establishing cell-to-cell communication through numerous gap junctions. Of the 2 cell layers forming the ciliary epithelium, the NPE cells are those that establish the blood–aqueous barrier by the presence of tight junctions proximal to the apical plasma membrane, thereby preventing the free passage of plasma proteins and other macromolecules from the stroma into the posterior chamber. In contrast, the PE cell layer is considered a leaky epithelium because it allows solutes to move through the intercellular space between the PE cells.

IOP is maintained by continuous aqueous formation and drainage, which allow the surrounding tissues to remove metabolic waste products. Inhibitors of enzymatic processes decrease aqueous inflow by varying amounts, providing additional evidence of active secretory processes. Carbonic anhydrase inhibitors and β-blockers are used systemically and topically in the treatment of glaucoma to reduce the rate of aqueous humor formation. For more information about glaucoma treatment, see Chapter 16 of this volume as well as BCSC Section 10, *Glaucoma*.

Composition of the Aqueous Humor

Table 9-1 summarizes the composition of the aqueous humor compared with that of plasma and vitreous. The electrolyte composition of aqueous is similar to that of plasma. Aqueous secretion, however, is not an ultrafiltrate of plasma (as was once speculated), because it is produced by energy-dependent processes in the epithelial layer of the ciliary body. This mode of production allows precise control to be maintained over composition of the fluid that bathes the structures essential for normal vision. The ionic composition of aqueous humor is determined by selective active-transport systems (eg, Na^+,K^+-$2Cl^-$ symport, Cl^--HCO_3^- and Na^+,H^+ antiports, cation channels, water channels, Na^+,K^+-ATPase,

Table 9-1 Composition of the Aqueous Humor

Components (mmol/kg H$_2$O)	Plasma	Aqueous	Vitreous
Na$^+$	146	163	144
Cl$^-$	109	134	114
HCO$_3^-$	28	20	20–30
Ascorbate	0.04	1.06	2.21
Glucose	6	3	3.4

From Macknight AD, MacLaughlin CW, Peart D, Purves RD, Carré DA, Civan MM. Formation of the aqueous humor. *Clin Exp Pharmacol Physiol.* 2000;27(1–2):100–106.

K$^+$ channels, Cl$^-$ channels, H$^+$-ATPase) that participate in secretion of aqueous humor by the ciliary epithelium. The systems' activities and cellular distributions along the cell membranes of PE and NPE cells determine unidirectional net secretion from the stroma to the posterior chamber, a process that involves 3 steps:

1. uptake of solute and water at the stromal surface by PE cells
2. transfer of solute and water from PE to NPE cells through gap junctions
3. transfer of solute and water by NPE cells into the posterior chamber

Likewise, it is thought that there is a mechanism for transporting solute and water from the posterior chamber back into the stroma. In this unidirectional reabsorption, another set of transporters may be involved in extruding Na$^+$, K$^+$, and Cl$^-$ back into the stroma. Molecular studies have shown that the secretory properties of the ciliary epithelium are not limited to ions and electrolytes but extend to a wide range of molecules with different molecular masses. Common features of many of these molecules are their local synthesis in the ciliary epithelium and their secretion by the NPE cells through the regulatory pathway into the aqueous humor. Among the proteins whose messenger RNA expression has been demonstrated are

- plasma proteins (eg, complement component C4, α_2-macroglobulin, selenoprotein P, apolipoprotein D, plasma glutathione peroxidases, angiotensinogen)
- proteinases (eg, cathepsin D, cathepsin O)
- a component of the visual cycle (eg, cellular retinaldehyde–binding protein, or CRALBP)
- a neurotrophic factor (eg, PE-derived factor)
- neuropeptide-processing enzymes (eg, carboxypeptidase E, peptidylglycine-α-amidating monoxygenase)
- neuroendocrine peptides (eg, secretogranin II, neurotensin, galanin)
- bioactive peptides and hormones (eg, atrial natriuretic peptide, brain natriuretic peptide)

These findings support the view that the ciliary epithelium exhibits neuroendocrine properties that are directly related to the makeup of the aqueous humor and its regulation. The aqueous humor composition is in dynamic equilibrium, determined both by its rate of production and outflow and by continuous exchanges with the tissues of the anterior segment. The aqueous contains the following:

- inorganic ions and organic anions
- carbohydrates
- glutathione and urea
- proteins
- growth-modulatory factors
- oxygen and carbon dioxide

Krupin T, Civan MM. Physiologic basis of aqueous humor formation. In: Ritch R, Shields MB, Krupin T, eds. *The Glaucomas.* 2nd ed. Vol 1. St Louis: Mosby; 1996:251–280.

Macknight AD, McLaughlin CW, Peart D, Purves RD, Carré DA, Civan MM. Formation of the aqueous humor. *Clin Exp Pharmacol Physiol.* 2000;27(1–2):100–106.

Inorganic Ions

The concentrations of sodium, potassium, and magnesium in the aqueous are similar to those in plasma, but the level of calcium is only half that of plasma. The 2 major anions are chloride and bicarbonate. Phosphate is also present in the aqueous (aqueous to plasma ratio, ~0.5 or lower), but its concentration is too low to have significant buffering capacity. Iron, copper, and zinc are all found in the aqueous humor at essentially the same levels as in plasma: approximately 1 mg/mL.

Organic Anions

Lactate is the most abundant organic anion in the aqueous, and its concentration there is always higher than that in plasma. Plasma and aqueous levels of lactate are directly related, and the contribution from the glycolytic metabolism of intraocular tissues is significant.

Ascorbic acid (vitamin C) is perhaps the most unusual constituent of the aqueous humor. In most mammalian species, its concentration ranges from 0.6 to 1.5 mmol/L, levels that are some 10–50 times higher than those in plasma.

Carbohydrates

Glucose concentration in the aqueous is roughly 70% of that in plasma. The rate of entry of glucose into the posterior chamber is much more rapid than would be expected from its molecular size and lipid solubility, suggesting that its passage across the ciliary epithelium occurs by facilitated diffusion. People with diabetes mellitus have increased glucose levels in aqueous, leading to higher concentrations in the lens and short-term refractive and longer-term cataract implications. Inositol, which is important for phospholipid synthesis in the anterior segment, is found at a concentration approximately 10 times that in plasma.

Glutathione and Urea

Glutathione, an important tripeptide with a reactive sulfhydryl group, is also found in the aqueous humor. Its concentration in primates ranges from 1 to 10 μmol/L. Blood contains a high concentration of glutathione, but virtually all glutathione resides within the erythrocytes, and plasma has a low concentration of only 5 μmol/L or less. Glutathione stabilizes the redox state of the aqueous by reconverting ascorbate to its functional form after oxidation, as well as by removing excess hydrogen peroxide. Glutathione also serves as a substrate in the enzymatic conjugation by cytosolic enzymes; this process is involved in the cellular detoxification of electrophilic compounds. These enzymes (glutathione S-transferases) are important in protecting tissues from oxidative damage and oxidative stress and are highly concentrated in the ocular ciliary epithelium.

The concentration of urea in the aqueous is between 80% and 90% of that in plasma. This compound is distributed passively across nearly all biological membrane systems, and its high aqueous to plasma ratio indicates that this small molecule (molecular weight, 60) readily crosses the epithelial barrier. Urea is effective in hyperosmotic infusion treatment for glaucoma. However, mannitol (molecular weight, 182) is preferred to urea because it crosses the epithelial barrier more easily.

Proteins

As stated, the nonpigmented ciliary epithelial cell layer establishes a blood–aqueous barrier that prevents the diffusion of plasma proteins from the stroma into the posterior chamber; nevertheless, plasma proteins do enter the aqueous humor, possibly through the root and anterior surface of the iris. Normal aqueous contains approximately 0.02 g of protein per 100 mL, as compared with the typical plasma level of 7 g per 100 mL. The most abundant plasma proteins identified in aqueous humor are albumin and transferrin, which together may account for 50% of the total protein content.

However, there is compelling evidence that the proteins that make up the aqueous humor might actually have been synthesized within the ciliary body and secreted directly into the aqueous humor. Molecular techniques (such as the screening of complementary DNA [cDNA] libraries constructed from intact human and bovine ciliary bodies) have enabled the isolation and identification of numerous protein-encoding genes. These studies, therefore, challenge the long-held view that plasma proteins in the aqueous humor are transported into the aqueous from outside the eye. Among the cDNA molecules isolated from the ciliary body–encoding plasma proteins are

- complement component C4, which participates in immune-mediated inflammation responses
- α_2-macroglobulin, a carrier protein that is involved in proteinase inhibition, clearance, and targeting, as well as the processing of foreign peptides
- apolipoprotein D, which binds and transports hydrophobic substances, including cholesterol, cholesteryl esters, and arachidonic acid (AA)
- selenoprotein P, which has antioxidant properties

Proteinases and inhibitors

Several proteinases and proteinase inhibitors have also been identified in the aqueous humor. The proteinases include cathepsin D and cathepsin O, which are synthesized and secreted by the ciliary epithelial cells. Cathepsin D is involved in the degradation of neuropeptides and peptide hormones and has been found in high levels in the cerebrospinal fluid of patients with Alzheimer disease. Less is known about cathepsin O, which may be involved in normal cellular protein degradation and turnover. Of the proteinase inhibitors, α_2-macroglobulin and α_1-antitrypsin are perhaps the most extensively studied. An imbalance in equilibrium between proteinases and proteinase inhibitors could alter aqueous humor composition, which may cause disease (eg, glaucoma).

Enzymes

Activators, proenzymes, and fibrinolytic enzymes are present in the aqueous and could play a role in the regulation of outflow resistance. Both plasminogen and plasminogen activator are found in human and monkey aqueous, but only traces of plasmin have been reported.

Neurotrophic and neuroendocrine proteins

The ciliary epithelia, which are derived from neuroectoderm, are functionally similar to neuroendocrine glands elsewhere in the body. Bioactive neuroendocrine markers, identified through human ciliary body cDNA subtraction studies, include neurotensin, angiotensin, endothelins, and natriuretic peptides; these markers are known to have systemic vascular hemodynamic effects and, by implication, may have similar roles in IOP regulation or aqueous secretion. Some authors have linked circadian IOP rhythms to these markers, but this hypothesis has not been proven because corneal biomechanical properties also fluctuate. The neuroendocrine properties of the ciliary epithelium may also determine the composition of the aqueous humor.

Growth-Modulatory Factors

The physical and chemical properties of the aqueous humor play a substantial role in modulating the proliferation, differentiation, functional viability, and wound healing of ocular tissues. These properties are largely influenced by several growth-promoting and differentiation factors that have been identified or quantified in aqueous humor, including

- transforming growth factor βs 1 and 2 (TGF-β_1 and -β_2)
- acidic and basic fibroblast growth factors (aFGF and bFGF)
- insulin-like growth factor I (IGF-I)
- insulin-like growth factor binding proteins (IGFBPs)
- vascular endothelial growth factors (VEGFs)
- transferrin

The growth factors in the aqueous humor perform diverse, synergistic, and sometimes opposite biological activities. Normally, the lack of significant mitosis of the corneal endothelium and trabecular meshwork in vivo is probably controlled by the complex coordination of effects and interactions among the different growth-modulatory substances present in the aqueous humor (see Part V, Ocular Pharmacology). Disruption in the balance among various growth factors, which occurs with the production of plasmoid aqueous humor, may explain the abnormal hyperplastic response of the lens epithelium and corneal endothelium observed in chronic inflammatory conditions and traumatic insults to the eye. Ultimately, however, the effect of a given growth factor on the aqueous humor is determined primarily by the growth factor's bioavailability. Bioavailability, in turn, depends on many factors, including the expression of receptors on target tissues, interactive effects of the growth factor with components of the extracellular matrix, and the levels of circulating and matrix-bound proteases.

The role of several growth factors has been studied in patients with diabetes mellitus. Levels of IGFBPs are elevated fivefold in patients with diabetes mellitus without retinopathy, and IGF-I levels are elevated in patients with diabetic retinopathy. These elevations suggest that the increase in vitreal IGFBPs is not the result of preexisting end-stage retinopathy but rather is an early ocular event in the diabetic process.

Vascular Endothelial Growth Factors

The VEGF family of glycoproteins includes VEGF-A, -B, -C, and -D, as well as placental growth factor (PlGF). VEGF-A, which has 9 isoforms, is the most thoroughly studied at present; it is the only VEGF family member induced by hypoxia, and it is a crucial regulator of angiogenesis and a potent inducer of vascular permeability. Three VEGF receptors (VEGFRs) have been identified:

1. VEGFR1, which has both positive and negative angiogenic effects
2. VEGFR2, which is the primary mediator of the mitogenic, angiogenic, and vascular permeability effects of VEGF-A
3. VEGFR3, which mediates the angiogenic effects on lymphatic vessels

Although most studied in relation to the vascular endothelium, VEGF-A and its receptors are also present in other tissues and organ systems, a finding that underscores other possible physiologic roles. VEGF may also be involved in retinal leukostasis and neuroprotection.

VEGF-A levels are increased not only in patients with active ocular neovascularization from proliferative diabetic retinopathy but also after occlusion of the central retinal vein and with iris neovascularization. The expression of VEGF-A is increased by hypoxia in retinal endothelial cells, retinal pericytes, Müller cells, and retinal pigment epithelium (RPE) cells. In addition, a soluble VEGF-dependent mechanism has been shown to mediate RPE barrier dysfunction in cocultures of RPE with endothelial cells (ECs). This EC–RPE contact-induced disruption of barrier properties occurs in ocular conditions such as choroidal neovascularization, wherein ECs pass through the Bruch membrane and contact the RPE. Also, aqueous VEGF-A levels increase in response to anterior segment ischemia in animal models, in addition to the well-described response to retinal hypoxia.

Bhisitkul RB. Vascular endothelial growth factor biology: clinical implications for ocular treatments. *Br J Ophthalmol.* 2006;90(12):1542–1547.

Oxygen and Carbon Dioxide

Oxygen is present in the aqueous humor at a partial pressure of approximately 55 mm Hg, roughly one-third of its concentration in the atmosphere. It is derived from the blood supply to the ciliary body and iris, as there is no net flux of oxygen from the atmosphere across the cornea. Indeed, the corneal endothelium depends critically on the aqueous oxygen supply for the active fluid-transport mechanism that maintains corneal transparency. The lens and the endothelial lining of the trabecular meshwork also derive their oxygen supply from the aqueous humor.

The carbon dioxide content of the aqueous humor ranges from about 40 to 60 mm Hg, contributing approximately 3% of the total bicarbonate. The relative proportions of carbon dioxide and bicarbonate determine the pH of the aqueous, which in most species ranges between 7.5 and 7.6. Carbon dioxide is continuously lost from the aqueous by diffusion across the cornea into the tear film and atmosphere. The Na^+,K^+-Cl^- cotransporter is also important both in the trabecular meshwork and for control of aqueous outflow.

Gong H, Tripathi RC, Tripathi BJ. Morphology of the aqueous outflow pathway. *Microsc Res Tech.* 1996;33(4):336–367.

Clinical Implications of Breakdown of the Blood–Aqueous Barrier

With compromise of the blood–aqueous barrier in conditions such as ocular insult (trauma or intraocular surgery), as well as uveitis and other inflammatory disorders, the protein content of aqueous humor may increase 10–100 times, especially in the high-molecular-weight polypeptides. The levels of inflammatory mediators, immunoglobulins, fibrin, and proteases rise, and the balance among the various growth factors is disrupted (see Chapter 16). The clinical sequelae include fibrinous exudate and clot (with or without a macrophage reaction and formation of cyclitic membranes) and synechiae formation (peripheral and posterior), as well as an abnormal neovascular response, which further exacerbates breakdown of the barrier. Chronic disruption of the blood–aqueous barrier is implicated in the abnormal hyperplastic response of the lens epithelium, corneal endothelium, trabecular meshwork, and iris, and in the formation of complicated cataracts. Degenerative and proliferative changes may occur in various ocular structures as well. The use of anti-inflammatory steroidal and nonsteroidal drugs, cycloplegics, protease activators or inhibitors, growth factor and anti–growth factor agents, and even surgical intervention may be necessary to combat these events.

Introduction to the Iris and Ciliary Body

The iris and ciliary body are the anterior parts of the *uveal tract*, which is continuous with the choroid posteriorly. The iris is a highly pigmented tissue that functions as a movable diaphragm between the anterior and posterior chambers of the eye to regulate the amount of light that reaches the retina. It is a delicate, dynamic structure that can make precise and rapid changes in pupillary diameter in response to both light and specific pharmacologic stimuli. The ciliary body produces and regulates the composition of the aqueous humor and thus directly influences the ionic environment and metabolism of the lens, cornea, and trabecular meshwork.

Unlike smooth muscle elsewhere in the body, which is derived from mesoderm, the smooth muscle in the iris and ciliary body is derived from neuroectoderm. The biochemistry of the smooth muscles of the iris is characterized by the following:

- contraction–relaxation
- receptor characteristics
- second-messenger formation and regulation
- protein phosphorylation
- phospholipid metabolism
- arachidonic acid release and eicosanoid biosynthesis

The ciliary body is the main pharmacologic target in the treatment of glaucoma. Many treatments employed to lower IOP in glaucoma, such as adrenergic and cholinergic drugs and PGs, work through receptors and their respective signal transduction pathways. The iris–ciliary body is rich in many types of receptors that bind to various agonists and antagonists, including adrenergic, muscarinic cholinergic, and peptidergic; PG; serotonin; platelet-activating factor; and growth factor receptors.

The following discussion concerns biochemical aspects of the iris–ciliary body such as eicosanoids and various receptors. Chapter 2 of this volume discusses and illustrates the various structures mentioned in this chapter.

Eicosanoids

Types and Actions

Eicosanoids, which include PGs, prostacyclin (also known as *prostaglandin I_2 [PGI_2]*), thromboxanes (eg, thromboxane A_2 [TXA_2]), and leukotrienes, are an important family of compounds with hormonal activity. They are synthesized as a result of PLA_2 stimulation, which causes the release of AA from membrane glycerolipids (Fig 9-1). These agents affect both male and female reproductive systems, the gastrointestinal system, the cardiovascular and renal systems, the nervous system, and the eye. PGI_2 and TXA_2 are natural biological antagonists. PGI_2, which is synthesized mainly in the endothelial cells of vascular tissues, is a potent vasodilator, a potent platelet-antiaggregating agent, and a stimulator of adenylate cyclase. In contrast, TXA_2, which is synthesized mainly by platelets, is a potent vasoconstrictor and a platelet-aggregating agent.

Prostaglandins have profound effects on inflammation in the eye, aqueous humor dynamics, and blood–ocular barrier functions. Arachidonic acid and PGs of the E and F subtypes, when administered intracamerally or topically at high concentrations, cause miosis, an elevation of IOP, an increase in aqueous protein content, and the entry of white cells into the aqueous and tear fluid. Evidence indicates that some antiglaucoma drugs, such as epinephrine, may affect IOP by influencing the production of PGs. Prostaglandins and their derivatives have been found to be useful as antiglaucoma agents. For example, several PGF_2 receptor agonists (latanoprost, bimatoprost, travoprost, and tafluprost) decrease IOP by 27%–35%. Unlike β-blockers, carbonic anhydrase inhibitors,

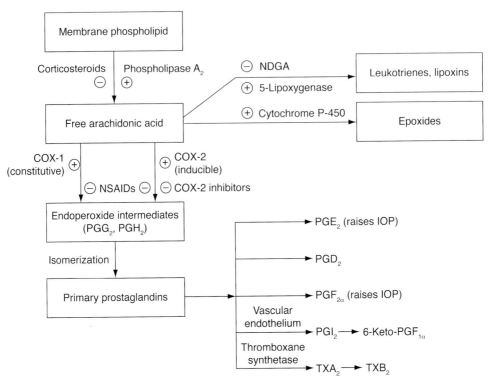

Figure 9-1 An outline of the synthesis of prostaglandins (PGs) and leukotrienes from arachidonic acid. In response to stimulation of a target cell with a relevant stimulus (eg, a cytokine, a neurotransmitter, various pharmacologic agents), phospholipase A_2 (PLA$_2$) is activated, and arachidonic acid is released from the *sn*-2 position of membrane phospholipids. Arachidonic acid is then converted by cyclooxygenase 1 (COX-1) or cyclooxygenase 2 (COX-2) to prostaglandin H_2 (PGH$_2$), and then PGH$_2$ is isomerized to biologically active prostanoid products. Arachidonic acid can also be metabolized through the 5-lipoxygenase and cytochrome P-450 pathways to generate leukotrienes and epoxides, respectively. PLA$_2$ can be inhibited by corticosteroids such as dexamethasone; COX-1, by nonsteroidal anti-inflammatory drugs (NSAIDs) such as indomethacin and aspirin; COX-2, by DUP697, SC58125, L-745-337, and NS398; and the 5-lipoxygenase pathway, by nordihydroguaiaretic acid (NDGA). IOP = intraocular pressure; PGD$_2$ = prostaglandin D$_2$; PGE$_2$ = prostaglandin E$_2$; PGF$_{1\alpha}$ = prostaglandin F$_{1\alpha}$; PGF$_{2\alpha}$ = prostaglandin F$_{2\alpha}$; PGG$_2$ = prostaglandin G$_2$; PGI$_2$ = prostaglandin I$_2$; TXA$_2$ = thromboxane A$_2$; TXB$_2$ = thromboxane B$_2$. *(Courtesy of Ata Abdel-Latif, PhD.)*

and α_2-agonists, PG analogues act on enhancement of outflow rather than on formation of aqueous humor.

Synthesis

Arachidonic acid can be released from plasma membrane phospholipids through a wide variety of stimuli: inflammatory, immunologic, neural, chemical, or simple mechanical agitation. Free AA reacts either with cyclooxygenase (also known as *PG synthetase*), the first enzyme of the PG biosynthetic sequence, or with lipoxygenase to generate hydroperoxy fatty acids (see Fig 9-1). Note that these enzymes are 2 isoforms of cyclooxygenase (COX-1 and COX-2). In the cyclooxygenase reaction, the released arachidonate is converted into endoperoxides (prostaglandin G_2 [PGG_2] and prostaglandin H_2 [PGH_2]) by the membrane-bound cyclooxygenase. The endoperoxides are then converted to TXA_2 by thromboxane synthetase or to various PGs by isomerase or reductase enzymes.

Most nonsteroidal anti-inflammatory drugs (NSAIDs), such as indomethacin and aspirin, can block PG biosynthesis from AA via the COX-1 reaction. The NSAIDs bind irreversibly to the cyclooxygenase enzyme. Topical NSAIDs have been used in the treatment of anterior segment inflammation, aphakic and pseudophakic cystoid macular edema, allergic conjunctivitis, and other sources of pain after refractive surgery. Topical NSAID drops such as flurbiprofen, 0.03%, and suprofen, 1%, are used preoperatively for the prevention of PG-mediated pupillary miosis during ocular surgery. Diclofenac, 0.1%, has been approved for the treatment of postoperative inflammation following cataract extraction. Ketorolac tromethamine, 0.5%, is indicated for the relief of itching from allergic conjunctivitis.

Prostaglandin biosynthesis, via the COX-2 reaction, can also be blocked by COX-2 inhibitors. Previously developed NSAIDs (eg, ibuprofen, naproxen) inhibit both COX-1 and COX-2 and compete with arachidonate in binding to the cyclooxygenase-active site. These compounds are effective anti-inflammatory drugs, but all of them are also quite ulcerogenic when administered systemically. In response, pharmaceutical companies have developed new cyclooxygenase inhibitors that selectively inhibit COX-2 while sparing inhibition of COX-1. These efforts were initially driven by 2 hypotheses that subsequently proved to be correct:

1. COX-2 is the relevant enzyme in inflammation (it is expressed at low levels under normal physiologic conditions and regulated only in response to pro-inflammatory signals).
2. Constitutively expressed COX-1 (but not COX-2) is present in various tissues (including the inner lining of the stomach).

COX-2 inhibitors are, indeed, anti-inflammatory and analgesic, and they lack gastrointestinal toxicity. Moreover, they provide time-dependent, reversible inhibition of the COX-2 enzyme. Oral COX-2 inhibitors, including rofecoxib, celecoxib, and valdecoxib, however, increase risks of cardiovascular toxicity and complications (eg, myocardial infarction).

Prostaglandin Receptors

There is a large family of G-protein–coupled, 7-transmembrane PG receptors. Complex specificity and regulatory functions arise because individual receptors have differing and overlapping specificities for individual PGs; they are specifically distributed among different cells and tissues; and there are different coupling mechanisms in different cells. Because of the variety of PGs and the variability in PG receptors, as explained earlier, the pathophysiologic functions for most PGs are very complicated and remain incompletely understood.

In general, PGs play key roles in

- regulation of smooth-muscle contractility
- mediation of pain and fever
- regulation of blood pressure and platelet aggregation
- other physiologic defense mechanisms, including immune and inflammatory responses

Inhibition of cyclooxygenases, and therefore PGs, is the mechanism underlying many of the analgesic, anti-inflammatory, antipyretic, and antithrombotic effects of NSAIDs.

Abdel-Latif AA. Release and effects of prostaglandins in ocular tissues. *Prostaglandins Leukot Essent Fatty Acids.* 1991;44(2):71–82.

Colin J. The role of NSAIDs in the management of postoperative ophthalmic inflammation. *Drugs.* 2007;67(9):1291–1308.

Drazen JM. COX-2 inhibitors—a lesson in unexpected problems. *N Engl J Med.* 2005;352(11): 1131–1132.

Ocular Receptors

Table 16-5 provides examples of ocular receptors, their subtypes, and their signal transduction mechanisms. Numerous reports have been published on the biochemical and pharmacologic characterization of these receptors. Understanding ocular receptors and their transduction mechanisms has played a significant role in the development of ocular pharmaceutical agents for the treatment of glaucoma. (See Chapter 16 for further discussion on this topic.) Current applications can be appreciated from the summary of the modes of action of various antiglaucoma agents provided in Table 16-7.

CHAPTER 10

Lens

The lens is a transparent, avascular body that, in concert with the cornea, focuses incident light onto the sensory elements of the retina. To do so, the lens must be transparent and must have an index of refraction higher than that of the surrounding fluids. Maintenance of transparency depends on the precise organization of the cellular structure of the lens. Transparency must be maintained while the lens changes shape during accommodation. The high refractive index is due to the presence of a high concentration of proteins—especially of the soluble proteins called *crystallins*—in the lens cells. Furthermore, because there is little if any turnover of protein in the central region of the lens (where the oldest, denucleated cells are found), the proteins of the human lens must be extremely stable to remain functionally viable for a lifetime. Considering the lens's mode of growth and the stresses to which the lens is chronically exposed, it is remarkable that in most people, lenses retain good transparency. However, humans typically do develop visually significant opacities by their sixth or seventh decade of life.

This chapter discusses the structure and composition of the lens, as well as aspects of membrane function, metabolism, and regulatory processes within the lens. BCSC Section 11, *Lens and Cataract,* provides additional information about both the lens and cataractogenesis.

Structure of the Lens

Capsule

The lens is enclosed in an elastic basement membrane called the *lens capsule* (Fig 10-1). The capsule is noncellular and is composed primarily of type IV collagen; it contains smaller amounts of other collagens and extracellular matrix components (including glycosaminoglycans, laminin, fibronectin, and heparan sulfate proteoglycan). The capsule is a very thick basement membrane, particularly on the anterior side of the lens, where the epithelial cells continue to secrete capsular material throughout life. On the posterior side of the lens, where there is no epithelium, the posterior fiber cells have limited capacity to secrete such material. The zonular fibers, from which the lens is suspended, insert into the capsule near the equator on both the anterior and posterior sides. The capsule is not a barrier to diffusion of water, ions, other small molecules, or proteins up to the size of serum albumin (which has a molecular weight of 68,000).

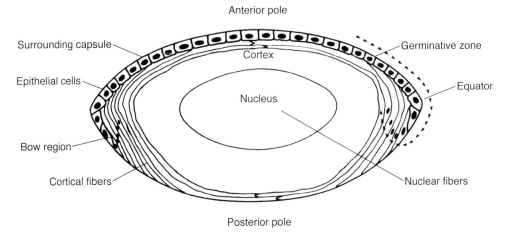

Figure 10-1 The mammalian lens in schematic cross section. The *small arrowheads* indicate the direction of cell migration from the epithelium to the cortex. *(Reproduced with permission from Anderson RE, ed.* Biochemistry of the Eye. *San Francisco: American Academy of Ophthalmology; 1983:112.)*

Epithelium

A single layer of epithelial cells covers the anterior surface of the lens. These cells have full metabolic capacity and play the primary role in regulating the water and ion balance of the entire lens. Although the cells of the central epithelium are not mitotically active, a germinative zone exists as a ring anterior to the equator, where the epithelial cells divide. The new cells migrate toward the equator and begin to differentiate into lens fibers.

Cortex and Nucleus

Aside from the single layer of epithelial cells on its anterior surface, the lens is composed of lens fibers, which are very long ribbonlike cells. All fibers are formed from epithelial cells at the lens equator; therefore, younger fibers are always exterior to older ones. The lens structure can be equated with the growth rings of a tree: the oldest cells are in the center, and the progressively younger layers, or shells, of fiber cells are toward the periphery. Unlike the case with many tissues, no cells are sloughed from the lens, and cells produced before birth remain at the center of the lens throughout life.

As new fiber cells elongate and differentiate into mature fibers, their cell nuclei form the *bow zone,* or *bow region,* at the lens equator. Elongating fibers substantially increase their volume and surface area and express large amounts of both lens crystallins and a lens-fiber–specific membrane protein called the *major intrinsic protein (MIP).* As the fibers become fully elongated and make sutures at each end with fibers that have elongated from the opposite side of the lens, they become mature, terminally differentiated fiber cells. The cell nuclei disintegrate, as do mitochondria and other organelles. This process occurs abruptly through mechanisms that remain obscure. What is understood is that the elimination of cellular organelles is necessary in the central portion of the lens because such bodies are sufficiently large to scatter light and thereby degrade visual acuity. Also, with the loss of cell nuclei, the mature fibers lose the machinery required for the synthesis of proteins. The fiber mass of the adult lens can be divided into the *cortex* (ie, the outer fibers, laid down after the age of approximately 20 years) and the *internal nucleus* (ie, the cells produced from embryogenesis through adolescence).

Chemical Composition of the Lens

Membranes

The chemical composition of lens-fiber plasma membranes suggests that they are both very stable and very rigid. A high content of saturated fatty acids, a high cholesterol to phospholipid ratio, and a high concentration of sphingomyelin all contribute to the tight packing and low fluidity of the membrane. Although lipids make up only about 1% of the total lens mass, they constitute approximately 55% of the plasma membrane's dry weight; cholesterol is the major neutral lipid. As the lens ages, the protein to lipid and cholesterol to phospholipid ratios increase as a result of phospholipid loss, especially in the nucleus.

Lens Proteins

The lens probably has the highest protein content of any tissue. In some species, more than 50% of lens weight is protein. Lens crystallins, a diverse group of proteins that are abundantly expressed in the lens-fiber cells and are thought to play crucial roles in providing the transparency and refractile properties essential to lens function, constitute 90%–95% of total lens protein. In addition to the crystallins, the lens has a full complement of enzymes and regulatory proteins that are present primarily in the epithelium and in immature fiber cells, where most metabolic activity occurs.

Crystallins

Crystallins are water-soluble proteins so named for their high abundance in the crystalline lens. Until the 1980s, crystallins were considered lens-specific proteins lacking biological activity; they were seen as highly evolved structural elements forming the transparent protein matrix of the lens. It is now clear that most crystallins are expressed in other tissues as well and have specific biological functions that are distinct from their roles in the lens as refractile elements.

All crystallins now appear to be "borrowed" proteins, recruited by the lens for a function that is completely distinct from their biological roles in other tissues. Although the specific criteria that make a protein suitable to function as a crystallin are not well understood, crystallins must have 2 obvious attributes:

1. They must be very stable structures because the proteins of the lens are probably the longest-lived proteins in the body.
2. Crystallins must remain soluble under conditions of high protein concentration without forming large aggregates, which would be light-scattering centers within the lens.

Crystallins can be divided into 2 groups. One group includes α-crystallin and the β,γ-crystallin family, both of which seem to be present in all vertebrate lenses. The second group consists of the taxon-specific crystallins, each of which is present only in phylogenetically restricted groups of species.

Andley UP. Crystallins in the eye: function and pathology. *Prog Retin Eye Res.* 2007;26(1): 78–98.

α-Crystallin α-Crystallin, the largest of the crystallins, has a native molecular mass ranging between 600 and 800 kD. It is composed of 2 subunits, αA and αB, which have a mass of approximately 20 kD and are nearly 55% identical in sequence. Native α-crystallin has a wide range of molecular masses, apparently because it is a dynamic structure wherein the number of subunits varies somewhat and subunit exchange occurs among the native multimers. Probably because of this molecular-mass variability, α-crystallin has thus far resisted attempts at crystallization, so a definitive 3-dimensional structure for this molecule has not been determined.

α-Crystallin is a member of the small heat-shock protein family; as such, the expression of αB is inducible by heat and other stresses. Both αA and αB have a chaperone-like activity through which they bind proteins that are beginning to denature and prevent further denaturation and aggregation. Zinc ions enhance the chaperone function and stability of α-crystallin. Because protein aggregates in the lens scatter light and cause loss of transparency, the antiaggregative function of α-crystallin is crucial to the long-term maintenance of transparency in the fibers of the lens nucleus, where synthesis of new protein is impossible and protein molecules must exist for decades.

β,γ-Crystallins Until the primary sequences of the various β- and γ-crystallins were determined, they were thought to be 2 unrelated families of proteins. However, the 2 groups are now known to be related members of the same protein superfamily. The β-crystallins, a complex group of oligomers composed of polypeptides, have molecular masses ranging from 23 to 32 kD.

The γ-crystallins are monomeric proteins with molecular masses near 20 kD. Most expression of γ-crystallins occurs early in development; thus, they tend to be most concentrated in the nuclear region of the lens. Given their compact and symmetric structures (which can pack very densely), γ-crystallins tend to be highly concentrated in aged, hard lenses, which have little to no accommodative ability.

Although no specific biological functions for the β- and γ-crystallins have been identified, at least some are expressed outside the lens, suggesting that such functions do exist. Members of the superfamily have also been identified in microorganisms, where they are expressed during spore or cyst formation (suggesting a possible role in stress response).

Taxon-specific crystallins In addition to the α-crystallin and β,γ-crystallins found in all vertebrate lenses, other proteins are abundantly expressed in various phylogenetic groups. Most taxon-specific crystallins are oxidoreductases, which bind pyridine nucleotides, and their presence in the lens significantly increases the concentration of the bound nucleotides. Reduced nucleotides absorb ultraviolet (UV) light and may protect the retina from UV-induced oxidation.

Cytoskeletal and membrane proteins

Although most proteins in the normal lens are water-soluble, several important structural proteins can be solubilized only in the presence of chaotropic agents or detergents. These water-soluble proteins include the cytoskeletal elements *actin* (actin filaments), *vimentin* (intermediated filaments), and *tubulin* (microtubules), as well as 2 additional proteins called *filensin* and *phakinin*. The last 2 proteins have been found only in lens-fiber cells and compose a cytoskeletal structure, the *beaded filament*, which is unique to the lens. The filamentous structures of the cytoskeleton provide structural support to the cells and play crucial roles in processes such as differentiation, motility and shape change, and organization of the cytoplasm.

Lens-fiber membranes have 1 quantitatively dominant protein, MIP (discussed earlier in this chapter), which has received a great deal of attention. MIP is expressed only in lens-fiber cells and was earlier thought to be a gap-junction protein; in fact, it is not a connexin but rather an aquaporin, a member of a large, diverse family of proteins involved in regulating water transport. Current data suggest that MIP functions as a water channel.

Posttranslational modifications to lens proteins

As indicated, the proteins of the lens are probably the longest-lived in the body; the oldest ones (in the center of the lens nucleus) are synthesized before birth. As would be expected, these proteins become structurally modified in various ways: oxidation of sulfur and aromatic residue side chains, inter- and intrapolypeptide crosslinking, glycation, racemization, phosphorylation, deamidation, and carbamylation. Many of these modifications occur early in life and are probably part of a programmed modification of the crystallins that is required for their long-term stability and functionality. There is evidence that certain of these processes (phosphorylation, thiol oxidation) are reversible and may serve a regulatory function, although this hypothesis remains to be proved.

What is known is that as the proteins age (particularly in some cataracts), certain oxidative modifications accumulate, which contributes to the crosslinking of crystallin polypeptides, alterations in fluorescent properties, and an increase in protein-associated pigmentation. In particular, the formation of disulfide crosslinks in the proteins of the lens nuclear region is associated with the formation of protein aggregates, light scattering, and cataract.

Physiologic Aspects of the Lens

Because of its avascularity and its mode of growth, the lens faces some unusual physiologic challenges. All nutrients must be obtained from the surrounding fluids. Likewise, all waste products must be released into those fluids. Most of the cells of the adult lens have reduced metabolic activity and lack the membrane machinery to regulate ionic homeostasis independently. Elucidating how the lens maintains ionic balance and how solutes move from cell to cell throughout the lens is crucial to understanding the normal biology of the organ as well as the process of cataractogenesis.

In the normal lens, sodium levels are low (~10 mmol/L) and potassium high (~120 mmol/L); in the aqueous humor, sodium levels are approximately 150 mmol/L and potassium approximately 5 mmol/L. When normal regulatory mechanisms are abrogated, potassium leaks out of the lens and sodium floods in, followed by chloride. Water then enters in response to the osmotic gradient, causing loss of transparency by disrupting the normally smooth gradient of refractive index. The ionic balance in the lens is maintained primarily by the Na^+,K^+-ATPase pump, an intrinsic membrane protein complex that hydrolyzes adenosine triphosphate (ATP) to transport sodium out of and potassium into the lens. Functional Na^+,K^+-ATPase pumps are found primarily at the anterior surface of the lens, in the epithelium and the outer, immature fibers. Studies using ouabain, a specific inhibitor of the pump, have established the pump's role as the primary determinant of the normal ionic state of the lens. Lens cells also contain membrane channels that pass ions; in particular, K^+-selective channels have been studied by patch-clamp techniques and found to be present primarily in the epithelial cells.

Communication between lens cells is provided by gap junctions, which are thought to account for most ion and small-molecule movement between cells. True gap junctions occur in the lens and are composed of members of the connexin family. Junctions between epithelial cells are composed of connexin 43; fiber–fiber gap junctions contain connexins 46 and 50. MIP also forms junctionlike structures, although these apparently do not provide direct communication from cell to cell.

Within the fiber mass, gap-junctional coupling is greatest in the outer layers of the lens, where the junctions can be uncoupled by lowering the pH. In the lens nuclear region, such uncoupling does not occur. This finding supports the idea that the lens nucleus may be a syncytium, resulting from membrane fusion between adjacent fibers.

Lens Metabolism and Formation of Sugar Cataracts

Energy Production

Energy, in the form of ATP, is produced in the lens primarily through anaerobic glycolysis in metabolically active cells in the anterior lens. This process is necessitated by the fact that the oxygen tension in the lens is much lower than that in other tissues, given that oxygen reaches the avascular lens only via diffusion from the aqueous humor.

Most of the glucose entering the lens is phosphorylated to glucose-6-phosphate by hexokinase, the rate-limiting enzyme of the glycolytic pathway. Under normal conditions, most glucose-6-phosphate passes through glycolysis, wherein 2 molecules of ATP are formed per original molecule of glucose. A small proportion of glucose-6-phosphate is metabolized through the pentose phosphate pathway (hexose monophosphate shunt). This pathway is activated under conditions of oxidative stress because it is responsible for replenishing the supply of nicotinamide adenine dinucleotide phosphate (NADPH) that becomes oxidized through the increased activity of glutathione reductase under such conditions.

Carbohydrate Cataracts

Much research on lens carbohydrate metabolism has been stimulated by interest in *"sugar" cataracts*, which are associated with diabetes mellitus and galactosemia. True diabetic cataract is a rapidly developing bilateral "snowflake" cataract (see BCSC Section 11, *Lens and Cataract*, Chapter 5, Fig 5-16) that appears in the lens cortex of patients with poorly controlled type 1 diabetes mellitus. People with type 2 diabetes mellitus do not typically develop this type of cataract but do have a higher prevalence of age-related cataract with a slightly earlier onset. It is likely that for these patients, the diabetes mellitus is simply an additional factor contributing to the development of age-related cataracts.

Defects in galactose metabolism also cause sugar cataracts. Classic galactosemia is caused by a deficiency of galactose-1-phosphate uridyltransferase. Infants with this inborn error of metabolism develop bilateral cataracts within a few weeks of birth unless milk (lactose) is removed from the diet. Cataracts are also associated with a deficiency of galactokinase. Under certain conditions in which sugar levels are elevated significantly, some glucose (or galactose) is metabolized through the polyol pathway (Fig 10-2). Aldose reductase is the key enzyme for the pathway, and it converts the sugars into the corresponding sugar alcohols. Because aldose reductase has a very high K_m (apparent affinity constant) value for glucose (or galactose), under normal conditions little or no activity occurs through this pathway. Under hyperglycemic conditions, however, aldose reductase competes with hexokinase for glucose (or galactose).

Studies using animal models have established the importance of the polyol pathway in experimental sugar cataracts. Animals with diabetes mellitus (either natural or induced) develop cataracts that are associated with the presence of sorbitol in the lens and with the influx of water. The osmotic hypothesis may account for these findings. This hypothesis considers the activity of aldose reductase central to the pathology by serving to increase the sorbitol content of the lens. Sorbitol is largely unable to penetrate cell membranes

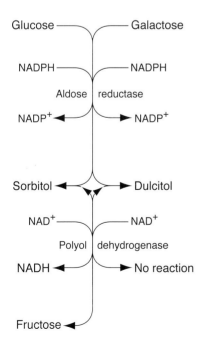

Figure 10-2 Polyol pathway for glucose and galactose metabolism. The reduction of glucose and galactose to sorbitol and dulcitol, respectively, is catalyzed by aldose reductase; the reduced form of nicotinamide adenine dinucleotide phosphate (NADPH) serves as cofactor. Subsequently, sorbitol (dulcitol is not a substrate) is oxidized to fructose, a reaction catalyzed by polyol dehydrogenase using nicotinamide adenine dinucleotide (NAD$^+$) as cofactor. This step is reversible in the human lens, as indicated by the *arrows*. NADH = reduced form of NAD$^+$; NADP$^+$ = nicotinamide adenine dinucleotide phosphate.

and thus is trapped inside the cells. Because its further conversion to fructose by polyol dehydrogenase is slow, sorbitol builds up in lens cells under conditions of hyperglycemia such that it creates an osmotic pressure that draws water into the lens, swelling the cells, damaging membranes, and causing cataract.

Mathias RT, Rae JL, Baldo GJ. Physiological properties of the normal lens. *Physiol Rev.* 1997; 77(1):21–50.

Piatigorsky J, Hejtmancik JF. In: Albert DM, Miller JW, Azar DT, Blodi BA, eds. *Albert & Jakobiec's Principles and Practice of Ophthalmology.* 3rd ed. Philadelphia: Elsevier Saunders; 2008:chap 105.

Quinlan RA, Sandilands A, Procter JE, et al. The eye lens cytoskeleton. *Eye.* 1999;13(Pt 3b): 409–416.

Slingsby C, Clout NJ. Structure of the crystallins. *Eye.* 1999;13(Pt 3b):395–402.

CHAPTER 11

Vitreous

The vitreous body is a specialized connective tissue whose postembryologic functions include

- serving as a transparent gel occupying the major volume of the globe
- acting as a conduit for nutrients and other solutes to and from the lens

The basic physical structure of the vitreous is that of a gel composed of a collagen framework interspersed with hydrated hyaluronan, also known as *hyaluronic acid,* molecules. The hyaluronan contributes to the viscosity of the vitreous humor and is thought to help stabilize the collagen network, although most of the hyaluronan can be removed enzymatically without collapse of the gel.

The relative amounts of collagen apparently determine whether the vitreous is a liquid or gel; the rigidity of the gel is greatest in regions of highest collagen concentration. The collagen fibrils confer resistance to tensile forces and give plasticity to the vitreous; the hyaluronan resists compression and confers viscoelastic properties.

Composition

The vitreous contains approximately 98% water and 0.15% macromolecules, including collagen, hyaluronan, and soluble proteins. The remainder of the solid matter consists of ions and low-molecular-weight solutes. In addition to the 2 major structural components of collagen and hyaluronan, several noncollagenous structural proteins and glycoproteins have been identified in the vitreous; these components include versican, link protein, fibulin-1, nidogen-1, fibronectin, and 2 novel glycoproteins—opticin and VIT1. Opticin and VIT1 were initially identified after extraction of a pellet of collagen fibrils obtained from bovine vitreous after centrifugation. The human vitreous also contains hyaluronidase and at least 1 matrix metalloproteinase (MMP-2, or *gelatinase*), suggesting that turnover of vitreous structural macromolecules can occur.

Collagen

Vitreous collagen fibrils are composed of 3 different collagen types:

1. *Type II,* which forms the major component of the fibrils
2. *Type IX,* which is located on the surface of the fibril
3. *Type V/XI,* which has an unconfirmed location that may allow its amino terminus to project from the surface of the fibril (Fig 11-1)

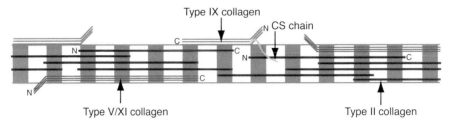

Figure 11-1 Model for the structure of a collagen fibril from the vitreous. Note that 3 different collagen types (II, IX, and V/XI) are assembled to form the fibril. Type II collagen, which forms the major structure of the vitreous, is staggered to form overlap and gap regions. Type IX collagen is located on the surface of the fibril and oriented such that part of the molecule projects from the surface. It is in an antiparallel direction compared with the type II collagen molecules. Type IX collagen also has a single chondroitin sulfate (CS) chain that may project from the surface of the fibril. Type V/XI collagen is also located close to the surface of the fibril with a part of the molecule projecting from the gap region. However, the location of this molecule is controversial; other models suggest it is located in the center of the fibril, where it may form a microfibril. C = carboxyl terminus; N = amino terminus. *(Adapted from Olsen BR. New insights into the function of collagens from genetic analysis.* Curr Opin Cell Biol. *1995;7(5):720–727.)*

At present, 19 types of collagen are known, and the genes for several more have been identified. Type V/XI collagen is unique to the vitreous in that native triple-helical molecules can be isolated that contain the α_1 (XI) and α_2 (V) chains. The vitreous collagens are closely related to the collagens of hyaline cartilage. They differ from the types I, III, XII, and XIV collagens commonly found in scar tissue and in tissues such as dermis, cornea, and sclera.

The collagen fibrils of the vitreous are only loosely attached to the internal limiting membrane (ILM) of the retina; however, at the vitreous base, the fibrils are firmly anchored to the peripheral retina and pars plana, as well as to the margins of the optic disc. Fibronectin and laminin mediate the interaction of cortical vitreous collagen with the ILM (Fig 11-2).

The origin of vitreous collagen in mammals is not well established. In vitro, human retinal Müller cell lines synthesize collagens of the vitreous–vitreoretinal interface. It has been shown in the chicken that during early development, the cells of the neural retina synthesize and probably secrete type II collagen. However, other cells (possibly hyalocytes) that are present within the vitreous cavity may also contribute. In the developing chicken eye, in situ hybridization of the retina initially yields positive results for type II collagen, whereas transcripts for type IX collagen are present only in the region of the ciliary body. Later in development, type II collagen mRNA also becomes localized only to the presumptive ciliary region. The origin of type V/XI collagen within the vitreous is unknown.

Hyaluronan

Hyaluronan is a polysaccharide (glycosaminoglycan) that has a repeating unit of glucuronic acid and N-acetylglucosamine. At physiologic pH, hyaluronan is a weak polyanion because of the ionization of the carboxyl groups present in each glucuronic acid residue; this ionization, together with the glycosaminoglycan residues, confers on hyaluronan its

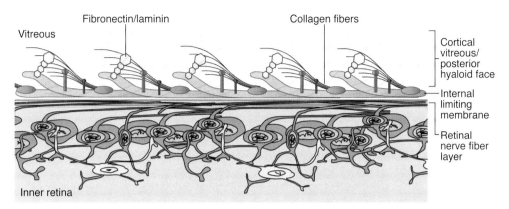

Figure 11-2 Condensed collagen fibers in the periphery form the cortical vitreous, also known as the *posterior hyaloid face.* The vitreoretinal interface lies between the collagen fibers of the posterior hyaloid face and the internal limiting membrane (ILM). Interaction between the cortical collagen fibers and the ILM occurs via several macromolecules, including laminin and fibronectin. Pharmacologic cleavage of these connections facilitates posterior vitreous detachment. *(From Barak Y, Ihnen MA, Schaal S. Spectral domain optical coherence tomography in the diagnosis and management of vitreoretinal interface pathologies. J Ophthalmol. 2012:876472. Epub 2012 Jun 4. http://dx.doi.org/10.1155/2012/876472. Accessed September 3, 2013.)*

affinity for water molecules. In free solution, hyaluronan occupies an extremely large volume relative to its weight and probably uses all of the space in the vitreous except for that occupied by the collagen fibrils. Hyaluronan molecules of the vitreous may undergo lateral interactions with each other, and such interactions may be stabilized by noncollagenous proteins. Link protein, which binds to hyaluronan in cartilage, is known to be present in the vitreous in small amounts. Hyaluronan is present in nearly all vertebrate connective tissues and is nontoxic, noninflammatory, and nonimmunogenic.

Both the concentration and the molecular weight of hyaluronan in the vitreous vary, depending on the species, location in the vitreous body, and type of analysis. Hyaluronan in human vitreous can achieve a molecular weight of greater than 1×10^6.

The source of hyaluronan is also poorly understood. In primate eyes, hyaluronan synthesis has been identified in the posterior pars plana, the neural retina, and the hyalocytes (macrophage-like cells) of the vitreous. Three forms of hyaluronan synthetase are known, but which isoform is responsible for synthesizing the hyaluronan of the vitreous has not been determined. In all animal species that have been analyzed, the hyaluronan concentration is highest in the posterior cortical layer near the retina and lowest in the anterior portion behind the lens.

Laurent TC, ed. *The Chemistry, Biology and Medical Applications of Hyaluronan and Its Derivatives.* Miami: Portland Press; 1998.

Soluble and Fibril-Associated Proteins

Many proteins remain in solution after the collagen fibrils and other insoluble elements present in the vitreous gel are removed by filtration or centrifugation. Serum albumin is the major soluble vitreous protein, followed by transferrin. Poorly defined glycoproteins make up 20% of the total vitreous protein and are thought to originate from surrounding tissues and not from blood. Other proteins include neutrophil elastase inhibitor (which may play a role in resisting neovascularization) and tissue plasminogen activator (which may have a fibrinolytic role in the event of vitreous hemorrhage). Serum albumin is thought to originate from the plasma, whereas transferrin at least partially originates from the region of the ciliary body. The concentration of soluble proteins estimated from a number of species is approximately 1.0 mg/mL. However, the concentration of serum proteins in the vitreous gel depends on the integrity of the retinal vasculature and the degree of any intraocular inflammation that may be present. Consequently, the concentration of soluble proteins within the vitreous cavity can rise dramatically if the blood–retina barrier is compromised.

Some structural proteins are specifically associated with the collagen fibrils and are isolated by extraction of collagen fibrils after centrifugation of the vitreous. These include a novel leucine-rich-repeat glycoprotein called *opticin,* which is produced in the posterior nonpigmented ciliary epithelium, and another novel glycoprotein called *VIT1.* Both opticin and VIT1 are thought to play key roles in the structure of the collagen fibril, and VIT1 may also interact with hyaluronan.

Zonular Fibers and Low-Molecular-Weight Solutes

Some zonular fibers are present in the anterior vitreous and can be observed by electron microscopy. However, most of these fibers form the zonular apparatus, which is the structural connection between the lens and the ciliary body. The major structural protein of these fibers is a large linear protein called *fibrillin,* which possesses unusually high cysteine content. Defects in fibrillin are present in patients with Marfan syndrome, some of whom experience spontaneous lens subluxation.

Ions and organic solutes originate from adjacent ocular tissues and blood plasma. The barriers that control entry into the vitreous include the vascular endothelium of retinal vessels, the retinal pigment epithelium (RPE), and the inner layer of the ciliary epithelium. The concentrations of Na^+ and Cl^- are similar to those in plasma, but the concentration of K^+ is somewhat higher than that in plasma.

Bishop PN. Structural macromolecules and supramolecular organisation of the vitreous gel. *Prog Retin Eye Res.* 2000;19(3):323–344.

Mayne R, Brewton RG, Ren Z-X. Vitreous body and zonular apparatus. In: Harding JJ, ed. *Biochemistry of the Eye.* London: Chapman & Hall Medical; 1997:135–143.

Biochemical Changes With Aging and Disease

Vitreous Liquefaction and Posterior Vitreous Detachment

The human vitreous gel undergoes progressive liquefaction with age, so that typically by the age of 80–90 years, more than half of the vitreous is liquid. Myopia is associated with faster vitreous liquefaction, which leads to early posterior vitreous detachment (PVD).

The process of vitreous liquefaction has, as a crucial component, the breakdown of the thin (12–15 nm) collagen fibrils into smaller fragments; implicated in this process is less "shielding" of type II collagen due to the age-related exponential loss of type IX collagen. Some proteolytic enzymes, such as plasminogen, may have elevated vitreous concentrations with increasing age, but others, such as MMP-2, do not. The fragments aggregate into thick fibers, or *fibrillar opacities,* which are visible with low-power, slit-lamp microscopy. As liquefaction proceeds, the collagen fibrils become condensed into the residual gel phase and are absent from (or in low concentration in) the liquid phase. In terms of hyaluronan concentration or molecular weight, there are no differences between the gel and liquid phases. With increasing age, there is a weakening of adhesion at the vitreoretinal interface between the cortical vitreous gel and the ILM. These combined processes eventually result in PVD in approximately 50% of the population.

PVD is a separation of the cortical vitreous gel from the ILM as far anteriorly as the posterior border of the vitreous base; the separation does not extend into the vitreous base owing to the unbreakable adhesion between the vitreous and retina in that zone. PVD is often a sudden event, during which liquefied vitreous from the center of the vitreous body passes through a hole in the posterior vitreous cortex and then dissects the residual cortical gel away from the inner limiting lamina. As the residual vitreous gel collapses anteriorly within the vitreous cavity, retinal tears sometimes occur at areas where the retina is more strongly attached to the vitreous than the surrounding retina can withstand, which subsequently can result in rhegmatogenous retinal detachment. A PVD can protect against proliferative diabetic retinopathy by denying a scaffold for fibrovascular proliferation emanating from the disc and the retina.

A PVD can be achieved surgically during macular hole surgery. However, it is now clinically recognized that in many eyes thought to have a PVD, collagen fibrils are still extensively attached to the ILM; and even after production of an acute PVD during vitreous surgery, some collagen fibrils typically remain adherent to the ILM. Removal of the ILM itself is now more frequently the goal in limiting the extent of traction maculopathy.

Myopia

When the axial length of the globe is greater than 26 mm, both collagen and hyaluronan concentrations are approximately 20%–30% lower than their concentrations in emmetropic eyes. In a model of negative power lens–induced myopic response in the tree shrew, hyaluronan was found to decrease rapidly when the lens was applied and to recover equally rapidly when the myopia-inducing lens was removed. Associated with these changes were biomechanical alterations in the sclera and increased axial length.

Vitreous as an Inhibitor of Angiogenesis

Numerous studies have shown that the normal vitreous is an inhibitor of angiogenesis. This inhibitory activity is decreased in diabetic vitreoretinopathy. However, the molecular basis of the phenomenon remains poorly understood. Known inhibitors of angiogenesis, such as thrombospondin 1 and pigment epithelium–derived factor, are present within the mammalian vitreous and may inhibit angiogenesis in normal eyes. Recently, the vitreous protein opticin has also been shown to suppress angiogenesis in mice models of retinal neovascularization. In contrast, vascular endothelial growth factor (VEGF), a promoter of angiogenesis, is markedly elevated in the vitreous of patients with proliferative diabetic vitreoretinopathy, in which the vitreous also acts as a scaffold for retinal neovascularization.

Le Goff MM, Lu H, Ugarte M, et al. The vitreous glycoprotein opticin inhibits preretinal neovascularization. *Invest Ophthalmol Vis Sci.* 2012;53(1):228–234.

Physiologic Changes After Vitrectomy

Both the normal vitreous and the vitreous cavity after vitrectomy are 99% water. Most of the changes in ocular physiology after vitrectomy result from altered viscosity in the vitreous cavity; when the vitreous is removed, the viscosity decreases between 300- and 2000-fold. Not only do growth factors and other compounds such as antibiotics transfer between the posterior and anterior segments more easily, but they are also cleared more quickly from the eye. This effect is proportional to the change in diffusion coefficient, which is of the same magnitude as the viscosity change. In addition, fluid currents may be present that may move solutes even more rapidly.

In particular, oxygen movement is more rapid, and the normal oxygen gradient between the well-oxygenated anterior segment and the posterior segment flattens significantly, with greatly increased oxygen tension at the retina. It has been proposed that increased oxygen tension at the posterior pole of the lens may be part of postvitrectomy cataractogenesis.

Holekamp NM, Shui YB, Beebe DC. Vitrectomy surgery increases oxygen exposure to the lens: a possible mechanism for nuclear cataract formation. *Am J Ophthalmol.* 2005;139(2):302–310.

Injury With Hemorrhage and Inflammation

If blood penetrates the vitreous cortex, platelets come into contact with vitreous collagen, aggregate, and initiate clot formation. The clot in turn stimulates a phagocytic inflammatory reaction, and the vitreous becomes liquefied in the area of a hemorrhage. The subsequent inflammatory reaction varies in degree for unknown reasons and may result in proliferative vitreoretinopathy (see also BCSC Section 12, *Retina and Vitreous*).

Streeten BAW, Wilson DJ. Disorders of the vitreous. In: Garner A, Klintworth GK, eds. *Pathobiology of Ocular Disease: A Dynamic Approach.* 2nd ed. 2 vols. New York: M. Dekker; 1994:701–742.

Involvement of Vitreous in Macular Hole Formation

With the development of optical coherence tomography (OCT) and, more recently, ultrahigh-resolution OCT, it is possible to directly visualize the vitreous cortex and the retina in the region of the macula. The results of studies using OCT suggest that macular holes sometimes originate from traction generated by attachment of the vitreous specifically to the fovea, with the subsequent generation of additional tangential tractional force along the ILM, causing hole enlargement. Lamellar macular holes may have a similar pathogenesis (see also BCSC Section 12, *Retina and Vitreous*).

Madreperla SA, McCuen BW, eds. *Macular Hole: Pathogenesis, Diagnosis, and Treatment.* Boston: Butterworth-Heinemann; 1998.

Witkin AJ, Ko TH, Fujimoto JG, et al. Redefining lamellar holes and the vitreomacular interface: an ultrahigh-resolution optical coherence tomography study. *Ophthalmology.* 2006; 113(3):388–397.

Genetic Disease Involving the Vitreous

In Stickler syndrome or Marshall syndrome, vitreous collapse is premature, which may induce retinal detachment (see BCSC Section 12, *Retina and Vitreous*). Mutations in both the α_1 (II) and α_1 (XI) collagen chains have been shown to be responsible for these syndromes. However, other families with hereditary hyaloideoretinopathies have also been identified in which the genetic basis is still not understood.

Snead MP, Yates JR. Clinical and molecular genetics of Stickler syndrome. *J Med Genet.* 1999; 36(5):353–359.

Enzymatic Vitreolysis

Considerable interest exists in enzyme preparations that may aid in the clearing of blood from the vitreous and in potentially performing noninvasive vitrectomy or inducing a PVD in young eyes (see BCSC Section 12, *Retina and Vitreous*). Enzymes that have been proposed for injection into the vitreous cavity include hyaluronidase, plasmin, dispase, and chondroitinase. Clinical trials with hyaluronidase and collagenase failed to induce a PVD. Ocriplasmin, which cleaves fibronectin and laminin, however, was able to induce a PVD (compared with placebo) and demonstrated efficacy in nonsurgical management of vitreomacular traction and macular holes.

Sebag J. Pharmacologic vitreolysis. *Retina.* 1998;18(1):1–3.

Stalmans P, Benz MS, Gandorfer A, et al. Enzymatic vitreolysis with ocriplasmin for vitreomacular traction and macular holes. *N Engl J Med.* 2012;367(7):606–615.

CHAPTER 12

Retina

The retina is composed of 2 laminar structures: an outer retinal pigment epithelium (RPE) and an inner neural retina. (This chapter discusses the neurosensory retina; the RPE is discussed in Chapter 13.) These laminar structures arise from an invagination of the embryonic optic cup that folds an ectodermal layer into apex-to-apex contact with itself, creating the subretinal space. The 2 layers form a hemispheric shell on which the visual image is focused by the anterior segment of the eye. The neural retinal cell types are as follows (Fig 12-1):

- photoreceptors—rods and 3 types of cones
- bipolar cells—rod on-bipolar cells and cone on- and off-bipolar cells
- interneurons—horizontal and amacrine cells
- ganglion cells and their axons, forming the optic nerve
- astroglia, oligodendroglia, Schwann cells, microglia, and vascular endothelium and pericytes

Neural Retina—The Photoreceptors

Rod Phototransduction

Catching light and converting its minute amount of energy into a neural response distinguishes the retina from all other neural structures, which it otherwise resembles. This combined process occurs within a specialized organelle of the photoreceptor cell, the *outer segment*. Most of our knowledge of phototransduction comes from information known about rods, which are sensitive nocturnal light detectors. Considerably more biochemical material can be obtained from rods than from cones because rods are much more numerous in most retinas. In addition, rods contain far more membrane than do cones, which contributes to the rods' higher sensitivity.

The outer segment of a rod is composed primarily of plasma-membrane material organized in an unusual way (see Fig 12-1; see also Chapter 2, Fig 2-29). Most of the membrane is in the form of membrane sacs flattened along the long axis of the outer segment. There are approximately 1000 sacs within a rod outer segment and 1 million membrane-bound rhodopsin molecules in each sac. The sacs float within the cytoplasm of the outer segment like a stack of coins disconnected from the plasma membrane. The sacs contain the protein machinery to capture and amplify light energy. This abundance

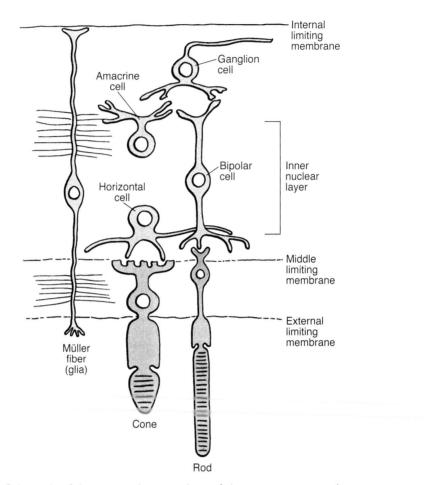

Figure 12-1 Schematic of the neuronal connections of the neurosensory retina. *(Redrawn from Federman JL, Fouras P, Schubert H, et al. Retina and vitreous. In: Podos SM, Yanoff M, eds.* Textbook of Ophthalmology. *Vol 9. London: Mosby; 1994.)*

of outer-segment membrane increases the number of rhodopsin molecules, which can absorb light. Some deep-sea fish, which need considerable sensitivity to detect the small amount of light available, have much longer rods than do humans.

Light is absorbed by rhodopsin concentrated in the outer-segment membrane of rods. Rhodopsin is a freely diffusible membrane protein similar to α- and β,-adrenergic receptors. It has 7 helical loops embedded in the lipid membrane (Fig 12-2). Phosphorylation sites exist on the cytoplasmic side of the protein, where rhodopsin is inactivated, and sugar is attached on the intradiscal side. At amino acid 296 on the seventh membrane loop, the 11-*cis*-retinal chromophore is bound to a lysine by a protonated Schiff base linkage. Each molecule responds to a single quantum of light. Rhodopsin absorbs green light best at wavelengths of approximately 510 nm. It absorbs blue and yellow light less well and is insensitive to longer wavelengths (red light). Rhodopsin is tuned to this part of the electromagnetic spectrum by its amino-acid sequence and by the binding of the 11-*cis* isomer of retinaldehyde, which creates a molecular antenna.

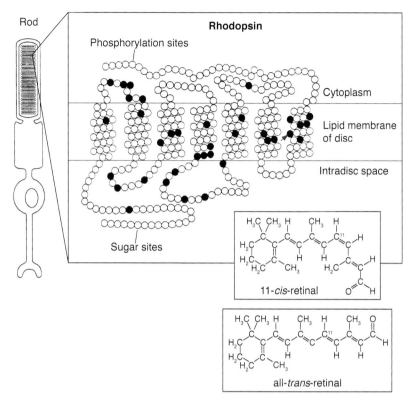

Figure 12-2 The rhodopsin molecule is embedded in the lipid membrane of the outer segment with 7 helical loops. Each circle represents an amino acid, and the highly conserved ones are shown in *black*. A *red arrow* shows the lysine to which the vitamin A chromophore is linked. Phosphorylation sites occur on the cytoplasmic and sugar attachment sites on the intradiscal (extracellular) ends of the rhodopsin molecule. Insets show the structures of 11-*cis*-retinal and all-*trans*-retinal. *(Courtesy of Peter Gouras, MD.)*

Once rhodopsin absorbs a quantum of light, the 11-*cis* double bond of retinal is broken (creating all-*trans*-retinal) and the opsin molecule undergoes a series of rapid configurational changes that lead to an activated state, *metarhodopsin II*. Activated rhodopsin starts a reaction that controls the inflow of cations into the rod outer segment (Fig 12-3). The target of this reaction is a cyclic guanosine monophosphate (cGMP)–gated cationic channel located on the outer membrane of the outer segment. This channel controls the flow of Na^+ and Ca^{2+} ions into the rod. In the dark, Na^+ and Ca^{2+} ions flow in through this channel, which is kept open by cGMP. Ionic balance is maintained by a Na^+,K^+-ATPase pump in the inner segment and a Na^+,K^+-Ca^{2+} exchanger in the outer-segment membrane, both of which require metabolic energy. Depolarization of the rod causes the transmitter glutamate to be released from its synaptic terminal. Light-activated rhodopsin drives a second molecule, transducin, by causing an exchange of guanosine diphosphate (GDP) for guanosine triphosphate (GTP) (see Fig 12-3A). One rhodopsin molecule can activate 100 transducin molecules, amplifying the reaction. Activated transducins excite a third protein, rod phosphodiesterase (rod PDE), which hydrolyzes cGMP to 5'-noncyclic GMP. The decrease in cGMP closes the gated channels, which

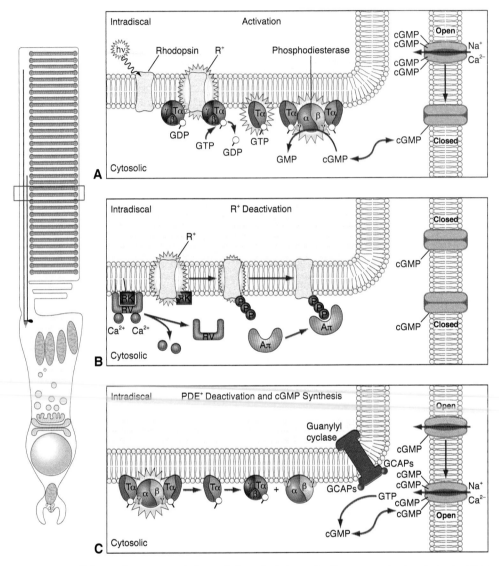

Figure 12-3 Schematic representation of the phototransduction cascade in photoreceptor outer segments. **A,** Light-activated rhodopsin (R⁺) causes levels of cyclic guanine monophosphate (cGMP) to be reduced via transducin-disinhibited phosphodiesterase (PDE), leading to closure of cGMP voltage-gated channels and subsequent hyperpolarization of the photoreceptor cell. **B,** R⁺ is deactivated through phosphorylation (indicated by Ps) and the binding of the protein arrestin (Arr). Phosphorylation is mediated by rhodopsin kinase (RK), which is regulated by recoverin (RV). RV dissociates from RK as calcium levels decrease following closure of cGMP voltage-gated channels. Arrestin binds to phosphorylated R⁺, completing the process. **C,** cGMP levels are restored through deactivation of transducin (T) via its intrinsic GTPase activity. Phosphodiesterase activity then reduces and guanylate cyclase activity increases, allowing cGMP levels to rise and opening the voltage-gated channels. GCAP = guanylate cyclase–activating protein; GDP = guanosine diphosphate; GTP = guanosine triphosphate; PDE = phosphodiesterase; T = transducin; T (α, β, γ) = subunits of transducin. *(Redrawn from Ryan SJ, Schachat AP, Wilkinson CP, Hinton DR, Sadda SR, Wiedemann P. Retina. 5th ed. London: Saunders/Elsevier; 2013:fig 14-4.)*

stops Na⁺ and Ca²⁺ entry and hyperpolarizes the rod. Hyperpolarization stops glutamate's release from the synaptic terminal.

When the light goes off, the rod returns to its dark state as the reaction cascade turns off. Rhodopsin is inactivated by phosphorylation at its C-terminal end by rhodopsin kinase, assisted by the binding of arrestin (see Fig 12-3B). Transducin is inactivated by the hydrolysis of GTP to GDP by transducin's intrinsic GTPase activity, which inactivates PDE. Guanylate cyclase, the enzyme that synthesizes cGMP from GTP, is activated by the decrease in intracellular Ca²⁺ caused by the channel closure; the enzyme's action is assisted by guanylate cyclase–assisting proteins (see Fig 12-3C). As cGMP levels increase, the gated channels close and the rod is re-depolarized. The corresponding rise in intracellular Ca²⁺ levels restores guanylate cyclase activity to its dark level. Calcium feedback may also regulate rhodopsin phosphorylation by recoverin as well as the sensitivity of the gated channel.

"Rim" proteins

Rod sacs differ from those of cones in that they are disconnected from the outer plasma membrane. The rim of each rod sac has a unique collection of proteins. Two such proteins are peripherin and rod outer segment protein 1 (ROM1), which play a role in the development and maintenance of the sac's curvature. Peripherin and ROM1 are also found in cone outer segments. A third protein is a member of the superfamily of adenosine triphosphate–binding cassette (ABC) transporters. This superfamily includes the cystic fibrosis transmembrane regulator (CFTR); P-glycoprotein, which is involved in multidrug resistance; the transporters associated with antigen processing, TAP1 and TAP2, which transport peptides in lymphocytes; prokaryotic permeases; and others. The ABC protein is unique to rod sacs and is not found in cones. It functions as a transporter of all-*trans*-retinal.

Biswas-Fiss EE. Functional analysis of genetic mutations in nucleotide binding domain 2 of the human retina specific ABC transporter. *Biochemistry.* 2003;42(36):10683–10696.

Outer-segment energy metabolism

Adenosine triphosphate (ATP) is necessary to drive the reactions that control the ionic current generators as well as the transporters in the outer segment. Because only the inner, and not the outer, segment contains mitochondria, oxidative metabolism is confined to the former. The outer segment is responsible for glycolysis, including the hexose monophosphate pathway and the phosphocreatine shuttle, which produces ATP and GTP and modulates nicotinamide adenine dinucleotide phosphate (NADPH). NADPH reduces retinal to retinol before it is returned to the RPE for isomerization, and it reduces glutathione, which protects against oxidative stress.

Cone Phototransduction

Qualitatively, the phototransduction of cones resembles that of rods. Light-activated cone opsins initiate an enzymatic cascade that hydrolyzes cyclic guanosine monophosphate (cGMP) and closes cone-specific cGMP–gated cation channels on the outer-segment membrane. Cone phototransduction is comparatively insensitive but fast and capable of adapting significantly to the ambient levels of illumination. The greater the ambient light level is, the faster and more temporally accurate is the response of a cone. Speed and temporal fidelity are important for all aspects of cone vision. This is one reason visual acuity improves progressively with increased illumination. Because of their ability to adapt, cones are indispensable to good vision. A person without cones loses the ability to read and see colors and can be legally blind. In comparison, lost rod function is less of a visual handicap.

Several factors contribute to light adaptation. For example, higher levels of illumination bleach away photopigments, making the outer segment less sensitive to light. As light levels increase, so does the noise level, which reduces sensitivity. Biochemical and neural feedback speed up the cone response. This feedback must be increased as light intensity increases and the cone absorbs more and more light. The biochemical processes responsible for this speedup have not yet been deciphered. All the processes that turn off the rod response are probably stronger in cones.

Cones also show neurally mediated negative feedback. Horizontal cells of the inner nuclear layer synapse antagonistically back onto cones, releasing γ-aminobutyric acid (GABA), an inhibitory transmitter. When light hyperpolarizes a cone, the cone hyperpolarizes neighboring horizontal cells. This effect inhibits the horizontal cells, stopping the release of GABA, which depolarizes (disinhibits) the cone by a recurrent synapse. This depolarization antagonizes the hyperpolarization produced by light and restores the cone to its resting state. Depolarization occurs with a synaptic delay so that its main effect is on the later response of the cone. Horizontal cell feedback occurs with strong stimuli, undoubtedly preventing the cone from being overloaded. The feedback also turns the cone response off more quickly, enabling the cone to respond more rapidly to a new stimulus. This process thus increases the flicker fusion frequency, which is much higher in cones (approximately 100 Hz) than in rods (approximately 30 Hz).

Trivariant color vision

To see colors, mammals must have at least 2 different spectral classes of cones. Most humans with normal vision have 3 types of cones and consequently a 3-variable color vision (3 cone opsins) system. Most mammals have divariant color vision with middle-wavelength-sensitive cones (termed *M cones*), which detect high-resolution achromatic (black and white) contrast, and short-wavelength-sensitive cones (termed *S cones*), which detect only color by comparing their signals with those of the M cones. This mechanism creates blue-yellow color vision. Because the S cones contribute only to color vision, they are much less numerous than M cones.

In primates, a third cone mechanism evolved to enhance color vision by splitting the high-resolution M cones into long (L)- and middle (M)-wavelength cones. This mechanism creates red-green color vision. Both L and M cones contribute to achromatic and chromatic contrast. Therefore, both are more numerous than S cones in the human retina.

Most color vision defects involve red-green discrimination and the genes coding for the L- and M-cone opsins. These genes are in tandem on the X chromosome. There is 1 copy of the L-cone opsin gene at the centromeric end of the X chromosome and 1–6 copies of the M-cone gene arranged in a head-to-tail tandem array. Normally, only the most proximal of these 2 genes is expressed. Most color vision abnormalities are caused by unequal crossing over between the L- and M-cone opsin genes. This inequality creates hybrid opsins that have different spectral absorption functions, which are usually less ideal than those of normal opsins. Some males have a serine-to-alanine substitution at amino acid 108 on the cone opsin gene, which allows more sensitivity to red light. Potentially, females with both the serine-containing and the alanine-containing opsins could have tetravariant color vision.

Rod-Specific Gene Defects

A number of mutations in rod-specific genes have been identified:

- *Rhodopsin:* More than 100 different mutations in the rhodopsin gene can cause autosomal dominant retinitis pigmentosa (ADRP). Mutations occur in different ways; they can alter transduction, protein folding, or localization of the protein. The most common mutation is P23H (responsible for 10% of RP cases in the United States), in which the protein does not fold properly and instead accumulates in the rough endoplasmic reticulum. Generally, mutations affecting the intradiscal area and amino-terminal end of rhodopsin are less severe than are mutations in the cytoplasmic region and the carboxyl tail. Alterations in the middle of the gene, coding for the transmembrane regions, result in moderately severe defects. Relatively uncommon mutations have been reported in the rhodopsin gene that cause autosomal recessive retinitis pigmentosa (ARRP) and a stationary form of nyctalopia.
- *Rod transducin:* A dominant G38D mutation produces Nougaret disease, the oldest known form of autosomal dominant stationary nyctalopia. With this mutation, transducin becomes continuously activated, an example of constitutively active rods that do not degenerate.
- *Rod cGMP phosphodiesterase:* Defects in either the α-subunit (PDEA) or β-subunit (PDEB) of cGMP phosphodiesterase (rod PDE) cause ARRP. These are nonsense mutations that truncate the catalytic domain of the protein. An H258D mutation in PDEB also causes dominant stationary nyctalopia. This mutation is near the binding site of the γ-subunit of PDE and may lead to constitutively active PDE, the downstream target of transducin.
- *Rod cGMP–gated channel:* Null mutations of the rod cGMP–gated channel β-subunit cause ARRP. No degeneration from the α- or γ-subunits has been reported.
- *Arrestin:* A homozygous defect in codon 309 of the gene for the protein arrestin causes Oguchi disease, a form of stationary nyctalopia. It produces a frameshift in and truncation of arrestin. There is genetic heterogeneity because defects in the rhodopsin kinase gene also cause Oguchi disease.
- *Rhodopsin kinase:* Null mutations of rhodopsin kinase cause Oguchi disease. These mutations also retard the turnoff of activated rhodopsin.
- *Guanylate cyclase:* Null mutations of the guanylate cyclase gene cause Leber congenital amaurosis (LCA), a childhood autosomal recessive form of RP. LCA shows genetic heterogeneity.
- *Rod ABC transporter:* Recessive defects of ABC transporter proteins cause Stargardt disease. There is allelic heterogeneity, which reflects the severity of the gene defects. Mild defects cause macular degeneration, intermediate ones cause cone–rod dystrophy, and severe ones cause RP. Heterozygous defects are also found in 4% of cases of age-related macular degeneration.

- *L-type calcium channel:* The L-type calcium channel gene codes for an α-subunit, and defects cause X-linked stationary nyctalopia. The protein seems to determine transmitter release from the rod synaptic terminal and may also affect cones.

Cone- and Rod-Specific Gene Defects

Gene defects specific to rods and cones have been identified and include the following:

- *Peripherin/RDS:* There is substantial allelic heterogeneity in the peripherin/RDS gene. Defects cause several dominantly inherited retinal degenerations that range from ADRP to macular degeneration, pattern macular dystrophy, vitelliform macular dystrophy, butterfly macular dystrophy, and fundus flavimaculatus. A null mutation of the homologous murine gene causes a semidominant form of degeneration, with failure of rod outer-segment development and slow degeneration.
- *ROM1:* Double-heterozygotic mutations in both the *ROM1* and the peripherin genes cause digenic RP. A *ROM1* gene defect alone has been reported in a patient with vitelliform macular dystrophy, but this gene is not responsible for Best macular dystrophy (discussed later in this chapter; for further discussion, see also BCSC Section 12, *Retina and Vitreous*).
- *Myosin VIIA:* Myosin VIIA is a protein found in cochlear hair cells and in the cilium connecting rod inner and outer segments. A heterozygous null mutation in a form of myosin VIIA causes Usher syndrome type I. Affected subjects have deafness and vestibular ataxia at birth and develop ARRP.

Cone-Specific Gene Defects

Gene defects specific to cones include the following:

- *Cone cGMP–gated channel:* A homozygous defect in the cone cGMP–gated channel α-subunit causes achromatopsia, loss of all cone function.
- *L- and M-cone opsins:* Two genetic steps involving both L- and M-cone opsins lead to blue-cone monochromatism. One genetic step reduces the tandem array of these genes to 1 gene, and the second step eliminates the residual gene. These defects occur in males because of the gene's location on the X chromosome. Defects in all 3 cone opsins lead to achromatopsia, also known as *rod-monochromatism.*
- *L- or M-cone opsins:* Defects in one or the other of the X-linked L- or M-cone opsin genes cause red-green color deficiencies, again almost exclusively in males.

RPE-Specific Gene Defects

Mutations specifically affecting the RPE include the following:

- *RPE65:* In addition to the null mutations of the guanylate cyclase gene mentioned earlier, other causes of LCA are homozygous defects in the gene *RPE65*. The RPE65 protein functions as an isomerohydrolase, converting all-*trans*-retinyl ester to 11-*cis*-retinol. This protein is the target of an active clinical trial using an adeno-associated virus to deliver the gene to the RPE of LCA patients.

- *Bestrophin:* Heterozygous missense mutations of the bestrophin gene produce Best disease, a dominantly inherited form of macular degeneration that involves the entire RPE layer but causes damage only in the macula. The gene codes for a chloride channel found on the basolateral surface of the RPE.
- *TIMP3:* Heterozygous point mutations of the *TIMP3* gene produce Sorsby macular dystrophy. The TIMP3 protein is an inhibitor of a metalloproteinase that regulates the extracellular matrix, where it acts as an antiangiogenesis factor. TIMP3 has also been shown to directly inhibit the action of vascular endothelial growth factor (VEGF).
- *CRALBP:* Homozygous defects of the gene *CRALBP* (cytoplasmic retinal-binding protein) cause retinitis punctata albescens. This protein facilitates 11-*cis*-retinal formation and shields the plasma membrane from the potential lytic effects of its aldehyde moiety.
- *11-*cis-*retinol dehydrogenase:* Homozygous defects in 11-*cis*-retinol dehydrogenase cause fundus albipunctus, a form of stationary nyctalopia. This enzyme forms 11-*cis*-retinal from 11-*cis*-retinol.
- *EFEMP1:* A single heterozygous, nonconservative mutation of the gene *EFEMP1* (EGF-containing fibrillin-like extracellular matrix protein) causes Malattia Leventinese (Doyne honeycombed retinal dystrophy), a dominant form of macular degeneration. It is uncertain whether the protein is unique to RPE.

Cideciyan AV, Jacobson SG, Beltran WA, et al. Human retinal gene therapy for Leber congenital amaurosis shows advancing retinal degeneration despite enduring visual improvement. *Proc Natl Acad Sci USA*. 2013;110(6):E517–525. Epub 2013 Jan 22.

Qi JH, Ebrahem Q, Moore N, et al. A novel function for tissue inhibitor of metalloproteinases-3 (TIMP3): inhibition of angiogenesis by blockage of VEGF binding to VEGF receptor-2. *Nat Med*. 2003;9(4):407–415. Epub 2003 Mar 24.

Ubiquitously Expressed Genes Causing Retinal Degenerations

Additional genetic links to retinal degenerations have been found:

- *REP-1:* REP-1 (Rab escort protein-1) is an X-linked gene that causes choroideremia. The protein is involved in prenylating Rab proteins, a process that facilitates their binding to cytoplasmic membranes and promoting vesicle fusion. Photoreceptors, RPE, and/or the choroid must be uniquely vulnerable for this process to occur.
- *OAT:* Homozygous defects of ornithine amino transferase (OAT) cause gyrate atrophy. The enzyme breaks down ornithine, which, in high concentrations, seems toxic to the RPE.
- *MTP:* Homozygous defects in microsomal triglyceride transfer protein (MTP) cause abetalipoproteinemia, or Bassen-Kornzweig syndrome, a condition characterized by ARRP and the patient's inability to absorb fat. The condition is treatable with fat-soluble vitamins.
- *PEX1:* Homozygous defects in the *PEX1* gene cause infantile Refsum disease, with RP, cognitive disabilities, and hearing deficits. Infantile Refsum disease represents the least severe disease in a spectrum of familial disorders involving mutations in the *PEX* genes. The *PEX* genes code for peroxins, proteins needed for peroxisome biogenesis.

- *PAHX:* Homozygous defects of *PAHX* cause Refsum disease, with RP, cerebellar ataxia, and peripheral polyneuropathy. The enzyme degrades phytanic acid and is located in peroxisomes. Elevated levels of phytanic acid are toxic to the RPE. Patients with Refsum disease may be treated with a phytanic acid–restricted diet.

Inner Nuclear Layer

The inner nuclear layer has 3 classes of neurons (bipolar, horizontal, and amacrine cells) and a glial cell (the Müller cell). There are separate bipolar cells for cones and rods and at least 2 distinctly different types of cone bipolar cells: *on-bipolar* and *off-bipolar* (Fig 12-4). The former are inhibited, the latter excited by the glutamate transmitter released by cones. Thus, when light hyperpolarizes the cones, the on-bipolar cell is excited (turned on) and the off-bipolar cell is inhibited (turned off). When a shadow depolarizes the cones, the reverse occurs.

Some cone bipolar cells synapse only with L cones and others only with M cones, a differentiation that is necessary for color vision. In the fovea, some cone bipolar cells synapse with a single L or M cone (Fig 12-5), which provides the highest spatial acuity. This cone selectivity is preserved throughout the ganglion cell layer. This selectivity for L- or M-cone inputs is transmitted by a tonic responding system of small ganglion cells. Separate L- and M-cone on-bipolar cells and off-bipolar cells transmit a faster, phasic signal to a parallel system of larger ganglion cells. Rods and probably S cones have only on-bipolar cells. Neither rods nor S cones are involved in high spatial resolution. The S cones are involved in color vision and the rods in twilight vision.

The horizontal cells are antagonistic interneurons that inhibit photoreceptors (see Fig 12-4) by releasing GABA when depolarized. The dendrites of horizontal cells synapse with cones. One class of horizontal cells modulates L and M cones, another class, mainly S cones. A thin axon terminal that emanates from the cell body of horizontal cells sends

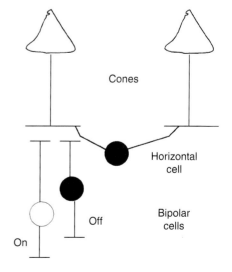

Figure 12-4 Basic circuitry of the cones. Separate on- and off-bipolar cells contact each cone. In the fovea, a cone has "midget" bipolar cells contacting only a single cone, and usually a single ganglion cell, for high spatial acuity. Horizontal cells are antagonistic neurons between cones. Absorbing light hyperpolarizes the cone; this in turn hyperpolarizes the horizontal cell, which resembles an off-bipolar cell. *(Courtesy of Peter Gouras, MD.)*

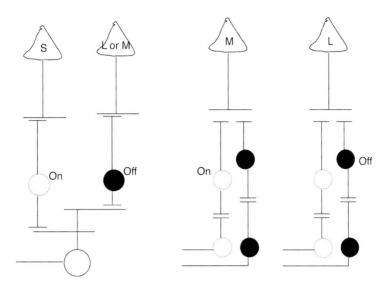

Figure 12-5 The tonic system transmits signals from the cones that are relatively maintained for the duration of the light or dark stimulus. This system provides the brain with information about a separate cone system, necessary for color vision. It preserves the polarity of the signal for each cone type. This process is shown here in the S-cone channel, which receives a signal of opposite polarity (off) from the L and M cones. *(Courtesy of Peter Gouras, MD.)*

dendrites to rods. The dendrites of horizontal cells receive glutamate from cones and rods and release GABA back onto cones and rods. This process provides negative feedback. When light causes the cone to hyperpolarize and stop its transmitter release, the horizontal cell is also hyperpolarized (turned off). This effect stops the release of GABA from the horizontal cell onto the cone, consequently depolarizing the cone.

Cone amacrine cells mediate antagonistic interactions among on-bipolar, off-bipolar, and ganglion cells. The rods have an unusual amacrine cell that receives the input of rod bipolar cells and delivers signals to on- and off-bipolar ganglion cells. Thus, rod signals undergo additional synaptic delays before they reach the ganglion cell output.

The retinal ganglion cells can be classified into 2 main types: *on* (center cells excited) and *off* (center cells inhibited by light in the center of their receptive field). A shadow initiates the opposite reaction in these 2 cell types. There are 3 main subgroups of retinal ganglion cells: tonic cells driven by L or M cones, tonic cells driven by S cones, and phasic cells.

Tonic cells driven by either L or M cones include small cells concentrated in the fovea (responsible for high acuity) and others located extrafoveally (see Fig 12-5). They project to the parvocellular layers of the lateral geniculate nucleus (the main relay station to the visual cortex) and mediate both high spatial resolution and color vision.

Tonic cells driven by S cones have a unique physiology designed to detect successive color contrast, for example, blue/yellow or gray/brown borders. These ganglion cells are excited by short waves entering and long waves leaving their receptive fields (see Fig 12-5). The phasic cells are larger, less concentrated in the fovea, and faster conducting than the ganglion cells (Fig 12-6). These phasic cells project to the magnocellular layers of the lateral geniculate nucleus and may be more important in movement detection.

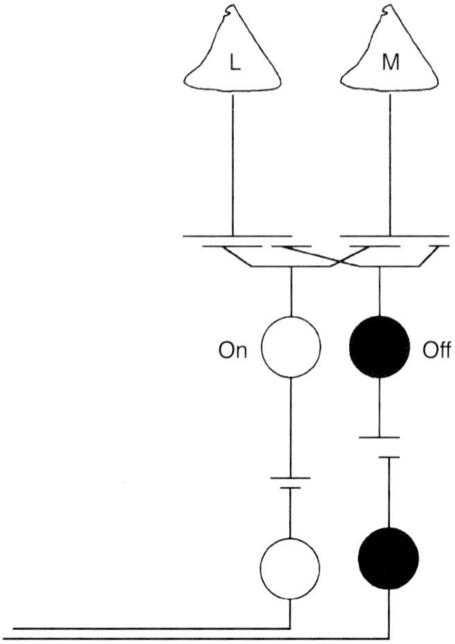

Figure 12-6 The phasic system transmits signals at the beginning or end of a light stimulus, producing a brief or transient response. L- and M-cone signals of the same polarity mix in driving the phasic system. *(Courtesy of Peter Gouras, MD.)*

Müller cells are the least understood of all the retinal cells. Nonneural, they play a supportive role to the neural tissue extending from the inner segments of the photoreceptors to the ILM, which is formed by their end-feet. They buffer the ionic concentrations in the extracellular space, seal off the subretinal space by forming the external limiting membrane (ELM), and may play a role in the vitamin A metabolism of cones.

The other nonneural, or neuroglial, cells of the retina are *macroglia* (astrocytes, oligodendroglia, and Schwann cells) and *microglia*. These cells provide physical support, respond to retinal cell injury, regulate the ionic and chemical composition of the extracellular milieu, participate in the blood–retina barrier, form the myelination of the optic nerve, guide neuronal migration during development, and exchange metabolites with neurons. Neuroglia have high-affinity transmitter-uptake systems and voltage-dependent and transmitter-gated ion channels; they can release transmitters, but their role in signaling, as in many other functions, is unclear.

In addition, the neural retina contains blood vessels with endothelial cells and pericytes. Pericytes play a role in the autoregulation of retinal blood vessels and are an early target in diabetes mellitus. Pericytes structurally support the endothelium and suppress proliferation, the loss of which leads to increased permeability and the development of microaneurysms.

Retinal Electrophysiology

Changes in the light flux on the retina produce electrical changes in all of the retinal cells, including the RPE and Müller cells, as well as neurons. These electrical changes result from ionic currents that flow when ion-specific channels are opened or closed. These currents reach the vitreous and the cornea, where they can be detected noninvasively by

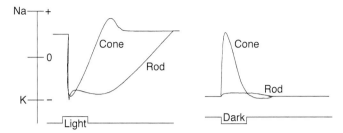

Figure 12-7 The responses of a rod and a cone to a pulse of light and a pulse of darkness. The light pulse hyperpolarizes both photoreceptors. The rod responses are prolonged. The cone responses turn off quickly, even while the pulse of light is on. Darkness depolarizes the cone rapidly but has only a small effect on the slower rod response.

an electroretinogram (ERG). The initiating process of the currents is the ionic response started in the rods and cones that influences the ionic current both *directly* by changes in Na^+ and K^+ fluxes and *indirectly* by synaptically modifying second-order retinal neurons.

The changes in the electrical potentials of the rods and cones are shown in Figure 12-7, which depicts the responses of rods and cones to a pulse of light and a pulse of darkness. Light hyperpolarizes cones and rods. The cone response is rapid; it turns off while the light is still on and overshoots the dark potential. The rod response is more prolonged and turns off very slowly. Dark depolarizes the cone and has little influence on the rod, which is saturated at high light levels and too slow to respond to the shadow. The ionic changes are due to shifts in the photoreceptors' conductivity of Na^+ and K^+ ions; this conductivity is facilitated by a cGMP-gated cation channel (see Fig 12-3). The concentration gradients for these ions are reversed across the membrane of the photoreceptors so that changes in the conductivity of these ions move currents in the opposite directions. (See also BCSC Section 12, *Retina and Vitreous.*)

Liou GI, Fei Y, Peachey NS, et al. Early onset photoreceptor abnormalities induced by targeted disruption of the interphotoreceptor retinoid-binding protein gene. *J Neurosci.* 1998;18(12): 4511–4520.

Molday RS. Photoreceptor membrane proteins, phototransduction, and retinal degenerative diseases. The Friedenwald Lecture. *Invest Ophthalmol Vis Sci.* 1998;39(13):2491–2513.

CHAPTER 13

Retinal Pigment Epithelium

The retinal pigment epithelium (RPE) is a single layer of cuboidal epithelial cells that constitutes the outermost layer of the retina. The RPE is located between the highly vascular choriocapillaris and the outer segments of photoreceptor cells (Fig 13-1). In humans, there are approximately 4–6 million RPE cells per eye. The ratio of photoreceptor cells to RPE cells is roughly 45:1. The RPE is derived embryologically from the same neural anlage as the sensory retina, but it differentiates into a secretory epithelium. Although it has no photoreceptive or neural function, the RPE is essential to the support and viability of photoreceptor cells.

Anatomical Description

The RPE cells are polarized epithelial cells. They have long microvillous processes on their apical surfaces that interdigitate with outer segments of photoreceptor cells. Their basal surface, which is adjacent to the Bruch membrane (an extracellular matrix between

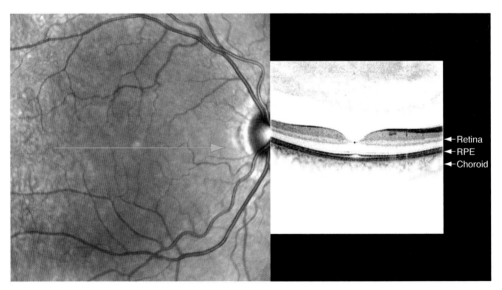

Figure 13-1 A spectral-domain optical coherence tomography (OCT) section of retina showing the relationship of the retinal pigment epithelium (RPE) to the retina and the choriocapillaris. *(Courtesy of Sandeep Grover, MD.)*

the RPE and choriocapillaris), has many infoldings that increase the surface area available for the exchange of solutes (Fig 13-2). RPE cells are joined near their apical side by tight junctions that block the passage of water and ions and constitute the outer blood–retina barrier. In addition to the organelles found in most cells (eg, the nucleus, Golgi apparatus, smooth and rough endoplasmic reticulum, and mitochondria), RPE cells also contain melanin granules and phagosomes, reflecting their role in light absorption and

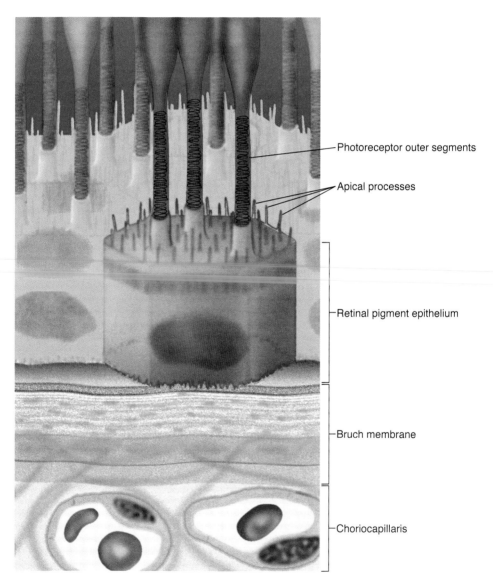

Figure 13-2 The RPE and Bruch membrane. The Bruch membrane separates the RPE from the choriocapillaris. Note the interdigitation of the apical processes of the RPE with the photoreceptor outer segments. *(Illustration by Daniel Casper, MD, PhD.)*

phagocytosis (discussed later in the chapter under Major Physiologic Roles of the RPE). The RPE is particularly rich in microperoxisomes, suggesting that it is quite active in detoxifying the large number of free radicals and oxidized lipids that are generated in this highly oxidative and light-rich environment.

Biochemical Composition

Biochemically, the RPE is a dynamic and complex cell. It must meet demands for its own active metabolism, its extraordinary phagocytic function, and its role as a biological filter for the neurosensory retina. These processes impose a very high energy requirement on the RPE; not surprisingly, the cells contain all the enzymes of the 3 major biochemical pathways: glycolysis, the Krebs cycle, and the pentose phosphate pathway. Glucose is the primary carbon source used for energy metabolism and for conversion to protein. Although the RPE does make a minor contribution to the glycosaminoglycan- and proteoglycan-containing interphotoreceptor matrix, glucose is not converted to glycogen in the RPE. Glucosamine, fucose, galactose, and mannose are all metabolized to some extent in the RPE, although mannose seems to be passed on almost directly to the photoreceptors.

Regarding the chemical composition of the RPE, more than 80% of its wet weight is contributed by water. Proteins, lipids, and nucleic acids contribute most of the remaining weight.

Proteins

Nearly 850 proteins have been identified in the RPE. Up to 200 acidic proteins are present, and approximately 180 plasma-membrane proteins have been identified. Many proteins found in other cells are also present in the RPE. For example, hydrolytic enzymes such as glutathione, peroxidase, catalase, and superoxide dismutase, which are important for detoxification, are present in the RPE. The cytoskeletal proteins actin, myosin, α-actinin, fodrin, and vinculin are also present.

Some proteins found in the RPE are localized differently from where they are found in other cells. A well-known example of such a protein is Na^+,K^+-ATPase, which has a unique location in RPE cells. Whereas most polarized epithelial cells localize Na^+,K^+-ATPase to their basolateral surface, the RPE places it on its apical surface. The sodium pump uses energy derived from adenosine triphosphate (ATP) hydrolysis to transport Na^+ and K^+ against their electrochemical gradients. It is thought that Na^+,K^+-ATPase is apically located in the RPE to maintain the balance of Na^+ and K^+ in the subretinal space. Additional proteins have been shown in RPE cells to have a reversed polarity compared with that in other polarized epithelial cells; examples include an isoform of neural cell adhesion molecule (NCAM-140) and folate receptor α. In addition, some proteins are expressed only in the RPE. One such protein, retinal pigment epithelium–specific protein 65 kDa (RPE65), is an obligate component of the isomerization and hydrolysis of vitamin A, which is required for regeneration of visual pigment (described later in Visual Pigment Regeneration).

Lipids

Lipids account for approximately 3% of the wet weight of the RPE; about half are phospholipids. Phosphatidylcholine and phosphatidylethanolamine make up more than 80% of the total phospholipid content. In general, levels of saturated fatty acids are higher in the RPE than in the adjacent outer segments. The saturated fatty acids palmitic acid and stearic acid are used for retinol esterification and for energy metabolism by the RPE mitochondria. The level of polyunsaturated fatty acids, such as docosahexaenoic acid (22:6, n–3), is much lower in the RPE than in the outer segments, although the level of arachidonic acid is relatively high. A number of studies have suggested that the retina may be spared the effects of essential fatty acid deficiency because the RPE efficiently sequesters fatty acids from the blood. The RPE actively conserves and efficiently reuses fatty acids, thus preventing their loss as waste products.

Nucleic Acids

Approximately 1% of the wet weight of the RPE is contributed by RNA. RNA is synthesized continually by the RPE—a result of the production of numerous enzymes needed for cell metabolism, phagocytosis of shed discs, and maintenance of the retinoid pathway and transport functions.

Major Physiologic Roles of the RPE

The RPE has a number of physiologic roles. Crucial among these functions are

- visual pigment regeneration
- phagocytosis of shed photoreceptor outer-segment discs
- transport of necessary nutrients and ions to photoreceptor cells and removal of waste products from photoreceptors
- absorption of scattered and out-of-focus light via pigmentation
- adhesion of the retina

These functions are discussed briefly in the following sections. Other important functions subserved by the RPE include its role in synthesis and remodeling of the interphotoreceptor matrix, formation of the outer blood–retina barrier, and elaboration of humoral and growth factors.

Visual Pigment Regeneration

Regeneration of the visual pigment rhodopsin, a process that has been studied extensively, involves both photoreceptors and the RPE. The RPE plays a major role in the uptake, storage, and mobilization of vitamin A for use in the visual cycle. Indeed, the RPE is second only to the liver in its concentration of vitamin A.

The basic function of the RPE cell in the visual process is to generate 11-*cis*-retinaldehyde, which is used in the formation of rhodopsin (Fig 13-3). As described in detail in Chapter 12, the photoreceptor cell synthesizes opsin, which uses 11-*cis*-retinaldehyde in the regeneration of rhodopsin. In the photoreceptor cell, rhodopsin is photolyzed and undergoes a *cis*-to-*trans* isomerization. All-*trans*-retinaldehyde is

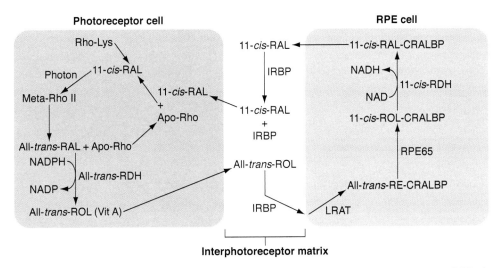

Figure 13-3 Role of the RPE in the visual cycle. All-*trans*-retinol is delivered to the RPE via interphotoreceptor retinoid-binding protein (IRBP). IRBP acts as a shuttle and also shields the cell membranes from the membranolytic retinol molecule. Once in the RPE, this molecule is esterified by lecithin retinol acyltransferase (LRAT). The ensuing retinyl ester is converted to 11-*cis*-retinol by the isomerohydrolase RPE65. Once the retinyl ester is converted, cellular retinal binding proteins (CRALBP) are utilized to shield the cell membranes from lytic intermediates. 11-*cis*-retinol is then converted to 11-*cis*-retinal by retinol dehydrogenase (RDH) and shuttled back to the photoreceptor outer segment to resume the visual cycle. The 11-*cis*-retinal chromophore attaches to a lysine residue on the rhodopsin. When the molecule absorbs light, it transforms into all-*trans*-retinal via photoisomerization. This process induces a conformational change in the attached rhodopsin molecule, activating the second-messenger system within the photoreceptor. Apo = aporhodopsin; Lys = lysine; Meta-Rho II = metarhodopsin II; NAD = nicotinamide adenine dinucleotide; NADH = reduced NAD; NADP = nicotinamide adenine dinucleotide phosphate; NADPH = reduced NADP; RAL = retinal; RE = retinyl ester; Rho = rhodopsin; ROL = retinol. *(Modified from Ryan SJ, Schachat AP, Wilkinson CP, Hinton DR, Sadda SR, Wiedemann P. Retina. 5th ed. London: Saunders/Elsevier; 2013:fig 16-9.)*

released and converted to all-*trans*-retinol by retinol dehydrogenase. The retinol is returned to the RPE in the presence of interphotoreceptor retinoid-binding protein (IRBP). In the RPE, retinol is converted to retinyl ester in the presence of the enzyme lecithin retinol acyltransferase. When needed for regeneration of rhodopsin, the retinyl ester is converted by an isomerohydrolase (isomerase) to 11-*cis*-retinol and is subsequently converted to 11-*cis*-retinal by a dehydrogenase. The 11-*cis*-retinal is returned to the photoreceptor cell along with IRBP. The protein RPE65 is the isomerohydrolase responsible for the conversion of all-*trans*-retinyl ester to 11-*cis*-retinol, the substrate of retinol dehydrogenase.

The RPE acquires vitamin A in 3 ways:

1. through release during bleaching of rhodopsin and return via the regeneration process of the visual cycle
2. from circulation, presumably through a receptor-mediated mechanism
3. via phagocytosis of shed photoreceptor outer-segment discs

The aldehyde and alcohol forms of vitamin A are membranolytic; hence, several retinoid-binding proteins mediate both vitamin A metabolism within the RPE and vitamin A's exchange with adjacent outer segments. A number of retinoid-binding proteins have been isolated and characterized in the RPE, subretinal space, and photoreceptors. The RPE esterifies retinol with available fatty acids (predominantly palmitic acid and, to a lesser extent, stearic and oleic acids) and stores retinol as a retinyl ester, a form no longer lytic to cell membranes. In conditions of hypervitaminosis A, toxicity to the RPE is minimal because of vitamin A storage as the ester.

Moiseyev G, Chen Y, Takahashi Y, Wu BX, Ma JX. RPE65 is the isomerohydrolase in the retinoid visual cycle. *Proc Natl Acad Sci USA*. 2005;102(35):12413–12418. Epub 2005 Aug 22.

Phagocytosis of Shed Photoreceptor Outer-Segment Discs

The RPE plays a crucial role in turnover of the photosensitive membrane of rod and cone photoreceptors. In the mid-1960s, autoradiography was used to establish that proteins were synthesized in the inner segment of the photoreceptor cells and were transported to the outer segment and incorporated into new discs forming at the base of the outer segment. The band of radioactive protein was displaced toward the apex of the cell over a period of approximately 9–11 days. The vital role of the RPE in phagocytosis of these discs was demonstrated when the radioactive distal tip of the outer segment arrived in the RPE cell and was subsequently phagocytosed.

The shed outer-segment discs are encapsulated in phagosomes, which in turn fuse with lysosomes and are digested. During degradation of the discs, building blocks are recycled into photoreceptors for use in the synthesis and assembly of new discs. The lipofuscin characteristic of the RPE is derived from photosensitive membranes and is responsible for generating the signal detected in fundus autofluorescence imaging (Fig 13-4). Each photoreceptor cell sheds approximately 100 outer-segment discs per day. Because many photoreceptors interdigitate with a single RPE cell, each RPE cell ingests/digests more than 4000 discs daily! The shedding event follows a circadian rhythm: in rods, shedding is most vigorous within 2 hours of light onset; in cones, shedding occurs most

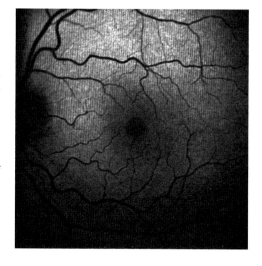

Figure 13-4 Example of fundus autofluorescence imaging, which is facilitated by lipofuscin molecules present within the RPE. Changes in fundus autofluorescence patterns reflect disorders of the RPE in the presence of hyperfluorescence and atrophic RPE in the presence of hypofluorescence (see BCSC Section 12, *Retina and Vitreous*). *(Courtesy of Vikram S. Brar, MD.)*

vigorously at the onset of darkness. Recent evidence suggests that the neurotransmitter dopamine acts within the photoreceptor–pigment epithelial complex to control disc shedding. Defects in the phagocytic function of the RPE are observed in the *Royal College of Surgeons rat* (animal model); these defects lead to degeneration of the photoreceptor cells.

Transport

The health and integrity of retinal neurons depend on a well-regulated extracellular environment. A crucial function of the RPE that contributes to this regulation is control of the volume and composition of fluid in the subretinal space through transport of ions, fluid, and metabolites. The distribution of transport proteins residing in the apical and basolateral membrane domains of the cell is clearly asymmetric, and this difference is what allows the epithelium to carry out vectorial transport. The membrane proteins remain in their proper location because of tight junction proteins. Intercellularly, asymmetry or polarity of the cell is maintained because of the intracellular molecular machinery that synthesizes new proteins and delivers them preferentially to the apical or basolateral cell membranes. Cytoskeletal proteins are fundamental in determining cell polarity and regulating transport.

The aqueous environment of the subretinal space is actively maintained by the ion-transport systems of the RPE. The active transport of a variety of ions (K^+, Ca^{2+}, Na^+, Cl^-, and HCO_3^-) across the RPE has been well documented. This transport is vectorial in most cases; for example, Na^+ is actively transported from the choriocapillaris toward the subretinal space, whereas K^+ is transported in the opposite direction. The apical membrane of the RPE appears to be the major locus of this transport. The ouabain-sensitive Na^+,K^+-ATPase is present at the apical, but not the basal, side. Similarly, an active bicarbonate-transport system appears to be located in this portion of the RPE membrane. High carbonic anhydrase activity seems to be associated with both the apical and basal sides of the cell.

Net ionic fluxes in the RPE are responsible for the transepithelial electrical potential that can be measured across the RPE apical membrane—a potential that is rapidly modified in the presence of a variety of metabolic inhibitors (eg, ouabain and dinitrophenol). In addition, the RPE apical membrane must be responsive to the changing conditions of phototransduction. For example, light evokes a decrease in K^+ ion concentration in the subretinal space, thus hyperpolarizing the RPE. Because the activity of Na^+,K^+-ATPase is controlled in part by K^+ ion concentration, light can affect the ionic composition of the subretinal space and the transport functions of the RPE. Active vectorial transport systems for other retinal metabolites (eg, taurine, methionine, and folate) have also been demonstrated. The RPE, therefore, appears to be important for maintaining the ionic environment of the subretinal space, which in turn is responsible for maintaining the integrity of the RPE–photoreceptor interface. The trans-RPE potential is the basis for the electro-oculogram (EOG), which is the most common electrophysiologic test for evaluating the RPE.

Pigmentation

A characteristic feature of the RPE is the presence of melanin pigment. Pigment granules are abundant in the cytoplasm of adult RPE cells, predominantly in the apical and mid-portions of the cell. During development, activation of the tyrosinase promoter triggers the onset of melanogenesis in this cell and marks the commitment of the neuroectoderm to become RPE. Although most melanogenesis occurs before birth, melanin production in the RPE does occur throughout life, albeit at a slow rate. As humans age, the melanin granules fuse with lysosomes; thus, the fundus of an older person is less pigmented than that of a young person.

The exact role of melanin inside cells remains speculative. One universally recognized function of melanin is to act as a neutral-density filter in scattering light. In so doing, melanin may have a protective role. In spite of the minimization of light scatter, visual acuity in the minimally pigmented fundus can be normal. Visual problems in individuals with albinism are attributable to foveal aplasia, not optical scatter. Genetic ocular disorders associated with melanin include varying forms of albinism. One form is oculocutaneous albinism (OCA), of which there are 10 types. The OCA1 and OCA2 types are due to defects in the tyrosinase gene and the pink-eyed dilution gene, respectively. When melanin levels are below a critical level, there is aberrant neuronal migration in the visual pathway, lack of foveal development, low vision, nystagmus, and strabismus (ocular albinism is characterized by a lack of pigment in the eye but relatively normal pigmentation of skin and hair). Melanin is thought to play a role in retinal development because albino mammals have underdeveloped central retinas, more contralateral projections of ganglion cells, and failure of foveal development. Melanin is a free-radical stabilizer and can bind many toxins. Some regard this feature as protective; others think that it contributes to tissue toxicity.

Retinal Adhesion

None of the aforementioned functions would be possible without another RPE function—the maintenance of retinal adhesion. The subretinal space is never bridged by tissue, and yet the neural retina remains rather firmly attached to the RPE throughout life. This adhesion is vital to the retina because detachment of the photoreceptors from the RPE can lead to permanent morphologic change in the tissue.

Numerous systems keep the retina in place. These factors include passive hydrostatic forces, interdigitation of outer segments and RPE microvilli, active transport of subretinal fluid, and the complex structure and binding properties of the interphotoreceptor matrix. In situations of pathology, retinal adhesion can diminish, and detachment of the retina occurs. Detachment does not occur simply because there is a hole in the retina or a leak in the RPE; there must be either positive traction pulling the neural retina or positive forces pushing fluid into the subretinal space.

The RPE in Disease

Clearly, the RPE is vital for normal visual function. Three retinal degenerations in humans appear to be caused by defects unique to the RPE: Sorsby fundus dystrophy and 2 forms of autosomal recessive retinitis pigmentosa (RP). There are 2 generalized retinal degenerations: Usher syndrome (type 1B) and sex-linked RP, in which the defective gene is expressed strongly in the RPE and weakly in neural retina. It has been suggested that some forms of macular degeneration, such as vitelliform macular degeneration ("Best disease") and malattia leventinese (dominant drusen), may be due to a primary defect in the RPE. Age-related macular degeneration and Stargardt disease appear to affect the RPE early in their course, although the genetic defects occur in the rods. Finally, choroideremia and gyrate atrophy produce blindness by their early impact on the RPE. In certain pathologic situations (including proliferative vitreoretinopathy and subretinal neovascularization), RPE cells detach from the basement membrane and become migratory. RPE cells undergo metaplasia, obtaining myofibroblast qualities, on contact with the vitreous and/or transforming growth factor beta (TGF-β). Efforts are now under way to determine effective methods of RPE transplantation that may ameliorate the functional deficits in these diseases.

Marmor MF, Wolfensberger TJ, eds. *The Retinal Pigment Epithelium: Function and Disease.* New York: Oxford; 1998:103–134.

Parapuram SK, Chang B, Li L, et al. Differential effects of TGFbeta and vitreous on the transformation of retinal pigment epithelial cells. *Invest Ophthalmol Vis Sci.* 2009;50(12):5965–5974. Epub 2009 Jul 2.

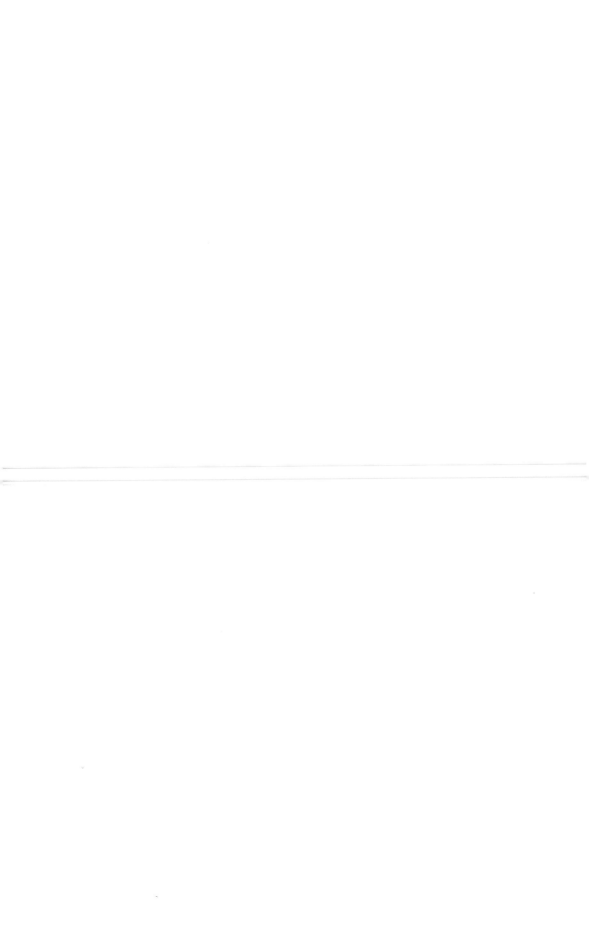

CHAPTER 14

Free Radicals and Antioxidants

The adverse effects of reactive forms of oxygen have been repeatedly proposed as causal factors in many types of visual impairment, including cataract, age-related macular degeneration (AMD), diabetic retinopathy, and glaucoma. Lipid peroxides are formed when free radicals or singlet oxygen molecules react with unsaturated fatty acids, which are present in cells largely as glyceryl esters in phospholipids or triglycerides. It has been hypothesized that the oxidation of membrane phospholipids increases the permeability of cell membranes and/or inhibits membrane ion pumps. This loss of barrier function is thought to lead to edema, disturbances in electrolyte balance, and elevation of intracellular calcium, all of which contribute to cell malfunction and potentially to cell lysis. Free radical–mediated DNA damage can also lead to cell death through induction of apoptosis.

Cellular Sources of Active Oxygen Species

The term *reactive oxygen intermediates (ROIs)* is used collectively to describe free radicals, hydrogen peroxide (H_2O_2), and singlet oxygen. *Free radicals* are molecules or atoms that possess an unpaired electron. This property makes them highly reactive toward other molecular species. Free radicals consist of superoxide anion (O_2^-), the hydroxyl radical (OH·), and the lipid peroxyl radicals. Some free-radical reactions are involved in normal cell functions; others are thought to be important mediators of tissue damage. Oxygen-derived free radicals and their metabolites are generated within aerobic organisms in several ways.

Oxygen necessary for normal metabolism usually undergoes tetravalent (4-electron) reduction by intracellular systems, such as the cytochrome oxidase complex in mitochondria, and is finally discarded as water without leakage of ROIs (Fig 14-1). However, a small percentage of the metabolized oxygen undergoes univalent reduction in four 1-electron steps. Oxygen accepts an electron from a reducing agent in each of these steps, and several ROIs are formed that are highly reactive.

Some of the reactive species leak out of their enzyme-binding sites and may damage other components of tissues, such as proteins, membrane lipids, and DNA, if they are not captured by detoxifying enzymes. Superoxide is not only produced in mitochondrial electron-transport systems but also formed in some enzymatic reactions, such as the xanthine/xanthine oxidase system. Hydrogen peroxide is produced directly in peroxisomes, as well as by enzyme-catalyzed dismutation of superoxide (see Fig 14-1). Any free iron (Fe^{2+})

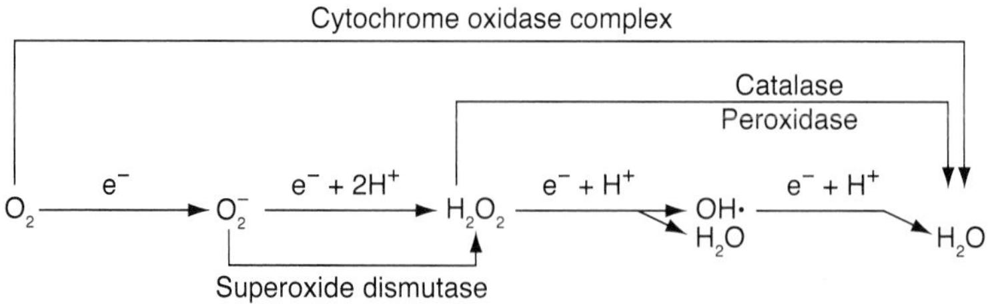

Figure 14-1 Enzymes involved in the metabolism of oxygen and in the detoxification of oxygen radicals generated by the univalent reduction of molecular oxygen. The univalent pathway involves a series of single-electron transfers, producing the superoxide free radical (O_2^-), hydrogen peroxide (H_2O_2), water, and the hydroxyl radical (OH·). Superoxide dismutase catalyzes the conversion of superoxide to hydrogen peroxide without oxidizing other molecules. Catalase and peroxidase catalyze the reduction of hydrogen peroxide to water without formation of the toxic hydroxyl radical. These enzyme systems are capable of preventing the buildup of toxic species produced from the univalent reduction of oxygen. The cytochrome oxidase complex appears to catalyze the tetravalent reduction of oxygen to water without leakage of reactive intermediates. *(Courtesy of F. J. G. M. van Kuijk, MD, PhD.)*

present may catalyze formation of the hydroxyl radical from superoxide and hydrogen peroxide. Iron and other catalytic metals such as copper may also be involved in generating these species by accelerating nonenzymatic oxidation of several molecules, including glutathione.

Other sources of activated oxygen species include products from the enzymatic synthesis of prostaglandins, leukotrienes, and thromboxanes (see Chapter 9, Fig 9-1). The nicotinamide adenine dinucleotide phosphate (NADPH) oxidase system of phagocytes yields activated oxygen species, especially during inflammation reactions. Oxygen-radical production is also associated with ionizing radiation and the metabolism of many chemicals and drugs, including carcinogenic compounds. Formation of reactive oxygen species—such as singlet oxygen by a light-mediated mechanism—is considered in the following section.

Superoxide and hydrogen peroxide are relatively stable in biological systems, whereas the hydroxyl radical is extremely reactive and capable of producing broad, nonspecific oxidative damage. However, free radicals and other active oxygen species also are important in many biological reactions that maintain normal cell functions, such as mitochondrial/microsomal electron-transport and second-messenger systems.

Sauer H, Wartenberg M, Hescheler J. Reactive oxygen species as intracellular messengers during cell growth and differentiation. *Cell Physiol Biochem.* 2001;11(4):173–186.

Mechanisms of Lipid Peroxidation

The mechanism by which random oxidation of lipids takes place is called *auto-oxidation*. This oxidation is a free-radical chain reaction usually described as a series of 3 processes: initiation, propagation, and termination. During the initiation step, the fatty acid is converted to an intermediate radical after removal of an allylic hydrogen. The propagation step follows immediately, and the fatty-acid radical intermediate reacts with oxygen at either end to produce fatty-acid peroxy radicals. Thus, a new fatty-acid radical is formed, which again can react with oxygen. As long as oxygen is available, a single free radical can lead to oxidation of thousands of fatty acids. A termination reaction, in which 2 radicals form a nonradical product, can interrupt the chain reaction. Auto-oxidation is also inhibited by free-radical scavengers such as vitamin E, which cause termination reactions.

Polyunsaturated fatty acids are susceptible to auto-oxidation because their allylic hydrogens are easily removed by several types of initiating radicals. The primary products of auto-oxidation formed during the propagation step are hydroperoxides (ROOH), which may decompose, especially in the presence of trace amounts of transition metal ions (eg, free iron or copper), to create peroxy radicals (ROO·); hydroxy radicals (HO·); and oxy radicals (RO·).

Photo-oxidation is a process by which oxygen is activated electronically by light to form singlet oxygen, which in turn reacts at a diffusion-controlled rate with unsaturated fatty acids or other cellular constituents. The mechanism of singlet-oxygen generation most widely accepted involves exposure of a photosensitizer to light in the presence of normal triplet oxygen ($^3O_2$). A photosensitizer is excited by absorption of light energy to an excited singlet state, which rapidly relaxes to an excited triplet state. In this state, the sensitizer may react with triplet oxygen ($^3O_2$) to form singlet oxygen ($^1O_2$). Photo-oxidation can be inhibited by singlet-oxygen quenchers such as carotenoids, which are discussed later in this chapter.

Lipid peroxidation causes not only direct damage to the cell membrane but also secondary damage in cells through its aldehydic breakdown products. Lipid hydroperoxides are unstable, and they break down to form many aldehydes, such as malondialdehyde and 4-hydroxyalkenals. These aldehydes can react quickly with proteins, inhibiting the proteins' normal functions. Both the lens and the retina are susceptible to such oxidative damage.

Oxidative Damage to the Lens

The lens is susceptible to challenge by various active species of oxygen because it contains low levels of molecular oxygen and trace amounts of transition metals such as copper and iron. It is thought that metal-catalyzed auto-oxidation reactions of various reducing agents in the lens can lead to the production of potentially damaging oxidants, such as oxidized glutathione (glutathione disulfide, or GSSG) and dehydroascorbic acid, as well as hydrogen peroxide, which can go on to produce hydroxyl radicals. In addition, ultraviolet radiation entering the lens can generate ROIs. Although most UVB radiation (<320 nm wavelength) striking the human eye is absorbed either by the cornea or by the high level of ascorbic acid in aqueous humor, a certain proportion is able to reach the lens epithelium, where it can cause damage. UVA light (320–400 nm wavelength) is able to reach more deeply into the lens, where it can react with various chromophores to generate hydrogen peroxide, superoxide anion, and singlet oxygen.

Although repair or regeneration mechanisms are active in the lens epithelium and super-ficial cortex, there are no such mechanisms in the deep cortex and the nucleus, where any damage to lens proteins and membrane lipids is irreversible. One result of this damage can be crosslinking and insolubilization of proteins, leading to loss of transparency (see Chapter 10). Certain types of human cataracts appear to initiate at the site of the fiber cell plasma membrane, possibly because oxygen is 5–7 times more soluble in membrane lipids than in cytoplasm.

To defend against oxidative stress, the young healthy lens possesses a variety of ef-fective antioxidant systems. These defenses include the enzymes glutathione peroxidase, catalase, and superoxide dismutase (SOD) (Fig 14-2). By means of the glutathione redox cycle, GSSG is reconverted to glutathione (GSH) by glutathione reductase via the pyridine nucleotide NADPH, which is provided by the hexose monophosphate shunt as the reduc-ing pathway. Thus, GSH acts as a major scavenger of active oxygen species in the lens. For reasons that are not well understood, the mammalian lens contains unusually high levels of protein sulfhydryl groups; however, it is clear that the groups must exist nearly completely in the reduced state for the tissue to remain transparent. The young human lens contains a high level of GSH, which is first synthesized in the epithelium and then migrates to the lens cortex and nucleus. With age, levels of GSH decline significantly in

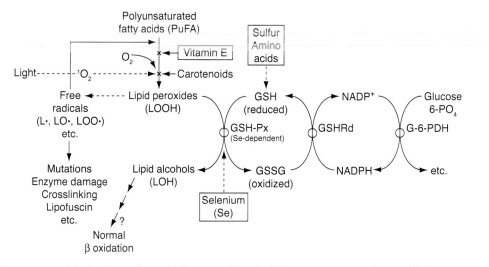

Figure 14-2 Mechanisms by which several antioxidants protect against oxidative dam-age. *Upper left,* Free radicals lead to the formation of lipid peroxides. Vitamin E inhibits this auto-oxidation process by scavenging free-radical intermediates. Carotenoids inhibit photo-oxidation by quenching singlet oxygen ($^1O_2$). *Center,* If lipid hydroperoxides are formed, they can be reduced by glutathione peroxidase (GSH-Px), which requires selenium as a cofactor. If these protective enzymes are not fully active, more free radicals are formed by the breakdown of lipid peroxides, which in turn leads to additional oxidation of polyunsaturated fatty acids. G-6-PDH = glucose-6-phosphate dehydrogenase; GSH = glutathione; GSHRd = glutathione reductase; GSSG = oxidized glutathione; NADP$^+$ = nicotinamide adenine dinucleotide phos-phate; NADPH = reduced NADP$^+$. *(Courtesy of F. J. G. M. van Kuijk, MD, PhD.)*

the human lens, particularly in the nucleus. Studies have indicated that a cortical–nuclear barrier may exist in the mature human lens, which inhibits the free flow of GSH to the nucleus. The result is that with age, the human lens nucleus becomes more susceptible to oxidative damage and cataract. Nuclear cataracts show high levels of oxidized cysteine and methionine in the lens proteins.

The free-radical scavengers ascorbic acid and vitamin E are also present in the lens. These scavengers work in conjunction with GSH and the glutathione redox cycle to protect against oxidative damage. Carotenoids that can quench singlet oxygen also exist in the lens. Epidemiologic (observational) studies have shown that people with higher levels of plasma antioxidants, particularly vitamin E, have a reduced risk of cataract, particularly nuclear cataract. However, 2 prospective, randomized, placebo-controlled clinical trials—the Age-Related Eye Disease Study (AREDS) and the Vitamin E, Cataract and Age-Related Maculopathy Trial (VECAT)—found that high-dose formulations of vitamin C, vitamin E, and beta carotene (AREDS), as well as vitamin E alone, neither prevented the development nor slowed the progression of age-related cataracts.

Age-Related Eye Disease Study Research Group. A randomized, placebo-controlled clinical trial of high-dose supplementation with vitamins C and E and beta carotene for age-related cataract and vision loss: AREDS report no. 9. *Arch Ophthalmol.* 2001;119(10):1439–1452. [Erratum appears in *Arch Ophthalmol.* 2008;126(9):1251.]

McNeil JJ, Robman L, Tikellis G, Sinclair MI, McCarty CA, Taylor HR. Vitamin E supplementation and cataract: randomized controlled trial. *Ophthalmology.* 2004;111(1):75–84.

Vulnerability of the Retina to Free Radicals

Experimental data have shown that retinal photoreceptors degenerate when they are exposed to oxidative challenges such as hyperbaric oxygen, iron overload, or injection of lipid hydroperoxides into the vitreous humor. The retina also degenerates when antioxidative defenses are reduced, which presumably elevates levels of lipid peroxidation in the absence of unusual oxidative stress. The retina is made vulnerable to damage from lipid peroxidation by several distinctive characteristics, 4 of which are considered here:

1. Vertebrate retinal rod outer segments are susceptible to damage by oxygen because of their high content of polyunsaturated fatty acids. Their phospholipids typically contain about 50 mol% docosahexaenoic acid, the most highly polyunsaturated fatty acid that occurs in nature. It is well established that polyunsaturated fatty acids are sensitive to peroxidation in proportion to their number of double bonds.

2. The rod inner segment is very rich in mitochondria, which may leak activated oxygen species.

3. The excellent oxygen supply through the choroid and the retinal vessels elevates the risk of oxidative damage. Vertebrate retinas maintained in vitro showed at least a sevenfold higher rate of oxygen consumption per milligram of protein compared with all other tissues tested (except the adrenal gland). The oxygen tension is highest at the choroid and drops toward the inner segments because of the high

metabolic demand of their mitochondria. Oxygen consumption has been reported to decrease when the retina is illuminated.

4. Light exposure may trigger photo-oxidative processes mediated by singlet oxygen, and the RPE may play a key role.

The RPE is tightly packed with endoplasmic reticulum and appears to be rich in anti-oxidant enzymes in most species tested. The RPE of pigmented animals contains melanin granules, which function as a light trap. Although melanin is commonly assumed to be photoprotective, its role in the prevention of light damage to ocular tissues is not clearly understood. Evidence suggests that the RPE is quite sensitive to dietary antioxidant deficiency, in which light-activated melanin may contribute to phototoxicity. If an RPE cell dies, then the numerous photoreceptors supported by that RPE cell may suffer severe damage or death.

Intense light at levels that may be encountered in daily life is phototoxic to the retina. Even though the cornea absorbs some UV radiation, the retinas of young people are exposed to a substantial amount of light in the range of 350–400 nm (young lenses transmit these wavelengths). The lens yellows with age, and the cutoff wavelength in older people moves up to approximately 430 nm. Because the adult lens absorbs nearly 100% of light below 400 nm, little or no UV light reaches the retina in older people.

In addition to UV light, blue light (400–500 nm) can be harmful to the retina (blue-light hazard). The photoreceptors in the retina are particularly susceptible to damage by blue light, a process that can lead to cell death and retinal disease. This damage is due to the formation of the phototoxic compound A2E. A2E (ie, A2E-epoxide) specifically targets cytochrome oxidase and induces irreversible DNA damage (apoptosis) of RPE cells. This molecular process is believed to be a precursor to the pathogenesis of AMD. Carotenoids (eg, lutein and zeaxanthin) present in the retina act as a blue-light filter, shielding the photoreceptors in the retina from this radiation, and in vitro studies have suggested that vitamin E and other antioxidants inhibit A2E-epoxide formation.

Shaban H, Richter C. A2E and blue light in the retina: the paradigm of age-related macular degeneration. *Biol Chem.* 2002;383(3–4):537–545.

Sparrow JR, Vollmer-Snarr HR, Zhou J, et al. A2E-epoxides damage DNA in retinal pigment epithelial cells. Vitamin E and other antioxidants inhibit A2E-epoxide formation. *J Biol Chem.* 2003;278(20):18207–18213. Epub 2003 Mar 19.

Wu Y, Yanase E, Feng X, Siegel MM, Sparrow JR. Structural characterization of bisretinoid A2E photocleavage products and implications for age-related macular degeneration. *Proc Natl Acad Sci USA.* 2010;107(16):7275–7280. Epub 2010 Apr 5.

Antioxidants in the Retina and RPE

Several antioxidant mechanisms have been established in biological systems, including free-radical scavenging, quenching of singlet oxygen, and enzymatic reduction of hydroperoxides. Antioxidants found in vertebrates include selenium, GSH, selenium-dependent glutathione peroxidase, non–selenium-dependent glutathione peroxidase (glutathione-S-transferase), vitamin E, carotenoids, SOD, and catalase; in addition, antioxidant roles for ascorbate and melanin have been reported. The relation between some of these antioxidants and the protective mechanisms is shown in Figure 14-2.

Yu BP. Cellular defenses against damage from reactive oxygen species. *Physiol Rev.* 1994; 74(1):139–162. [Erratum appears in *Physiol Rev.* 1995;75(1):preceding 1.]

Selenium, Glutathione, Glutathione Peroxidase, and Glutathione-S-Transferase

A number of enzymes have been identified that can provide antioxidant protection by a peroxide-decomposing mechanism. For example, selenium-dependent glutathione peroxidase (GSH-Px) and several enzymes of the glutathione-S-transferase (GSH-S-Ts) group can reduce organic hydroperoxides. GSH-Px is also active with H_2O_2 as a substrate, although the GSH-S-Ts group cannot act on H_2O_2. All of these enzymes require GSH, which is converted to GSSG during the enzymatic reaction. The hexose monophosphate shunt enzymes produce NADPH, which is needed for reduction of GSSG by GSH reductase. Both GSH-Px and GSH-S-Ts activities have been measured in human retinas. The highest concentration of selenium in the human eye is present in the RPE: 100–400 ng in the RPE cells of a single human eye, up to 10 times more than in the retina (40 ng). In addition, the amount of selenium appears to be similar in both eyes of the same individual. The selenium level in the human retina is constant with age; in the human RPE, however, the level increases with age.

Vitamin E

Vitamin E acts by scavenging free radicals, thus terminating the propagation steps and leading to interruption of the auto-oxidation reaction. Reports on the vitamin E content of the retina of the adult rat raised on a normal chow diet show values ranging from 215 to 325 ng. A detailed study on the vitamin E content of microdissected parts of vertebrate eyes showed that the RPE is rich in vitamin E relative to the photoreceptors and that photoreceptors are rich in vitamin E relative to most other cells in the eye. Studies on vitamin E in postmortem human eyes also found that the level of vitamin E is higher in the RPE than in the retina. Furthermore, vitamin E levels in human retinal tissues increase with age until the sixth decade of life and then decrease. This decrease coincides with the age at which the incidence of AMD increases in the population.

Friedrichson T, Kalbach HL, Buck P, van Kuijk FJ. Vitamin E in macular and peripheral tissues of the human eye. *Curr Eye Res.* 1995;14(8):693–701.

Superoxide Dismutase and Catalase

Superoxide dismutase catalyzes the dismutation of superoxide to hydrogen peroxide, which is further reduced to water by catalase or peroxidase. Two types of SOD are usually isolated from mammalian tissues: Cu-Zn SOD, the cytoplasmic enzyme, which is inhibited by cyanide; and Mn SOD, the mitochondrial enzyme, which is not inhibited by cyanide.

Catalase catalyzes the reduction of hydrogen peroxide to water. Information on catalase activity in the retina is currently rather limited. Total retinal catalase activity was found to be very low but detectable in rabbits. A protective role for catalase has been reported in rats with experimental allergic uveitis as well as in rats with retinal reperfusion injury.

Ascorbate

Ascorbate (vitamin C) is thought to function synergistically with vitamin E to terminate free-radical reactions. It has been proposed that vitamin C can react with the vitamin E radicals formed when vitamin E scavenges free radicals. Vitamin E radicals are then regenerated to native vitamin E. The vitamin C radicals resulting from this regeneration can be reduced by nicotinamide adenine dinucleotide (NADH) reductase, with NADH as the electron acceptor. Ascorbic acid is found throughout the eye of many species in concentrations that are high relative to those in other tissues.

Delamere NA. Ascorbic acid and the eye. In: Harris JR, ed. *Subcellular Biochemistry.* New York: Plenum Press; 1996. *Ascorbic Acid: Biochemistry and Biomedical Cell Biology;* vol 25:313–329.

Carotenoids

Various roles have been proposed for carotenoids (xanthophylls) in biological systems, including limiting chromatic aberration at the fovea of the retina and the quenching of singlet oxygen. β-Carotene is the precursor of vitamin A and can act as a free-radical trap at low oxygen tension. In postmortem human retinas, carotenoids have been shown to make up the yellow pigment in the macula. A mixture of the 2 carotenoids *lutein* and *zeaxanthin* is present in the macula and located in the Henle fiber layer. It has been demonstrated that in humans, zeaxanthin is concentrated primarily in the fovea, whereas lutein is dispersed in the retina. Interestingly, little β-carotene is present in the human eye. Furthermore, carotenoids are present only in the retina and not at all in the RPE. In the peripheral retina, lutein and zeaxanthin are also concentrated in the photoreceptor outer segments and may act as antioxidants to protect the macula against short-wavelength visible light. Figure 14-3A shows the localization of antioxidants in the human macula and peripheral retina; Figure 14-3B shows their localization in a cross section of the peripheral retina.

Chew EY, Clemons TE, Agrón E, et al; Age-Related Eye Disease Study Research Group. Long-term effects of vitamins C and E, β-carotene, and zinc on age-related macular degeneration: AREDS report no. 35. *Ophthalmology.* 2013;120(8):1604–1611. Epub 2013 Apr 10.

Khachik F, Bernstein PS, Garland DL. Identification of lutein and zeaxanthin oxidation products in human and monkey retinas. *Invest Ophthalmol Vis Sci.* 1997;38(9):1802–1811.

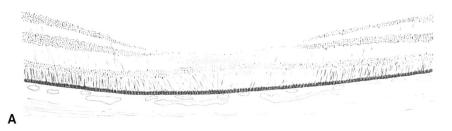

A

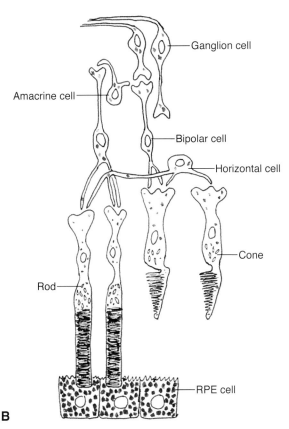

Ganglion cell

Amacrine cell

Bipolar cell

Horizontal cell

Cone

Rod

RPE cell

B

Figure 14-3 **A,** The localization of antioxidants in the human macula and peripheral retina. Vitamin E (represented by *blue*) and selenium (represented by *red*) are primarily concentrated in the RPE. In the macula, carotenoids *(yellow)* are present in the fibers of Henle; in the peripheral retina, they are also present in the rods. **B,** The localization in a cross section of the peripheral retina. Vitamin E and selenium remain primarily concentrated in the RPE but are also enriched in the rod outer segments. Carotenoids have been found in rod outer segments in the peripheral retina. *(Illustrations by J. Woodward, MD; courtesy of F. J. G. M. van Kuijk, MD, PhD.)*

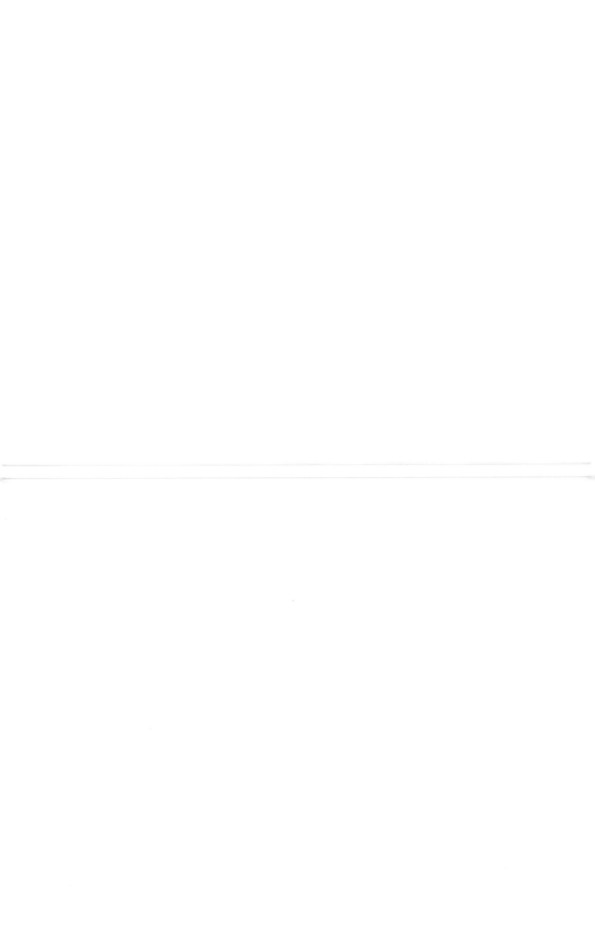

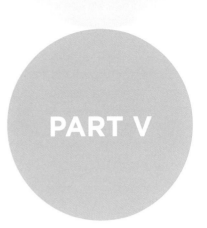

PART V

Ocular Pharmacology

CHAPTER 15

Pharmacologic Principles

Introduction

Pharmacology is the study of the interactions of living organisms with therapeutic substances through biochemical processes. In other words, it is the study of drug action. A drug can be defined as a chemical substance used in the treatment, cure, prevention, or diagnosis of disease or used to enhance physical or mental well-being. The 2 main branches of pharmacology are pharmacokinetics and pharmacodynamics. Pharmacokinetics studies how the chemical substances cycle through the biological system, whereas pharmacodynamics examines the biological and chemical effects of the chemical on the biological system. Pharmacotherapeutics is the study of how to achieve desirable effects or avoid or minimize adverse effects or toxicity of the drug. This chapter begins with a review of general principles of pharmacology, including attention to special features of the eye that facilitate or impede ocular therapy.

Pharmacokinetics

Pharmacokinetics concerns the cycle of a drug through the body, including the absorption, distribution, metabolism, and excretion of that drug. To achieve a therapeutic effect, a drug must reach its site of action in sufficient concentration. The concentration at the site of action is a function of the route of administration, the amount administered, the extent and rate of absorption at the administration site, the distribution and binding in tissues, the movement by bulk flow in circulating fluids, the transport between compartments, biotransformation, and excretion. Pharmacokinetics and dose together determine *bioavailability,* or concentration of the active drug at the therapeutic site.

Pharmacodynamics

Pharmacodynamics refers to the biological activity and clinical effects of a drug. It is the drug action after pharmacokinetics has distributed the active agent to the therapeutic site. Included within the area of pharmacodynamics are the tissue receptor for the drug and the intracellular changes initiated by binding of the active drug with the receptor. The pharmacodynamic action of a drug is often described using the receptor for that drug; for example, a drug may be categorized as an α-adrenergic agonist or β-adrenergic antagonist.

Pharmacotherapeutics

Pharmacotherapeutics is the administration of a drug so as to reach a given clinical endpoint, such as the prevention or treatment of disease. The therapeutic dose may vary for any patient and is related to the patient's age, sex, race, other currently prescribed medications, and preexisting medical conditions. Pharmacotherapeutics is covered in Chapter 16.

Toxicity

Toxicity refers to the adverse effects of either medications or environmental chemicals, including poisoning. Toxicity may be influenced by pharmacokinetics and/or pharmacodynamics. For example, topically applied ophthalmic medications are readily absorbed through the mucous membranes of the eye and nasopharynx, as well as through the iris and ciliary body. Topical absorption avoids the first-pass metabolism of the liver and increases systemic bioavailability. The systemic toxicity of these medications may therefore be more than expected relative to the total topical dose. Drug metabolism and excretion are less developed in neonates and infants than in adults. For example, in early neonatal life, the drug-metabolizing activities of the cytochrome P450–dependent, mixed-function oxidases and the conjugating enzymes are approximately 50%–70% of adult values. A second example is in glucuronide formation, which does not reach adult levels until the third and fourth years of life. Similarly, glomerular filtration rate reaches the adult value by 6–12 months of life. Therefore, drug doses and dosing schedules must be adjusted appropriately in pediatric populations to avoid toxicity.

Local toxicity of topical drugs is more common than is systemic toxicity. Local toxicity may be a type I immunoglobulin E (IgE)–mediated hypersensitivity reaction or may represent a delayed reaction to either the medication or the preservatives.

Preservatives common in ophthalmic preparations include quaternary cationic surfactants such as benzalkonium chloride and benzododecinium bromide; mercurials such as thimerosal, chlorobutanol, and parahydroxybenzoates; and aromatic alcohols. Preservatives used in ophthalmic solutions can be toxic to the ocular surface following topical administration and can enhance the corneal permeability of various drugs.

Newer preservatives have been developed to reduce the toxic effect on the ocular surface. One method allows the preservative to dissipate upon exposure to light or to the ions in the tear film. Two examples of this method are stabilized oxychloro complex, which breaks down to sodium chloride and water, and sodium perborate, which breaks down to hydrogen peroxide before becoming oxygen and hydrogen. These "disappearing preservatives" theoretically should have no toxicity to the corneal surface.

Other, newer preservative systems may be less toxic to the ocular surface than quaternary cationic surfactants such as benzalkonium chloride. One such system is an ionic buffer containing borate, sorbitol, propylene glycol, and zinc that breaks down into innate elements upon encountering the cations in the tear film of the eye. Another preservative system, polyquaternium-1, is a cationic polymer of quaternary ammonium structures that lacks a hydrophobic region. Although it is a detergent, human corneal epithelial cells tend to repel the compound. In order to completely eliminate toxicity from preservatives, some topical ocular products are currently available in preservative-free, single-use containers.

Pharmacologic Principles in Elderly Patients

Pharmacologic principles apply differently to elderly patients. Compared with younger patients, elderly patients have less lean body mass due to a decrease in muscle bulk, less body water and albumin, and an increased relative percentage of adipose tissue. These physiologic differences alter tissue binding and drug distribution. Human renal function decreases 50% with age; both hepatic perfusion and enzymatic activity are variably affected as well. Older patients tend to take more medications for chronic conditions than do younger people, and many of the drugs they use are processed simultaneously by their already-compromised metabolic systems.

The pharmacokinetic processing of drugs in elderly patients is therefore significantly altered, extending the effective half-life of most medications. The pharmacodynamic action of a drug is often independently potentiated in these patients. The increase in both drug effect and adverse effects occurs even if the dose is decreased in consideration of these pharmacokinetic differences. Thus, the pharmacotherapeutic effects and toxicity of a medication may be altered simply by the aging process, independent of drug dosage. Accordingly, the selection of a specific therapeutic agent should be guided by the general health, age, and concomitant medication taken by the individual patient.

Pharmacokinetics: The Route of Drug Delivery

Topical Administration

Eyedrops

Most ocular medications are administered topically as eyedrops. This route of administration maximizes the anterior segment concentrations while minimizing systemic toxicity. The drug gradient from the concentrated tear reservoir to the relatively barren corneal and conjunctival epithelium forces a passive route of absorption.

Amount administered Some features of topical ocular therapy limit treatment effectiveness. Very little of an administered drop is retained by the eye. When a 50-µL drop is delivered from the usual commercial dispenser, the volume of the tear lake rises from 7 µL to only 10 µL in the blinking eye of an upright patient. Thus, at most, 20% of the administered drug is retained (10 µL/50 µL). A rapid turnover of fluid also occurs in the tear lake—16% per minute in the undisturbed eye—with even faster turnover if the drop elicits reflex tearing. Consequently, for slowly absorbed drugs, at most only 50% of the drug that was initially retained in the tear reservoir (50% of the 20% of the delivered medication, or 10%) remains 4 minutes after instillation ($0.84^4 = 0.50$), and only 17% remains after 10 minutes, or 3.4% of the original dose. The amount of time that a drug remains in the tear reservoir and tear film is called the *residence time* of a medication. This time is affected not only by drug formulation but also by the timing of subsequent medication, tear production, and drainage.

Some simple measures have been shown to improve ocular absorption of materials that do not traverse the cornea rapidly. Patients using more than one topical ocular medication should be instructed to allow 5 minutes between drops; otherwise, the second drop may simply wash out the first. Blinking also diminishes a drug's effect by activating the nasal lacrimal pump mechanism, forcing fluid from the lacrimal sac into the nasopharynx, and creating a negative sac pressure that empties the tear lake (see BCSC Section 7, *Orbit, Eyelids, and Lacrimal System*). Patients can circumvent this loss of drug reservoir by either compressing the nasolacrimal duct with digital pressure at the medial canthus or closing the eyelids for 5 minutes after instillation of each drop. These 2 measures will prevent emptying of the tear lake and will reduce systemic toxicity by decreasing absorption through the nasal mucosa. Nasolacrimal occlusion will increase the absorption of topically applied materials (Fig 15-1) and decrease the systemic absorption and potential toxicity. Tear reservoir retention and drug contact time can also be extended either by increasing the viscosity of the vehicle or by using drug delivery objects such as contact lenses, collagen shields, and inserts.

Topical medications that are absorbed by the nasal mucosa can attain significant levels in the blood. One to 2 drops of a topical medication may provide a significant systemic dose of that drug. For example, a 1% solution of atropine has 1 g/100 mL, or 10 mg/1 mL. A simpler way of remembering this conversion is to add a 0 to the drug percentage to change the value to mg/mL. As there are 20 drops per milliliter (up to 40 in some newer, small-tip dispensers), there is ¼–½ mg of 1% atropine per drop. If this drop is given bilaterally, there is up to 1 mg of active agent available for systemic absorption, though the actual amount absorbed is limited by dilution and the wash-out effect of tears.

Because the contact time of topical medication is short, the rate of transfer from the tear fluid into the cornea is crucial. The corneal epithelium and endothelium have tight intercellular junctions that limit passage of molecules in the extracellular space. Topically applied medication must first pass through hydrophobic/lipophilic cell membranes in the epithelium, then through the hydrophilic/lipophobic corneal stroma, and finally through the hydrophobic/lipophilic cell membranes in the endothelium in order to enter the anterior segment. Topical ophthalmic drug formulations must therefore be both lipophilic and hydrophilic. As nonionic particles are more lipophilic than ionic particles are, they pass through the cellular phospholipid membranes more readily. The pH of the medication can be manipulated to increase the percentage of the drug in an uncharged or nonionized

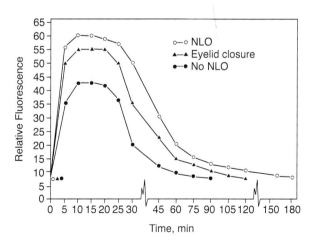

Figure 15-1 Fluorescein concentration in the anterior chamber at various times after application: with nasolacrimal occlusion (NLO), with 5 minutes of eyelid closure, or with no intervention (no NLO).

form. Mechanical disruption of the epithelial barrier in corneal abrasion or infection also increases the rate of intraocular drug penetration.

Similar considerations apply to the conjunctiva. The permeability of the conjunctiva to small water-soluble molecules is thought to be 20 times that of the cornea. Perilimbal conjunctiva offers an effective transscleral route for delivery of drugs to anterior segment structures.

The factors determining the amount of medication that can penetrate the cornea are concentration and solubility in the delivery vehicle, viscosity, lipid solubility, and the drug's pH, ionic and steric form, molecular size, chemical structure and configuration, vehicle, and surfactants. In addition, reflex tearing and the binding of the active medication to proteins in tears and tissue affect drug bioavailability.

Drug concentration and solubility To get a sufficient amount of a drug through the corneal barriers, it may be necessary to load the tear reservoir with concentrated solutions (eg, by selecting pilocarpine 4% instead of pilocarpine 1%). A practical limit to exploiting these high concentrations is reached when the high tonicity of the resulting solutions elicits reflex tearing or when drugs that are poorly water-soluble reach their solubility limits and precipitate. A drug with adequate solubility in an aqueous solution can be formulated as a solution, whereas a drug with poor solubility may need to be provided in a suspension. A suspension requires agitation so that the active medication is redistributed prior to administration. Suspensions may be more irritating to the ocular surface than solutions are, a factor that may affect the choice of drug formulation.

The units of concentration or dilution of solution are not standardized. Students of pharmacology need to familiarize themselves with the conversions between different units. The solution's labeled percentage (%) represents the amount of active ingredient in the number of grams per 100 mL of solution (eg, 1% = 1 g/100 mL, or 1000 mg/100 mL, or 10 mg/mL). The solution concentration may also be presented in a dilution ratio. For example, a 1:1000 solution has 1 g of active ingredient per 1000 mL solution, or 1000 mg/1000 mL, or 1 mg/1 mL. Converting this ratio to a percentage, a 1:1000 solution equals a concentration of 0.1 g/100 mL, or 0.1%.

Viscosity The addition of high-viscosity substances such as methylcellulose and polyvinyl alcohol (PVA) to a drug increases drug retention in the inferior cul-de-sac, aiding drug penetration. For example, the gel form of timolol maleate contains a heteropolysaccharide that thickens on contact with the tear film, maintaining therapeutic levels while decreasing the dosing to once daily.

Improvement in ocular drug delivery is observed over the viscosity range from 1 to 15 centipoise (cP), and it is suggested that the optimal viscosity should be 12–15 cP. Further increases in viscosity above this level do not appear to proportionally increase the drug concentration in aqueous. In fact, formulations with higher levels of viscosity cause ocular surface irritation, resulting in reflex blinking, lacrimation, and increased drainage of the applied formulation. High viscosity levels may also inhibit product–tear mixing and distort the ocular surface. Products with viscosity levels that are too high may impart a sticky feeling and are uncomfortable for patients to use.

Lipid solubility Studies of the permeability of isolated corneas to families of chemical compounds show that lipid solubility is more important than water solubility in promoting penetration. To determine the solubility of a drug or group of drugs, researchers ascertain the ratio of lipid solubility to water solubility for each compound in the series by (1) measuring the phase separation of a drug between 2 solvents—1 lipid-soluble and 1 water-soluble (eg, octanol and water); and (2) calculating the ratio of the drug concentration in the 2 compartments (partition coefficient). Drugs with greater relative lipid solubility have a higher partition coefficient.

For example, the permeability coefficient is 70 times higher for substituted ethoxzolamides with high lipid solubility than for those of low lipid solubility. Drugs with higher levels of lipid solubility and higher partition coefficients have increased penetration of cell membranes. However, compounds with excessively high partition coefficients are often poorly soluble in tears. Experimental studies of substituted compounds need to account for the effects of the substituents on potency, solubility, and the permeability coefficient.

pH and ionic charge Many eye medications are alkaloids, or weak bases. Such drugs as tropicamide, cyclopentolate, atropine, and epinephrine exist in both charged and uncharged forms at the slightly alkaline pH of tears (pH 7.4). The partition coefficients, and therefore the drug penetration, can be increased by raising the pH of the water phase, thereby increasing the proportion of drug molecules in the more lipid-soluble, uncharged form. However, a large difference between the pH of the topical solution and the pH of tears may result in ocular irritation and stimulate reflex tearing that dilutes or washes away the topical drops.

Surfactants Many preservative agents used in topical drops to prevent bacterial contamination are surface-active agents that alter cell membranes in the cornea as well as in bacteria. They reduce the barrier effect of the corneal epithelium and increase drug permeability. For example, a 0.1% carbachol solution containing 0.03% benzalkonium chloride can elicit the same miotic response as a 2% solution without the preservative.

Reflex tearing Ocular irritation and secondary tearing wash out the drug reservoir in the tear lake and reduce the contact time of the drug with the cornea. Reflex tearing occurs when topical medications are not isotonic and when they have a nonphysiologic pH or contain irritants.

Tissue binding of medication Tear and surface proteins, as well as ocular melanin, may bind topical or systemic medication, making the drug unavailable or creating a slow release reservoir. This binding may alter the lag time, or onset of action, of a medication as well as the peak effect and duration of action, and it can cause a delayed local toxicity despite discontinuation of the medication. One example of this effect is the retinal toxicity that progresses even after discontinuation of the aminoquinoline antimalarial drugs chloroquine and hydroxychloroquine.

Ointments

Another strategy for increasing the contact time of ocular medications is through the use of ointments. Commercial oil-based ointments usually consist of petrolatum and mineral oil. The mineral oil allows the ointment to melt at body temperature. Both ingredients are also effective lipid solvents. However, most water-soluble medications are insoluble in the ointment and are present as microcrystals. Only those microcrystals on the surface of the ointment dissolve in the tears; the rest are trapped until the ointment melts. Such protracted, slow release may prevent the drug from reaching a therapeutic level in the tears. Only if the drug has high lipid solubility (which allows it to diffuse through the ointment) and some water solubility will it escape from the ointment into both the corneal epithelium and the tears. Fluorometholone, chloramphenicol, and tetracycline are examples of drugs that achieve higher aqueous levels when administered as ointment than as drops.

Local Administration

Periocular injections

Injection of medication beneath the conjunctiva or the Tenon capsule allows drugs to bypass the conjunctival and corneal epithelial barriers and absorb passively down a concentration gradient into the sclera and intraocular tissues. Subconjunctival, sub-Tenon, and retrobulbar injections all allow medications to reach therapeutic levels behind the lens–iris diaphragm. This approach is especially useful for drugs with low lipid solubility (such as penicillin), which do not penetrate the eye adequately if they are given topically. Injections can also be helpful in delivering medication closer to the local site of action— for example, posterior sub-Tenon injections of steroids for cystoid macular edema (CME) or subconjunctival injection of 5-fluorouracil after trabeculectomy. Retrobulbar and peribulbar anesthesia techniques for ocular surgery are covered in BCSC Section 11, *Lens and Cataract*. Other examples of local, injectable medications are botulinum toxin, which is used in the treatment of benign essential blepharospasm and hemifacial spasm and for cosmesis; and retrobulbar alcohol as therapy for chronic pain in blind eyes.

Intraocular medications

The intraocular injection of drugs instantly delivers effective concentrations at the target site. Although this route may reduce systemic adverse effects, ocular adverse effects may be more pronounced. For instance, a significant increase in intraocular pressure may persist for a long duration after intraocular injection of corticosteroids. Other ocular adverse effects may include uveitis, hypopyon, and infection. Great care must be taken to avoid using preserved medication and to control the concentration of intraocular drugs so that the delicate internal structures of the eye are protected from toxicity. To avoid infection, strict adherence to standard aseptic technique is required for the preparation and injection of intraocular medication. There are 2 types of intraocular injections: intracameral injections into the anterior chamber and intravitreal injections into the vitreous cavity. Some examples of substances and medications delivered via intraocular routes are summarized in Table 15-1.

Ho AC, Scott IU, Kim SJ, et al. Anti-vascular endothelial growth factor pharmacotherapy for diabetic macular edema: a report by the American Academy of Ophthalmology. *Ophthalmology.* 2012;119(10):2179–2188. Epub 2012 Aug 20.

Wen JC, McCannel CA, Mochon AB, Garner OB. Bacterial dispersal association with speech in the setting of intravitreous injections. *Arch Ophthalmol.* 2011;129(12):1551–1554. Epub 2011 Aug 8.

Yeh S, Albini TA, Moshfeghi AA, Nussenblatt RB. Uveitis, the Comparison of Age-Related Macular Degeneration Treatments Trials (CATT), and intravitreal biologics for ocular inflammation. *Am J Ophthalmol.* 2012;154(3):429–435.

Table 15-1 Medications Delivered by Intracameral and Intravitreal Routes

Route of Administration	Clinical Application
Intracameral	
Acetylcholine Carbachol	Constrict pupil in intraocular surgery
Balanced salt solution Viscoelastic material	Intraocular surgery, re-formation of anterior chamber
Epinephrine	Dilate pupil in intraocular surgery
Lidocaine (preservative free)	Intraocular surgery, anesthesia
Methylene blue	Staining of anterior capsule in cataract surgery
Tissue plasminogen activator (tPA; off-label use)	Assist fibrinolysis of fibrin in anterior chamber and subretinal hemorrhage
Intravitreal	
Anti–vascular endothelial growth factor (anti-VEGF; eg, bevacizumab, ranibizumab)	Chorioretinal neovascularization, proliferative diabetic retinopathy, diabetic macular edema
Corticosteroids (eg, triamcinolone acetonide; sustained-release intraocular implants such as dexamethasone in polylactic acid–coglycolic acid matrix and fluocinolone acetonide in a polyvinyl acetate/silicone laminate)	Cystoid macular edema, retinal vein occlusion, posterior uveitis
Ganciclovir injection or implant	Cytomegalovirus retinitis
Silicone oil Intraocular gases Perfluorocarbon	Vitreoretinal surgery
Various antibiotics	Intraocular bacterial infection

Systemic Administration

Just as the intercellular tight junctions of the corneal epithelium and endothelium limit anterior access to the interior of the eye, similar barriers limit access through vascular channels. The vascular endothelium of the retina, like that of the brain, is nonfenestrated and knitted together by tight junctions. Although both the choroid and the ciliary body have fenestrated vascular endothelia, the choroid is effectively sequestered by the retinal pigment epithelium; and the ciliary body, by its nonpigmented epithelium.

Drugs with higher lipid solubilities more readily penetrate the blood–ocular barrier. Thus, chloramphenicol, which is highly lipid-soluble, penetrates 20 times better than does penicillin, which has poor lipid solubility.

The ability of systemically administered drugs to gain access to the eye is also influenced by the degree to which they are bound to plasma proteins. Only the unbound form can cross the blood–ocular barrier. Sulfonamides are lipid-soluble but penetrate poorly because, at therapeutic levels, more than 90% of the medication is bound to plasma proteins. Similarly, compared with methicillin, oxacillin has reduced penetration because of its increased binding of plasma protein. Because bolus administration of a drug exceeds the binding capacity of plasma proteins and leads to higher intraocular drug levels than can be achieved by a slow intravenous drip, this approach is used for the administration of antibiotics in order to attain high peak intraocular levels.

Sustained-release oral preparations

The practical value of sustained-release preparations is substantial. For example, a single dose of acetazolamide will reduce intraocular pressure for up to 10 hours, whereas a single dose of sustained-release acetazolamide will produce a comparable effect lasting 20 hours. Sustained-release medications offer a more steady blood level of the drug, avoid marked peaks and valleys, and reduce the frequency of administration.

Intravenous injections

Intravenous medication can be administered for either diagnostic or therapeutic effect. Two diagnostic agents, sodium fluorescein and indocyanine green, are used for retinal angiography to aid in the diagnosis of retinal and choroidal diseases. Edrophonium chloride is used intravenously in the diagnosis of myasthenia gravis.

Intravenous medications are also used therapeutically in ophthalmology. Although intravitreal injections have replaced intravenous therapy for postoperative endophthalmitis, continuous intravenous administration of an antibiotic is an effective way of maintaining intraocular levels in endogenous infection (see BCSC Section 12, *Retina and Vitreous*).

The barriers and reservoir effects of the eye affect the ocular pharmacodynamics of antibiotics such as ampicillin, chloramphenicol, and erythromycin. These drugs penetrate the eye with higher initial intraocular levels and maintain comparable bioavailability for 4 hours when given as a single intravenous bolus rather than by continuous infusion. Medication may have better intraocular penetration in the inflamed eye than in the healthy eye due to the disruption of the blood–aqueous and blood–retina barriers. This disruption is demonstrated by the leakage of fluorescein from inflamed retinal vessels into the vitreous during angiography.

Studies in rabbit eyes found that the bioavailability of intravenous ampicillin, tetracycline, and dexamethasone is different in various structures of the rabbit eye, with the highest levels of these medications found in the sclera and conjunctiva, followed by the iris and ciliary body, and finally the cornea, aqueous humor, choroid, and retina. Very low levels appeared in the lens and vitreous. The drugs showed no marked differences in their vascular distribution, however. The tissue bioavailability is determined by the vascularity of the tissue and the barriers that exist between the blood and that tissue.

Intramuscular injections

In ophthalmology, intramuscular drugs are used less frequently than are topical, oral, or intravenous medications. Notable exceptions include the use of prostigmine in the diagnosis of myasthenia gravis and local therapeutic use of botulinum toxin in facial dystonias.

Methods of Ocular Drug Design and Delivery

New ocular drugs are designed with a focus on specificity and safety, with delivery systems aimed at improving convenience and patient adherence. Each of the following approaches responds to a specific problem in ocular pharmacokinetics.

Prodrugs

Ophthalmic prodrugs are therapeutically inactive derivatives of drug molecules that are designed to be activated by enzymatic systems within the eye. These derivatives are usually synthesized by conjugation of a specific promoiety to the parent drug via ester or amide. The ester and amide ophthalmic prodrugs are hydrolyzed by esterase and amidases to the active molecules as they permeate through the cornea or conjunctiva. Permeability across the cornea is also improved by the increased lipid solubility of the prodrug. Prostaglandin analogues are successful examples of this drug-delivery strategy. Prostaglandin analogues used as prodrugs currently available internationally include latanoprost, travoprost, unoprostone, and tafluprost as ester prodrugs, and bimatoprost as an amide prodrug.

Valacyclovir HCl is an antiviral prodrug that is easily absorbed through the gastrointestinal system and quickly converted to the active form of acyclovir. Likewise, famciclovir is a prodrug of the active antiviral penciclovir.

Sustained-release delivery

Eyedrop therapy involves periodic delivery of relatively large quantities of a drug to overcome low ocular bioavailability due to various factors, such as tearing and blinking, nasolacrimal drainage, conjunctival blood and lymph flow, metabolic degradation, and corneal and blood–aqueous barriers. The high peak drug levels attained in bolus dosing can cause local and systemic side effects, such as miosis and induced accommodation following the use of pilocarpine. In addition, significant variation can occur in the concentration of a drug in the eye due to variations in application technique and patient adherence to dosing amounts and schedules. There is a need for an efficient delivery system that can provide controlled release of a drug with a reduced dosing frequency.

Devices have been developed that deliver an adequate supply of medication at a steady-state level, thus achieving beneficial effects with fewer adverse effects. The Ocusert delivery system, designed to deliver pilocarpine at a steady rate of 40 µg/hr, was the therapeutic equivalent of 2% pilocarpine used 4 times a day. However, because the total daily dose of pilocarpine was only 960 µg (24 hours × 40 µg/hr) when delivered with the device as compared with 4000 µg (4 doses × 2000 mg/100 mL × 0.05 mL/dose) with administration via eyedrops, miosis was less marked, and the induced accommodation was reduced. The Ocusert device was discontinued as the use of pilocarpine decreased, but it remains an interesting example of steady-state drug delivery. This device may be resurrected in the future for use with other medications.

Another sustained-release intraocular device is surgically implanted and delivers a steady source of ganciclovir for 5–8 months. An ethylene vinyl acetate disc with polyvinyl alcohol coating serves as the drug reservoir. The thickness of the polyvinyl alcohol lid regulates the delivery of ganciclovir to the target tissue. Similarly, fluocinolone acetonide intravitreal implants are used for the slow, targeted delivery of corticosteroids to the vitreous cavity for treatment of posterior uveitis. A dexamethasone intravitreal implant is a biodegradable polymer matrix loaded with dexamethasone for injection into the vitreous cavity. The polymer degrades, and dexamethasone is slowly released inside the vitreous cavity.

Collagen cornea shields

In the design of collagen cornea shields, porcine scleral tissue is extracted and molded into contact lens–like shields that are useful as a delivery system to prolong the contact between the drug and the cornea. Drugs can be incorporated into the collagen matrix during the manufacturing process, absorbed into the shield during rehydration, or applied topically while the shield is in the eye. Because the shield dissolves in 12, 24, or 72 hours, depending on the manufacturing process for collagen crosslinking, the drug is released gradually into the tear film, and high concentrations are maintained on the corneal surface and in the conjunctival cul-de-sac.

The shields have been used for the early management of bacterial keratitis, as well as for antibiotic prophylaxis. They have also been used to promote epithelial healing after ocular surgery, trauma, or spontaneous erosion. Despite these therapeutic benefits, collagen shields are poorly tolerated because they are very uncomfortable.

New technologies in drug delivery

Ongoing research approaches for contact lens drug-delivery systems focus on improving the residence time of the drug at the surface of the eye to enhance bioavailability and provide more convenient and efficacious therapy. Drug incorporation to the lens body is achieved using various techniques. These techniques include soaking of the lens in drug solution, incorporation of monomers able to interact with target drugs into the contact lens hydrogels, incorporation of drug-loaded colloidal nanoparticles into the matrix of the contact lens, and use of a molecular imprinting technique in which the components of the hydrogel network are organized such that high-affinity binding sites for the drug are created. These contact lens systems need to be designed so they also preserve the transparency and oxygen permeability required for vision and health of the cornea.

Various punctal plug–mediated ocular delivery systems are currently under clinical investigation. The design of these delivery systems generally includes a central cylindrical polymeric core loaded with the drug compound, an impermeable shell, and a cap (or head portion of the plug exposed to the tear film) with pores from which the drug is released by diffusion. Most examples of punctal plug systems show near zero-order drug-release rates for drug molecules. Delivery of drugs by punctal plug has several potential advantages over administration via eyedrops, including dose reduction, controlled release of the drug at an optimum rate, and improved patient adherence. Limitations include ocular irritation, itchiness, discomfort, increased lacrimation, and spontaneous extrusion of the plug.

Encapsulated-cell technology has been applied to the delivery of therapeutic agents intravitreally for treatment of retinal diseases. This technology uses cells encapsulated within a semipermeable polymer capsule that secretes the therapeutic material into the vitreous.

Liposomes are synthetic lipid microspheres that serve as multipurpose vehicles for the topical delivery of drugs, genetic material, and cosmetics. They are produced when phospholipid molecules interact to form a bilayer lipid membrane in an aqueous environment. The interior of the bilayer consists of the hydrophobic fatty-acid tails of the phospholipid molecule, whereas the outer layer is composed of hydrophilic polar-head groups of the molecule. A water-soluble drug can be dissolved in the aqueous phase of the interior compartment; a hydrophobic drug can be intercalated into the lipid bilayer itself. However, the routine use of liposome formulation for topical ocular drug delivery is limited by these products' short shelf life, limited drug-loading capacity, and difficulty with stabilizing the preparation.

The application of nanotechnology to protect active molecules and provide sustained drug delivery is being actively pursued. Methods used to transport hydrophilic and lipophilic drugs and genes include the use of biodegradable nanoparticles such as nanospheres, nanocapsules, and nanomicelles; the colloidal dispersion of nanoparticles as nanosuspension; and the use of nanoemulsion. These methods are modeled after the molecular structure of viruses.

The physical process of moving charged molecules by an electrical current is called *iontophoresis.* This procedure places a relatively high concentration of a drug locally, where it can achieve maximum benefit with little waste or systemic absorption. Animal studies have demonstrated that iontophoresis increases penetration of various antibiotics and antiviral drugs across ocular surfaces into the cornea and the interior of the eye. However, patient discomfort, ocular tissue damage, and necrosis restrict the popularity of this mode of drug delivery.

Pharmacodynamics: The Mechanism of Drug Action

Most drugs act by binding to and altering the function of regulatory macromolecules, usually neurotransmitter receptors, hormone receptors, or enzymes. Binding may be a reversible association mediated by electrostatic and/or van der Waals forces, or it may involve formation of a covalent intermediate. If the drug–receptor interaction stimulates the receptor's natural function, the drug is termed an *agonist.* Stimulation of an opposing effect characterizes an *antagonist.* Corresponding effectors of enzymes are termed *activators* and *inhibitors.* This terminology is crucial to understanding the next chapter.

The relationship between the initial drug–receptor interaction and the drug's clinical dose-response curve may be simple or complex. In some cases, the drug's clinical effect closely reflects the degree of receptor occupancy on a moment-to-moment basis. Such is usually the case for drugs that affect neural transmission or for drugs that are enzyme inhibitors. In contrast, some drug effects lag hours behind receptor occupancy or persist long after the drug is gone. Such is the case with many drugs acting on hormone receptors, because their effects are often mediated through a series of biochemical events.

In addition to differences in timing of receptor occupancy and drug effects, the degree of receptor occupancy can differ considerably from the corresponding drug effect. For example, because the amount of carbonic anhydrase present in the ciliary processes is 100 times that required to support aqueous secretion, more than 99% of the enzyme must be inhibited before secretion is reduced. On the other hand, some maximal hormone responses occur at concentrations well below that required for receptor saturation, indicating the presence of "unbound receptors."

Cholkar K, Patel SP, Vadlapudi AW, Mitra AK. Novel strategies for anterior ocular drug delivery. *J Ocular Pharmacol Ther.* 2013;29(2):106–123. Epub 2012 Dec 5.

Gaudana R, Ananthula HK, Parenky A, Mitra AK. Ocular drug delivery. *AAPS J.* 2010;12(3): 348–360. Epub 2010 May 1.

Guzman-Aranguez A, Colligris B, Pintor J. Contact lenses: promising devices for ocular drug delivery. *J Ocular Pharmacol Ther.* 2013;29(2):189–199. Epub 2012 Dec 5.

CHAPTER 16

Ocular Pharmacotherapeutics*

Legal Aspects of Medical Therapy

The US Food and Drug Administration (FDA) has statutory authority to approve the marketing of prescription drugs and to specify the uses of these drugs. The FDA has created a 3-step process to regulate human testing of new drugs before they are approved for marketing. After animal and in vitro studies, *phase 1* testing begins; this process involves tests on 10–80 people for toxicology and pharmacokinetic data concerning dosage range, absorption, metabolism, and toxicity. *Phase 2* testing involves randomized, controlled clinical trials on a minimum of 50–100 affected people to determine safety and effectiveness. *Phase 3* testing uses controlled and uncontrolled trials to evaluate the overall risk–benefit relationship and to provide an adequate basis for physician labeling. The data gathered from these tests are then submitted as part of a new drug application for marketing. The FDA's approval of each drug and its specific uses is based on documentation submitted by manufacturers that supports the safety and efficacy of specific drug applications. Although the FDA has developed distinct approaches to making drugs available as rapidly as possible, the process of bringing new products to market requires tremendous research and development efforts that span many years and consume millions of dollars.

Once approved for any use, a drug may be prescribed by individual physicians for any indication in all ages without violating federal law. However, physicians remain liable to malpractice actions. In particular, a nonapproved use that does not adhere to an applicable standard of care places a practitioner in a difficult legal position. If a respectable minority of similarly situated physicians prescribes in the same manner, a standard of care could be met in most jurisdictions. Informed consent in equivocal cases is helpful.

---

*This chapter may include information on pharmaceutical applications that are not considered community standard, that are approved for use only in restricted research settings, or that reflect indications not included in approved US Food and Drug Administration (FDA) labeling (off-label use). For example, many ophthalmic uses of systemic medications, including most systemic antibiotics and antifungal drugs compounded for treatment of ocular infections such as keratitis and endophthalmitis, are off-label. Many antifungal drugs are used with an off-label application based on in vitro and animal data because human data for unusual infectious agents are often limited. **The FDA has stated that it is the responsibility of the physician to determine the FDA status of each drug or device he or she wishes to use and to use it with appropriate, informed patient consent in compliance with applicable law. (The legal aspect of medical therapy varies in different countries and regions. For example, the General Medical Council [GMC] in the United Kingdom recognizes that a physician has a moral duty toward all his or her patients, which may affect decision making when choosing the appropriate medical therapy under tight budgetary restrictions.)**

Many common drugs are used off-label in ophthalmology. These drugs include (but are not limited to) the following:

- bevacizumab, an antiangiogenic drug used off-label in intravitreal injections for numerous neovascular ocular diseases
- acetylcysteine (10% or 20%), used as a mucolytic drug in filamentary keratopathy and as an anticollagenase drug in severe alkali injuries
- tissue plasminogen activator (tPA), used as an intravitreal injection for thrombolysis and fibrinolysis
- fluorouracil (5-FU), used to improve the outcomes of glaucoma filtration surgery
- mitomycin, used to improve the outcomes of glaucoma filtration surgery and to treat ocular surface neoplasia
- cyclosporine A, used off-label as a 2% compounded solution in high-risk corneal transplants and in severe vernal, ligneous, and autoimmune keratopathies
- doxycycline, used for ocular rosacea
- edetate disodium (salt of ethylenediaminetetraacetic acid, EDTA), used for band keratopathy
- hyaluronic acid, used as a viscoelastic material for re-formation of the anterior chamber
- fibrin sealant, used to adhere the conjunctival graft to the scleral bed in pterygium resection

One of the most commonly used medications, topical prednisolone, has not been approved by the FDA specifically for postoperative care. When used postoperatively for cataract surgery, it is an off-label application. The FDA has established clear guidelines for the use of investigational drugs, which must meet specified commercial and investigative requirements.

Compounding Pharmaceuticals

Compounded pharmaceuticals are used to treat numerous ophthalmologic diseases both in surgical settings and for diagnostic office procedures. The Pharmacy Compounding Accreditation Board (PCAB) accredits pharmacies that provide evidence of adherence to quality standards for pharmacy compounding. The PCAB requires proper licensure with state and federal regulatory authorities, appropriate training of personnel, and facilities and methods that permit aseptic compounding of sterile preparations and meet the US Pharmacopeia (USP) guidelines.

In light of the 2011 outbreaks of infectious endophthalmitis associated with compounded bevacizumab used for intravitreal injections, the American Academy of Ophthalmology (AAO) issued the following 2 recommendations for the sourcing of bevacizumab for intravitreal injections:

1. Select a compounding pharmacy that is accredited by the PCAB and adheres to quality standards for aseptic compounding of sterile medications (USP Chapter 797 guidelines; see www.pcab.org/accredited-pharmacies).
2. Record the lot number of the medication vial and the lot number of the syringes in the patient record or a log, in case they need to be tracked.

Although ensuring the safety and sterility of the compounded products is certainly important, maintaining practitioner access to essential compounded products for office use is crucial. Practicing ophthalmologists should stay up-to-date with current state and federal pharmacy regulations concerning compounding pharmaceuticals. The AAO and many subspecialty societies provide e-mail alerts and updates on regulation and legislation to their members.

Cholinergic Drugs

Several commonly used ophthalmic medications affect the activity of acetylcholine receptors in synapses of the somatic and autonomic nervous systems (Fig 16-1). Such receptors are found in

- the motor end plates of the extraocular and levator palpebrae superioris muscles (supplied by somatic motor nerves)
- the cells of the superior cervical (sympathetic) ganglion and the ciliary and sphenopalatine (parasympathetic) ganglia (supplied by preganglionic autonomic nerves)

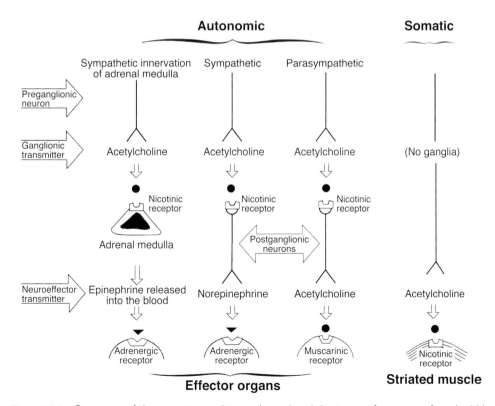

Figure 16-1 Summary of the neurotransmitters released and the types of receptors found within the autonomic and somatic nervous systems. *(Reproduced with permission from Mycek MJ, Harvey RA, Champe PC, eds. Pharmacology. 2nd ed. Lippincott's Illustrated Reviews. Philadelphia: Lippincott-Raven; 1997:32.)*

- parasympathetic effector sites in the iris sphincter and ciliary body and in the lacrimal, accessory lacrimal, and meibomian glands (supplied by postganglionic parasympathetic nerves)

Although all cholinergic receptors are by definition responsive to acetylcholine, they are not homogeneous and can be classified by their responses to 2 drugs: muscarine and nicotine (Table 16-1). *Muscarinic receptors* are found in the end organs of the parasympathetic autonomic system. *Nicotinic receptors* are found in the postganglionic neurons of both the sympathetic and parasympathetic systems, in striated muscle (the end organ of the somatic system), and in the adrenal medulla. Cholinergic drugs may be further divided into the following groups (Fig 16-2):

- direct-acting agonists, which act on the receptor to elicit an excitatory postsynaptic potential
- indirect-acting agonists, which increase endogenous acetylcholine levels at the synaptic cleft by inhibiting acetylcholinesterase
- antagonists, which block the action of acetylcholine on the receptor

Muscarinic Drugs

Direct-acting agonists

Topically applied, direct-acting agonists have 3 actions. First, they cause contraction of the iris sphincter, which not only constricts the pupil *(miosis)* but also changes the anatomical relationship of the iris to both the lens and the chamber angle. Second, they cause contraction of the circular fibers of the ciliary muscle, relaxing the zonular tension on the lens equator and allowing the lens to shift forward and assume a more spherical shape *(accommodation)*. Third, they cause contraction of the longitudinal fibers of the ciliary muscle, producing tension on the scleral spur (opening the trabecular meshwork) and facilitating

Table 16-1 Cholinergic and Adrenergic Receptors*

Receptors	Agonists	Blocking Agents
Cholinergic (sphincter)	Acetylcholine	
Muscarinic	Muscarine	Atropine
Nicotinic	Nicotine	d-Tubocurarine
Adrenergic (dilator)	Norepinephrine	
Alpha†	Phenylephrine	Phentolamine and phenoxybenzamine
α_1	Phenylephrine	Prazosin, thymoxamine, dapiprazole
α_2	Apraclonidine	Yohimbine
Beta	Isoproterenol	Propranolol and timolol
β_1	Tazolol	Betaxolol
β_2	Albuterol	Butoxamine

*The cholinergic agonists and the adrenergic blockers listed cause miosis; the adrenergic agonists and the cholinergic blockers listed cause dilation.

†The prefixes α_1 and α_2 have been proposed for post- and presynaptic α-adrenoceptors, respectively. According to the present view, the classification into α_1 and α_2 subtypes is based exclusively on the relative potencies and affinities of agonists and antagonists, regardless of their function and localization.

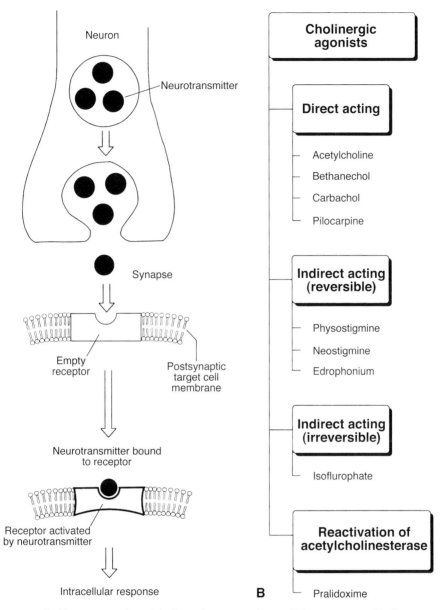

Figure 16-2   A, Neurotransmitter binding triggers an intracellular response. **B,** Summary of cholinergic agonists. *(Reproduced with permission from Harvey RA, Champe PC, eds.* Pharmacology. *Lippincott's Illustrated Reviews. Philadelphia: Lippincott; 1992:30, 35.)*

aqueous outflow. Contraction of the ciliary musculature also produces tension on the peripheral retina, occasionally resulting in a retinal tear or even rhegmatogenous detachment.

Acetylcholine does not penetrate the corneal epithelium well, and it is rapidly degraded by acetylcholinesterase (Fig 16-3). Thus, it is not used topically. Acetylcholine, 1%, and carbachol, 0.01%, are available for intracameral use in anterior segment surgery. These drugs produce prompt and marked miosis.

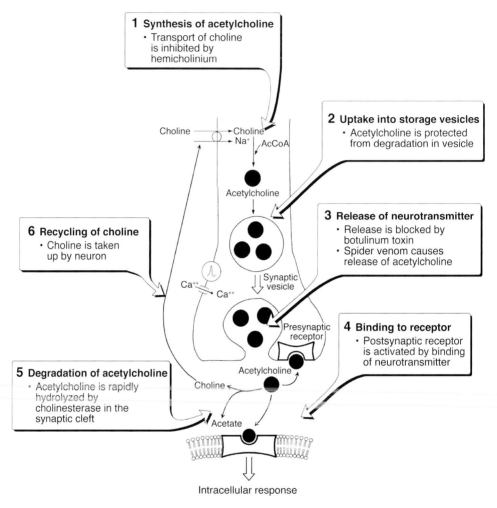

Figure 16-3 Synthesis and release of acetylcholine from the cholinergic neuron. AcCoA = acetyl coenzyme A. *(Reproduced with permission from Mycek MJ, Harvey RA, Champe PC, eds. Pharmacology. 2nd ed. Lippincott's Illustrated Reviews. Philadelphia: Lippincott-Raven; 1997:37.)*

Intracameral acetylcholine, 1%, has a more rapid onset than that of intracameral carbachol; it acts within seconds of instillation, but the effect is short-lived. Acetylcholine is not stable in aqueous form and is rapidly broken down by acetylcholinesterase in the anterior chamber. Intracameral carbachol, 0.01%, is 100 times more effective and longer lasting than is acetylcholine administered similarly. Maximal miosis is achieved within 5 minutes and lasts for 24 hours. In addition, carbachol, 0.01%, is an effective hypotensive drug and lowers intraocular pressure (IOP) during the crucial 24-hour period after surgery.

Pilocarpine, 0.12%, is used diagnostically to confirm an Adie tonic pupil, a condition in which the parasympathetic innervation of the iris sphincter and ciliary muscle is defective because of the loss of postganglionic fibers. Denervated muscarinic smooth-muscle fibers in the affected segments of the iris exhibit supersensitivity and respond well to this weak miotic, whereas the normal iris does not.

Pilocarpine, 0.25%, 0.5%, 1%, 2%, 3%, 4%, or 6% (4 times daily), and carbachol, 1.5% or 3% (2 times daily), are used in the treatment of *primary open-angle glaucoma (POAG)* because they lower IOP by increasing outflow facility (Table 16-2). Use of pilocarpine, 4%, is contraindicated in acute attacks of angle-closure glaucoma because this strong miotic may induce intense anterior movement of the lens–iris diaphragm, closing the angle completely. Miotic therapy can be used (1) to treat elevated IOP in patients with primary angle-closure glaucoma in which the anterior chamber angle remains occludable despite laser iridotomy and (2) for prophylaxis for angle closure prior to iridotomy, but it should not be used as long-term treatment to substitute for laser iridotomy (also see BCSC Section 10, *Glaucoma,* for additional information).

Miosis, cataractogenesis, and induced myopia are generally unwelcome side effects of muscarinic therapy. Although the broad range of retinal dark adaptation usually compensates sufficiently for the effect of miosis on vision during daylight hours, patients may be visually incapacitated in dim light. In addition, miosis often compounds the effect of axial lenticular opacities; many patients with cataracts are unable to tolerate miotics. Older patients with early cataracts have visual difficulty in scotopic conditions; the miosis induced by cholinergic drugs may increase the risk of falls.

Younger patients may have difficulty with miotics as well. Induced myopia and induced accommodation occur because of the drug-induced contraction of the ciliary body, which increases the convexity of the lens and shifts the lens forward. Patients younger than 50 years may manifest disabling myopia and induced accommodation from this adverse effect. Other complications observed with use of higher concentrations of miotics include miotic iris cysts and an increased incidence of retinal detachment due to ciliary body contraction and traction on the pars plana.

Systemic adverse effects of muscarinic agonists include salivation, diarrhea, urinary urgency, vomiting, bronchial spasm, bradycardia, and diaphoresis. However, systemic adverse effects following topical use of direct-acting agonists are rare. A slowly dissolving pilocarpine gel used at bedtime minimizes the unwanted side effects of pilocarpine and is useful for younger patients, patients with symptoms of variable myopia or intense miosis, older patients with lens opacities, and patients who have difficulty adhering to more frequent dosing regimens.

Ciliary muscle stimulation can be desirable for managing accommodative esotropia. The near response is a synkinesis of accommodation, miosis, and convergence. As

Table 16-2 Miotics

Generic Name	Trade Name	Strengths
Cholinergic drugs		
Carbachol	Isopto Carbachol	1.5%, 3%
Pilocarpine HCl	Isopto Carpine	0.25%, 1%, 2%, 4%
	Available generically	0.5%, 1%, 2%, 3%, 4%, 6%
Pilocarpine HCl ointment	Pilopine HS gel	4%
Cholinesterase inhibitors		
Physostigmine	Available generically	1 mg/mL ampule
Echothiophate iodide	Phospholine Iodide	0.125%

discussed previously, muscarinic agonists contract the ciliary body and induce accommodation as an adverse effect. Therefore, the patient does not need to accommodate at near, which decreases not only the synkinetic convergence response but also the degree of accommodative esotropia.

Indirect-acting agonists

Topically applied, indirect-acting muscarinic agonists (cholinesterase inhibitors) have the same actions as direct-acting muscarinic agonists, although they have a longer duration of action and are frequently more potent. Twice-daily treatment is sufficient. These medications react with the active serine hydroxyl site of cholinesterases, forming an enzyme–inhibitor complex. Thus, they render the enzyme unavailable for hydrolyzing spontaneously released acetylcholine. The duration of inhibitory action is determined by the strength of the bond between the inhibitor and the enzyme. Inhibitors that are organic derivatives of phosphoric acid (organophosphates, such as echothiophate) undergo initial binding and hydrolysis by the enzyme, forming a phosphorylated active site. Such a covalent phosphorus–enzyme bond is extremely stable and hydrolyzes very slowly. The duration of inhibitory action is much longer than that of inhibitors with a quaternary ammonium group (eg, edrophonium) and carbamates (eg, neostigmine). Because of the marked differences in duration of action, organophosphate inhibitors are referred to as *irreversible inhibitors.* The 2 classes of cholinesterase inhibitors are

1. *reversible inhibitors,* such as physostigmine (available as powder for compounding and as solution for injection), neostigmine, and edrophonium
2. *irreversible inhibitors,* such as echothiophate (phospholine iodide, no longer available for ophthalmic use in the United States); diisopropyl phosphorofluoridate (DFP; no longer available for ophthalmic use in the United States), which phosphorylates both the acetylcholinesterase of the synaptic cleft and the butyrylcholinesterase (pseudocholinesterase) of plasma; and demecarium bromide (no longer available for ophthalmic use in the United States)

The action of phosphorylating cholinesterase inhibitors can be reversed on an acute basis by treatment with oxime-containing compounds that remove the dialkylphosphate moiety from the enzyme. This treatment must take place rapidly, before the spontaneous elimination of 1 of the alkyl residues (half-life, or $t_{1/2}$, is 20 minutes for butyrylcholinesterase and 270 minutes for acetylcholinesterase), which renders the monoalkylphosphate intermediate no longer susceptible to regeneration by oxime. Thus, the oxime pralidoxime (2-PAM)—although useful in the treatment of acute organophosphate poisoning (eg, insecticide exposure)—is of little value in reversing the marked reduction of plasma butyrylcholinesterase activity that occurs with long-term, irreversible cholinesterase-inhibitor therapy.

Patients receiving long-term, irreversible cholinesterase-inhibitor therapy such as echothiophate may experience toxic reactions from systemic absorption of local anesthetics containing ester groups (eg, procaine) that are normally inactivated by plasma cholinesterase. Administration of the muscle relaxant succinylcholine during induction of general anesthesia would also be hazardous in such patients, because the drug would not be metabolized and would result in prolonged respiratory paralysis.

Phosphorylating cholinesterase inhibitors may also cause local ocular toxicity. Children may develop cystlike proliferations of the iris pigment epithelium at the pupil margin that can block the pupil. For unknown reasons, cyst development can be minimized by concomitant use of phenylephrine (2.5%) drops. In adults, cataracts may develop or preexisting opacities may progress. Interestingly, such cataracts are rare in children, and significant epithelial cysts are rare, if they occur at all, in adults.

Therapy with cholinesterase inhibitors should not be combined with direct-acting cholinergic agonists. This combination is less effective than either drug given alone.

Because cholinesterase inhibitors are potent insecticides, they were used in the past as treatment for lice infestations of the eyelashes. Physostigmine, echothiophate, DFP, and demecarium bromide are no longer commercially available for ophthalmic use in the United States (also see BCSC Section 8, *External Disease and Cornea*).

Antagonists

Topically applied muscarinic antagonists, such as atropine, react with postsynaptic muscarinic receptors and block the action of acetylcholine. Paralysis of the iris sphincter, coupled with the unopposed action of the dilator muscle, causes pupillary dilation, or *mydriasis* (Table 16-3). Mydriasis facilitates examination of the peripheral lens, ciliary body, and retina; it is approved for therapeutic use in the treatment of iritis in adults because it reduces contact between the posterior iris surface and the anterior lens capsule, thereby preventing the formation of iris–lens adhesions, or *posterior synechiae.* Topically applied muscarinic antagonists reduce permeability of the blood–aqueous barrier and are useful for treating ocular inflammatory disease. Atropine and cyclopentolate have been approved by the FDA for use in pediatric patients but not for all indications.

Muscarinic antagonists also paralyze the ciliary muscles, which helps relieve pain associated with iridocyclitis, inhibit accommodation for accurate refraction in children (cyclopentolate, atropine), and treat ciliary block (malignant) glaucoma. However, use of cycloplegic drugs to dilate the pupils of patients with POAG may elevate IOP, especially in patients who require miotics for pressure control. Therefore, it is advisable to use short-acting medications and to consider monitoring IOP in patients with severe optic nerve damage.

In situations requiring complete cycloplegia, such as in the treatment of iridocyclitis (scopolamine, homatropine, or atropine for adults) or the full refractive correction of accommodative esotropia, more potent drugs are preferred. Although a single drop of atropine has some cycloplegic effect that will last for days, 2 or 3 instillations a day may be required to maintain full cycloplegia to relieve pain in iritis. It may become necessary to change medications if atropine elicits a characteristic local irritation with swelling and maceration of the eyelids and conjunctival hyperemia. When mydriasis alone is necessary to facilitate examination or refraction, drugs with a shorter residual effect are preferred, because they allow faster return of pupil response and reading ability.

Systemic absorption of topically administered muscarinic antagonists can produce dose-related toxicity, especially in children, for whom the dose is distributed within a smaller body mass. Flushing, fever, tachycardia, constipation, urinary retention, and even delirium can result from a combination of central and peripheral effects. Mild cases may require only discontinuation of the drug, but severe cases can be treated with intravenous

Table 16-3 **Mydriatics and Cycloplegics**

Generic Name	Trade Name	Strengths	Onset	Duration of Action
Phenylephrine HCl	AK-Dilate	Solution, 2.5%, 10%	30–60 min	3–5 h
	Altafrin	Solution, 2.5%, 10%		
	Mydfrin	Solution, 2.5%		
	Neofrin	Solution, 2.5%		
	Neo-Synephrine	Solution, 2.5%		
	Available generically	Solution, 2.5%, 10%		
Hydroxyamphetamine hydrobromide, 1%		Available as powder for compounding	30–60 min	3–5 h
Atropine sulfate	Atropine-Care	Solution, 1%	45–120 min	7–14 days
	Isopto Atropine	Solution, 1%		
	Available generically	Solution, 1%		
		Ointment, 1%		
Cyclopentolate HCl	AK-Pentolate	Solution, 1%	30–60 min	2 days
	Cyclogyl	Solution, 0.5%–2%		
	Cylate	Solution, 1%		
	Available generically	Solution, 1%, 2%		
Homatropine hydrobromide	Isopto Homatropine	Solution, 2%, 5%	30–60 min	3 days
	Homatropaire	Solution, 5%		
Scopolamine hydrobromide	Isopto Hyoscine	Solution, 0.25%	30–60 min	4–7 days
Tropicamide	Mydral	Solution, 0.5%, 1%	20–40 min	4–6 h
	Mydriacyl	Solution, 1%		
	Tropicacyl	Solution, 0.5%, 1%		
	Available generically	Solution, 0.5%, 1%		
Cyclopentolate HCl/ phenylephrine HCl*	Cyclomydril	Solution, 0.2%/1%	30–60 min	1–2 days
Hydroxyamphetamine hydrobromide/ tropicamide†	Paremyd	Solution, 1%/0.25%	20–40 min	4–6 h

*A dilute combination agent for infant examinations.
†Used for dilating the pupil and cannot be used to test for Horner syndrome.

physostigmine (approved for adults and children), slowly titrated, until the symptoms subside. Physostigmine is used because it is a tertiary amine (uncharged) and can cross the blood–brain barrier.

Systemic administration of atropine blocks the oculocardiac reflex, a reflex bradycardia that is sometimes elicited during ocular surgery by manipulation of the conjunctiva, the globe, or the extraocular muscles. The reflex can also be prevented at the afferent end by retrobulbar anesthesia, although it can occur during administration of the retrobulbar block.

Nicotinic Drugs

Indirect-acting agonists

The only cholinesterase inhibitor that ophthalmologists administer in a dose sufficient to allow it to work as an indirect-acting nicotinic agonist is edrophonium. Edrophonium is a short-acting competitive inhibitor of acetylcholinesterase that binds to the enzyme's active site but does not form a covalent link with it. It is used in the diagnosis of myasthenia gravis, a neuromuscular disease caused by autoimmunity to acetylcholine receptors (nicotinic receptors) in the neuromuscular junction and characterized by muscle weakness and marked fatigability of skeletal muscles. This disease may manifest primarily as ptosis and diplopia. In patients with myasthenia gravis, the inhibition of acetylcholinesterase by edrophonium allows acetylcholine released into the synaptic cleft to accumulate to levels that are adequate to act through the reduced number of acetylcholine receptors. Because edrophonium also augments muscarinic transmission, muscarinic adverse effects (vomiting, diarrhea, urination, and bradycardia) may occur unless 0.4–0.6 mg of atropine is coadministered intravenously (also see BCSC Section 5, *Neuro-Ophthalmology*). Neostigmine methylsulfate is a longer-acting intramuscular drug that is also used in the diagnosis of myasthenia gravis. The longer duration of activity allows the examiner time to specifically assess a complex endpoint, such as orthoptic measurements.

Antagonists

Nicotinic antagonists are administered as neuromuscular blocking agents to facilitate intubation for general anesthesia (Table 16-4). There are 2 types of nicotinic antagonists:

1. *nondepolarizing agents,* including curare-like drugs such as gallamine and pancuronium, which bind competitively to nicotinic receptors on striated muscle but do not cause contraction
2. *depolarizing agents,* such as succinylcholine and decamethonium, which bind competitively to nicotinic receptors and cause an initial receptor depolarization and muscle contraction

In singly innervated *(en plaque)* muscle fibers, depolarization and contraction are followed by prolonged unresponsiveness and flaccidity. However, these drugs produce sustained contractions of multiply innervated fibers, which make up one-fifth of the muscle fibers of extraocular muscles. Such contractions of extraocular muscles (a nicotinic agonist action) exert force on the globe, an undesirable effect in cases in which IOP is to be measured. The use of these drugs in the induction of general anesthesia should be avoided in operations on lacerated eyes, because the force of the muscles on the globe could expel intraocular contents.

Table 16-4 **Cholinergic Antagonists**

Category	Examples
Muscarinic receptor–blocking drugs	Atropine Scopolamine
Ganglion-blocking drugs	Nicotine Trimethaphan Mecamylamine
Neuromuscular blocking drugs	Tubocurarine Pancuronium Gallamine Succinylcholine

Adrenergic Drugs

Several ophthalmic medications affect the activity of adrenergic receptors (also called *adrenoceptors*) in synapses of the peripheral nervous system (Table 16-5). Such receptors are found in the following locations:

- the cell membranes of the iris dilator muscle, the superior palpebral smooth muscle of Müller, the ciliary epithelium and processes, the trabecular meshwork, and the smooth muscle of ocular blood vessels (supplied by postganglionic autonomic fibers from the superior cervical ganglion)
- the presynaptic terminals of some sympathetic and parasympathetic nerves, where they have feedback-inhibitory actions

Although adrenergic receptors were originally defined by their response to epinephrine (adrenaline), the transmitter of most sympathetic postganglionic fibers is actually norepinephrine. Adrenergic receptors are subclassified into 5 categories—α_1, α_2, β_1, β_2, and β_3—on the basis of their profile of responses to natural and synthetic catecholamines (Fig 16-4; see Table 16-5). α_1-Receptors generally mediate smooth-muscle contraction, whereas α_2-receptors mediate feedback inhibition of presynaptic sympathetic (and sometimes parasympathetic) nerve terminals. β_1-Receptors are found predominantly in the heart, where they mediate stimulatory effects; β_2-receptors mediate relaxation of smooth muscle in most blood vessels and in the bronchi; and β_3-receptors are found on fat cells mediating lipolysis.

Systemic absorption of ocular adrenergic drugs is frequently sufficient to cause systemic effects, which are manifested in the cardiovascular system, the bronchial airways, and the brain. Adrenergic drugs may be direct-acting agonists, indirect-acting agonists, or antagonists at 1 or more of the 5 types of receptors.

Table 16-5 Ocular Receptor Subtypes and Their Signal Transduction Mechanisms

Receptor	Receptor Subtypes and Their Signal Transduction Mechanisms			
β-Adrenoceptor	β_1 cAMP ↑	β_2 cAMP ↑	β_3 cAMP ↑	
α_1-Adrenoceptor	α_1A $IP_3/Ca^{2+}/DAG$	α_1B $IP_3/Ca^{2+}/DAG$	α_1D $IP_3/Ca^{2+}/DAG$	
α_2-Adrenoceptor	α_2A cAMP ↓	α_2B cAMP ↓	α_2C cAMP ↓	α_2D cAMP ↓
Muscarinic cholinergic	M_1 $IP_3/Ca^{2+}/DAG$	M_2 cAMP ↓	M_3 $IP_3/Ca^{2+}/DAG$	M_4 cAMP ↓
Calcitonin gene-related peptide (CGRP)	$CGRP_1$ cAMP ↑	$CGRP_2$ cAMP ↑		
Endothelin (ET)	ET_A $IP_3/Ca^{2+}/DAG$ cAMP ↓	ET_B $IP_3/Ca^{2+}/DAG$		
Prostaglandin	DP, EP (EP_1, EP_2, EP_3, EP_4), FP, IP, TP Increase in cAMP or IP_3 depending on the receptor subtype			

cAMP = cyclic adenosine monophosphate; DAG = diacylglycerol.

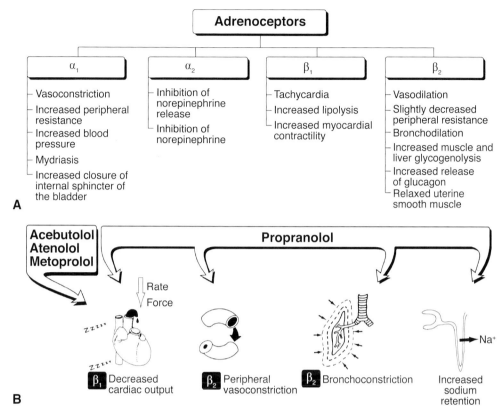

Figure 16-4 **A,** Major effects mediated by α- and β-adrenoceptors. **B,** Actions of propranolol and β₁-blockers. *(Reproduced with permission from Mycek MJ, Harvey RA, Champe PC, eds. Pharmacology. 2nd ed. Lippincott's Illustrated Reviews. Philadelphia: Lippincott-Raven; 1997:60, 75.)*

α-Adrenergic Drugs

Direct-acting α₁-adrenergic agonists

The primary clinical use of direct-acting α₁-adrenergic agonists, such as phenylephrine, is stimulation of the iris dilator muscle to produce mydriasis. Because the parasympathetically innervated iris-sphincter muscle is much stronger than the dilator muscle, the dilation achieved with phenylephrine alone is largely overcome by the pupillary light reflex during ophthalmoscopy. Coadministration of a cycloplegic drug allows sustained dilation.

Systemic absorption of phenylephrine may elevate systemic blood pressure. This effect is clinically significant if the patient is an infant or has an abnormally increased sensitivity to α-agonists, which occurs with orthostatic hypotension and in association with the use of drugs that accentuate adrenergic effects (eg, reserpine, tricyclic antidepressants, cocaine, monoamine oxidase [MAO] inhibitors—discussed later). Even with lower doses of phenylephrine (2.5%), infants may exhibit a transient rise in blood pressure, because the dose received in an eyedrop is high for their weight. Phenylephrine, 10%, should be used cautiously, particularly in pledget application and in patients with vasculopathic risk factors. A 10% solution contains 5 mg of drug per drop, and ocular medications passing through the canalicular system are available for systemic absorption through the vascular nasal mucosa (see Chapter 15). In contrast, the typical systemic dose of phenylephrine for hypotension is 50–100 μg given all at once. The ophthalmic use of phenylephrine, 10%, has been associated with stroke, myocardial infarction, and cardiac arrest. Vascular baroreceptors are particularly sensitive to phenylephrine. An increase in blood pressure after topical application may therefore cause a significant drop in pulse rate that can be particularly dangerous in an individual with vasculopathy who is already on a β-blocking systemic medication.

$α_2$-Adrenergic agonists

Apraclonidine hydrochloride (*para*-aminoclonidine) is a selective $α_2$-adrenergic agonist and a clonidine derivative that prevents release of norepinephrine at nerve terminals (Tables 16-6, 16-7). It decreases aqueous production as well as episcleral venous pressure and improves trabecular outflow. However, its true ocular hypotensive mechanism is not fully understood. When administered pre- and postoperatively, the drug effectively diminishes the acute increase in IOP that follows argon laser iridectomy, argon or selective

Table 16-6 Adrenergic Agonists

Generic Name	Trade Name	Strengths
$β_2$-Adrenergic agonists		
Dipivefrin HCl	Propine	0.1%
	Available generically	0.1%
Epinephrine HCl	Not available in the United States	0.5%, 1%, 2%
$α_2$-Selective agonists		
Apraclonidine HCl	Iopidine	0.5%, 1% (single-use container)
Brimonidine tartrate	Alphagan P	0.1%, 0.15%
	Available generically	0.2%
Brimonidine tartrate/timolol maleate	Combigan	0.2%/0.5%

Table 16-7 Mode of Action of Antiglaucoma Drugs That Act Through Receptors

Primary Mechanism of Action	Drug Class	Examples
Decrease aqueous humor production	1. β-Adrenergic antagonists	Timolol, betaxolol, carteolol, levobunolol
	2. $α_2$-Adrenergic agonists	Apraclonidine, brimonidine
Increase trabecular outflow	1. Miotics	Pilocarpine
	2. Adrenergic agonists	Epinephrine, dipivalyl epinephrine
Increase uveoscleral outflow	1. Prostaglandins	Latanoprost, bimatoprost, travoprost, tafluprost
	2. α-Adrenergic agonists	Apraclonidine, brimonidine

laser trabeculoplasty, Nd:YAG laser capsulotomy, and cataract extraction (see BCSC Section 10, *Glaucoma,* for additional information on apraclonidine). Apraclonidine hydrochloride may be effective for the short-term reduction of IOP, but the development of topical sensitivity and tachyphylaxis often limits its long-term use.

Brimonidine tartrate is another selective α_2-adrenergic agonist. Compared with apraclonidine, brimonidine tartrate is more α_2 selective, is more lipophilic, and causes less tachyphylaxis during long-term use. The rate of allergic reactions, such as follicular conjunctivitis and contact blepharodermatitis, is also lower (less than 15% for brimonidine but up to 40% for apraclonidine). Cross-sensitivity to brimonidine in patients with known hypersensitivity to apraclonidine is minimal.

Brimonidine's mechanism of lowering IOP is thought to involve both decreased aqueous production and increased uveoscleral outflow. Similar to the case with β-blockers, a central mechanism may account for part of the IOP reduction from brimonidine, 0.2%: a 1-week trial of treatment for a single eye caused a statistically significant reduction of 1.2 mm Hg in the fellow eye. Brimonidine is available in a 0.2% solution preserved with benzalkonium chloride, a 0.15% solution preserved with polyquaternium-1, and 0.15% and 0.1% solutions with sodium chlorite as the preservative. Brimonidine tartrate, 0.15%, is comparable to brimonidine, 0.2%, when given 3 times daily. Because brimonidine is more lipophilic than apraclonidine, its penetration of the blood–brain barrier is presumably higher. Central nervous system adverse effects include fatigue and drowsiness. Severe systemic toxicity, with hypotension, hypothermia, and bradycardia, has been reported in infants after use of topical ocular brimonidine. This drug is contraindicated in infants and should be used with caution in small children.

Brimonidine's peak IOP reduction is approximately 26%. At peak (2 hours postdose), its IOP reduction is comparable to that of a nonselective β-blocker and superior to that of the selective β-blocker betaxolol, although at trough (12 hours postdose), the reduction is only 14%–15%, which makes brimonidine at trough less effective than the nonselective β-blockers but comparable to betaxolol. Brimonidine may also have neuroprotective properties, as shown in animal models of optic nerve and retinal injury that are independent of IOP reduction. The proposed mechanism of neuroprotection is upregulation of a neurotrophin, basic fibroblast growth factor, and cellular regulatory genes.

Ophthalmologists should exercise caution when using apraclonidine or brimonidine in patients taking MAO inhibitors or tricyclic antidepressants and in patients with severe cardiovascular disease. Use of these drugs concomitantly with β-blockers (ophthalmic and systemic), antihypertensives, and cardiac glycosides also requires prudence. Although effective for rapid lowering of IOP in angle-closure glaucoma, these drugs may also induce vasoconstriction that can prolong iris-sphincter ischemia and reduce the efficacy of concurrent miotics. Apraclonidine has a much greater affinity for α_1-receptors than does brimonidine and is therefore more likely to produce vasoconstriction in the eye. Brimonidine does not induce vasoconstriction in the posterior segment or the optic nerve.

Ligand binding to α_2-receptors in other systems mediates inhibition of the enzyme adenylate cyclase. Adenylate cyclase is present in the ciliary epithelium and is thought to have a role in aqueous production.

Indirect-acting adrenergic agonists

Indirect-acting adrenergic agonists (cocaine, 4% or 10%, and hydroxyamphetamine, 1%, currently available only through compounding pharmacies) are used to test for and localize defects in sympathetic innervation to the iris dilator muscle. Normally, pupil response fibers originating in the hypothalamus pass down the spinal cord to synapse with cells in the intermediolateral columns. In turn, preganglionic fibers exit the cord through the anterior spinal roots in the upper thorax to synapse in the superior cervical ganglion in the neck. Finally, postganglionic adrenergic fibers terminate in a neuroeffector junction with the iris dilator muscle. The norepinephrine released is inactivated primarily by reuptake into secretory granules in the nerve terminal (Fig 16-5). Approximately 70% of released norepinephrine is recaptured (see the discussion of Horner syndrome in BCSC Section 5, *Neuro-Ophthalmology*).

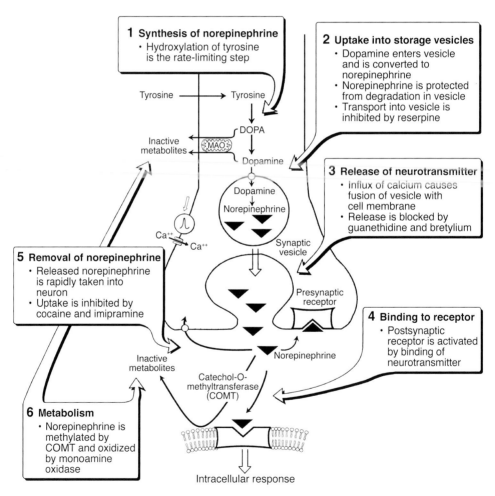

Figure 16-5 Synthesis and release of norepinephrine from the adrenergic neuron. DOPA = dihydroxyphenylalanine; MAO = monoamine oxidase inhibitor. *(Reproduced with permission from Mycek MJ, Harvey RA, Champe PC, eds.* Pharmacology. *2nd ed. Lippincott's Illustrated Reviews. Philadelphia: Lippincott-Raven; 1997:57.)*

Antagonists

Thymoxamine hydrochloride (moxisylyte), an α_1-adrenergic blocking agent, acts by competitively inhibiting norepinephrine at the receptor site. Thymoxamine inhibits α-adrenergic receptors of the dilator muscle of the iris and causes pupil constriction; however, it has no significant effect on ciliary muscle contraction and therefore does not induce substantial changes in anterior chamber depth, facility of outflow, IOP, or accommodation in POAG. In patients with an increase of IOP secondary to primary angle closure, thymoxamine may widen the peripheral angle and reduce IOP. Thymoxamine is useful in differentiating angle-closure glaucoma from POAG with narrow angles and in reversing the pupil dilation caused by phenylephrine. However, this drug is not commercially available in the United States, although it has been widely used in Europe for years.

Dapiprazole hydrochloride (no longer available in the United States) is an α-adrenergic blocking agent that reverses, in 30 minutes, the mydriasis produced by phenylephrine and tropicamide but not by cycloplegics. It affects the dilator muscle but not ciliary muscle contraction (anterior chamber depth, facility of outflow, or accommodation).

β-Adrenergic Drugs

β_2-Adrenergic agonists

β_2-Adrenergic agonists lower IOP by improving trabecular outflow and possibly by increasing uveoscleral outflow. The beneficial effect on outflow more than compensates for a small increase in aqueous inflow as detected by fluorophotometry. The effect on outflow facility seems to be mediated by β_2-receptors.

β_2-Receptors linked to adenylate cyclase are present in the ciliary epithelium and processes as well as in the trabecular meshwork (see Table 16-5). Treatment with L-epinephrine, a nonselective mixed α- and β-agonist, increases intracellular levels of cyclic adenosine monophosphate (cAMP) in these tissues and in the aqueous humor. In other tissues, β-receptor–mediated generation of cAMP in turn activates cAMP-dependent enzymes, which results in responses such as glycogenolysis and gluconeogenesis in the liver and lipolysis in adipose tissue. However, the biochemical mechanisms responsible for lowering IOP remain to be determined.

Topical L-epinephrine is no longer commercially available in the United States or used in most countries (see Table 16-6). Local and systemic adverse effects are common (see BCSC Section 10, *Glaucoma*, Chapter 7). Clinically, nonselective adrenergic drugs have been replaced by the selective α_2-adrenergic agonists because of their improved efficacy and adverse-effect profiles. In an animal model, long-term therapy with epinephrine has been shown to downregulate the number of β-receptors. This phenomenon may underlie the loss of some of the drug's therapeutic effectiveness over time (tachyphylaxis).

β-Adrenergic antagonists

β-Adrenergic antagonists, also known as *β-blockers,* lower IOP by reducing aqueous humor production by as much as 50% (Table 16-8). Six drugs are approved for use in the treatment of glaucoma: betaxolol, carteolol, levobunolol, metipranolol, timolol maleate, and timolol hemihydrate. Although it is likely that the site of action resides in the ciliary body, it is not known whether the vasculature of the ciliary processes or the pumping

Table 16-8 β-Adrenergic Antagonists

Generic Name	Trade Name	Strengths
Betaxolol HCl	Betoptic S	0.25%
	Available generically	0.5%
Carteolol HCl	Ocupress	1%
	Available generically	1%
Levobunolol HCl	Betagan	0.25%, 0.5%
	Available generically	0.25%, 0.5%
Metipranolol HCl	OptiPranolol	0.3%
	Available generically	0.3%
Timolol hemihydrate	Betimol	0.25%, 0.5%
Timolol maleate	Istalol	0.5%
	Timoptic in Ocumeter or Ocumeter Plus container	0.25%, 0.5%
	Available generically	0.25%, 0.5%
	Timoptic-XE in Ocumeter or Ocumeter Plus container (gel)	0.25%, 0.5%
	Available generically as Timolol gel forming solution	0.25%, 0.5%
Timolol maleate (preservative-free)	Timoptic in OcuDose	0.25%, 0.5%
Timolol maleate/brimonidine tartrate	Combigan	Timolol maleate, 0.5%/ brimonidine tartrate, 0.2%
Timolol maleate/dorzolamide HCl	Cosopt Ocumeter Plus	Timolol, 0.5%/dorzolamide, 2%
	Available generically	Timolol, 0.5%/dorzolamide, 2%
Timolol maleate/dorzolamide HCl (preservative-free)	Cosopt in Ocudose	Timolol, 0.5%/dorzolamide, 2%

mechanism of the ciliary epithelium is primarily affected. A possible mechanism may be an effect on the β-adrenergic receptor–coupled adenylate cyclase of the ciliary epithelium (see Table 16-5). Although systemic administration of β-blockers has been reported to elevate blood lipid levels, such elevation has not been demonstrated with topical β-blockers such as timolol. All β-blockers can inhibit the increase in pulse and blood pressure that is exhibited in response to exertion. For this reason, they may be poorly tolerated in elderly patients during routine activities, as well as in young, physically active individuals. Nonselective β-blockers inhibit the pulmonary β$_2$-receptors that dilate the respiratory tree. The induced bronchospasm may be significant in patients with asthma or chronic obstructive lung disease. In patients with bradycardia and second- or third-degree atrioventricular block, the underlying cardiac condition may be exacerbated with use of these drugs.

The traditional teaching that β-blockers are contraindicated in patients with congestive heart failure is being challenged. Indeed, current cardiologic evidence strongly demonstrates that β-blockage is an important component of treatment for heart failure. However, β-blockage also affects the contractility of the cardiac muscle, and patients' medical conditions change with age (especially in elderly patients). Therefore, ophthalmologists should maintain continuous communication with patients' internists or cardiologists regarding the systemic effects of the ophthalmologic therapy.

Timolol maleate, 0.25% or 0.5%, and levobunolol, 0.25% or 0.5%, are mixed β_1/β_2-antagonists. Tests of more-specific β-blockers suggest that β_2-antagonists have a greater effect on aqueous secretion than do β_1-antagonists. For example, comparative studies have shown that the specific β_1-antagonist betaxolol, 0.5%, is approximately 85% as effective in lowering IOP as timolol.

Metipranolol hydrochloride is a nonselective β_1- and β_2-adrenergic receptor–blocking drug. As a 0.3% topical solution, it is similar in effect to other topical nonselective β-blockers and is effective in reducing IOP.

Carteolol hydrochloride demonstrates intrinsic sympathomimetic activity; in other words, while acting as a competitive antagonist, it also causes a slight to moderate activation of receptors. Thus, even though carteolol produces β-blocking effects, these effects may be tempered, reducing the effect on cardiovascular and respiratory systems. Carteolol may also be less likely than other β-blockers to adversely affect the systemic lipid profile.

Betaxolol is a selective β_1-antagonist that is substantially safer than the nonselective β-blockers when pulmonary, cardiac, central nervous system, or other systemic conditions are considered. Betaxolol may be useful in patients with a history of bronchospastic disorders, although other therapies should be tried in lieu of betaxolol (β selectivity is only relative and not absolute, and some β_2 effect can therefore remain). In general, the IOP-lowering effect of betaxolol is less than that of the nonselective β-adrenergic antagonists. Betaxolol is available as a generic 0.5% solution and as a 0.25% suspension. The 0.25% suspension causes less irritation on instillation yet maintains its clinical efficacy compared with the brand-name 0.5% solution (now discontinued), a finding that is generally extrapolated to the generic 0.5% solution currently available.

Prodrugs of nonselective β-blockers are being developed. They may offer the benefit of the higher potency of β_1/β_2-blocking medications while reducing their potential systemic adverse effects.

Curiously, both β-agonist and β-antagonist drugs can lower IOP. This paradox is compounded by the observation that β-agonist and β-antagonist drugs have slightly additive effects in lowering IOP.

Carbonic Anhydrase Inhibitors

Aqueous humor is secreted into the posterior chamber by the epithelium of the ciliary processes. This secretion depends largely on active transport of sodium by Na^+,K^+-ATPase on the surface of nonpigmented epithelial cells. Unidirectional secretion of aqueous requires the uptake of Na^+ and Cl^- by the pigmented epithelial cells through antiports and symports, the transfer of NaCl to nonpigmented epithelial cells through gap junctions, and finally the release Na^+ and Cl^- largely through Cl^- channels and Na^+,K^+-ATPase. The osmotic gradient that is established produces a driving force of water transport from the stroma of ciliary processes to the posterior chamber (Fig 16-6). Na^+ transport and fluid flow seem to be partially linked to HCO_3^- formation in the ciliary epithelium. Carbonic anhydrase catalyzes the hydration of dissolved CO_2 to H_2CO_3, which ionizes into HCO_3^- and H^+. HCO_3^- is then available to accompany secreted Na^+ to the posterior chamber. HCO_3^- formation can be substantially reduced by inhibition of the enzyme carbonic

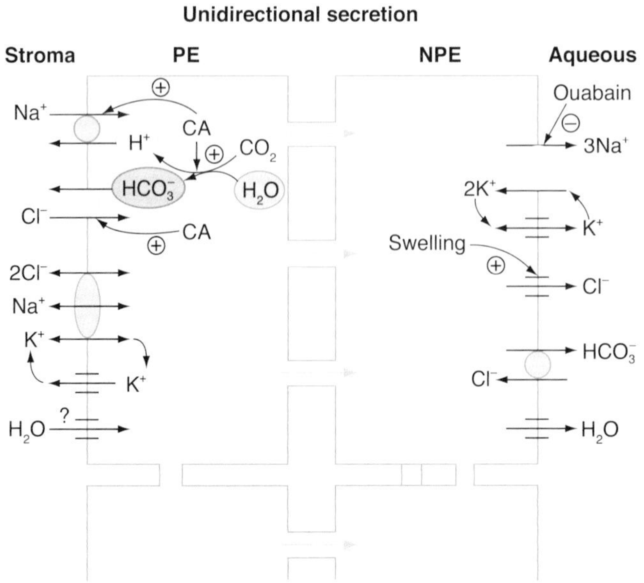

Figure 16-6 Secretion of aqueous humor arises primarily from ciliary epithelial transfer of NaCl from the stroma of the ciliary processes to the posterior chamber of the eye, establishing an osmotic driving force for secondary water transport. CA = carbonic anhydrase; NPE = non-pigmented epithelium; PE = pigmented epithelium. *(Reproduced with permission from McLaughlin CW, Zellhuber-McMillan S, Macknight AD, Civan MM. Electron microprobe analysis of rabbit ciliary epithelium indicates enhanced secretion posteriorly and enhanced absorption anteriorly. Am J Physiol Cell Physiol. 2007;293(5):C1455–1466.)*

anhydrase (Table 16-9). Carbonic anhydrase inhibitors (CAIs) such as acetazolamide and methazolamide are approved for the treatment of glaucoma in adults and may also be effective in treating cystoid macular edema (CME) and pseudotumor cerebri.

The amount of carbonic anhydrase is much higher than needed to supply the amount of HCO_3^- transported. Calculations based on the K_{cat} (catalysis constant) and K_m (apparent affinity constant) of the enzyme and on the concentrations of substrates and product indicate that the amount of enzyme present in the ciliary body is 100 times greater than needed. Correspondingly, in clinical use, the enzyme must be more than 99% inhibited to significantly reduce aqueous flow. The amount of enzyme in the kidney, which is 1000-fold greater than needed, must be more than 99.9% inhibited to affect the usual pathway for HCO_3^- reabsorption. With the inhibitor methazolamide, the difference between the concentration of carbonic anhydrase in the ciliary body and that in the kidney can be exploited to lower IOP without incurring renal HCO_3^- loss, and unpleasant metabolic acidosis can be avoided. Even though renal stone formation has been reported with use of methazolamide, the incidence is significantly lower than with other drugs because of this specific property. In contrast, acetazolamide is actively secreted into the renal tubules, and renal effects are unavoidable.

The topical forms of CAIs—dorzolamide and brinzolamide—are also available for the long-term treatment of glaucoma. They penetrate the cornea easily, are water soluble, and are specially formulated for topical ophthalmic use. When administered as solution 3 times per day, these drugs effectively inhibit carbonic anhydrase II and avoid

Table 16-9 **Carbonic Anhydrase Inhibitors**

Generic Name	Trade Name	Strengths	Onset	Duration of Action
Systemic				
Acetazolamide	Diamox Sequels	500 mg (time-release)	1–1.5 h, 2 h	8–12 h, 18–24 h
	Available generically	125, 250 mg, 500 mg (time-release)	1–1.5 h	8–12 h
Acetazolamide sodium	Available generically	500 mg, 5–10 mg/kg^3	2 min	4–5 h
Methazolamide	Available generically	25, 50 mg	2–4 h	10–18 h
Topical				
Brinzolamide	Azopt	1% suspension	2 h	8–12 h
Dorzolamide HCl	Trusopt Ocumeter Plus	2% solution	5 min	8 h
	Available generically	2% solution	5 min	8 h
Combination Drugs				
Dorzolamide HCl/timolol maleate	Cosopt Ocumeter Plus	Dorzolamide HCl, 2%/timolol, 0.5%	2 h	1 h
	Available generically	Dorzolamide HCl, 2%/timolol, 0.5%	2 h	1 h
Dorzolamide HCl/timolol maleate (preservative-free)	Cosopt in Ocudose	Dorzolamide HCl, 2%/timolol, 0.5%	2 h	1 h

the systemic adverse effects of oral administration. Both medications are equally effective and reduce IOP by 14%–17%. The hypotensive effects of topical and oral CAIs are probably not additive when adequate doses of each are used. Adverse effects of topical CAIs include burning on instillation, punctate keratitis, local allergy, and bitter taste. Dorzolamide hydrochloride and timolol maleate are available as a combination drug, which provides superior antihypertensive action compared with either drug administered alone, although clinical trials showed that the combination is slightly less effective than both drugs administered concomitantly. However, the use of a single combined medication may improve patient adherence and therefore lead to an equivalent efficacy in clinical practice.

The systemic CAIs are administered orally and/or parenterally. The longer half-life of methazolamide allows it to be used twice daily; acetazolamide is also available in a sustained-release, 500-mg form used twice daily. None of these compounds has the ideal combination of high potency (low binding affinity, K_i) good ocular penetration (high penetration percentage in the nonionized form and high lipid solubility to facilitate passage through the blood–ocular barrier), high proportion of the drug present in the blood in the unbound form, and long plasma half-life. In addition to lowering IOP by inhibiting ciliary body carbonic anhydrase, each drug at high doses further lowers IOP by causing renal metabolic acidosis. The mechanism by which acidosis lowers secretion is uncertain, but it probably involves reduction in HCO_3^- formation and activity of Na^+,K^+-ATPase.

At the onset of acidosis, renal effects cause alkaline diuresis, with loss of Na^+, K^+, and HCO_3^-. In patients receiving CAI therapy concurrently with diuretics, steroids, or adrenocorticotropic hormone (ACTH), severe hypokalemia can result. This situation may be dangerous for patients using digitalis, in whom hypokalemia may elicit arrhythmias. Such patients receiving long-term CAI therapy should have their potassium levels checked at regular intervals, preferably by their primary care physicians.

Acidosis prompts a renal mechanism for HCO_3^- reabsorption unrelated to carbonic anhydrase; this mechanism limits the degree of acidosis and halts both the diuresis and K^+ loss after the first few days of treatment. However, dichlorphenamide also acts as a chloruretic agent and may cause continued K^+ loss. Dichlorphenamide is no longer available in the United States.

CAI therapy may interact unfavorably with certain systemic conditions. Alkalinization of the urine, present during initial CAI treatment, prevents excretion of NH_4^+, a factor to consider in patients with cirrhosis of the liver. Metabolic acidosis may exacerbate diabetic ketoacidosis. In patients with severe chronic obstructive pulmonary disease, respiratory acidosis may be caused by impairment of CO_2 transfer from the pulmonary vasculature to the alveoli. Elderly patients have physiologically reduced renal function, which predisposes them to severe metabolic acidosis with the use of systemic CAIs.

The use of acetazolamide has been linked to the formation of stones in the urinary tract. A retrospective case-control series showed that the incidence of stones was 11 times higher in patients using this drug than in those not using it. The increased risk occurred primarily during the first year of therapy. Continued use after occurrence of a stone was associated with a high risk of recurrent stone formation. However, a history of spontaneous stone formation more than 5 years prior to acetazolamide therapy did not appear to be associated with particular risk. The mechanisms responsible for such stone formation may be related to metabolic acidosis and associated pH changes, as well as to decreased excretion of citrate.

Nearly 50% of patients are intolerant of systemic CAIs because of central nervous system and gastrointestinal adverse effects. Adverse effects include numbness and tingling of the hands, feet, and lips; malaise; metallic taste when drinking carbonated beverages; anorexia and weight loss; nausea; somnolence; impotence and loss of libido; and depression. When the clinical situation allows, it is wise to begin therapy at low doses (eg, 125 mg acetazolamide 4 times daily or 25–50 mg methazolamide twice daily) because the incidence and severity of adverse effects may be reduced. Patients should be informed of the potential adverse effects of these drugs; otherwise, they may fail to associate their systemic symptoms with the use of a medication prescribed by their ophthalmologists.

Rare adverse effects from this class of drugs include those common to other members of the sulfonamide family, such as transient myopia, hypersensitive nephropathy, skin rash, Stevens-Johnson syndrome, and thrombocytopenia. One potential adverse effect, aplastic anemia, is idiosyncratic. White blood cell counts do not identify susceptible patients. CAIs have been associated with teratogenic effects (forelimb deformity) in rodents, and their use is not advised during pregnancy. However, these systemic adverse effects are rare with topical CAIs.

Prostaglandin Analogues

Prostaglandin (PG) analogues are the newest class of ocular hypotensive drugs (Table 16-10). Currently, 5 PG analogues have been approved by the FDA for clinical use. Latanoprost, bimatoprost, travoprost, and tafluprost are administered once daily, with nighttime dosing; unoprostone is used twice daily. Tafluprost is available preservative-free in single-use containers.

Latanoprost is a prodrug of prostaglandin $F_{2\alpha}$ ($PGF_{2\alpha}$); it penetrates the cornea and becomes biologically active after being hydrolyzed by corneal tissue esterase. It appears to lower IOP by enhancing uveoscleral outflow and may reduce the pressure by 6–9 mm Hg (25%–35%). A potential advantage of this drug is once-daily dosing. Other advantages include the lack of cardiopulmonary adverse effects and the additivity to other antiglaucoma medications.

An ocular side effect that is unusual for this class of drugs is the darkening of the iris and periocular skin as a result of increased numbers of melanosomes (increased melanin content, or melanogenesis) within the melanocytes. The risk of iris pigmentation correlates with baseline iris pigmentation. Light-colored irides may experience increased pigmentation in 10%–20% of eyes in the initial 18–24 months of therapy, whereas nearly 60% of eyes that are light brown or 2-toned may experience increased pigmentation over the same time period. The long-term sequelae of this side effect are unknown. Other adverse effects reported in association with the use of a topical PG analogue include conjunctival hyperemia, hypertrichosis of the eyelashes, CME, and uveitis. CME and uveitis are more common in eyes with preexisting risk factors for either condition. Reported systemic reactions include flulike symptoms, skin rash, and possible uterine bleeding in postmenopausal women. Reactivation of herpetic keratitis has been reported with use of latanoprost. Topical PGs are classified as category C according to the FDA's use-in-pregnancy ratings. Although elimination of topically applied PGs from human plasma

Table 16-10 Prostaglandin Analogues

Generic Name	Trade Name	Strengths
Bimatoprost	Lumigan	0.01%, 0.03%
Latanoprost	Xalatan	0.005%
	Available generically	0.005%
Travoprost	Travatan	0.004%
	Travatan Z	0.004%
Unoprostone isopropyl	Rescula	0.15%
Tafluprost	Zioptan in single-use containers (preservative-free)	0.0015%
Bimatoprost/timolol maleate	Ganfort (not available in the United States)	Bimatoprost, 0.03%/ timolol, 0.5%
Latanoprost/timolol maleate	Xalacom (not available in the United States)	Latanoprost, 0.005%/ timolol, 0.5%
Travoprost/timolol maleate	DuoTrav (not available in the United States)	Travoprost, 0.004%/ timolol, 0.5%

is rapid, PGs are known to cause contraction of the uterus. Topical PGs should be used with caution in pregnant patients.

Combined Medications

Medications that are combined and placed in a single bottle have the potential benefits of improved efficacy, convenience, and patient adherence, as well as reduced cost. FDA guidelines require the fixed combination to be more efficacious than either drug given alone. Before a patient uses the combination drug, each component should be checked for its effect on that patient's IOP (see BCSC Section 10, *Glaucoma*).

Osmotic Drugs

Actions and Uses

Increased serum osmolarity reduces IOP and vitreous volume by drawing fluid out of the eye across vascular barriers. The osmotic activity of a drug depends on the number of particles in solution and the maintenance of an osmotic gradient between the plasma and the intraocular fluids. This activity is independent of the molecular weight. Low-molecular-weight agents such as urea that penetrate the blood–ocular barrier produce a small increase in IOP after an initial reduction because of a reversal of the osmotic gradient when the kidneys clear the blood of excess urea. Osmotic drugs are approved for the short-term management of acute glaucoma in adults and may be used to reduce vitreous volume prior to cataract surgery.

Specific Osmotic Drugs

Osmotic drugs should be used with care in patients in whom cardiovascular overload might occur with moderate vascular volume expansion, such as patients with a history of congestive heart failure, angina, systemic hypertension, or recent myocardial infarct. The hyperosmotic drugs glycerin, mannitol, and urea are currently available for ophthalmic use in the United States (Table 16-11).

Intravenous drugs

Mannitol must be administered intravenously because it cannot be absorbed from the gastrointestinal tract. This drug may be given as either an intravenous infusion or an intravenous push. For an intravenous infusion, mannitol may be given as a 20% premixed solution (concentration, 200 mg/mL) over 30–60 minutes. For an intravenous push, a 25% solution may be injected over 3–5 minutes. A too-rapid infusion of mannitol may shift intracellular water into the extracellular space, causing cellular dehydration with a high risk of hyponatremia, congestive heart failure, pulmonary edema, and intracranial bleeding.

Urea is unpalatable and thus is used intravenously. Use of urea has fallen out of favor because of rebound (see the earlier section Actions and Uses) and because of its tendency to cause tissue necrosis if it extravasates during administration. Intravenous administration produces a rapid onset of action, which is usually desirable, but both mannitol and urea

Table 16-11 Hyperosmotic Drugs

Generic Name	Trade Name	Strengths	Dose	Route	Onset	Duration of Action
Glycerin	Available generically		1–1.5 g/kg	Oral	10–30 min	5 h
Mannitol	Osmitrol	5%–20%	0.5–2 g/kg	Intravenous	30–60 min	4–8 h
	Available generically	5%–25%	0.5–2 g/kg	Intravenous	30–60 min	4–8 h
Urea	Available generically	Powder	0.5–2 g/kg	Intravenous	30–45 min	5–6 h

have been associated with subarachnoid hemorrhage attributed to rapid volume overload of the blood vessels and/or rapid shrinkage of the brain with traction of the subarachnoid vessels. This shrinkage is of particular concern in elderly patients, who may already have brain shrinkage from microischemic disease and are therefore at increased risk of bleeding.

These drugs are cleared by the kidneys and produce marked osmotic diuresis that may be troublesome during surgery. Conscious patients should void shortly before surgery, and a urinal or bed pan should be available. If general anesthesia is employed, an indwelling urethral catheter may be required to prevent bladder distension.

Oral drugs

Glycerin, 50%, was discontinued in the United States in 2004; it can be compounded, however, by diluting the 100% solution. This frequently used oral osmotic drug is given over cracked ice to minimize its nauseating sweet taste. The nonmetabolized sugar isosorbide was preferred in diabetic patients but has been discontinued in the United States.

Lichter PR. Glaucoma clinical trials and what they mean for our patients. *Am J Ophthalmol.* 2003;136(1):136–145.

Netland PA. *Glaucoma Medical Therapy: Principles and Management.* 2nd ed. Ophthalmology Monograph 13. San Francisco: American Academy of Ophthalmology; 2008.

Anti-inflammatory Drugs

Ocular inflammation can be treated with medications administered topically, by local injection, by ocular implantation, or systemically. These drugs may be classified as glucocorticoids, nonsteroidal anti-inflammatory drugs, mast-cell stabilizers, antihistamines, or antifibrotics.

Glucocorticoids

Corticosteroids, or *steroids,* are applied topically to prevent or suppress ocular inflammation in trauma and uveitis, as well as after most ocular surgical procedures (Table 16-12). Subconjunctival and retrobulbar injections of steroids are used to treat more severe cases of ocular inflammation. Systemic steroid therapy is used to treat systemic immune diseases such as giant cell arteritis, vision-threatening capillary hemangiomas in childhood, and severe ocular inflammations that are resistant to topical therapy. Intravenous methylprednisolone is an option in the treatment of demyelinating optic neuritis; see BCSC Section 5, *Neuro-Ophthalmology,* for further discussion of this issue.

Table 16-12 Topical Anti-inflammatory Drugs

Generic Name	Trade Name	Strengths
Corticosteroids		
Dexamethasone sodium phosphate	Maxidex	Suspension, 0.1%
	Maxidex, Ocu-Dex	Ointment, 0.05%
	Available generically	Solution, 0.1%
Difluprednate	Durezol	Emulsion, 0.05%
Fluorometholone	FML S.O.P.	Ointment, 0.1%
	FML Liquifilm	Suspension, 0.1%
	FML Forte Liquifilm	Suspension, 0.25%
	Fluor-Op	Suspension, 0.1%
	Available generically	Suspension, 0.1%
Fluorometholone acetate	Flarex	Suspension, 0.1%
Loteprednol etabonate	Alrex	Suspension, 0.2%
	Lotemax	Suspension, 0.5%
	Lotemax	Ointment, 0.5%
Medrysone	HMS	Suspension, 1%
Prednisolone acetate	Econopred Plus	Suspension, 1%
	Omnipred	Suspension, 1%
	Pred Forte	Suspension, 1%
	Available generically	Suspension, 1%
	Pred Mild	Suspension, 0.12%
Prednisolone sodium phosphate	Inflamase Forte	Solution, 1%
	Prednisol	Solution, 1%
	Available generically	Solution, 1%, 0.125%
Rimexolone	Vexol	Suspension, 1%
Nonsteroidal Anti-inflammatory Drugs		
Bromfenac sodium	Xibrom, Bromday	Solution, 0.09%
	Prolensa	Solution, 0.07%
Diclofenac sodium	Voltaren	Solution, 0.1%
	Available generically	Solution, 0.1%
Flurbiprofen sodium	Ocufen	Solution, 0.03%
	Available generically	Solution, 0.03%
Ketorolac tromethamine	Acular, Acular PF	Solution, 0.5%
	Acular LS	Solution, 0.4%
	Acuvail	Solution, 0.45%
	Available generically	Solution, 0.5%
Nepafenac	Nevanac	Suspension, 0.1%

Glucocorticoids induce cell-specific effects on lymphocytes, macrophages, polymorphonuclear leukocytes, vascular endothelial cells, fibroblasts, and other cells. In each of these types of cells, glucocorticoids must

- penetrate the cell membrane
- bind to soluble receptors in the cytosol
- allow the translocation of the glucocorticoid receptor complex to nuclear binding sites for gene transcription
- induce or suppress the transcription of specific messenger RNAs (mRNAs)

The proteins produced in the eye under the control of these mRNAs are not known, and only resultant effects have been described.

At the tissue level, glucocorticoids prevent or suppress local hyperthermia, vascular congestion, edema, and pain of initial inflammatory responses, whether the cause is traumatic (radiant, mechanical, or chemical), infectious, or immunologic. They also suppress the late inflammatory responses of capillary proliferation, fibroblast proliferation, collagen deposition, and scarring.

At the biochemical level, the most important effect of anti-inflammatory drugs may be the inhibition of arachidonic acid release from phospholipids (see Part IV, Biochemistry and Metabolism). Liberated arachidonic acid is otherwise converted into PGs, PG endoperoxides, leukotrienes, and thromboxanes, which are potent mediators of inflammation. Glucocorticoids also suppress the liberation of lytic enzymes from lysozymes.

The effects of glucocorticoids on immune-mediated inflammation are complicated. Glucocorticoids do not affect the titers of either immunoglobulin E (IgE), which mediates allergic mechanisms, or immunoglobulin G (IgG), which mediates autoimmune mechanisms. Also, glucocorticoids do not appear to interfere with the normal processes in the afferent limb of cell-mediated immunity, as in graft rejection. Instead, they interfere with the efferent limb of the immune response. For example, glucocorticoids prevent macrophages from being attracted to sites of inflammation by interfering with the macrophages' response to lymphocyte-released migration-inhibiting factor. Systemically administered glucocorticoids cause sequestration of lymphocytes, especially the T lymphocytes that mediate cellular immunity. However, the posttranscriptional molecular mechanisms of these responses remain unknown. BCSC Section 9, *Intraocular Inflammation and Uveitis*, discusses immune responses in detail.

Adverse effects

Glucocorticoids may cause several adverse effects in the eye and elsewhere in the body. Complications in the eye include

- glaucoma
- posterior subcapsular cataracts
- exacerbation of bacterial and viral (especially herpetic) infections through suppression of protective immune mechanisms
- fungal infection
- ptosis
- mydriasis
- scleral melting
- eyelid skin atrophy
- pseudohypopyon from intraocular injection
- central serous retinopathy

In the body, oral doses can cause

- suppression of the pituitary–adrenal axis
- gluconeogenesis resulting in hyperglycemia, muscle wasting, and osteoporosis
- redistribution of fat from the periphery to the trunk
- central nervous system effects, such as euphoria
- insomnia
- aseptic necrosis of the hip

- peptic ulcer
- diabetes mellitus
- occasionally, psychosis

Elderly patients have particular difficulty taking long-term systemic steroids. For example, the side effect of proximal muscle wasting may make it difficult for these patients to climb stairs. Another adverse effect of glucocorticoids, osteoporosis, exacerbates the risk of falls and fractures for these patients, who are generally at an increased risk of both. Elderly patients with inflammatory diseases may require a steroid-sparing regimen with methotrexate due to steroid-induced complications. The systemic adverse effects of steroids are discussed in BCSC Section 1, *Update on General Medicine.*

Steroid-induced elevation in IOP may occur with topical, intraocular, periocular, nasal, and systemic glucocorticoid therapy. Individuals differ in their responsiveness: approximately 4% develop pressures higher than 31 mm Hg after 6 weeks of therapy with topical dexamethasone. High levels of response are generally reproducible. The mechanism by which steroids decrease the facility of aqueous outflow through the trabecular meshwork remains unknown. The IOP response to topical prednisolone in a normotensive cat model is comparable to that of topical dexamethasone.

Individual response to steroids is highly dependent on the duration, strength, and frequency of therapy and the potency of the drug used. Steroid-induced IOP elevation almost never occurs in less than 5 days and is infrequent in less than 2 weeks of use. It is not generally appreciated that late responses to therapy are common and that failure of IOP to rise after 6 weeks of therapy does not ensure that a patient will maintain normal IOP after several months of therapy. For this reason, IOP monitoring is required at periodic intervals during the entire course of long-term steroid therapy to prevent iatrogenic glaucomatous nerve damage. Steroid-induced elevations in IOP are usually reversible by discontinuing therapy if the drug has not been used longer than 1 year, but permanent elevations of pressure are common if therapy has continued for 18 months or more.

Table 16-13 lists the anti-inflammatory and pressure-elevating potencies of 6 steroids used in ophthalmic therapy. These anti-inflammatory potencies were determined by an in vitro assay of inhibition of lymphocyte transformation, and the IOP effects were determined by tests in individuals already known to be highly responsive to topical dexamethasone. However, until all these drugs are compared in a model of ocular inflammation relevant to human disease, no conclusion can be reached about the observed dissociation of effects. The lower-than-expected effect on pressure of some of these drugs may be explained by more rapid metabolism of fluorometholone in the eye compared with dexamethasone and by the relatively poor penetration of medrysone. The efficacy of these drugs for intraocular inflammation may be similarly reduced.

When a steroid-induced pressure rise is suspected but continued steroid therapy is warranted, the physician faces the following choices:

- continue the same treatment and closely monitor the status of the optic nerve
- attempt to offset the pressure rise with other drugs or treatments
- reduce the potency, concentration, or frequency of the steroid used, while monitoring both pressure and inflammation

Table 16-13 Comparison of Anti-inflammatory* and IOP-Elevating† Potencies

Glucocorticoid	Relative Potency	Rise in IOP (mm Hg)
Dexamethasone, 0.1%	24	22
Fluorometholone, 0.1%‡	21	6
Prednisolone acetate, 1%	2.3	10
Medrysone, 1%§	1.7	1
Tetrahydrotriamcinolone, 0.25%	1.4	2
Hydrocortisone, 0.5%	1.0	3

*Anti-inflammatory potency determined by in vitro assay of inhibition of lymphocyte transformation. Anti-inflammatory potency of difluprednate, 0.05%, is equal to or stronger than betamethasone, 0.1%, which has a 6-fold anti-inflammatory potency when compared with prednisolone or equivalent to dexamethasone. In clinical trials on uveitis, a significant increase in intraocular pressure (IOP) occurred in 6% of patients treated with difluprednate, 0.05%, emulsion compared with 5% of those treated with prednisolone acetate, 1%.

†IOP effects determined in topical dexamethasone responders.

‡Rapid metabolism of fluorometholone in the eye compared with dexamethasone.

§Relatively poor ocular penetration of medrysone.

Immunomodulatory therapy (IMT) is an important component of the management of ocular inflammation, sparing the toxicity associated with long-term corticosteroid therapy. IMT drugs can be classified as antimetabolites, inhibitors of T-cell signaling, alkylating agents, and biologic response modifiers. Biologic response modifiers inhibit various cytokines, which are active in inflammation. BCSC Section 9, *Intraocular Inflammation and Uveitis*, discusses IMT in detail.

Specific drugs and regimens

Selecting appropriately from the available corticosteroid drugs and dosage regimens remains somewhat empirical. Steroids can be used topically (iritis), intravenously (optic neuritis), intravitreally (endophthalmitis), or periocularly (uveitis) (Table 16-14). All

Table 16-14 Usual Route of Corticosteroid Administration in Ocular Inflammation

Condition	Route
Blepharitis	Topical
Conjunctivitis	Topical
Endophthalmitis	Systemic/periocular, intravitreal
Keratitis	Topical
Macular edema, cystoid	Topical, periocular, intravitreal injection or implant
Macular edema, diabetic	Periocular, intravitreal
Optic neuritis	Systemic
Scleritis	Topical, regional, and/or systemic
Scleritis-Epi (Episcleritis)	Topical
Sympathetic ophthalmia	Systemic, periocular topical, intravitreal
Temporal arteritis	Systemic
Uveitis, anterior	Topical and/or periocular, systemic
Uveitis, posterior	Systemic and/or periocular, intravitreal injection or implant

corticosteroids may exacerbate bacterial, viral, mycobacterial, and fungal diseases of the eye and should be used with caution in these conditions. Prolonged use may result in secondary glaucoma, cataract formation, and secondary ocular infections following suppression of the host response and/or perforation of the globe. Recent research in corticosteroids aims to develop drugs with less effect on IOP as well as medications that can be used intraocularly and periocularly.

Rimexolone, 1%, is a synthetic topical steroid designed to minimize IOP elevations, similar to fluorinated steroids. Elevated IOP has been reported, but it is rare. Ocular adverse effects still include secondary glaucoma and posterior subcapsular cataracts. Systemic adverse effects, including headache, hypotension, rhinitis, pharyngitis, and taste perversion, occur in fewer than 2% of patients.

Loteprednol etabonate, 0.5%, is structurally similar to other steroids but lacks a ketone group at position 20. Studies have shown that in corticosteroid responders, patients treated with loteprednol demonstrate a low incidence of clinically significant, increased IOP. Loteprednol etabonate, 0.2%, is marketed for the temporary treatment of allergic conjunctivitis. The combination drug loteprednol etabonate (0.5%)/tobramycin (0.3%) is approved for superficial bacterial infection of the eye with inflammation.

The fluocinolone acetonide implant was approved in 2005 for intraocular implantation in the vitreous cavity for treatment of chronic noninfectious uveitis. A 40-mg/mL, preservative-free triamcinolone acetonide injectable suspension was approved for intraocular use in 2007. FDA-approved indications include visualization during vitrectomy and treatment of sympathetic ophthalmia, temporal arteritis, uveitis, and ocular inflammatory conditions that do not respond to topical corticosteroids.

Armaly MF. Effect of corticosteroids on intraocular pressure and fluid dynamics. I. The effect of dexamethasone in the normal eye. *Arch Ophthalmol.* 1963;70(4):482–491.

Armaly MF. Effect of corticosteroids on intraocular pressure and fluid dynamics. II. The effect of dexamethasone in the glaucomatous eye. *Arch Ophthalmol.* 1963;70(4):492–499.

Mulki L, Foster CS. Difluprednate for inflammatory eye disorders. *Drugs Today (Barc).* 2011; 47(5):327–333.

Nonsteroidal Anti-inflammatory Drugs

Derivatives

Derivatives of arachidonic acid, a 20-carbon essential fatty acid, mediate a wide variety of biological functions, including regulation of smooth-muscle tone (in blood vessels, bronchi, uterus, and gut), platelet aggregation, hormone release (growth hormone, ACTH, insulin, renin, and progesterone), and inflammation. The synthetic cascade that produces a wide variety of derivatives (depending on the stimulus and tissue) begins with stimulation of phospholipase A_2, the enzyme that liberates arachidonic acid from phospholipids of the cell membrane. (Phospholipase A_2 is inhibited by corticosteroids.) Arachidonic acid is then converted either into cyclic endoperoxides by cyclooxygenase (PG synthase) or into hydroperoxides by lipoxygenase. Subsequent products of the endoperoxides include the PGs, which mediate inflammation and other responses; prostacyclin, a vasodilator and platelet antiaggregant; and thromboxane, a vasoconstrictor and platelet aggregant. The hydroperoxides form a chemotactic agent and the leukotrienes C_4, D_4, and E_4, previously known as the slow-reacting substance of anaphylaxis.

Specific drugs

Table 16-15 lists several nonsteroidal anti-inflammatory drugs (NSAIDs), along with their starting adult oral dosages. Aspirin and other NSAIDs inhibit the local signs of inflammation (heat, vasodilation, edema, swelling), as well as pain and fever. They have complex effects on clotting. At low doses (300 mg every other day), aspirin permanently inhibits the cyclooxygenase in platelets that is essential for the conversion of arachidonic acid to prostaglandin G_2 (PGG_2) and thromboxane. Inhibition of thromboxane production, in turn, prevents coagulation. Whereas nucleated cells can replenish their cyclooxygenase, anucleate platelets cannot. The anticoagulant effect of aspirin therefore lasts for 7–10 days, mirroring the life span of the inhibited platelets, despite the discontinuation of aspirin therapy. Other NSAIDs inhibit clotting in a reversible fashion, and their use does not need to be discontinued as far in advance before elective surgery. Aspirin has been associated with Reye syndrome in children when used during febrile viral infections, although no causal link has been proved. The National Reye's Syndrome Foundation, the US Surgeon General, the FDA, the Centers for Disease Control and Prevention, and the American Academy of Pediatrics recommend that aspirin and combination products containing aspirin not be taken by anyone younger than 19 years during fever-causing illnesses. The British Medicines and Healthcare Products Regulatory Agency recommends that aspirin labels state that the drug is not intended for use in

Table 16-15 Nonsteroidal Anti-inflammatory Drugs

Drug (Generic Name)	Starting Oral Dosage (Adult)
Aspirin	650 mg, 4 times daily
Celecoxib	100 mg, 2 times daily
Diclofenac	50 mg, 3 times daily
Diflunisal	500 mg, 2 times daily
Etodolac	300 mg, 2 times daily
Fenoprofen	200 mg, 4 times daily
Flurbiprofen	300 mg, 3 times daily
Ibuprofen	400 mg, 4 times daily
Indomethacin	25 mg, 3 times daily
Ketoprofen	75 mg, 3 times daily
Ketorolac	10 mg, 4 times daily
Meloxicam	7.5 mg, 4 times daily
Nabumetone	1000 mg, 4 times daily
Naproxen	250 mg, 2 times daily
Oxaprozin	1200 mg, 4 times daily
Piroxicam	20 mg, 4 times daily
Sulindac	150 mg, 2 times daily
Tolmetin	400 mg, 3 times daily

children younger than 16 years unless recommended by a physician. Other NSAIDs are effective antipyretics and are not associated with the constellation of symptoms observed in Reye syndrome.

The relative risks and benefits of aspirin therapy should be assessed specifically for each patient. Aspirin therapy for postoperative pain or for pain associated with traumatic hyphema may increase the risk of hemorrhage because of the antiaggregant effect on platelets. The same side effect may benefit patients with platelet emboli, as in some cases of amaurosis fugax. Diversion of arachidonic acid to the lipoxygenase pathway by inhibition of cyclooxygenase may explain why aspirin use can be associated with asthma attacks and hypersensitivity reactions (mediated by leukotrienes C_4, D_4, and E_4) in susceptible people. Systemic acidosis associated with concomitant use of CAIs may shift a higher proportion of aspirin molecules into the more lipid-soluble nonionized form, which penetrates the blood–brain barrier more readily and potentiates the central nervous system toxicity of aspirin.

Aspirin and other cyclooxygenase inhibitors are less effective than steroids in the treatment of scleritis and uveitis. NSAIDs such as indomethacin can be effective for orbital inflammatory diseases. The prophylactic use of indomethacin in patients with cataract surgery has been reported to reduce the incidence of angiographically detected CME, but an effect on visually significant CME has yet to be determined. Topical NSAIDs have been used to treat ocular inflammation and to prevent and treat postoperative CME.

Flurbiprofen sodium, 0.03% (generic available), was the first commercially available topical ocular NSAID. When applied preoperatively, it reduces PG-mediated intraoperative miosis. Topical diclofenac sodium, 0.1% (generic available), has been approved by the FDA for postoperative prophylaxis and treatment of ocular inflammation and has also been used successfully to prevent and treat CME (see Table 16-12).

Ketorolac tromethamine (0.4%, 0.45%, 0.5%, and generic 0.5%) has been approved by the FDA for the treatment of postoperative inflammation and allergic conjunctivitis. Ketorolac blocks the metabolism of arachidonic acid by cyclooxygenase. Arachidonic acid metabolites are present in greater quantities in the tears of patients with ocular allergies. Two double-masked studies have revealed that such patients who were treated with ketorolac tromethamine had significantly less conjunctival inflammation, ocular itching, and tearing than did those given placebo. Ketorolac does not have a decongestant effect and does not relieve redness. The recommended dose of ketorolac is 1 drop (0.4%, 0.45%, or 0.5%) 4 times per day. The most common adverse effects are stinging and burning on instillation (40%).

Nepafenac, 0.1%, was approved in 2005 for 3-times-daily dosing for pain and inflammation 1 day before and 2 weeks after cataract surgery. Bromfenac sodium, 0.09%, was approved in 2006 for twice-daily dosing from 24 hours to 2 weeks after cataract surgery for pain and inflammation.

Topical NSAIDs may be used for their topical analgesic properties following corneal abrasion and after anterior segment surgery and refractive surgical procedures. All NSAIDs are associated with corneal complications, including melting and corneal perforation; these complications have been observed both in postoperative patients and in cases of uveitis, usually in patients with preexisting diabetes mellitus and ocular surface disorders. Most of these patients were found to be taking generic diclofenac.

Topical cyclosporin emulsion, 0.05%, is an immunomodulator with anti-inflammatory effects. The drug is indicated to increase tear production in patients in whom tear production is presumed to be suppressed because of ocular inflammation associated with keratoconjunctivitis sicca (see the section Medications for Dry Eye for further discussion).

Congdon NG, Schein OD, von Kulajta P, Lubomski LH, Gilbert D, Katz J. Corneal complications associated with topical ophthalmic use of nonsteroidal antiinflammatory drugs. *J Cataract Refract Surg.* 2001;27(4):622–631.

Flach AJ. Corneal melts associated with topically applied nonsteroidal anti-inflammatory drugs. *Trans Am Ophthalmol Soc.* 2001;99:205–210.

Antiallergic Drugs: Mast-Cell Stabilizers and Antihistamines

The human eye has approximately 50 million mast cells. Each cell contains several hundred granules that in turn contain preformed chemical mediators. Allergic conjunctivitis is an immediate hypersensitivity reaction in which triggering antigens couple to reaginic antibodies (IgE) on the cell surface of mast cells and basophils, causing the release of histamine, PG, leukotrienes, and chemotactic factors from secretory granules. The released histamine causes capillary dilatation and increased permeability and, therefore, conjunctival injection and swelling. It also stimulates nerve endings, causing pain and itching. Drugs that interfere at different points along this pathway can treat ocular allergy. Corticosteroids are very effective, but adverse effects limit their application for this chronic condition. Mast-cell stabilizers, NSAIDs, antihistamines, and decongestants have fewer and less-dangerous adverse effects and can be used singly or in combination. Table 16-16 lists drugs that relieve allergic conjunctivitis.

Patients may achieve short-term relief of mild allergic symptoms with over-the-counter preparations of topical antihistamines such as antazoline and pheniramine, which are usually combined with the decongestant naphazoline. Specific H_1-antagonists include emedastine, levocabastine, and azelastine.

Emedastine difumarate, 0.05%, is a relatively selective H_1-receptor antagonist indicated for temporary relief of signs and symptoms of allergic conjunctivitis. Recommended dosing is 1 drop up to 4 times per day. The most common adverse effect reported is headache (11%). Unpleasant taste, blurred vision, burning or stinging, corneal infiltrates, dry eye, rhinitis, and sinusitis are other noted adverse effects.

Levocabastine HCl has an onset of action that occurs within minutes and lasts for at least 4 hours; it is as effective as cromolyn sodium. The usual dosage of levocabastine, 0.05%, is 1 drop 4 times per day for up to 2 weeks. This drug has been discontinued in the United States.

Azelastine HCl is effective and well tolerated at a strength of 0.05%. This drug is also available as a nasal spray for the treatment of allergic rhinitis. Ketorolac tromethamine,

Table 16-16 Drugs for Allergic Conjunctivitis

Generic Name	Trade Name	Class
Alcaftadine	Lastacaft	H$_1$-antagonist/mast-cell inhibitor
Azelastine HCl	Optivar, available generically	H$_1$-antagonist/mast-cell inhibitor
Bepotastine besilate	Bepreve	H$_1$-antagonist/mast-cell inhibitor
Cromolyn sodium	Crolom, available generically	Mast-cell inhibitor
Emedastine difumarate	Emadine	H$_1$-antagonist
Epinastine HCl	Elestat, available generically	H$_1$-antagonist/mast-cell inhibitor
Ketorolac tromethamine	Acular, Acular PF, Acular LS Acuvail, ketorolac, 0.5%, available generically	NSAID
Ketotifen fumarate	Zaditor (OTC), Alaway (OTC), available generically	H$_1$-antagonist/mast-cell inhibitor
Levocabastine HCl	Discontinued in the United States	H$_1$-antagonist
Lodoxamide tromethamine	Alomide	Mast-cell inhibitor
Loteprednol etabonate	Alrex	Corticosteroid
Naphazoline HCl	Ak-Con, Albalon, available generically	Decongestant
Naphazoline HCl/antazoline phosphate	Vasocon-A (OTC)	Antihistamine/decongestant
Naphazoline HCl/pheniramine maleate	Naphcon-A (OTC), Opcon-A (OTC), Visine-A (OTC)	Antihistamine/decongestant
Nedocromil sodium	Alocril	Mast-cell inhibitor
Olopatadine HCl	Patanol, 0.1%, Pataday, 0.2%	H$_1$-antagonist/mast-cell inhibitor
Pemirolast potassium	Alamast	Mast-cell inhibitor

NSAID = nonsteroidal anti-inflammatory drug; OTC = over-the-counter.

a topical NSAID, is used to prevent itching and has a rapid onset of action but does not relieve conjunctival hyperemia.

Mast-cell stabilizers were previously thought to prevent calcium influx across mast-cell membranes, thereby preventing mast-cell degranulation and mediator release. Traditional mast-cell stabilizers such as cromolyn sodium, lodoxamide, and pemirolast prevent mast-cell degranulation but take days to weeks to reach peak efficacy. They have little or no antihistamine effect and do not provide immediate relief from allergic symptoms. They are used for allergic, vernal, and atopic conjunctivitis.

Lodoxamide has been shown to stabilize the mast-cell membrane 2500 times as effectively as cromolyn sodium does. In treating allergic conjunctivitis, its onset of action is more rapid, with less stinging, than that observed with cromolyn sodium. A multicenter, double-masked study showed that lodoxamide was superior to cromolyn sodium in treating vernal keratoconjunctivitis. However, as with all mast-cell stabilizers, lodoxamide does not become clinically effective for several weeks. Therefore, it may be necessary to use topical steroids or H$_1$-antagonists concurrently with mast-cell stabilizers for the first several weeks, until these drugs are fully effective. The usual dose of lodoxamide, 0.1%, for adults and children older than 2 years is 1–2 drops in the affected eye 4 times daily for up to 3 months. The most frequently reported adverse reactions are burning, stinging, and discomfort upon instillation (15%).

Pemirolast potassium, 0.1%, is used to prevent itching due to allergic conjunctivitis. In clinical studies, the most common adverse effects were headache, rhinitis, and cold and flu symptoms, which were generally mild.

Some drugs, including olopatadine, ketotifen, nedocromil, epinastine, azelastine, and alcaftadine have a mast-cell–stabilizing effect as well as H_1-antagonism. These drugs provide immediate relief against released histamine and prevent the future degranulation of mast cells. Olopatadine HCl, 0.1%, has a rapid onset and a duration of action lasting at least 8 hours. Recommended dosing is 1–2 drops in the affected eye 2 times per day at an interval of 6–8 hours. This drug is now also available for once-a-day dosing as olopatadine, 0.2%. Adverse reactions of ocular burning, stinging, dry eye, foreign-body sensation, hyperemia, keratitis, eyelid edema, pruritus, asthenia, cold syndrome, pharyngitis, rhinitis, sinusitis, and taste perversion were all reported at an incidence of less than 5%. For ketotifen fumarate, 0.025%, recommended dosing is 1 drop every 8–12 hours. This medication is now available without a prescription. Adverse effects of conjunctival injection, headaches, and rhinitis were reported at an incidence of 10%–25%.

Nedocromil sodium, 2%, is a mast-cell stabilizer with a twice-daily dosing regimen. Alcaftadine, 0.25%, is approved for once-daily use for prevention of itching associated with allergic conjunctivitis. Comparisons between different mast-cell stabilizers and antihistamines are limited, and no clinical evidence indicates that any particular product is superior to others in treating ocular allergies.

Corticosteroids are very effective for treating ocular allergies but are prone to overuse and have a more dangerous adverse-effect profile. Loteprednol etabonate, 0.2%, a steroid designed to cause less IOP elevation, can be used for the temporary treatment of ocular allergies. Recalcitrant cases of severe allergic, vernal, and atopic conjunctivitis may require the short-term use of stronger topical steroids, but these cases should be carefully monitored and patients switched to one of the previously mentioned drugs as soon as clinically prudent.

Foulks GN, Nichols KK, Bron AJ, Holland EJ, McDonald MB, Nelson JD. Improving awareness, identification, and management of meibomian gland dysfunction. *Ophthalmology.* 2012;119(Suppl 10):S1–S12.

Geerling G, MacLennan S, Hartwig D. Autologous serum eye drops for ocular surface disorders. *Br J Ophthalmol.* 2004;88(11):1467–1474.

Greiner JV, Edwards-Swanson K, Ingerman A. Evaluation of alcaftadine 0.25% ophthalmic solution in acute allergic conjunctivitis at 15 minutes and 16 hours after instillation versus placebo and olopatadine 0.1%. *Clin Ophthalmol.* 2011;13(5):87–93.

Kunert KS, Tisdale AS, Gipson IK. Goblet cell numbers and epithelial proliferation in the conjunctiva of patients with dry eye syndrome treated with cyclosporine. *Arch Ophthalmol.* 2002;120(3):330–337. [Erratum appears in *Arch Ophthalmol.* 2002;120(8):1099.]

Kunert KS, Tisdale AS, Stern ME, Smith JA, Gipson IK. Analysis of topical cyclosporine treatment of patients with dry eye syndrome: effect on conjunctival lymphocytes. *Arch Ophthalmol.* 2000;118(11):1489–1496.

La Rosa M, Lionetti E, Reibaldi M, et al. Allergic conjunctivitis: a comprehensive review of the literature. *Ital J Pediatr.* 2013;14(39):18.

Pflugfelder SC. Antiinflammatory therapy for dry eye. *Am J Ophthalmol.* 2004;137(2):337–342.

Tong L, Petznick A, Lee S, Tan J. Choice of artificial tear formulation for patients with dry eye: where do we start? *Cornea.* 2012;31(Suppl 1):S32–S36.

Verin P. Treating severe eye allergy. *Clin Exp Allergy.* 1998;28(Suppl 6):44–48.

Antifibrotic Drugs

Antiproliferative medications, also known as *antimetabolites,* are occasionally required for the treatment of severe ocular inflammatory diseases, such as Behçet syndrome and sympathetic ophthalmia, or of ocular diseases that are part of a systemic vasculitis. Systemic therapy with such drugs is best carried out in consultation with a chemotherapist. The uses and adverse effects of these drugs are discussed in BCSC Section 9, *Intraocular Inflammation and Uveitis.*

Fluorouracil (5-FU) is a fluorinated pyrimidine nucleoside analogue that blocks production of thymidylate synthase and interrupts normal cellular DNA and RNA synthesis. Its primary action may be to cause cellular thymine deficiency and resultant cell death. The effect of fluorouracil is most pronounced on rapidly growing cells, and its use as an antiviral drug is related primarily to the destruction of infected cells (eg, warts) by topical application. The drug is also thought to inhibit the cellular proliferation that could otherwise occur in response to inflammation. Two randomized clinical trials compared use of low-molecular-weight heparin with 5-FU infusion and placebo during vitrectomy to prevent proliferative vitreoretinopathy; one trial was conducted in patients at high risk of developing postoperative proliferative vitreoretinopathy and the other in unselected cases of rhegmatogenous retinal detachment. The results were inconclusive concerning the effects of these 2 agents. In high-risk patients, including young glaucoma patients (≤40 years), the initial trabeculectomy with adjunctive 5-FU had a higher success rate than did surgery without the adjunct. Fluorouracil is used postoperatively as a subconjunctival injection and intraoperatively as a topical application to the trabeculectomy site.

Mitomycin C is a compound isolated from the fungus *Streptomyces caespitosus.* The parent compound becomes a bifunctional alkylating agent after enzymatic alteration within the cell; it then inhibits DNA synthesis by DNA cross-linkage. Mitomycin's immunosuppressive properties are fairly weak; however, it is a potent inhibitor of fibroblast proliferation. Mitomycin C is used as a single topical application during glaucoma filtering operations to impede scarring and prevent surgical failure. Complications of therapy are wound leakage, hypotony, and localized scleral melting. Severe toxicity has been reported in an animal model with intraocular instillation of mitomycin C, resulting in irreversible progressive bullous keratopathy in 3 of 4 rabbits (see BCSC Section 10, *Glaucoma*).

Both mitomycin and fluorouracil have been used to treat conjunctival intraepithelial neoplasia. Topical mitomycin C has also been recommended both as a single-dose therapy and as postoperative drops for use in the prevention of recurrence of pterygia after pterygium excision. Recommended dosage is 0.02%–0.04% 4 times daily for 1–2 weeks after surgery. The recurrence rate with such therapy has been reported to be as low as 0%–11%. However, several adverse effects—such as corneal edema, corneal and scleral perforation, corectopia, iritis, cataract, and intractable pain—have been reported. A primary conjunctival graft after pterygium removal may offer similar low recurrence rates without these serious complications. Mitomycin has been commonly used to reduce haze in phototherapeutic keratectomy (PTK) patients. (For additional information on uses of mitomycin and fluorouracil, see BCSC Section 8, *External Disease and Cornea*).

Anderson Penno E, Braun DA, Kamal A, Hamilton WK, Gimbel HV. Topical thiotepa treatment for recurrent corneal haze after photorefractive keratectomy. *J Cataract Refract Surg.* 2003;29(8):1537–1542.

Khaw PT. Advances in glaucoma surgery: evolution of antimetabolite adjunctive therapy. *J Glaucoma.* 2001;10(5 Suppl 1):S81–S84.

Sundaram V, Barsam A, Virgili G. Intravitreal low molecular weight heparin and 5-fluorouracil for the prevention of proliferative vitreoretinopathy following retinal reattachment surgery. *Cochrane Database Syst Rev.* 2010;7:CD006421.

Wormald R, Wilkins MR, Bunce C. Post-operative 5-fluorouracil for glaucoma surgery. *Cochrane Database Syst Rev.* 2001;3:CD001132.

Yamamoto N, Ohmura T, Suzuki H, Shirasawa H. Successful treatment with 5-fluorouracil of conjunctival intraepithelial neoplasia refractive to mitomycin-C. *Ophthalmology.* 2002; 109(2):249–252.

Medications for Dry Eye

Artificial tear preparations (demulcents) and emollients form an occlusive film over the corneal surface to lubricate and protect the eye from drying. The active ingredients in demulcent preparations are polyvinyl alcohol, cellulose, and methylcellulose as well as their derivatives: hydroxypropyl cellulose, hydroxyethylcellulose, hydroxypropyl methylcellulose (HPMC), and carboxymethylcellulose. Other ingredients used for formulation include glycerin, polysorbate 80, polyethylene glycol (PEG)-400, dextran 70, povidone, and propylene glycol.

The viscosity of artificial tears varies in part due to the concentration of the wetting agent. For example, carboxymethylcellulose is available in 0.25%, 0.5%, and 1% solutions; higher-viscosity solutions are used to treat increasingly severe dry eye symptoms.

Some data support the hypothesis that changes in tear osmolality trigger corneal and conjunctival epithelial damage and initiation of dry eye. Artificial tear products with lower osmolality may relieve dry eye symptoms to a greater extent, but clinical results thus far have not been conclusive.

The pH of commercially available artificial tear products varies widely. A patient may experience a stinging sensation after eyedrop use because of a mismatch between the pH of the instilled eyedrops and that of the patient's tear. Patients who report a stinging sensation following eyedrop use may try another product with a different pH.

Multidose preparations contain preservatives, including benzalkonium chloride, EDTA (ethylenediaminetetraacetic acid), methylparaben, polyquad (polyquaternium 1), potassium sorbate, propylparaben, sodium chlorite, sodium perborate, and sorbic acid. Although early preservatives such as thimerosal and benzalkonium chloride were highly toxic, the newest generation of ophthalmic preservatives is less harmful to the ocular surface. Nonpreserved unit-dose preparations eliminate the cytotoxic effects of preservatives.

Ocular emollients are ointments prepared with sterile petrolatum, liquid lanolin, mineral oil, methylparaben, and polyparaben. Ophthalmic lubricating ointments help ease the symptoms of severe dry eye and exposure keratopathy and are suitable for nighttime use in dry eye and nocturnal lagophthalmos.

Some principles can help guide the choice of artificial tear preparation for a particular patient in the presence of the wide variety of commercially available products. Generally, a more viscous tear lubricant should be used as the severity of the dry eye increases. A trial-and-error approach may be necessary that involves titration of the frequency of instillation according to the patient's daily activities, the use of tear substitutes with different mechanisms of action or properties, and even a combination of different lubricants. Preservative-free products should be recommended if frequent instillation is required, such as for severe dry eye. Nonpreserved preparations are at risk of microbial contamination and therefore should be discarded within a few hours of use, even though the vial may be recapped after opening.

Topical cyclosporine, 0.05%, targets the inflammatory etiology of dry eye. Because cyclosporine is poorly water soluble, it is prepared in an emulsion composed of glycerin, castor oil, and polysorbate 80. Biopsies have demonstrated a measurable repopulation of goblet cells and a decrease in both conjunctival epithelial cell turnover and the number of lymphocytes. This agent is available in a multi-dose bottle and a preservative-free single-use package.

Lifitegrast 5% preservative-free topical solution, a lymphocyte function-associated antigen-1 (LFA-1) antagonist used twice daily, was approved by the FDA in 2016 for the treatment of dry eye. It inhibits binding of intercellular adhesion molecule-1 (ICAM-1) to LFA-1 and has been shown to be effective in reducing ocular surface inflammation.

Autologous serum eye drops are beneficial for the treatment of ocular surface diseases such as persistent epithelial defects, superior limbic keratoconjunctivitis, keratoconjunctivitis sicca, and neurotrophic keratopathy. They are formulated by compounding to a 20% solution packaged into sterile dropper bottles. Reported complications include peripheral corneal infiltrate and ulcer, eyelid eczema, microbial keratitis, ocular discomfort or epitheliopathy, bacterial conjunctivitis, scleral vasculitis and melting in patients with rheumatoid arthritis, and immune complex deposition with 100% serum.

Two dry eye products currently under investigation are diquafosol tetrasodium and rebamipide. Diquafosol tetrasodium is a $P2Y_2$ purinergic receptor agonist that activates $P2Y_2$ receptors on the ocular surface, causing rehydration through activation of the fluid pump mechanism of the accessory lacrimal glands on the conjunctival surface. Rebamipide is a derivative of quinolone-class antibiotics that enhances the secretion of mucin to support tear-film adhesion and slow tear-film breakup time.

Tauber J, Karpecki P, Latkany R, et al; OPUS-2 Investigators. Lifitegrast ophthalmic solution 5.0% versus placebo for treatment of dry eye disease: results of the randomized phase III OPUS-2 study. *Ophthalmology.* 2015;122(12):2423–2431.

Ocular Decongestants

Common drugs such as naphazoline, oxymetazoline, tetrahydrozoline, and phenylephrine hydrochloride are used as topical drops to cause temporary vasoconstriction of conjunctival vessels. This effect is mediated by α_1-receptors. Possible adverse effects include rebound vasodilation and conjunctival hyperemia. The mechanisms of the adverse effects are unclear; possibilities include receptor desensitization and damage to the ocular surface as a result of vasoconstriction of nutrient arteries, which may involve activation of

α_2-receptors, and toxicity of preservatives. These medications can be abused by patients and may cause ocular surface toxicity. Systemic absorption of ocular adrenergic drugs is frequently sufficient to cause systemic effects, which are manifested in the cardiovascular system, the bronchial airways, and the brain (see the earlier section Adrenergic Drugs). Although ocular decongestants are available as over-the-counter preparations, patients should be instructed not to use them on a long-term basis.

Antimicrobial Drugs

Penicillins and Cephalosporins

The penicillins and cephalosporins are β-lactam–containing antibacterial drugs that react with and inactivate a particular bacterial transpeptidase that is essential for bacterial cell-wall synthesis (Table 16-17). Some bacteria are resistant to the action of penicillins and cephalosporins. The lipopolysaccharide outer coat of many gram-negative bacteria may prevent certain hydrophilic antibiotics from reaching their cytoplasmic membrane sites of action. Furthermore, some bacteria produce β-lactamases (penicillinase), enzymes capable of cleaving the critical amide bond within these antibiotics. The different penicillins and cephalosporins vary in susceptibility to the β-lactamases produced by different bacterial species.

The penicillins and cephalosporins penetrate the blood–ocular and blood–brain barriers poorly and are actively transported out of the eye by the organic-acid transport system of the ciliary body. However, their penetration into the eye increases with inflammation and with coadministration of probenecid.

Serious and occasionally fatal hypersensitivity (anaphylactoid) reactions can occur in association with penicillin and cephalosporin therapy. A history of immediate allergic response (anaphylaxis or rapid onset of hives) to any penicillin is a strong contraindication to the use of any other penicillin. Approximately 10% of people who are allergic to a penicillin will have cross-reactivity to cephalosporins.

Kelkar PS, Li JT. Cephalosporin allergy. *N Engl J Med*. 2001;345(11):804–809.

Penicillins

There are 5 classes of penicillins, which differ in their spectrum of antibiotic activity and in their resistance to penicillinase:

1. Penicillin G, penicillin V, and phenethicillin are highly effective against most gram-positive and gram-negative cocci, many anaerobes, and *Listeria, Actinomyces, Leptospira,* and *Treponema* organisms. However, most strains of *Staphylococcus aureus* and many strains of *S epidermidis,* anaerobes, and *Neisseria gonorrhoeae* are now resistant, often through production of penicillinase. Resistance by enterococci often arises from altered penicillin-binding proteins. Penicillin V and phenethicillin are absorbed well orally, whereas penicillin G is better absorbed when administered intravenously because it is inactivated by stomach acid. These penicillins are excreted rapidly by the kidneys and have short half-lives unless they are given in depot forms (ie, procaine penicillin G) or administered with probenecid, which competitively inhibits excretion by the kidneys.

Table 16-17 Principal Antibiotics and Their Administration*

Drug Name	Topical	Subconjunctival	Intravitreal	Intravenous (Adult)
Amikacin sulfate	10 mg/mL	25 mg	400 µg	15 mg/kg daily in 2–3 doses
Ampicillin sodium	50 mg/mL	50–150 mg	500 µg	4–12 g daily in 4 doses
Bacitracin zinc	10,000 units/mL	5000 units	NA	NA
Carbenicillin disodium	4–6 mg/mL	100 mg	250–2000 µg	8–24 g daily in 4–6 doses
Cefazolin sodium	50 mg/mL	100 mg	2250 µg	2–4 g daily in 3–4 doses
Ceftazidime	50 mg/mL	200 mg	2000 µg	1 g daily in 2–3 doses
Ceftriaxone	50 mg/mL	125 mg	2000 µg	1–2 g daily
Clindamycin	50 mg/mL	15–50 mg	1000 µg	900–1800 mg daily in 2 doses
Colistimethate sodium	10 mg/mL	15–25 mg	100 µg	2.5–5.0 mg/kg daily in 2–4 doses
Erythromycin	50 mg/mL	100 mg	500 µg	NA
Gentamicin sulfate	8–15 mg/mL	10–20 mg	100–200 µg	3–5 mg/kg daily in 2–3 doses
Imipenem/cilastatin sodium	5 mg/mL	NA	NA	2 g daily in 3–4 doses
Kanamycin sulfate	30–50 mg/mL	30 mg	500 µg	15 mg/kg daily in 2–3 doses
Methicillin sodium	50 mg/mL	50–100 mg	1000–2000 µg	6–10 g daily in 4 doses
Neomycin sulfate	5–8 mg/mL	125–250 mg	NA	NA
Penicillin G	100,000 units/mL	0.5–1.0 million units	300 units	12–24 million units daily in 4 doses
Polymyxin B sulfate	10,000 units/mL	100,000 units	NA	NA
Ticarcillin disodium	6 mg/mL	100 mg	NA	200–300 mg/kg daily
Tobramycin sulfate	8–15 mg/mL	10–20 mg	100–200 µg	3–5 mg/kg daily in 2–3 doses
Vancomycin HCl	12.5–50 mg/mL	25 mg	1000 µg	15–30 mg/kg daily in 1–2 doses

*Most penicillins and cephalosporins are physically incompatible when combined in the same bottle or syringe with aminoglycosides.

NA = not applicable.

2. The penicillinase-resistant penicillins include methicillin sodium, nafcillin, oxacillin sodium, cloxacillin sodium, dicloxacillin sodium, and floxacillin. They are less potent than penicillin G against susceptible organisms but are the drugs of choice for infections that are caused by penicillinase-producing *S aureus* and that are not methicillin resistant. Methicillin and nafcillin are acid labile; therefore, they are given either parenterally or by subconjunctival injection. The other medications in this group have reasonable oral absorption. When they are given systemically, co-administration of probenecid reduces renal excretion and outward transport from the eye.

3. The broad-spectrum penicillins such as ampicillin, amoxicillin, and bacampicillin HCl have antibacterial activity that extends to such gram-negative organisms as *Haemophilus influenzae, Escherichia coli, Salmonella* and *Shigella* species, and *Proteus mirabilis.* Resistant strains of *H influenzae* are becoming more common. These drugs are stable in acid and may be given orally. They are not resistant to penicillinase or to the broader-spectrum β-lactamases that are increasingly common among gram-negative bacteria.

4. Carbenicillin and ticarcillin have antimicrobial activity that extends to *Pseudomonas* and *Enterobacter* species and indole-positive strains of *Proteus.* These drugs are given parenterally or subconjunctivally, although the indanyl ester of carbenicillin may be given orally. They are not resistant to penicillinase and are less active against gram-positive bacteria and *Listeria* species.

5. Piperacillin sodium, mezlocillin sodium, and azlocillin are particularly potent against *Pseudomonas* and *Klebsiella* species and retain a strong gram-positive coverage and activity against *Listeria* species. They are administered parenterally or subconjunctivally, and they are not resistant to penicillinase.

Cephalosporins

Bacterial susceptibility patterns and resistance to β-lactamases have determined the classification of the cephalosporins as first, second, third, or fourth generation, although fifth- and sixth-generation drugs are under development.

1. *First generation.* Cephalothin, cefazolin, cephalexin, cefadroxil, and cephradine have strong antimicrobial activity against gram-positive organisms, especially *Streptococcus* species and *S aureus.* They retain moderate activity against gram-negative organisms. Cephalothin is the most resistant of these drugs to staphylococcal β-lactamase and is used in severe staphylococcal infections. Because cephalothin is painful when given intramuscularly, it is used only intravenously. In contrast, cefazolin is more sensitive to β-lactamase but has somewhat greater activity against *Klebsiella* species and *E coli.* Cefazolin has a longer half-life and is tolerated both intramuscularly and intravenously; thus, it is used more frequently than the other first-generation cephalosporins. Cephalexin, cefadroxil, and cephradine are stable in gastric acid and are available in oral forms.

2. *Second generation.* These medications were developed to expand the activity against gram-negative organisms while retaining much of their gram-positive spectrum of activity. Cefamandole, cefoxitin, and cefuroxime display greater activity against *H influenzae, Enterobacter aerogenes,* and *Neisseria* species. Cefamandole has increased activity against *Enterobacter* and indole-positive *Proteus* species, *H influenzae,* and *Bacteroides* species. Cefoxitin is active against indole-positive *Proteus* and *Serratia* organisms, as well as against *Bacteroides fragilis.* Cefuroxime is valuable in the treatment of penicillinase-producing *N gonorrhoeae* and ampicillin-resistant *H influenzae,* and its penetration of the blood–brain barrier is adequate for initial treatment of suspected pneumococcal, meningococcal, or *H influenzae* meningitis.

3. *Third generation.* The third-generation cephalosporins have further enhanced activity against gram-negative bacilli, specifically the β-lactamase–producing

members of the Enterobacteriaceae family, but they are inferior to first-generation cephalosporins with regard to their activity against gram-positive cocci. Commonly used drugs include cefotaxime, cefoperazone sodium, ceftriaxone sodium, ceftazidime, and ceftizoxime sodium. These drugs have a similar spectrum of activity against gram-positive and gram-negative organisms; anaerobes; *Neisseria, Serratia,* and *Proteus* species; and some *Pseudomonas* isolates. Cefoperazone and ceftazidime are particularly effective against *Pseudomonas* but lose more coverage of the gram-positive cocci. Cefotaxime penetrates the blood–brain barrier better than the other cephalosporins can, and it presumably also penetrates the blood–ocular barrier.

4. *Fourth generation.* Cefepime HCl and cefpirome have a spectrum of gram-negative coverage similar to that of the third-generation cephalosporins, but these drugs are more resistant to some β-lactamases.

No cephalosporin provides coverage for enterococci, *Listeria* and *Legionella* species, or methicillin-resistant *S aureus.*

Other Antibacterial Drugs

Tables 16-18 and 16-19 list ophthalmic antibacterial drugs and ophthalmic combination anti-inflammatory/antibiotic drugs, respectively.

Fluoroquinolones

Fluoroquinolones are synthetic fluorinated derivatives of nalidixic acid. The most commonly used ophthalmic fluoroquinolones include ofloxacin, levofloxacin, ciprofloxacin, moxifloxacin, gatifloxacin, and besifloxacin. These drugs are highly effective, broad-spectrum antimicrobials with potent activity against common gram-positive and gram-negative ocular pathogens. Their mechanism of action targets bacterial DNA supercoiling through the inhibition of bacterial topoisomerase II (DNA gyrase) and topoisomerase IV, 2 of the enzymes responsible for replication, genetic recombination, and DNA repair. Mutations in the bacterial genes for these enzymes allow the development of resistance to fluoroquinolone drugs. There is increased incidence of resistance to these drugs, as well as evidence of cross-resistance among them. Fluoroquinolone resistance has been reported in *Mycobacterium chelonae, S aureus,* coagulase-negative *Staphylococcus* species, *Pseudomonas aeruginosa, Clostridium difficile, Salmonella enterica, E coli,* and *Helicobacter pylori.*

In vitro studies have demonstrated that the fluoroquinolones, especially ciprofloxacin and temafloxacin, inhibit 90% of common bacterial corneal pathogens and have a lower minimum inhibitory concentration than that of the aminoglycosides gentamicin and tobramycin and the cephalosporin cefazolin. They are also less toxic to the corneal epithelium than are the aminoglycosides. Methicillin-susceptible strains of *S aureus* are generally susceptible to fluoroquinolones, but methicillin-resistant strains of staphylococci are often resistant to them.

The older generations of fluoroquinolones have good potency against gram-negative bacteria, and the newer generations were designed to broaden the spectrum of coverage and increase the potency against gram-positive bacteria. For example, the second-generation

Table 16-18 Ophthalmic Antibacterial Drugs

Generic Name	Trade Name	Strength
Individual Drugs		
Azithromycin	AzaSite	1% solution
Bacitracin zinc	Ak-Tracin, available generically	Ointment (500 units/g)
Besifloxacin	Besivance	0.6% suspension
Chloramphenicol	Powder available for compounding	0.5% solution, 1% ointment
Ciprofloxacin HCl	Ciloxan, available generically	0.3% solution, 0.3% ointment
Erythromycin	Romycin, available generically	0.5% ointment
Gatifloxacin	Zymar, Zymaxid	0.3% solution, 0.5% solution
Gentamicin sulfate	Garamycin	0.3% solution, 0.3% ointment
	Genoptic	0.3% solution
	Gentasol	0.3% solution
	Gentak	0.3% solution, 0.3% ointment
	Available generically	0.3% solution, 0.3% ointment
Levofloxacin	Quixin	0.5% solution
Moxifloxacin HCl	Vigamox, Moxeza	0.5% solution
Ofloxacin	Ocuflox	0.3% solution
	Available generically	0.3% solution
Sulfacetamide sodium	Bleph-10	10% solution, 10% ointment
	Available generically	10% solution, 10% ointment
Tobramycin sulfate	Ak-Tob	0.3% solution
	Tobrasol	0.3% solution
	Tobrex	0.3% solution, 0.3% ointment
	Available generically	0.3% solution
Combination Drugs		
Polymyxin B sulfate/bacitracin zinc	Ak-Poly-Bac	Ointment (10,000 units/g, 500 units/g)
	Polycin-B	Ointment (10,000 units/g, 500 units/g)
	Available generically	Ointment (10,000 units/g, 500 units/g)
Polymyxin B sulfate/neomycin sulfate/bacitracin zinc	Available generically	Solution (10,000 units, 1.75 mg, 0.025 mg/mL), ointment (10,000 units/g, 3.5 mg/base, 400 units/g)
Polymyxin B sulfate/neomycin sulfate/gramicidin	Neosporin, available generically	Solution (10,000 units/mL, 1.75 mg/base mL, 0.025 mg/mL)
Polymyxin B sulfate/oxytetracycline	Terak	Ointment (10,000 units/g, equivalent to 5 mg base/g)
Polymyxin B sulfate/trimethoprim sulfate	Polytrim, available generically	Solution (10,000 units/mL, equivalent to 1 mg base/mL)

fluoroquinolone ciprofloxacin may be more effective against *P aeruginosa* than the newer drugs.

Six currently available fluoroquinolones are ofloxacin ophthalmic solution, 0.3%, ciprofloxacin, 0.3%, levofloxacin, 0.5%, gatifloxacin, 0.3% and 0.5%, moxifloxacin, 0.5%, and besifloxacin, 0.6%. They are used to treat corneal ulcers caused by susceptible strains of *S aureus*, *S epidermidis*, *Streptococcus pneumoniae*, *P aeruginosa*, *Serratia marcescens*

Table 16-19 Combination Ocular Anti-inflammatory and Antibiotic Drugs

Generic Name	Trade Name	Preparation and Concentration
Dexamethasone/neomycin sulfate/polymyxin B sulfate	Ak-Trol, Poly-Dex, Dexacidin, Dexasporin, Maxitrol, available generically	Suspension, 0.1%; equivalent to 3.5 mg base/mL; 10,000 units/mL
	Maxitrol, Ak-Trol, Poly-Dex, available generically	Ointment, 0.1%; equivalent to 3.5 mg base/g; 10,000 units/g
Dexamethasone/tobramycin	Tobradex, available generically	Suspension, 0.1%, 0.3%
	Tobradex	Ointment, 0.1%, 0.3%
Fluorometholone/ sulfacetamide	FML-S	Suspension, 0.1%, 10%
Hydrocortisone/neomycin sulfate/polymyxin B sulfate	Cortisporin suspension, available generically	Suspension, 1%; equivalent to 3.5 mg base/mL; 10,000 units/mL
Hydrocortisone/neomycin sulfate/polymyxin B sulfate/bacitracin zinc	Ak-Spore, Cortisporin ointment, available generically	Ointment, 1%; equivalent to 3.5 mg base/g; 5000 units/g; 400 units/g
Loteprednol etabonate/ tobramycin	Zylet	Suspension, 0.5%, 0.3%
Neomycin sulfate/polymyxin B sulfate/prednisolone acetate	Poly-Pred, available generically	Suspension; equivalent to 0.35% base; 10,000 units/mL; 0.5%
Prednisolone acetate/ gentamicin sulfate	Pred-G	Suspension; equivalent to 0.3% base; 1%
	Pred-G S.O.P.	Ointment; equivalent to 0.3% base; 0.6%
Prednisolone acetate/ sulfacetamide sodium	Blephamide, available generically	Suspension, 0.2%, 10%
	Blephamide S.O.P.	Ointment, 0.2%, 10%
Prednisolone sodium phosphate/sulfacetamide sodium	Vasocidin, available generically	Solution, 0.25%, 10%
	Ak-Cide	Ointment, 0.5%, 10%

(efficacy studied in fewer than 10 infections), and *Propionibacterium acnes*. They are also indicated for bacterial conjunctivitis due to susceptible strains of *S aureus*, *S epidermidis*, *S pneumoniae*, *Enterobacter cloacae*, *H influenzae*, *P mirabilis*, and *P aeruginosa*. These fluoroquinolones have a high rate of penetration into ocular tissue. Their sustained tear concentration levels exceed the minimum inhibitory concentrations of key ocular pathogens for 12 hours or more after 1 dose. They also deliver excellent susceptibility kill rates; one in vitro study confirmed eradication of 87%–100% of indicated pathogenic bacteria, including *P aeruginosa*. Ofloxacin has a high intrinsic solubility that enables it to be formulated at a near-neutral pH of 6.4. Ciprofloxacin is formulated at a pH of 4.5, gatifloxacin at a pH of 6.0, and moxifloxacin at a pH of 6.8. The most frequently reported drug-related adverse reaction is transient ocular burning or discomfort. Other reported reactions include stinging, redness, itching, chemical conjunctivitis/keratitis, periocular/facial edema, foreign-body sensation, photophobia, blurred vision, tearing, dry eye, and eye pain. Although rare, dizziness has also been reported. Both norfloxacin and ciprofloxacin have been reported to cause white, crystalline corneal deposits of medication, which resolve after discontinuation of the drug.

Case reports of tendonitis and tendon rupture have been associated with systemic fluoroquinolone use. The possibility of damage to growth-plate cartilage poses a safety concern for the use of fluoroquinolones in children. However, larger cohorts and comparative studies did not show an increased risk of musculoskeletal disorders in children treated with systemic fluoroquinolones. There is no evidence that the ophthalmic administration of fluoroquinolones has any effect on weight-bearing joints in the pediatric population.

Sulfonamides

Sulfonamides are derivatives of *para*-aminobenzenesulfonamide. They are structural analogues of *para*-aminobenzoic acid (PABA) and competitive antagonists of dihydropteroate synthase for the bacterial synthesis of folic acid. Unlike mammals, bacteria cannot use exogenous folic acid but must synthesize it from PABA. Sulfonamides are bacteriostatic only. They are more effective when administered with trimethoprim or pyrimethamine, each of which is a potent inhibitor of bacterial dihydrofolate reductase; together, they block successive steps in the synthesis of folic acid. Systemic pyrimethamine, sulfadiazine, and folinic acid are used in the treatment of toxoplasmosis. Folinic acid is coadministered to minimize bone-marrow suppression. Chlamydial infection requires a 3-week course of systemic sulfonamide therapy.

Sulfacetamide ophthalmic solution (10%–30%) and ointment (10%) penetrate the cornea well but may sensitize the patient to sulfonamide medication. Susceptible organisms include *S pneumoniae*, *Corynebacterium diphtheriae*, *H influenzae*, *Actinomyces* species, and *Chlamydia trachomatis*. Local irritation, itching, periorbital edema, and transient stinging are some common adverse effects from topical administration. As for all sulfonamide preparations, severe sensitivity reactions such as toxic epidermal necrolysis and Stevens-Johnson syndrome have been reported. The incidence of adverse reactions to all sulfonamides is approximately 5%.

The cross-allergenicity between sulfonamide antibiotics and nonantibiotic sulfonamide-containing drugs complicates drug therapy. The immunologic determinant of type I immediate hypersensitivity reaction to sulfonamide antibiotics is the N1-heterocyclic ring. Nonantibiotic sulfonamides do not contain this structural feature. Non–type I hypersensitivity responses to sulfonamide antibiotics are largely attributable to reactive metabolites formed at the N4 amino nitrogen of the sulfonamide antibiotics, a structure that is also not found on any nonantibiotic sulfonamide drugs. Therefore, cross-reactivity between sulfonamide antibiotics and nonantibiotic sulfonamide-containing drugs is unlikely. However, a T-cell–mediated immune response to the parent sulfonamide structure appears to be responsible for the hypersensitivity that occurs in a small subset of patients. Thus, cross-reactivity remains possible, at least theoretically. Sulfate refers to the bivalent SO_4 group of a compound. There is no cross-allergenicity between sulfonamide and the sulfate group.

Brackett CC, Singh H, Block JH. Likelihood and mechanisms of cross-allergenicity between sulfonamide antibiotics and other drugs containing a sulfonamide functional group. *Pharmacotherapy.* 2004;24(7):856–870.

Tetracyclines

The tetracycline family includes agents produced by *Streptomyces* species (chlortetracycline, oxytetracycline, demeclocycline), as well as the semisynthetically produced medications tetracycline, doxycycline, and minocycline. Tetracyclines enter bacteria by active transport across the cytoplasmic membrane. They inhibit protein synthesis by binding to the 30S ribosomal subunit, thereby preventing access of aminoacyl transfer RNA (tRNA) to the acceptor site on the mRNA–ribosome complex. Host cells are less affected because they lack an active-transport system. Doxycycline and minocycline are more lipophilic and thus more active by weight. As bacteriostatic drugs, tetracyclines may inhibit bactericidal medications such as the penicillins; therefore, these drugs should not be used concurrently. The use of tetracyclines may decrease the efficacy of oral contraceptives. Patients should be instructed to use an additional form of birth control during administration of tetracyclines and for 1 month after discontinuation of their use.

Tetracyclines are broad-spectrum bacteriostatic antibiotics that are active against many gram-positive and gram-negative bacteria and against *Rickettsia* species, *Mycoplasma pneumoniae*, and *Chlamydia* species. However, many strains of *Klebsiella* and *H influenzae* and nearly all strains of *Proteus vulgaris* and *P aeruginosa* are resistant. These medications demonstrate cross-resistance. Tetracycline is poorly water soluble but is soluble in eyedrops containing mineral oil; it readily penetrates the corneal epithelium. Chlortetracycline was previously used in ophthalmic preparation, but neither chlortetracycline nor tetracycline is currently available for ophthalmic use in the United States. Oxytetracycline is available in combination with polymyxin as an ophthalmic ointment.

Systemic therapy with the tetracyclines is used to treat chlamydial infections; because these drugs are excreted into oil glands, they are also used to treat staphylococcal infections of the meibomian glands. Tetracyclines have anti-inflammatory properties that include suppression of leukocyte migration, reduced production of nitric oxide and reactive oxygen species, inhibition of matrix metalloproteinases, and inhibition of phospholipase A2. They are used to treat meibomian gland dysfunction and rosacea (see BCSC Section 8, *External Disease and Cornea*). They chelate to calcium in milk and antacids and are best taken on an empty stomach. Because tetracyclines may cause gastric irritation, they may be taken with nondairy foods to improve patient adherence. Tetracyclines should not be given to children or pregnant women because they may be deposited in growing teeth, causing permanent discoloration of the enamel, and they may deposit in bone and inhibit bone growth. Tetracyclines depress plasma prothrombin activity and thereby potentiate warfarin. They have been implicated as a cause of pseudotumor cerebri, a condition discussed in BCSC Section 5, *Neuro-Ophthalmology*. The use of tetracyclines also causes photosensitivity; consequently, patients taking tetracycline should avoid extended exposure to sunlight. Degraded or expired tetracyclines may cause renal toxicity, also called Fanconi syndrome.

Chloramphenicol

Chloramphenicol, a broad-spectrum bacteriostatic drug, inhibits bacterial protein synthesis by binding reversibly to the 50S ribosomal subunit, preventing aminoacyl tRNA from binding to the ribosome. Chloramphenicol is effective against most *H influenzae*, *Neisseria meningitidis*, and *N gonorrhoeae*, as well as all anaerobic bacteria. It has some activity against *S pneumoniae, S aureus, Klebsiella pneumoniae, Enterobacter* and *Serratia* species, and *P mirabilis. Pseudomonas aeruginosa* is resistant.

Chloramphenicol penetrates the corneal epithelium well during topical therapy and penetrates the blood–ocular barrier readily when given systemically. However, the use of this medication is limited because it has been implicated in an idiosyncratic and potentially lethal aplastic anemia. Although most cases of this type of anemia have occurred after oral administration, some have been associated with parenteral and even topical ocular therapy. Chloramphenicol is available as a powder for compounding, but it should not be used if an alternative drug with less potential toxicity is available.

Aminoglycosides

The aminoglycosides consist of amino sugars in glycosidic linkage. They are bactericidal agents that are transported across the cell membrane into bacteria, where they bind to the 30S and 50S ribosomal subunits, interfering with initiation of protein synthesis. The antibacterial spectrum of these drugs is determined primarily by the efficiency of their transport into bacterial cells. Such transport is energy dependent and may be reduced in the anaerobic environment of an abscess. Resistance to aminoglycosides may be caused by failure of transport, low affinity for the ribosome, or a plasmid-transmitted ability to enzymatically inactivate the drug. The coadministration of drugs such as penicillin that alter bacterial cell-wall structure can markedly increase aminoglycoside penetration, resulting in a synergism of antibiotic activity against gram-positive cocci, especially enterococci. One such aminoglycoside, amikacin, is remarkably resistant to enzymatic inactivation.

Gentamicin, tobramycin, kanamycin, and amikacin have antibacterial activity against aerobic, gram-negative bacilli such as *P mirabilis; P aeruginosa;* and *Klebsiella, Enterobacter,* and *Serratia* species. Gentamicin and tobramycin are also active against gram-positive *S aureus* and *S epidermidis.* Kanamycin is generally less effective than the others against gram-negative bacilli. Resistance to gentamicin and tobramycin has gradually increased as a result of a plasmid-transmitted ability to synthesize inactivating enzymes. Thus, amikacin, which is generally impervious to these enzymes, is particularly valuable in treating such resistant organisms. It is effective against tuberculosis, as well as atypical mycobacteria, and can be compounded for topical use against mycobacterial infection.

Aminoglycosides are not absorbed well orally but are given systemically, either intramuscularly or intravenously. They do not readily penetrate the blood–ocular barrier but may be administered as eyedrops, ointments, or periocular injections. Gentamicin and carbenicillin should not be mixed for intravenous administration because the carbenicillin inactivates the gentamicin over several hours. Similar incompatibilities exist in vitro between gentamicin and other penicillins and cephalosporins.

The use of streptomycin is now limited to *Streptococcus viridans* bacterial endocarditis, tularemia, plague, and brucellosis. Neomycin is a broad-spectrum antibiotic that is effective against *Enterobacter* species, *K pneumoniae, H influenzae, N meningitidis, C diphtheriae,* and *S aureus.* It is given topically in ophthalmology and orally as a bowel preparation for surgery. Topical allergy to ocular use of neomycin occurs in approximately 8% of cases. Neomycin can cause punctate epitheliopathy and retard re-epithelialization of abrasions.

All aminoglycosides can cause dose-related vestibular and auditory dysfunction and nephrotoxicity when they are given systemically. Dosage adjustments must be made to prevent accumulation of drug and toxicity in patients with renal insufficiency.

Miscellaneous antibiotics

Vancomycin is a tricyclic glycopeptide produced by *Streptococcus orientalis.* It is bactericidal for most gram-positive organisms through the inhibition of glycopeptide polymerization in the cell wall. Vancomycin is useful in the treatment of staphylococcal infections in patients who are allergic to or have not responded to the penicillins and cephalosporins. It can also be used in combination with aminoglycosides to treat S *viridans* or *Streptococcus bovis* endocarditis. Oral vancomycin is poorly absorbed but is effective in the treatment of pseudomembranous colitis caused by *C difficile.* Vancomycin resistance has increased in isolates of *Enterococcus* and *Staphylococcus,* and antibiotic resistance is transmitted between pathogens by a conjugative plasmid.

Vancomycin may be used topically or intraocularly to treat sight-threatening infections of the eye, including infectious keratitis and endophthalmitis caused by methicillin-resistant staphylococci or streptococci. It has been used within the irrigating fluid of balanced salt solution during intraocular surgery. There is controversy concerning the contribution of this prophylactic use of vancomycin to the emergence of resistant bacteria, as well as to an increased risk of postoperative CME. Vancomycin is a preferred substitute for a cephalosporin used in combination with an aminoglycoside in the empirical treatment of endophthalmitis. See BCSC Section 8, *External Disease and Cornea,* and Section 9, *Intraocular Inflammation and Uveitis,* for further discussion.

The intravenous dosage of vancomycin in adults with normal renal function is 500 mg every 6 hours or 1 g every 12 hours. Dosing must be adjusted in patients with renal impairment. Topical vancomycin may be compounded and given in a concentration of 50 mg/mL in the treatment of infectious keratitis. Intravitreal vancomycin combined with amikacin has been used for initial empirical therapy for exogenous bacterial endophthalmitis. Ceftazidime has largely replaced amikacin in clinical practice, primarily because of concerns of potential aminoglycoside retinal toxicity. A vancomycin dose of 1 mg/0.1 mL establishes intraocular levels that are significantly higher than the minimum inhibitory concentration for most gram-positive organisms.

Unlike for systemic treatment, topical vancomycin and intraocular vancomycin have not been associated with ototoxicity or nephrotoxicity. Hourly use of 50 mg of vancomycin per milliliter delivers a dose of 36 mg/day, which is well below the recommended systemic dose. In addition to the ototoxicity and nephrotoxicity associated with systemic therapy, possible complications include chills, rash, fever, and anaphylaxis. Further, rapid intravenous infusion may cause "red-man syndrome" due to flushing.

Erythromycin is a macrolide (many-membered lactone ring attached to deoxy sugars) antibiotic that binds to the 50S subunit of bacterial ribosomes and interferes with protein synthesis. It is bacteriostatic against gram-positive cocci such as *Streptococcus pyogenes* and S *pneumoniae,* gram-positive bacilli such as *C diphtheriae* and *Listeria monocytogenes,* and a few gram-negative organisms such as *N gonorrhoeae.* It may be bactericidal, in sufficient dosing, against susceptible organisms.

Drug resistance to erythromycin is rising and is as high as 40% among *Streptococcus* isolates. There are 4 mechanisms of resistance:

1. esterases from Enterobacteriaceae
2. mutations that alter the 50S ribosome
3. enzyme modification of the ribosomal binding site
4. active pumping to extrude the drug

Macrolide antibiotics such as erythromycin are the treatment of choice for *Legionella pneumophila,* the agent of Legionnaires' disease, as well as for *M pneumoniae.* Erythromycin is administered orally as enteric-coated tablets or in esterified forms to avoid inactivation by stomach acid. It can also be administered parenterally or topically as an ophthalmic ointment. The drug penetrates the blood–ocular and blood–brain barriers poorly.

Clarithromycin and azithromycin are semisynthetic macrolides with a spectrum of activity similar to that of erythromycin. Clarithromycin is more effective against staphylococci, streptococci, and *Mycobacterium leprae,* and azithromycin is more active against *H influenzae, N gonorrhoeae,* and *Chlamydia* species. Both drugs have enhanced activity against *Mycobacterium avium-intracellulare,* atypical mycobacteria, and *Toxoplasma gondii.* Azithromycin, 1%, has been approved by the FDA for bacterial conjunctivitis caused by CDC (Centers for Disease Control and Prevention) coryneform group G, *H influenzae, S aureus,* the *Streptococcus mitis* group, and *S pneumoniae.*

Polymyxin B sulfate is a mixture of basic peptides that function as cationic detergents to dissolve phospholipids of bacterial cell membranes, thereby disrupting cells. It is used topically or by local injection to treat corneal ulcers. Gram-negative bacteria including *Enterobacter* and *Klebsiella* species and *P aeruginosa* are susceptible; bacterial sensitivity is related to the phospholipid content of the cell membrane, and resistance may occur if a cell wall prevents access to the pathogen cell membrane. Topical hypersensitivity is uncommon. Systemic use of this medication has been abandoned due to severe nephrotoxicity. One commercially available topical antibiotic contains polymyxin B sulfate and trimethoprim sulfate. Sulfonamide allergy does not preclude the use of products with trimethoprim or with a sulfate group.

Bacitracin is a mixture of polypeptides that inhibit bacterial cell-wall synthesis. It is active against *Neisseria* and *Actinomyces* species, *H influenzae,* most gram-positive bacilli and cocci, and most but not all strains of methicillin-resistant *S aureus.* It is available as an ophthalmic ointment either alone or in various combinations with polymyxin, neomycin, and hydrocortisone. The primary adverse effect is local hypersensitivity, although it is not commonly observed.

Topical povidone-iodine solution, 5%, exhibits broad-spectrum antimicrobial activity when used to prepare the surgical field and to rinse the ocular surface; it is approved by the FDA for this purpose. It is the only drug that has been shown to have a significant effect on postsurgical endophthalmitis. Povidone-iodine scrub may be used periocularly, but it is contraindicated in the eye because it is damaging to the corneal epithelium.

Topical povidine-iodine solution has been traditionally considered contraindicated in patients with hypersensitivity to iodine or to intravenous contrast dye. However, a reported allergy to seafood or contrast media is probably not a contraindication to the use of topical povidine-iodine solution. Iodine is a simple molecule that is widely believed to lack the complexity required for antigenicity. Instead, patients are probably developing hypersensitivity reactions to specific proteins of the food itself (eg, seafood) or to the contrast media, rather than to the iodine in the compound.

Ciulla TA, Starr MB, Masket S. Bacterial endophthalmitis prophylaxis for cataract surgery: an evidence-based update. *Ophthalmology.* 2002;109(1):13–24.

Isenberg SJ, Apt L, Yoshimori R, Khwarg S. Chemical preparation of the eye in ophthalmic surgery. IV. Comparison of povidine-iodine on the conjunctiva with a prophylactic antibiotic. *Arch Ophthalmol.* 1985;103(9):1340–1342.

Kollef MH. Limitations of vancomycin in the management of resistant staphylococcal infections. *Clin Infect Dis.* 2007;45(Suppl 3):S191–S195.

Scoper SV. Review of third- and fourth-generation fluoroquinolones in ophthalmology: in-vitro and in-vivo efficacy. *Adv Ther.* 2008;25(10):979–994.

Werner G, Klare I, Fleige C, Witte W. Increasing rates of vancomycin resistance among *Enterococcus faecium* isolated from German hospitals between 2004 and 2006 are due to wide clonal dissemination of vancomycin-resistant enterococci and horizontal spread of vanA clusters. *Int J Med Microbiol.* 2008;298(5–6):515–527.

Wykoff CC, Flynn HW, Han DP. Allergy to povidone-iodine and cephalosporins: the clinical dilemma in ophthalmic use. *Am J Ophthalmol.* 2011;151(1):4–6.

Antifungal Drugs

Table 16-20 summarizes common antifungal drugs encountered in ophthalmology practice.

Polyenes

The polyene antibiotics are named for a component sequence of 4–7 conjugated double bonds. That lipophilic region allows these antibiotics to bind to sterols in the cell membrane of susceptible fungi, an interaction that results in damage to the membrane and leakage of essential nutrients. Other antifungals (such as flucytosine and the imidazoles) and even other antibiotics (such as tetracycline and rifampin) can enter through the damaged membrane, yielding synergistic effects.

Natamycin and amphotericin B are 2 examples of polyene macrolide antibiotics. Natamycin is available as a 5% suspension for topical ophthalmic use (once per hour). Local hypersensitivity reactions of the conjunctiva and eyelid and corneal epithelial toxicity may occur. Amphotericin B may be reconstituted at 0.25%–0.5% in sterile water (with deoxycholate to improve solubility) for topical use (every 30 minutes). It may also be administered systemically for disseminated disease, although careful monitoring for renal and other toxicities is required. Both drugs penetrate the cornea poorly. They have been used topically against various filamentous fungi, including species of *Aspergillus, Cephalosporium, Curvularia, Fusarium,* and *Penicillium,* as well as the yeast *Candida albicans.* Systemic amphotericin B has been reported as useful in treating systemic *Aspergillus, Blastomyces, Candida, Coccidioides, Cryptococcus,* and *Histoplasma* infections.

Table 16-20 **Antifungal Drugs**

Generic (Trade) Name	Route	Dosage	Indication (Additional Reports of Use)
Polyenes			
Amphotericin B (Fungizone, available generically)	Topical	0.1%–0.5% solution; dilute with water for injection or dextrose 5% in water	*Aspergillus* *Candida* *Cryptococcus* *(Blastomyces)* *(Coccidioides)* *(Colletotrichum)* *(Histoplasma)*
	Subconjunctival	0.8–1.0 mg	
	Intravitreal	5 µg	
	Intravenous	Because of possible adverse effects and toxicity, dose needs to be carefully adjusted.	
Natamycin (Natacyn)	Topical	5% suspension	*Fusarium* *(Aspergillus)* *(Candida)* *(Cephalosporium)* *(Curvularia)* *(Penicillium)*
Imidazoles			
Ketoconazole (Nizoral, available generically)	Oral	200 mg daily, up to 400 mg for severe or incomplete response	*Blastomyces* *Candida* *Coccidioides* *Histoplasma*
Miconazole nitrate (available as powder for compounding)	Topical	1% solution	*Aspergillus* *Candida* *Cryptococcus*
	Subconjunctival	5 mg	
	Intravitreal	10 µg	
Triazoles			
Fluconazole (Diflucan)	Oral	200 mg daily	*Candida* *Cryptococcus* *(Acremonium)*
Itraconazole (Sporanox)	Oral	200 mg daily	*Aspergillus* *Blastomyces* *Histoplasma* *(Candida)* *(Curvularia)* *(nonsevere Fusarium)*
	Intravenous		
Voriconazole (Vfend)	Topical	1% (made from intravenous solution)	*Aspergillus* *Blastomyces* *Candida* *Cryptococcus* *Fusarium* *Histoplasma* *Penicillium* *Scedosporium*
	Oral	200 mg orally twice daily	
	Intravenous	3–6 mg/kg intravenously every 12 h	
Fluorinated Pyrimidine			
Flucytosine (Ancobon)	Oral	50–150 mg/kg daily divided every 6 h	*Candida* *Cryptococcus* *(Aspergillus)*
	Topical	1% solution	

Imidazoles and triazoles

The imidazole- and triazole-derived antifungal drugs also increase fungal cell-membrane permeability and interrupt membrane-bound enzyme systems. The triazoles have less effect on human sterol synthesis, as well as a longer half-life, than the imidazoles, and they are being more actively developed. The imidazole miconazole is available in a 1% solution that may be injected subconjunctivally (5 mg/0.5 mL, once or twice daily) or applied topically. Miconazole penetrates the cornea poorly.

Ketoconazole is available in 200-mg tablets for oral therapy (once or twice daily). Ketoconazole normally penetrates the blood–brain barrier and, presumably, the blood–ocular barrier poorly, but therapeutic levels can be achieved in inflamed eyes. The triazole itraconazole, with an expanded antifungal spectrum and less systemic toxicity, has largely replaced ketoconazole. However, there is an extensive and growing list of potentially dangerous drug interactions with itraconazole that should be consulted prior to instituting systemic therapy. Fluconazole, another triazole, may also increase the plasma concentrations of other medications. Oral voriconazole is rapidly replacing other antifungals because of its excellent intraocular penetration and broad-spectrum coverage. The imidazole and triazole antifungals act against various species of *Aspergillus, Coccidioides, Cryptococcus,* and *Candida.*

Flucytosine

Flucytosine (5-fluorocytosine) is converted by some species of fungal cells to 5-fluorouracil by cytosine deaminase, and then to 5-fluorodeoxyuridylate. This last compound inhibits thymidylate synthase, an important enzyme in DNA synthesis. Host cells lack cytosine deaminase activity and are less affected. Only fungi that have both a permease to facilitate flucytosine penetration and a cytosine deaminase are sensitive to flucytosine. Flucytosine is taken orally at 50–150 mg/kg daily, divided every 6 hours. Although the drug is well absorbed and penetrates the blood–ocular barrier well, most *Aspergillus* and half of *Candida* isolates are resistant to it. Flucytosine is used primarily as an adjunct to systemic amphotericin B therapy.

Antiviral Drugs

Table 16-21 summarizes information on common antiviral drugs.

Topical antiviral drugs

Idoxuridine, trifluridine, and vidarabine compete with natural nucleotides for incorporation into viral and mammalian DNA and have been used to treat herpes simplex virus (HSV) keratitis. Idoxuridine (5-iodo-2′-deoxyuridine) and trifluridine are structural analogues of thymidine and work in a similar manner; vidarabine is an analogue of adenine. Trifluridine (1% drops, every 2–4 hours) is more soluble than the other drugs and can be used in drop form, providing adequate penetration of diseased corneas to treat herpetic iritis. Trifluridine is currently marketed in the United States, but vidarabine ophthalmic ointment (3%) is not. Idoxuridine and vidarabine powder are available for compounding.

Table 16-21 Antiviral Drugs

Generic Name	Trade Name	Topical Concentration/ Ophthalmic Solution	Systemic Dosage
Trifluridine	Viroptic, available generically	1%	NA
Idoxuridine	Available as powder for compounding	0.1%	NA
Vidarabine monohydrate	Vira-A, available as powder for compounding	3% (ophthalmic ointment)	NA
Acyclovir sodium*	Zovirax, available generically	NA	Oral: herpes simplex virus (HSV) keratitis 200–400 mg 5 times daily for 7–10 days Oral: herpes zoster virus (HZV) ophthalmicus 600–800 mg 5 times daily for 10 days; intravenous if patient is immunocompromised
	Zovirax ointment (not available in the United States)	3% (ophthalmic ointment)	NA
Zidovudine	Retrovir, available generically	NA	Dosage variable per source consulted; dosing per internal medicine consultation recommended
Cidofovir*†	Vistide	NA	Intravenous induction: 5 mg/ kg constant infusion over 1 h once weekly for 2 consecutive weeks Maintenance: 5 mg/kg constant infusion over 1 h administered every 2 weeks
Famciclovir*†	Famvir HZV	NA	500 mg 3 times daily for 7 days
Foscarnet sodium	Foscavir, available generically	NA	Intravenous induction: By controlled infusion only, either by central vein or by peripheral vein induction: 60 mg/kg (adjusted for renal function) given over 1 h every 8 h for 14–21 days Maintenance: 90–120 mg/kg given over 2 h once daily
Ganciclovir	Vitrasert	NA	Intravitreal: 4.5 mg sterile intravitreal insert designed to release the drug over a 5–8-mo period

(Continued)

Table 16-21 *(continued)*

Generic Name	Trade Name	Topical Concentration/ Ophthalmic Solution	Systemic Dosage
Ganciclovir sodium*†	Cytovene IV	NA	Intravenous induction: 5 mg/kg every 12 h for 14–21 days Maintenance: 5 mg/kg daily (7 days per week) or 6 mg/kg once daily (5 days per week)
	Zirgan	0.15% ophthalmic gel	NA
Valacyclovir HCl*‡	Valtrex HZV	NA	1 g 3 times daily for 7–14 days
Valganciclovir	Valcyte	NA	Induction: 900 mg every 12 h for 21 days Maintenance: 900 mg once a day

*Dose adjustment is recommended for geriatric and renal patients or with concomitant nephrotoxic medications.

†Because of potential adverse and toxic effects with systemic dosage, the possible dosage adjustments and warnings should be followed properly.

‡At high doses, valacyclovir has been associated with thrombotic thrombocytopenic purpura/hemolytic uremic syndrome (TTP/HUS) in immunocompromised patients.

NA = not applicable.

Vidarabine can be used if a drug with a different mechanism of action is required. Cross-resistance does not seem to occur among these medications.

Acyclovir is activated by HSV thymidase kinase to inhibit viral DNA polymerase. The 3% ophthalmic ointment is not commercially available in the United States, and the 5% dermatologic ointment is not approved for ophthalmic use. Ganciclovir is activated by triphosphorylation to inhibit viral DNA polymerase. It is available as 0.15% ophthalmic gel approved for treatment of HSV keratitis. It has been shown to be moderately effective in treating CMV corneal endotheliitis and anterior uveitis.

Systemic antiviral drugs

Acyclovir is a synthetic guanosine analogue that requires phosphorylation by viral thymidine kinase to become active. Because the viral thymidine kinase in HSV types 1 and 2 has much more affinity to acyclovir than does host thymidine kinase, high concentrations of acyclovir monophosphate accumulate in infected cells. Acyclovir monophosphate is then further phosphorylated to the active compound acyclovir triphosphate, which cannot cross cell membranes and accumulates further.

Acyclovir-resistant thymidine kinase HSVs have evolved. They occur primarily in patients receiving multiple courses of therapy or in patients with human immunodeficiency virus (HIV) infection. Thymidine kinase mutants are susceptible to vidarabine and foscarnet. Changes in viral DNA polymerase structures can also mediate resistance to acyclovir.

Oral acyclovir is only 15%–30% bioavailable, and food does not affect absorption. For unknown reasons, bioavailability is lower in patients with transplants. The drug is well distributed; cerebrospinal fluid (CSF) and brain concentrations equal approximately 50% of serum values. Concentrations of acyclovir in zoster vesicle fluid are equivalent to those in plasma. Aqueous humor concentrations are 35% those of plasma, and salivary concentrations are 15%. Vaginal concentrations are equivalent to those of plasma, and breast-milk concentrations exceed them.

The plasma half-lives for adults and neonates with normal renal function are 3.3 and 3.8 hours, respectively. The half-life increases to 20 hours in anuric patients. Acyclovir may interfere with the renal excretion of drugs that are eliminated through the renal tubules (eg, methotrexate); probenecid significantly decreases the renal excretion of acyclovir. This drug is effectively removed by hemodialysis (60%) but only minimally removed by peritoneal dialysis. A commonly used intravenous dosage for acyclovir is 1500 mg/m²/day.

Acyclovir is used off-label for ocular HSV and herpes zoster virus (HZV) but has proved effective in preventing the recurrence of HSV epithelial and stromal keratitis with twice-daily oral doses of 400 mg. Although this prophylactic dosage was originally studied over a 1-year treatment period, clinicians are now using this dosage indefinitely to decrease the likelihood of disease recurrence. Similar dosing of acyclovir has proved beneficial in reducing the likelihood of recurrent herpetic eye disease after corneal transplantation. However, oral acyclovir was not found to be beneficial when used with topical steroids and trifluridine in the treatment of active HSV stromal keratitis. The addition of oral acyclovir to a regimen of topical antiviral drugs may be considered for patients with HSV iridocyclitis. Although the benefit of this drug did not reach statistical significance in one study, participant enrollment had been halted due to inadequate numbers of patients. Acyclovir is well tolerated in oral form, but parenteral acyclovir can cause renal toxicity due to crystalline nephropathy. Neurotoxicity may also occur with intravenous use.

Valacyclovir is currently approved for management of HZV infections in immunocompetent persons but not for HSV. It is an amino-acid ester prodrug of acyclovir; its bioavailability is much higher than that of acyclovir (54% vs 20%, respectively). Valacyclovir has been associated with nephrotoxicity and thrombocytopenia in immunocompromised patients.

Famciclovir is the prodrug of penciclovir and is currently approved for the management of uncomplicated acute HZV. It has demonstrated efficacy in relieving acute zoster signs and symptoms and reducing the duration of postherpetic neuralgia when administered during acute HZV.

Ganciclovir (9-2-hydroxypropoxymethylguanine) is a synthetic guanosine analogue active against many herpesviruses. It is approved for cytomegalovirus (CMV) retinitis and for CMV prophylaxis in patients with advanced HIV infection and in transplant patients. Like acyclovir, it must be phosphorylated to become active. Infection-induced kinases, viral thymidine kinase, or deoxyguanosine kinase of various herpesviruses can catalyze this reaction. After monophosphorylation, cellular enzymes convert ganciclovir to the triphosphorylated form, and the triphosphate inhibits viral DNA polymerase rather than cellular DNA polymerase. Because of ganciclovir's toxicity and the availability of acyclovir for treatment of many herpesvirus infections, the use of ganciclovir is currently restricted to treatment of CMV retinitis, predominantly as an intraocular implant.

Systemic ganciclovir is used primarily intravenously, because less than 5% of an oral dose is absorbed. CSF concentrations are approximately 50% those of plasma; peak plasma concentrations reach 4–6 µg/mL. The plasma half-life is 3–4 hours in people with normal renal function, increasing to more than 24 hours in patients with severe renal insufficiency. More than 90% of systemic ganciclovir is eliminated unchanged in urine, and dose modifications are necessary for individuals with compromised renal function. Ganciclovir is approximately 50% removed by hemodialysis. Bone-marrow suppression is the primary adverse effect of systemic therapy. Periodic complete blood counts and platelet counts are required during the course of treatment. Oral ganciclovir may be used to suppress CMV retinitis after initial control is obtained with parenteral therapy. Ganciclovir can be administered intravitreally or as a sustained-release intraocular device.

Valganciclovir is a prodrug for ganciclovir. After oral administration, it is rapidly converted to ganciclovir by intestinal and hepatic esterases.

Foscarnet (phosphonoformic acid) inhibits DNA polymerases, RNA polymerases, and reverse transcriptases. In vitro, it is active against herpesviruses, influenza virus, and HIV. Foscarnet is approved for the treatment of HIV-infected patients with CMV retinitis and for acyclovir-resistant mucocutaneous HSV infections in immunocompromised patients. Foscarnet acts by blocking the pyrophosphate receptor site of CMV DNA polymerase. Viral resistance is attributable to structural alterations in this enzyme. Foscarnet inhibits herpesviruses and CMVs that are resistant to acyclovir and ganciclovir. It is administered intravenously in doses adjusted for renal function and with hydration to establish sufficient diuresis.

Foscarnet bioavailability is approximately 20%. Because it can bind with calcium and other divalent cations, foscarnet becomes deposited in bone and may be detectable for many months; 80%–90% of the administered dose appears unchanged in the urine. Dosage adjustment is required for persons with impaired renal function. Treatment may be limited by nephrotoxicity in up to 50% of patients; other adverse effects include hypocalcemia and neurotoxicity.

Cidofovir is a third medication approved by the FDA for the treatment of CMV retinitis, and it is approved only for that use. Cidofovir is a cytidine nucleoside analogue that is active against herpesviruses, poxviruses, polyomaviruses, papillomaviruses, and adenoviruses. The mechanism of action is inhibition of DNA synthesis, and resistance is through mutations in DNA polymerase. The prolonged intracellular half-life of an active metabolite allows once-weekly dosing during induction, with dosing every 2 weeks thereafter. The primary adverse effect is renal toxicity, which can be decreased by intravenous prehydration and by both pretreatment and posttreatment with high-dose probenecid. Ocular adverse effects include uveitis and irreversible hypotony. Cidofovir does not have direct cross-resistance with acyclovir, ganciclovir, or foscarnet, although some virus isolates may have multiple resistances and even develop triple resistance. In a small series of patients, cidofovir was shown to inhibit CMV replication when administered intravitreally. Long-lasting suppression of CMV retinitis was observed; the average time to progression was 55 days. Cidofovir is the second-line therapy for complications after smallpox vaccination (vaccinia virus) and has been used in selected studies for varicella-zoster retinitis, as well as adenoviral keratoconjunctivitis.

Zidovudine is a thymidine nucleoside analogue with activity against HIV. Zidovudine becomes phosphorylated to monophosphate, diphosphate, and triphosphate forms by cellular kinases in infected and uninfected cells. It has 2 primary methods of action:

1. The triphosphate acts as a competitive inhibitor of viral reverse transcriptase.
2. The azido group prevents further chain elongation and acts as a DNA chain terminator.

Zidovudine inhibits HIV reverse transcriptase at much lower concentrations than those needed to inhibit cellular DNA polymerases. Since the introduction of zidovudine in the 1980s, numerous antiretroviral drugs have been approved for the treatment of HIV infection. They are divided into 6 classes: nucleoside reverse transcriptase inhibitors (NRTIs), non-nucleoside reverse transcriptase inhibitors (NNRTIs), protease inhibitors (PIs), fusion inhibitors, entry inhibitors, and integrase strand transfer inhibitors. The current standard antiretroviral therapy (ART) consists of a combination of antiretroviral drugs.

Fluorouracil is discussed previously in the section Antifibrotic Drugs.

Herpetic Eye Disease Study Group. Acyclovir for the prevention of recurrent herpes simplex virus eye disease. *N Engl J Med.* 1998;339(5):300–306.

Herpetic Eye Disease Study Group. Oral acyclovir for herpes simplex virus eye disease: effect on prevention of epithelial keratitis and stromal keratitis. *Arch Ophthalmol.* 2000;118(8): 1030–1036.

Medications for *Acanthamoeba* Infections

Acanthamoeba is a genus of ubiquitous, free-living amoebae that inhabit soil, water, and air. Their appearance as corneal pathogens has increased due to several factors, including the increased use of contact lenses. The species responsible for corneal infections, which include *A polyphaga, A castellanii, A hatchetti,* and *A culbertsoni,* exist as both trophozoites and double-walled cysts. Because of the variations among species of *Acanthamoeba,* no single drug is effective in treating all cases of *Acanthamoeba* keratitis. Polyhexamethylene biguanide (PHMB, 0.02% solution) is a non–FDA-approved disinfectant and the first-line agent with the lowest minimal amebicidal concentration. Effective medications include chlorhexidine; neomycin; polymyxin B–neomycin–gramicidin mixtures; natamycin, 5% topical suspension; imidazoles such as miconazole (powder compounded to 1% topical solution); systemic imidazoles and triazoles; propamidine isethionate, 0.1% drops (not approved in the United States); and topical dibromopropamidine, 0.15% ointment (not approved in the United States). Combination therapy is commonly required. See BCSC Section 8, *External Disease and Cornea,* for further discussion of treatment recommendations.

Dart JK, Saw VP, Kilvington S. Acanthamoeba keratitis: diagnosis and treatment update 2009. *Am J Ophthalmol.* 2009;148(4):487–499.

Seal DV. *Acanthamoeba* keratitis update—incidence, molecular epidemiology and new drugs for treatment. *Eye.* 2003;17(8):893–905.

Local Anesthetics

Overview

Local anesthetics are used extensively in ophthalmology. Topical preparations yield corneal and conjunctival anesthesia for comfortable performance of examination techniques such as tonometry, gonioscopy, removal of superficial foreign bodies, corneal scraping for bacteriologic studies, and paracentesis, as well as for use of contact lenses associated with fundus examination and laser procedures. Topical and intracameral anesthesia has gained increasing acceptance in cataract, pterygium, and glaucoma surgery. Local retrobulbar, peribulbar, and eyelid blocks yield excellent anesthesia and akinesia for intraocular and orbital surgery (Tables 16-22, 16-23).

The local anesthetic drugs used in ophthalmology are tertiary amines linked by either ester or amide bonds to an aromatic residue. Because the protonated form is far more soluble and these compounds undergo hydrolysis more slowly in acidic solutions, local anesthetic drugs are supplied in the form of their hydrochloride salts. When exposed to tissue fluids at pH 7.4, approximately 5%–20% of the anesthetic agent molecules will be in the unprotonated form, as determined by the pK_a value (8.0–9.0), of the individual drug. The more lipid-soluble unprotonated form penetrates the lipid-rich myelin sheath and cell membrane of axons. Once inside, most of the molecules are again protonated. The protonated form gains access to and blocks the sodium channels on the inner wall of the cell membrane and increases the threshold for electrical excitability. As increasing numbers of sodium channels are blocked, nerve conduction is impeded and finally blocked.

After administration of a local anesthetic, small or unmyelinated nerve fibers are blocked the most quickly because their higher discharge rates open sodium channel gates

Table 16-22 Regional Anesthetics

Generic Name (Trade Name)	Concentration (Maximum Dose)	Onset of Action	Duration of Action	Major Advantages/ Disadvantages
Bupivacaine* (Sensorcaine, Marcaine)	0.25%–0.75%	5–11 min	480–720 min (with epinephrine)	Long duration of action/increased toxicity to the extraocular muscles
Lidocaine* (Xylocaine, Anestacaine)	0.5%–2% (500 mg)	4–6 min	40–60 min; 120 min (with epinephrine)	Spreads readily without hyaluronidase
Mepivacaine* (Carbocaine)	2% (500 mg)	3–5 min	120 min	Duration of action greater without epinephrine
Procaine† (Novocain)	1%–2% (500 mg)	7–8 min	30–45 min; 60 min (with epinephrine)	Short duration; poor absorption from mucous membranes

*Amide-type compound.
†Ester-type compound.

Table 16-23 Topical Anesthetic Drugs

Generic Name	Trade Name	Strength
Cocaine		1%–4%
Fluorescein sodium/benoxinate	Fluress	0.25%
	Flurox	0.25%
	Available generically	0.25%
Fluorescein sodium/proparacaine	Fluoracaine	0.25%/0.1%
	Flucaine	0.25%/0.1%
Lidocaine	Topical solution	4%
	Viscous gel	2%
Proparacaine	Alcaine	0.5%
	Parcaine	0.5%
	Ophthetic	0.5%
	Available generically	0.5%
Tetracaine	Altacaine	0.5%
	Tetravisc	0.5%
	Available generically	0.5%

more frequently and because conduction can be prevented by the disruption of a shorter length of axon. The action potential in unmyelinated fibers spreads continuously along the axon; in myelinated fibers, the action potential spreads by saltation. Therefore, only a short length of an unmyelinated fiber need be functionally interrupted, whereas one or more nodes must be blocked in a myelinated fiber. In larger myelinated fibers, the nodes are farther apart.

Clinically, local anesthetics first block the poorly myelinated and narrow parasympathetic fibers (as evidenced by pupil dilation) and sympathetic fibers (vasodilation), followed by sensory fibers (pain and temperature), and finally the larger and more myelinated motor fibers (akinesia). The optic nerve, enclosed in a meningeal lining, is often not blocked by retrobulbar injections.

Amide local anesthetics are preferred to ester drugs for retrobulbar blocks because the amides have a longer duration of action and less systemic toxicity. However, this duration of action is limited by diffusion from the site of injection because amide drugs are not metabolized locally but rather are metabolized and inactivated in the liver, primarily by dealkylation.

Ester anesthetics are susceptible to hydrolysis by serum cholinesterases in ocular vessels as well as by metabolism in the liver. Toxicity of ester anesthetics may occur at lower doses when serum cholinesterase levels are low because of treatment with echothiophate eyedrops or a hereditary serum cholinesterase deficiency.

The toxic manifestations of local anesthetics are generally related to dose. However, patients with severe hepatic insufficiency may have symptoms of toxicity with either amide or ester local anesthetics, even at lower doses. These manifestations include restlessness and tremor that may proceed to convulsions, and respiratory and myocardial depression. Central nervous system stimulation can be counteracted by intravenous diazepam; respiratory depression calls for ventilatory support.

Because local anesthetics block sympathetic vascular tone and dilate vessels, a 1:200,000 concentration of epinephrine is frequently added to shorter-acting drugs to retard vascular absorption. Such use of epinephrine raises circulating catecholamine levels and may cause systemic hypertension and cardiac arrhythmias.

Topically applied anesthetics disrupt intercellular tight junctions, resulting in increased corneal epithelial permeability to subsequently administered drugs (ie, dilating drops). They also interfere with corneal epithelial metabolism and repair and thus cannot be used for chronic pain relief. Because topical anesthetics can become drugs of abuse that can eventually lead to chronic pain syndromes and vision loss, they should not be dispensed to patients.

Lidocaine is an amide local anesthetic used in strengths of 0.5%, 1%, and 2% (with or without epinephrine) for injection, of 2% as gel, and of 4% as solution for topical mucosal anesthesia, although its use is off-label for topical cataract surgery. It yields a rapid (5-minute) retrobulbar or eyelid block that lasts 1–2 hours. The topical solution, applied to the conjunctiva with a cotton swab for 1–2 minutes, reduces the discomfort of subconjunctival injections. Topical lidocaine is preferable to cocaine or proparacaine for conjunctival biopsy because it has less effect on epithelial morphology. Lidocaine is also extremely useful for suppressing cough during ocular surgery. The maximum safe dose of the 2% solution for local injection is 15 mL in adults. A common adverse effect is drowsiness.

Mepivacaine is an amide drug used in strengths of 1%–3% (with or without a vasoconstrictor). It has a rapid onset and lasts approximately 2–3 hours. The maximum safe dose is 25 mL of a 2% solution.

Bupivacaine is an amide anesthetic that has a slower onset of action than that of lidocaine. It may yield relatively poor akinesia but has the advantage of a long duration of action, up to 8 hours. It is available in 0.25%–0.75% solutions (with or without epinephrine) and is frequently administered in a mixture with lidocaine or mepivacaine to achieve a rapid, complete, and long-lasting effect. The maximum safe dose is 25 mL of a 0.75% solution.

Hyaluronidase catalyzes the hydrolysis of hyaluronic acid, a constituent of the extracellular matrix; it temporarily lowers the viscosity of the extracellular matrix and increases tissue permeability. Hyaluronidase can be combined with local injection of anesthetics to increase the dispersion of the anesthetic drug(s) for intraocular or orbital surgery. Increased dispersion of the anesthetic drug may reduce the pressure rise in the limited orbital space and IOP, produce less distortion of the surgical site, decrease the risk of postoperative strabismus and myotoxicity, and increase akinesia of the globe and lid; lower volumes of anesthetic may be employed.

Hyaluronidase products approved by the FDA include those derived from bovine and ovine sources, as well as a recombinant human product. Due to a lack of reliable animal sources and a shortage of supply from manufacturers, compounded formulations of hyaluronidase from animal-derived active pharmaceutical ingredients have been used in ophthalmology. FDA regulations for compounding pharmacies are not as stringent as are regulations for pharmaceutical products, and concerns have been raised about the potency and purity of compounded products. There have been reports of hypersensitivity reactions to retrobulbar or peribulbar blocks associated with use of animal-derived hyaluronidase. For retrobulbar or peribulbar injection, 1 mL of hyaluronidase

(150 USP units/mL, single-dose vial of recombinant human product) can be added to a syringe of the anesthetic to be administered.

Several other drugs are commonly used for topical anesthesia of the ocular surface. Because of their higher lipid solubilities, these medications have a more rapid onset than others; thus, the initial discomfort caused by the drops is reduced. Proparacaine is an ester topical anesthetic available as a 0.5% solution. The least irritating of the topical anesthetics, it has a rapid onset of approximately 15 seconds and lasts approximately 20 minutes. Used without a preservative, proparacaine reportedly does not inhibit the growth of *Staphylococcus, Candida,* or *Pseudomonas,* so it may be preferred to other drugs for corneal anesthesia prior to obtaining a scraping for culture from a corneal ulcer. Its structure is different enough from that of other local anesthetics that cross-sensitization apparently does not occur.

Benoxinate (also known as *oxybuprocaine*) is an ester topical anesthetic available in a 0.4% solution with fluorescein for use in tonometry. Its onset and duration are similar to those of proparacaine. Benoxinate is also available alone as a topical anesthetic in Europe.

Tetracaine is an ester topical anesthetic that is available in 0.5% solution and is approved for short-duration ocular surface procedures. Its onset of action and duration of action are longer than those of proparacaine, and it causes more extensive corneal epithelial toxicity.

Topical Anesthetics in Anterior Segment Surgery

The first modern use of topical anesthetics was Koller's use of cocaine in 1884. Since then, synthetic drugs have become available; cocaine is no longer used because of the potential risk of adverse effects and drug abuse. Tetracaine, 0.5% or 1% (amethocaine), and proparacaine, 0.5%, are short-acting (20 minutes) drugs and are the least toxic of the regional and topical anesthetics to the corneal epithelium. Lidocaine, 4%, for injection can be used topically, as can lidocaine jelly, 2%. Bupivacaine, 0.5% and 0.75%, has a longer duration of action but an increased risk of associated corneal toxicity.

Technique

The aim of topical anesthetic use is to block the nerves that supply the superficial cornea and conjunctiva—namely, the long and short ciliary, nasociliary, and lacrimal nerves. Patients should be warned that they will experience some stinging upon application of the drops onto the surface of the cornea. Because visual perception is not lost, the patient is asked to focus on the source of the light, the intensity of which is subsequently reduced.

Topical anesthetics may be combined with subconjunctival anesthetics. Such combinations are well tolerated by patients and allow subconjunctival and scleral manipulations to be carried out. Topical anesthetics can be augmented with a blunt cannula sub-Tenon infusion of anesthetic as a primary anesthetic or intraoperatively in patients who become intolerant of topical anesthetics.

Intraocular lidocaine

Recently, intraocular lidocaine has been used to provide analgesia during surgery. The solution used is 0.3 mL of 1% isotonic, nonpreserved lidocaine administered intracamerally.

No adverse effects have been reported, except for possible transient retinal toxicity if lidocaine is injected posteriorly in the absence of a posterior capsule. Lidocaine obviates the need for intravenous and regional anesthetic supplementation in most patients. Adequate anesthesia is obtained in approximately 10 seconds. As with topical techniques, patient cooperation during surgery is desirable. Contrasting studies have shown no difference in the degree of cooperation whether or not intracameral lidocaine is used as a supplement to topical anesthetics. Because of unreliable patient cooperation, topical and intracameral anesthetics should be used cautiously, if at all, in patients with deafness, dementia, and severe photophobia.

Crandall AS. Anesthesia modalities for cataract surgery. *Curr Opin Ophthalmol.* 2001;12(1): 9–11.

Kansal S, Moster MR, Gomes MC, Schmidt CM Jr, Wilson RP. Patient comfort with combined anterior sub-Tenon's, topical, and intracameral anesthesia versus retrobulbar anesthesia in trabeculectomy, phacotrabeculectomy, and aqueous shunt surgery. *Ophthalmic Surg Lasers.* 2002;33(6):456–462.

Mindel JS. Pharmacology of local anesthetics. In: Tasman W, Jaeger EA, eds. *Duane's Foundations of Clinical Ophthalmology.* Vol 3. Philadelphia: Lippincott Williams & Wilkins; 2006: chap 35.

Purified Neurotoxin Complex

Botulinum toxin type A is produced from cultures of the Hall strain of *Clostridium botulinum.* It blocks neuromuscular conduction by binding to receptor sites on motor nerve terminals, entering the nerve terminals, and inhibiting the release of acetylcholine. Botulinum toxin type A injections provide effective relief of the excessive, abnormal contractions associated with benign essential blepharospasm and hemifacial spasm. Cosmetic use of botulinum toxin, specifically in the treatment of glabellar folds, has gained popularity as well. Botulinum is approved for the treatment of strabismus; it may function by inducing an atrophic lengthening of the injected muscle and a corresponding shortening of the muscle's antagonist (also see BCSC Section 7, *Orbit, Eyelids, and Lacrimal System*).

Dutton JJ, Fowler AM. Botulinum toxin in ophthalmology. *Focal Points: Clinical Modules for Ophthalmologists.* San Francisco: American Academy of Ophthalmology; 2007, module 3.

Harrison AR. Chemodenervation for facial dystonias and wrinkles. *Curr Opin Ophthalmol.* 2003;14(5):241–245.

Hyperosmolar Drugs

Hyperosmolar drugs are used to decrease corneal and epithelial edema. One such drug is sodium chloride, which is available without a prescription in a 2% or 5% solution or as an ointment. Such products are used to treat corneal edema from Fuchs dystrophy, other causes of endothelial dysfunction, prolonged edema postoperatively, and recurrent erosion syndrome.

Irrigating Solutions

Sterile isotonic solutions are for general ophthalmic use. Depending on the solution, non-prescription ocular irrigating solutions may contain sodium chloride, potassium chloride, calcium chloride, magnesium chloride, sodium acetate, sodium citrate, boric acid, sodium borate, and sodium phosphate. They are preserved with EDTA, benzalkonium chloride, and sorbic acid. Sterile, physiologically balanced, preservative-free salt solutions are isotonic to eye tissues and are used for intraocular irrigation during surgical procedures. Glucose glutathione bicarbonate solution causes the least change in the corneal endothelial morphology postoperatively and augments the postoperative endothelial pump function. It is not routinely used due to cost concerns, but it may be used in patients who have compromised corneas preoperatively.

Diagnostic Agents

Solutions commonly used in the examination and diagnosis of external ocular diseases include fluorescein, 2%; lissamine green, 1%; and rose bengal, as impregnated paper strips. The first 2 stains outline defects of the conjunctival and corneal epithelium, whereas rose bengal indicates abnormal devitalized epithelial cells. A stinging sensation with instillation of these eyedrops is common. For the study of retinal and choroidal circulation as well as abnormal changes in the retinal pigment epithelium (RPE), sodium fluorescein solution in a concentration of 5%, 10%, or 25% is injected intravenously. Fundus fluorescein angiography is helpful in diagnosing various vascular diseases and neoplastic disorders. Fluorescein dye can also be used in anterior segment angiography to demonstrate anterior segment vascular disorders. Adverse effects range from localized skin reactions to hypersensitivity and allergic reactions.

Rose bengal has significant antiviral activity. Therefore, diagnostic use of rose bengal prior to viral culture may preclude a positive result, and its use to grade keratitis in the study of new antiviral drugs is discouraged.

Indocyanine green, a tricarbocyanine dye, is approved for the study of choroidal vasculature in a variety of choroidal and retinal disorders. Typically, 25 mg of dye is injected as an intravenous solution. Indocyanine green angiography is particularly helpful in identifying and delineating poorly defined choroidal neovascular membranes in age-related macular degeneration (AMD). Indocyanine green is mildly toxic; adverse effects include localized skin reactions, sore throat, and hot flushes. Individual cases have been reported of severe adverse effects such as anaphylactic shock, hypotension, tachycardia, dyspnea, and urticaria. Indocyanine green and trypan blue dye are useful for delineating the anterior capsule during phacoemulsification of mature cataracts. Whereas the FDA has approved trypan blue for use as an anterior capsule stain during surgery, using indocyanine green for this purpose constitutes an off-label use. Indocyanine green, trypan blue, and triamcinolone acetonide are also used to facilitate internal membrane peeling in macular-hole repair, although use of indocyanine green and trypan blue in this way is off-label. Despite considerable literature raising concerns about the toxicity of indocyanine green dye to the retina and RPE, good surgical and visual results have been reported. The toxicity of indocyanine green on cultured RPE cells may be related to the hypoosmolarity of the solvent. Short exposure of trypan blue was not found to have a toxic effect on cultured RPE cells. However, trypan blue does not appear to stain the internal limiting membrane as effectively as indocyanine green does. The exposure of the dye to the retina and pooling at the macular hole should be minimized to reduce concerns about toxicity to the retina.

Korb DR, Herman JP, Finnemore VM, Exford JM, Blackie CA. An evaluation of the efficacy of fluorescein, rose bengal, lissamine green, and a new dye mixture for ocular surface staining. *Eye Contact Lens.* 2008;34(1):61–64.

McDermott M, Snyder R, Slack J, Holley G, Edelhauser H. Effects of intraocular irrigants on the preserved human corneal endothelium. *Cornea.* 1991;10(5):402–407.

Saini JS, Jain AK, Sukhija J, Gupta P, Saroha V. Anterior and posterior capsulorhexis in pediatric cataract surgery with or without trypan blue dye: randomized prospective clinical study. *J Cataract Refract Surg.* 2003;29(9):1733–1737.

Werner L, Pandey SK, Escobar-Gomez M, Hoddinott DS, Apple DJ. Dye-enhanced cataract surgery. Part 2: learning critical steps of phacoemulsification. *J Cataract Refract Surg.* 2000; 26(7):1060–1065.

Viscoelastic Agents

Viscoelastic materials possess certain chemical and physical properties, which include the capacity to resist flow and deformation. Viscoelastics for ophthalmic use must also be inert, isosmotic, sterile, nonpyrogenic, nonantigenic, and optically clear. In addition, they must be sufficiently hydrophilic to allow easy dilution and irrigation from the eye. Naturally occurring and synthetic compounds available in various concentrations include sodium hyaluronate, chondroitin sulfate, hydroxypropyl methylcellulose, and polyacrylamide. Combined chondroitin sulfate/sodium hyaluronate materials are also available. Viscoelastic agents protect ocular tissues, such as the corneal endothelium and epithelium, from surgical trauma; help maintain intraocular space; and facilitate tissue manipulation. Thus, they are indispensable tools in cataract or glaucoma surgery, penetrating keratoplasty, anterior segment reconstruction surgery, and retinal surgery.

The 2 basic categories of viscoelastic materials are cohesive and dispersive. Cohesive viscoelastic material has a higher molecular weight and surface tension and tends to cohere to itself. Dispersive viscoelastic material has a lower molecular weight and surface tension and tends to coat the intraocular structures. Available viscoelastic products form a continuum on the basis of their cohesive and dispersive properties. The products Healon, Healon-GV, and Healon-5 (Abbott Medical Optics, Abbott Park, IL) are mostly cohesive, and Ocucoat (Bausch + Lomb, Rochester, NY) and Viscoat (Alcon, Fort Worth, TX) are mostly dispersive. (Also see the discussions of hyaluronic acid and vitreous collagen crosslinking in Chapter 11 and in BCSC Section 11, *Lens and Cataract.*)

Riedel PJ. Ophthalmic viscosurgical devices. *Focal Points: Clinical Modules for Ophthalmologists.* San Francisco: American Academy of Ophthalmology; 2012, module 7.

Fibrinolytic Agents

Tissue plasminogen activator (tPA), urokinase, and streptokinase are all fibrinolytic agents. tPA is a naturally occurring serine protease with a molecular mass of 68 kD. Because tPA is normally present at a higher concentration in the aqueous humor of the human eye than it is in blood, it is less toxic to ocular tissues and is specific for dissolution of fibrin clots. tPA has been used successfully to resolve fibrin clots after vitrectomy, keratoplasty, and glaucoma filtering procedures. These drugs are not approved by the FDA for ocular use and are therefore utilized off-label.

> Zalta AH, Sweeney CP, Zalta AK, Kaufman AH. Intracameral tissue plasminogen activator use in a large series of eyes with valved glaucoma drainage implants. *Arch Ophthalmol.* 2002;120(11):1487–1493.

Thrombin

Thrombin, a sterile protein substance, is approved for the control of hemorrhage from accessible capillaries and small venules, as would be observed with standard surface incisions. Its use in maintaining hemostasis during complicated intraocular surgery is off-label because such use requires injection. Intravitreal thrombin has been used to control intraocular hemorrhage during vitrectomy. The addition of thrombin (100 units/mL) to the vitrectomy infusate significantly shortens intraocular bleeding time, and thrombin produced by DNA recombinant techniques minimizes the degree of postoperative inflammation. Thrombin causes significant ultrastructural corneal endothelial changes when human corneas are perfused with 1000 units/mL.

Fibrin sealant is a biological tissue adhesive that includes a fibrinogen component and a thrombin component, both of which are prepared from pooled human plasma. When activated by thrombin, a solution of human fibrinogen imitates the final stages of the coagulation cascade. Fibrin sealant has been used widely in ophthalmic surgeries, including as a substitute for suturing in conjunctival or corneal wound closures, in fixing conjunctival autografts during pterygium surgery, for closing or preventing corneal perforation, during amniotic membrane transplantation, and in a variety of oculoplastic surgeries. The use of fibrin sealant in ophthalmic surgery is off-label. It has the advantage of reducing the total surgical time. The incidence of allergic reactions is low, but anaphylactic reactions following its application have been reported. The tissue sealant is applied as a thin layer to ensure that the amount applied is sufficient to cover the intended application area entirely. Preparation of this product for application must adhere to the instructions provided by the manufacturer.

Antifibrinolytic Agents

Antifibrinolytic drugs, such as ε-aminocaproic acid and tranexamic acid, inhibit the activation of plasminogen. These medications may be used systemically to treat patients with hemorrhage secondary to excessive fibrinolysis and to prevent recurrent hyphema, which most commonly occurs 2–6 days after the original hemorrhage. These agents are contraindicated in the presence of active intravascular clotting, such as diffuse intravascular coagulation (DIC), because they can increase the risk of thrombosis. They should not be used in pregnant patients, in patients with coagulopathies or on platelet inhibition therapy, or in patients with renal or hepatic disease. Patients with larger hyphemas and those with delayed presentation are at high risk of rebleeding, but patients with early presentation and those with smaller hyphemas are at low risk of rebleeding. The use of ε-aminocaproic acid is usually reserved for patients at higher risk of rebleeding.

ε-Aminocaproic acid is used in a dosage of 50–100 mg/kg every 4 hours, up to 30 g daily. Possible adverse reactions include nausea, vomiting, muscle cramps, conjunctival suffusion, nasal congestion, headache, rash, pruritus, dyspnea, tonic toxic confusional states, cardiac arrhythmias, and systemic hypotension. Gastrointestinal adverse effects are similar with doses of either 50 or 100 mg/kg. The drug should be continued for a full 5–6 days to achieve maximal clinical effectiveness. Topical ε-aminocaproic acid may be an attractive alternative to systemic delivery in the treatment of traumatic hyphema, but the efficacy of topical treatment has been questioned. Optimal topical concentration to maximize aqueous levels and minimize corneal epithelial toxicity is 30% ε-aminocaproic acid in 2% carboxypolymethylene.

Tranexamic acid is another antifibrinolytic drug used off-label to reduce the incidence of rebleeding after traumatic hyphema. It is 10 times more potent in vitro than is ε-aminocaproic acid. The usual dosage is 25 mg/kg of tranexamic acid 3 times daily for 3–5 days. Gastrointestinal adverse effects are rare.

Karkhaneh R, Naeeni M, Chams H, Abdollahi M, Mansouri MR. Topical aminocaproic acid to prevent rebleeding in cases of traumatic hyphema. *Eur J Ophthalmol.* 2003;13(1):57–61.

Vitamin Supplements and Antioxidants

Nonprescription vitamin supplements have enjoyed increased popularity because of their antioxidant properties and are used for intermediate-to-severe AMD. The Age-Related Eye Disease Study (AREDS) is discussed in depth in BCSC Section 12, *Retina and Vitreous.* Omega-3 fatty acid supplements seem to have some beneficial effect in treating meibomian gland dysfunction (see BCSC Section 8, *External Disease and Cornea*).

Interferon

A naturally occurring species-specific defense against viruses, interferon is synthesized intracellularly and increases resistance to viral infection. Synthetic analogues such as polyinosinic acid–polycytidylic acid have been used to induce patients to form their own interferon.

Topically administered interferon is ineffective in the treatment of epidemic keratoconjunctivitis caused by adenovirus. In patients with herpes simplex keratitis, however, interferon used in conjunction with acyclovir yielded significantly faster healing time than treatment with acyclovir alone (5.8 vs 9.0 days). Interferon also speeds the healing of an epithelial defect when used in combination with trifluridine. The dosage of interferon (30 million IU/mL) is 2 drops per day for the first 3 days of treatment. Interferon alone has little effect on the treatment of herpes simplex keratitis. In combination, however, it seems to act as a topical adjuvant to traditional antiviral therapy in resistant herpes simplex keratitis.

Interferon also has been shown to inhibit vascular endothelial cell proliferation and differentiation. It is particularly effective in the treatment of juvenile pulmonary hemangiomatosis, which was fatal before the development of interferon. Interferon-α_{2b}, administered subconjunctivally or intralesionally and topically, is a treatment option for conjunctival intraepithelial neoplasia and invasive squamous cell carcinoma (see BCSC Section 8, *External Disease and Cornea*). Intralesional administration of interferon is reported to be especially effective in ocular Kaposi sarcoma.

Growth Factors

Growth factors are a diverse group of proteins that act at autocrine and paracrine levels to affect various cellular processes, including metabolic regulation, tissue differentiation, cell growth and proliferation, maintenance of viability, and changes in cell morphology. Growth factors are synthesized in a variety of cells and have a spectrum of target cells and tissues. Various growth factors have been found in retina, vitreous humor, aqueous humor, and corneal tissues. These include

- epidermal growth factor
- fibroblast growth factors
- transforming growth factor βs
- vascular endothelial growth factor (VEGF)
- insulin-like growth factors

These growth factors are capable of diverse, synergistic, and sometimes antagonistic biological activities.

Under normal physiologic conditions, the complex and delicate coordination of both the effects of and the interactions among growth factors maintains the homeostasis of intraocular tissues. The net effect of a growth factor depends on its bioavailability, which is determined by its concentration; its binding to carrier proteins; the level of its receptor in the target tissue; and the presence of complementary or antagonistic regulatory factors.

Pathologically, the breakdown of the blood–ocular barrier disrupts the balance among growth factors in the ocular media and tissues and may result in various abnormalities. The disruption in the balance among isoforms of transforming growth factor βs, basic fibroblast growth factor, VEGF, and insulin-like growth factors is suspected to cause ocular neovascularization. Transforming growth factor βs and platelet-derived growth factor are implicated in the pathogenesis of proliferative vitreoretinopathy and in the excessive proliferation of Tenon capsule fibroblasts, which can result in scarring of the glaucoma filtration bleb. Increased concentrations of insulin-like growth factors in plasmoid aqueous humor may be responsible for the abnormal hyperplastic response of the lens epithelium and corneal endothelium observed in inflammatory conditions and in traumatic insults to the eye.

Identifying growth factors and understanding their mechanisms of action in the eye offer great potential for providing the ophthalmologist with new methods for manipulation of and intervention in ocular disorders. Epidermal growth factor and fibroblast growth factor can accelerate corneal wound repair after surgery, chemical burns, or ulcers and can increase the number of corneal endothelial cells. Fibroblast growth factor also has been shown to delay the process of retinal dystrophy in Royal College of Surgeons rats.

VEGF, also known as *vasculotropin,* deserves special mention. It is a dimeric, heparin-binding polypeptide mitogen and has 4 isoforms that are generated from alternative splicing of mRNA. The *VEGF* gene is widely expressed in actively proliferating vascular tissue and is implicated in the pathogenesis of various neovascular retinopathies, such as that in diabetes mellitus and in age-related choroidal neovascularization (CNV).

Intravitreal injections of VEGF inhibitors are used in the treatment of wet macular degeneration. Patients with CNV who have been treated with anti-VEGF have shown a slower loss of vision, especially moderate (>3 lines of vision lost) to severe (>6 lines lost) vision loss and, in some cases, an improvement in vision. Pegaptanib, the first approved drug, requires intravitreal injections every 6 weeks for up to 2 years and decreases in efficacy in the second year of treatment. Newer drugs have largely supplanted pegaptanib.

Bevacizumab, a full-length antibody against VEGF that is approved for the intravenous treatment of advanced carcinomas, has been used extensively in ophthalmology for exudative AMD, diabetic retinopathy, retinal vein occlusions, retinopathy of prematurity, and other chorioretinal vascular disorders. Ranibizumab is a monoclonal antibody fragment (Fab) derived from the same parent mouse antibody as bevacizumab. Pegaptanib and ranibizumab were developed for intraocular use, for which they are approved by the FDA. Although these drugs exhibit excellent safety profiles, ocular and systemic complications, particularly thromboembolic events, remain a concern for patients receiving therapy.

Aflibercept is a novel recombinant fusion protein engineered to bind all isoforms of VEGF-A, VEGF-B, and placental growth factor, and it has been approved for the treatment of neovascular AMD. It may have a longer duration of action than other anti-VEGF therapies; a monthly loading dose is administered for 3 months, after which the drug is given every 2 months (see BCSC Section 12, *Retina and Vitreous*).

Bartlett JD, Jaanus SD, eds. *Clinical Ocular Pharmacology.* 5th ed. St Louis: Butterworth-Heinemann/Elsevier; 2008.

Brunton LL, Lazo JS, Parker KL, eds. *Goodman & Gilman's The Pharmacological Basis of Therapeutics: Digital Edition.* 11th ed. New York: McGraw-Hill; 2006.

Fraunfelder FT, Fraunfelder FW. *Drug-Induced Ocular Side Effects.* 5th ed. Boston: Butterworth-Heinemann; 2001.

Murray L, ed. *Physicians' Desk Reference.* 58th ed. Montvale, NJ: Thomson PDR; 2004.

Physicians' Desk Reference for Ophthalmic Medicines. 35th ed. Montvale, NJ: Thomson PDR; 2007.

U.S. Food and Drug Administration website. Drugs@FDA: FDA Approved Drug Products. Available at www.accessdata.fda.gov/scripts/cder/drugsatfda/. Accessed October 15, 2013.

Basic Texts

Anatomy

Bron AJ, Tripathi RC, Tripathi BJ, eds. *Wolff's Anatomy of the Eye and Orbit.* 8th ed. London: Chapman & Hall; 1997.

Dutton JJ. *Atlas of Clinical and Surgical Orbital Anatomy.* 2nd ed. Philadelphia: Saunders; 2011.

Miller NR, Newman NJ, Biousse V, Kerrison JB, eds. *Walsh and Hoyt's Clinical Neuro-Ophthalmology.* 6th ed. Philadelphia: Lippincott Williams & Wilkins; 2004.

Rootman J. *Orbital Surgery: A Conceptual Approach.* 2nd ed. Philadelphia: Lippincott Williams & Wilkins; 2013.

Snell RS, Lemp MA. *Clinical Anatomy of the Eye.* 2nd ed. Malden, MA: Wiley-Blackwell; 1998.

Tasman W, Jaeger EA, eds. *Duane's Ophthalmology on DVD-ROM, 2013 Edition.* Philadelphia: Lippincott Williams & Wilkins; 2013.

Zide BM, ed. *Surgical Anatomy Around the Orbit: The System of Zones.* Philadelphia: Lippincott Williams & Wilkins; 2006.

Embryology

Jakobiec FA, ed. *Ocular Anatomy, Embryology, and Teratology.* Philadelphia: Harper & Row; 1982.

O'Rahilly R, Müller F. *Human Embryology and Teratology.* 3rd ed. New York: Wiley-Liss; 2001.

Genetics

Merin S. *Inherited Eye Diseases: Diagnosis and Management.* 2nd ed. Boca Raton, FL: Taylor & Francis; 2005.

Nussbaum RL, McInnes RR, Huntington FW. *Thompson & Thompson Genetics in Medicine.* 7th ed. Philadelphia: Elsevier/Saunders; 2007.

Traboulsi EI, ed. *Genetic Diseases of the Eye.* New York: Oxford University Press; 1998.

Biochemistry and Metabolism

Kaufman PL, Alm A, eds. *Adler's Physiology of the Eye.* 10th ed. Philadelphia: Elsevier/Mosby; 2003.

Tombran-Tink J, Barnstable CJ. *Retinal Degenerations: Biology, Diagnostics, and Therapeutics.* Totowa, NJ: Humana Press; 2007.

Ocular Pharmacology

Bartlett JD, Jaanus SD, eds. *Clinical Ocular Pharmacology.* 5th ed. St Louis: Elsevier/ Butterworth-Heinemann; 2008.

Brunton LL, ed. *Goodman and Gilman's The Pharmacological Basis of Therapeutics.* 11th ed. New York: McGraw-Hill; 2006.

Zimmerman TJ, Karanjit K, Mordechaie S, Fechtner RD, eds. *Textbook of Ocular Pharmacology.* 3rd ed. Philadelphia: Lippincott Williams & Wilkins; 1997.

Related Academy Materials

The American Academy of Ophthalmology is dedicated to providing a wealth of high-quality clinical education resources for ophthalmologists.

Print Publications and Electronic Products

For a complete listing of Academy products related to topics covered in this BCSC Section, visit our online store at http://store.aao.org/clinical-education/topic/comprehensive-ophthalmology.html. Or call Customer Service at 866.561.8558 (toll free, US only) or +1 415.561.8540, Monday through Friday, between 8:00 AM and 5:00 PM (PST).

Online Resources

Visit the Ophthalmic News and Education (ONE®) Network at aao.org/onenetwork to find relevant videos, online courses, journal articles, practice guidelines, self-assessment quizzes, images and more. The ONE Network is a free Academy-member benefit.

Access free, trusted articles and content with the Academy's collaborative online encyclopedia, EyeWiki, at aao.org/eyewiki.

Requesting Continuing Medical Education Credit

The American Academy of Ophthalmology is accredited by the Accreditation Council for Continuing Medical Education (ACCME) to provide continuing medical education for physicians.

The American Academy of Ophthalmology designates this enduring material for a maximum of 15 *AMA PRA Category 1 Credits™*. Physicians should claim only the credit commensurate with the extent of their participation in the activity.

To claim *AMA PRA Category 1 Credits™* upon completion of this activity, learners must demonstrate appropriate knowledge and participation in the activity by taking the posttest for Section 2 and achieving a score of 80% or higher.

To take the posttest and request CME credit online:

1. Go to www.aao.org/cme-central and log in.
2. Click on "Claim CME Credit and View My CME Transcript" and then "Report AAO Credits."
3. Select the appropriate media type and then the Academy activity. You will be directed to the posttest.
4. Once you have passed the test with a score of 80% or higher, you will be directed to your transcript. *If you are not an Academy member, you will be able to print out a certificate of participation once you have passed the test.*

CME expiration date: June 1, 2019. *AMA PRA Category 1 Credits™* may be claimed only once between June 1, 2014, and the expiration date.

For assistance, contact the Academy's Customer Service department at 866-561-8558 (US only) or +1 415-561-8540 between 8:00 AM and 5:00 PM (PST), Monday through Friday, or send an e-mail to customer_service@aao.org.

Study Questions

Please note that these questions are *not* part of your CME reporting process. They are provided here for your own educational use and identification of any professional practice gaps. The required CME posttest is available online (see "Requesting CME Credit"). Following the ques-, tions are a blank answer sheet and answers with discussions. Although a concerted effort has been made to avoid ambiguity and redundancy in these questions, the authors recognize that differences of opinion may occur regarding the "best" answer. The discussions are provided to demonstrate the rationale used to derive the answer. They may also be helpful in confirming that your approach to the problem was correct or, if necessary, in fixing the principle in your memory. The Section 2 faculty thanks the Self-Assessment Committee for reviewing these self-assessment questions.

1. If all the nerves passing through the annulus of Zinn were transected, what nerve would continue to function?
    a. superior division of cranial nerve III
    b. cranial nerve IV
    c. nasociliary branch of cranial nerve V (V_1)
    d. optic nerve

2. Which extraocular muscle originates from the annulus of Zinn?
    a. levator palpebrae superioris
    b. superior oblique
    c. lateral rectus
    d. inferior oblique

3. What is the ratio of optic nerve axons that cross at the optic chiasm to those that do not cross at the optic chiasm?
    a. 67:33
    b. 50:50
    c. 30:70
    d. 53:47

4. A patient presents with left-sided ophthalmoplegia and forehead numbness. The lesion is most likely to be located at the
    a. brainstem
    b. cavernous sinus
    c. superior orbit
    d. intraconal space

5. The first cells to develop in the embryonic retina are the
   a. ganglion cells
   b. photoreceptors
   c. amacrine cells
   d. bipolar cells

6. Which disorder is associated with a defect in a nonmitochondrial gene?
   a. Leber hereditary optic neuropathy
   b. chronic progressive external ophthalmoplegia
   c. neuropathy, ataxia, and retinitis pigmentosa
   d. retinoblastoma

7. What characteristic of retinoblastoma may facilitate its diagnosis as a familial condition?
   a. It may be associated with chromosome 11 short-arm deletion syndrome and Wilms tumor.
   b. It affects approximately 1 per 100,000 live births in the United States.
   c. Approximately 90% of patients with hereditary retinoblastoma have a family history of the disease.
   d. The hereditary pattern in familial retinoblastoma is autosomal dominant, but the defect is mitochondrial at a cellular level.

8. Mutations in the rhodopsin gene are associated with what inherited ocular disease?
   a. juvenile glaucoma
   b. Leber hereditary optic neuropathy
   c. retinitis pigmentosa
   d. Stargardt disease

9. Mitochondrial inheritance is transmitted by what route?
   a. paternal mitochondria
   b. maternal mitochondria
   c. acquired mitochondria
   d. de novo mitochondria

10. Mutations of *PAX6* are associated with what disorder?
    a. aniridia
    b. retinal coloboma
    c. renal hypoplasia
    d. corneal granular dystrophy

11. An unaffected woman has a brother, maternal uncle, and son affected with retinitis pigmentosa. What is the most likely mode of inheritance?

a. autosomal dominant

b. X-linked recessive

c. autosomal recessive

d. sporadic

12. What is the basis for complex genetic diseases?

a. a single recessive gene

b. X-linked genes

c. a single spontaneous genetic mutation

d. the resultant effect of many genes, in combination with health habits and environmental factors

13. What structure, if inflamed, would be considered a sign of uveitis?

a. optic nerve

b. Descemet membrane

c. choroid

d. retinal pigment epithelium

14. What pair accurately matches a cell-type origin with the correct tear-layer product?

a. goblet cells–lipid layer

b. meibomian glands–mucin layer

c. glands of Krause–aqueous layer

d. glands of Wolfring–mucin layer

15. What option most accurately describes the immunoglobulin(s) that can be found in the tear film?

a. IgA only

b. IgA and IgG only

c. IgG and IgM only

d. IgA, IgG, IgM, and IgD

16. What intraocular structure is a true basement membrane (basal lamina)?

a. Bowman layer

b. zonule of Zinn

c. Descemet membrane

d. anterior border layer of iris

17. What is the principal structural protein in the Descemet membrane?
    a. type I collagen
    b. type II collagen
    c. type III collagen
    d. type IV collagen

18. What mechanism holds the flap created during laser in situ keratomileusis (LASIK) in place after surgery?
    a. endothelial–Descemet membrane interaction
    b. endothelial pump
    c. Bowman layer–stromal adhesions
    d. stromal collagen adhesions

19. What property of the retina renders it susceptible to oxidative stress?
    a. high content of polyunsaturated fatty acids in photoreceptor outer segments
    b. high concentration of carotenoids compared with other intraocular structures
    c. presence of vitamin E
    d. absence of retinal vessels in the foveal avascular zone

20. What pigment within the retinal pigment epithelium is responsible for the signal generated in fundus autofluorescence imaging?
    a. melanin
    b. lipofuscin
    c. rhodopsin
    d. lutein

21. The retinal pigment epithelium is the first site of melanogenesis in the body. Ocular melanin has been shown to participate in what process?
    a. pathogenesis of retinitis pigmentosa
    b. vitamin A metabolism
    c. retinal adhesion
    d. retinal development and neuronal migration

22. Age-related loss of type IX collagen has been implicated in what process related to the vitreous?
    a. vitreous hemorrhage
    b. angiogenesis
    c. increased diffusion of oxygen from the anterior segment into the posterior segment
    d. vitreous liquefaction

23. What vitamin is most critical for the photoreceptor response to light?
    a. A
    b. B
    c. C
    d. E

24. In prescribing for elderly patients, what pharmacologic adjustments must be considered?
    a. Hepatic perfusion and enzymatic activity increase with age.
    b. Renal function decreases with age.
    c. Elderly patients have more albumin relative to weight.
    d. Elderly patients have more body water relative to weight.

25. What technique or strategy improves the ocular absorption of eyedrops?
    a. rapid instillation of eyedrops one after the other without interruption
    b. application of digital pressure at the lateral canthus to prevent the eyedrop from escaping
    c. keeping the eye open and rolling the eye around after instillation of each drop
    d. increasing the viscosity of the delivery vehicle

26. Atropine, 1%, has how many milligrams of drug per drop, assuming 20 drops per milliliter?
    a. 1 mg
    b. 0.5 mg
    c. 0.1 mg
    d. 0.05 mg

27. How much epinephrine is present in 1 mL of the 1:10,000 epinephrine solution?
    a. 1 mg of epinephrine
    b. same amount of epinephrine as in 1 mL of 0.01% epinephrine
    c. same amount of epinephrine as in 1 mL of 1:1000 epinephrine
    d. same amount of epinephrine as in 1 mL of 0.1% epinephrine

28. Direct-acting muscarinic agents (miotics) have what clinical effect?
    a. hyperopic shift in refraction
    b. increased range of accommodation
    c. central anterior chamber deepening
    d. increased night vision

29. What management strategy has been shown to reduce postsurgical endophthalmitis?
    a. preoperative preparation of the eye with topical povidone-iodine
    b. intracameral vancomycin
    c. intracameral aminoglycosides
    d. subconjunctival fluoroquinolones

30. What property of latanoprost may limit its usefulness?

    a. It is a prodrug of prostaglandin $E_{2\alpha}$.

    b. It reduces intraocular pressure by increasing trabecular meshwork outflow.

    c. It can cause darkening of the iris and periocular skin and hypertrichosis of the eyelashes.

    d. It increases the number of melanocytes.

31. What systemic side effect may result from treatment with oral carbonic anhydrase inhibitors?

    a. insomnia

    b. weight gain

    c. hyperkalemia

    d. aplastic anemia

32. What is a clinically important property of brimonidine?

    a. Brimonidine is a selective α_1-adrenergic agonist.

    b. Brimonidine is more lipophilic than apraclonidine.

    c. Brimonidine has been associated with tachycardia and hyperventilation when used in infants.

    d. Rates of tachyphylaxis and allergic reaction are higher in brimonidine than in apraclonidine.

Answer Sheet for Section 2 Study Questions

Question	Answer	Question	Answer
1	a b c d	17	a b c d
2	a b c d	18	a b c d
3	a b c d	19	a b c d
4	a b c d	20	a b c d
5	a b c d	21	a b c d
6	a b c d	22	a b c d
7	a b c d	23	a b c d
8	a b c d	24	a b c d
9	a b c d	25	a b c d
10	a b c d	26	a b c d
11	a b c d	27	a b c d
12	a b c d	28	a b c d
13	a b c d	29	a b c d
14	a b c d	30	a b c d
15	a b c d	31	a b c d
16	a b c d	32	a b c d

Answers

1. **b.** Cranial nerve IV passes through the superior orbital fissure but not through the annulus of Zinn.

2. **c.** The lateral rectus muscle originates from the annulus of Zinn. The superior, inferior, medial, and lateral rectus muscles all arise from the annulus of Zinn.

3. **d.** Anatomical studies demonstrate that more axonal fibers cross at the optic chiasm than do not cross, in a 53:47 ratio.

4. **b.** The cavernous sinus is where the trigeminal nerve (ophthalmic branch) and the nerves controlling eye movement are in proximity to one another.

5. **a.** The ganglion cells are the first cells to differentiate in the embryonic eye.

6. **d.** The hereditary pattern in familial retinoblastoma is autosomal dominant and associated with a mutation in the nuclear tumor-suppressor gene on chromosome 13 (the retinoblastoma, or *RB1,* gene). The other conditions named have been associated with mutations in mitochondrial genes.

7. **c.** The retinoblastoma gene is located on the long arm of chromosome 13. The aniridia gene, *PAX6,* and the Wilms tumor gene are adjacent on chromosome 11; their proximity is important to recognize, as children with aniridia need to be screened for Wilms tumor. Retinoblastoma occurs at a rate of approximately 1 per 15,000–20,000 live births. Most cases of retinoblastoma are unilateral and not inherited. Of people who inherit the gene mutation, 90% will develop retinoblastoma (90% penetrance).

8. **c.** More than 100 different mutations in the rhodopsin gene are known to cause retinitis pigmentosa. Juvenile glaucoma is associated with myocilin mutations, Leber hereditary optic neuropathy is associated with mitochondrial DNA mutations, and Stargardt disease is associated with *ABCA4* gene mutations.

9. **b.** A significant number of disorders associated with the eye or visual system involve mitochondrial deletions or mutations. Because a fertilized embryo receives most of its mitochondria from the egg (maternal side), mitochondrial disease should be considered whenever the inheritance pattern of a trait suggests maternal transmission.

10. **a.** A *PAX6* mutation is associated with aniridia. The *PAX6* gene product is a transcription factor that is required for normal development of the eye. Almost all cases of aniridia are the result of *PAX6* mutations.

11. **b.** Three affected males connected through an unaffected female suggest an X-linked inheritance. The other modes are possible but much less likely.

12. **d.** Many common eye diseases are complex genetic diseases involving the effects of multiple genes. Examples include glaucoma, age-related macular degeneration, and myopia. The combined effects of many genes, along with health habits and environmental factors, result in the disease.

13. **c.** The optic nerve, cornea, and retinal pigment epithelium are not part of the uvea. The uveal tract is the main vascular compartment of the eye and consists of the iris, ciliary body, and choroid.

14. **c.** Goblet cells produce the mucin layer, and meibomian glands form the lipid layer. Glands of Krause and Wolfring produce the aqueous layer.

15. **d.** Proteins in the tear film include immunoglobulin A (IgA) and secretory IgA (sIgA). IgA is formed by plasma cells in interstitial tissues of the main and accessory lacrimal glands and by the substantia propria of the conjunctiva. The secretory component is produced within lacrimal gland acini, and sIgA is secreted into the lumen of the main and accessory lacrimal glands. IgA plays a role in local host-defense mechanisms of the external eye, as shown by increased levels of IgA and IgG in human tears associated with ocular inflammation. Other immunoglobulins in tears are IgM, IgD, and IgE. Vernal conjunctivitis causes elevated tear and serum levels of IgE, increased IgE-producing plasma cells in the giant papillae of the superior tarsal conjunctiva, and elevated histamine levels.

16. **c.** The Descemet membrane is a true basement membrane produced by the basolateral surfaces of the basal layer of the corneal endothelium.

17. **d.** The Descemet membrane is a 10–12-μm-thick basement membrane between the endothelium and the posterior corneal stroma. Type IV collagen is the most abundant collagen in the Descemet membrane. Type I collagen, however, is the major collagen component of the corneal stroma.

18. **b.** The endothelial pump is responsible for generating the negative hydrostatic pressure that is necessary for holding the laser in situ keratomileusis (LASIK) flap in place after surgery.

19. **a.** Polyunsaturated fatty acids have increased numbers of carbon–carbon double bonds, which enhances their susceptibility to lipid peroxidation. Other aspects of the retina that increase its susceptibility to oxidative stress include an increased concentration of mitochondria, a high oxygen tension, and photo-oxidation triggered by light exposure.

20. **b.** Lipofuscin molecules are the fine yellow-brown pigment granules of the retina. They are thought to be "wear-and-tear" deposits resulting from phagosomal activity. Histologically, lipofuscin stains with Sudan stain and exhibits autofluorescence.

21. **d.** Melanin acts as a neutral-density filter on all wavelengths of light. Patients with oculocutaneous albinism have foveal hypoplasia and more contralateral projections of the retinal ganglion cells, thought to be due to reduced melanin levels resulting from defects in the tyrosinase gene. Additional functions of melanin include stabilization of free radicals and detoxification.

22. **d.** Vitreous liquefaction, also known as *syneresis,* begins with the breakdown of collagen fibrils into smaller fragments. This liquefaction is thought to occur because of a loss of "shielding" of type II collagen by type IX collagen. This process has no direct effect on the development of vitreous hemorrhage unless it leads to the development of posterior vitreous detachment (PVD). A PVD can protect against retinal neovascularization by eliminating the scaffold for fibrovascular proliferation. Oxygen tension increases in the posterior chamber in postvitrectomized eyes.

23. **a.** 11-*cis*-retinal is a vitamin A derivative. Vitamins C and E play antioxidant roles in the retina but do not participate in the light response of the retina.

24. **b.** Compared with younger patients, older patients have less lean body mass because of decreased muscle bulk, less body water, decreased albumin, and increased relative adipose tissue. These physiologic differences alter tissue binding and drug distribution. Human renal function decreases with age. Hepatic perfusion and enzymatic activity decrease with age.

25. **d.** Increased viscosity of the vehicle generally increases drug retention in the inferior cul-de-sac, aiding drug penetration.

26. **b.** A 1% solution has 1 g/100 mL, or 1000 mg/100 mL, of active ingredient. Assuming there are 20 drops/mL, 1 drop contains 0.05 mL of drug. Multiplying 1000 mg/100 mL × 0.05 mL yields 0.5 mg per drop of atropine available for systemic absorption.

27. **b.** A 1:10,000 dilution has 1 g of drug in 10,000 mL (or 1000 mg/10,000 mL). This concentration is equivalent to a 0.01% solution (0.01 g/100 mL, or 10 mg/100 mL). One milliliter of the 1:10,000 dilution of epinephrine contains 0.1 mg of epinephrine. If the concentration of the solution increases to 1:1000, 0.1 mL of it contains the same amount of epinephrine as in 1 mL of the 1:10,000 solution.

28. **b.** Miotic agents constrict the pupillary sphincter and the ciliary muscle. Ciliary muscle contraction results in increased myopia and a decreased central anterior chamber. Pupillary constriction causes decreased night vision but increases the range of accommodation (pinhole effect).

29. **a.** Topical povidone-iodine solution, 5%, exhibits broad-spectrum antimicrobial activity when used to prepare the surgical field and rinse the ocular surface. It has been shown to have a significant effect on postsurgical endophthalmitis.

30. **c.** Latanoprost is a prodrug of prostaglandin $F_{2\alpha}$ that reduces the intraocular pressure primarily by increasing the uveoscleral outflow. It increases the number of melanosomes (increased melanin content, or melanogenesis) within the melanocytes but has not been shown to cause melanocytosis (increased number of melanocytes).

31. **d.** Use of oral carbonic anhydrase inhibitors can cause paresthesias, imbalance, anorexia, weight loss, hypokalemia, somnolence, kidney stones, metabolic acidosis, and aplastic anemia.

32. **b.** Brimonidine is a selective α_2-adrenergic agonist. It is more lipophilic than apraclonidine and penetrates the blood–brain barrier better. Its use in infants is contraindicated, and it should be used with caution in small children because of severe systemic toxicities, in particular bradycardia and apnea. Brimonidine has lower rates of tachyphylaxis and allergic reaction than apraclonidine.

Index

(*f* = figure; *t* = table)

A2E, photoreceptor light damage and, 286
AA. *See* Arachidonic acid
AAVs. *See* Adeno-associated viruses
ABC transporters. *See* ATP binding cassette (ABC)
    transporters
Abducens nerve. *See* Cranial nerve VI
Abetalipoproteinemia
    microsomal triglyceride transfer protein (MTP)
        defects causing, 265
    vitamin supplements in management of, 203
Acanthamoeba, 361
    treatment of infection caused by, 361
Accessory lacrimal glands, 22*f*, 23*t*, 29, 215*f*, 216
    of Krause, 20*f*, 22*f*, 23*t*, 29, 216
    of Wolfring, 20*f*, 22*f*, 23*t*, 29, 216
Accommodation, 63
    aging affecting, 63
    muscarinic drugs affecting, 308, 311
    near reflex and, 96
    zonular fibers in, 64*f*, 66
Accommodative esotropia, muscarinic agents for
    management of, 313
Acebutolol, 317*f*
Acetazolamide, 324, 325, 325*t*, 326
    sustained-release oral preparation for, 301, 325
Acetylcholine, 308*t*, 309–310, 309*f*
    clinical use of, 309–310
    intracameral administration of, 300*t*, 309, 310
    receptors for, drugs affecting, 307–315, 307*f*, 308*t*, 309*f*,
        310*f*, 311*t*, 314*t*, 315*t*. *See also* Cholinergic agents
    synthesis/release/degradation of, 309, 309*f*, 310, 310*f*
    in tear secretion, 216, 218, 218*f*
Acetylcholinesterase
    in acetylcholine degradation, 309, 309*f*, 310*f*
    defective, succinylcholine effects and, 201–202
Acetylcysteine, off-label use of, 306
Acetyltransferase, in isoniazid pharmacogenetics, 201
Ach. *See* Acetylcholine
Achromatopsia (monochromatism)
    blue-cone, 264
        ocular findings in carriers of, 199*t*
    gene defects causing, 264
    with myopia, racial and ethnic concentration of, 197
    rod, 264
Acidic fibroblast growth factor. *See also* Fibroblast
    growth factor
    in aqueous humor, 234
Acidosis, carbonic anhydrase inhibitors
    causing, 325–326
    aspirin interactions and, 336
Acinar cells, lacrimal gland, 28, 28*f*
ACTH (adrenocorticotropic hormone), in tear
    secretion, 219
Actin, 245
    in retinal pigment epithelium, 273
Actin filaments, 245
α-Actinin, in retinal pigment epithelium, 273

Activators (drug), 304
Active transport/secretion
    across retinal pigment epithelium, 273, 277
    in aqueous humor dynamics, 230, 323, 324*f*
    in lens ionic balance, 246
Acular. *See* Ketorolac
Acuvail. *See* Ketorolac
Acyclovir, 357*t*, 358–359
    off-label use of, 359
Adaptation, light, 262
Adeno-associated viruses (AAVs), as vectors in gene
    therapy, 169
Adenylyl/adenylate cyclase
    adrenoceptor binding and, 319, 321, 322
    tear secretion and, 219, 219*f*
Adie tonic pupil, pharmacologic testing for, 310
Adnexa. *See* Ocular adnexa
Adrenaline. *See* Epinephrine
Adrenergic drugs, 308*t*, 316–323, 316*t*, 317*f*, 318*t*, 320*f*,
    322*t*
    for glaucoma
        agonists, 318–319, 318*t*
        antagonists/β-blockers, 230, 318*t*, 321–323, 322*t*
    as miotics, 308, 308*t*, 309, 310, 311, 311*t*
    as mydriatics, 314*t*, 317–318
Adrenergic receptors (adrenoceptors), 308*t*, 316*t*, 317*f*.
    See also specific type
    drugs affecting, 308*t*, 316–323, 316*t*, 317*f*, 318*t*, 320*f*,
        322*t*. *See also* Adrenergic drugs
    effects mediated by, 316, 317*f*
    locations of, 316
    signal transduction and, 316*t*
    in tear secretion, 218, 218*f*, 219, 219*f*
Adrenoceptors. *See* Adrenergic receptors
Adrenocorticotropic hormone (ACTH), in tear
    secretion, 219
ADRP. *See* Autosomal dominant retinitis pigmentosa
Afferent fibers
    somatic, 103
    visceral, 103
Afferent pupillary pathway, 96
aFGF. *See* Acidic fibroblast growth factor
Aflibercept, 372
Age/aging
    accommodative response/presbyopia and, 63
    carbonic anhydrase inhibitor use and, 326
    ciliary muscle affected by, 58
    corticosteroid use and, 332
    Descemet membrane/corneal endothelium affected
        by, 41, 42, 227
    drug toxicity and, 294, 295
    facial bones and, 7
    lens changes associated with, 63
    lens proteins affected by, 245
    mitochondrial DNA diseases and, 157
    parental, chromosomal abnormalities/Down
        syndrome and, 188, 190

pharmacologic principles affected by, 295
telomeric DNA and, 150
trabecular meshwork and, 49, 51
vitreous changes and, 80, 252–255
Age-related cataracts, in diabetes mellitus, 247
Age-Related Eye Disease Study (AREDS), 285, 370
Age-related macular degeneration/maculopathy
genetic factors in, genome-wide association studies
(GWAS) and, 165, 167f
retinal pigment epithelium abnormalities associated
with, 279
Agonist (drug), 304
Aicardi syndrome, 180–181
Air–tear-film interface, 38–39, 39f
Ak-Cide. See Prednisolone, in combination preparations
Ak-Con. See Naphazoline
Ak-Dilate. See Phenylephrine
Ak-Mycin. See Erythromycin
Ak-Pentolate. See Cyclopentolate
Ak-Poly-Bac. See Polymyxin B, in combination
preparations
Ak-Spore. See Hydrocortisone, in combination
preparations
Ak-Tob. See Tobramycin
Ak-Tracin. See Bacitracin
Ak-Trol. See Dexamethasone, in combination
preparations
Alamast. See Pemirolast
Alaway. See Ketotifen
Albalon. See Naphazoline
Albinism, 174, 175t, 278
defective melanin synthesis and, 174, 278
enzyme defect in, 175t
genetic heterogeneity and, 185
ocular
ocular findings in carriers of, 198–200, 199f, 199t
X-linked (Nettleship-Falls), ocular findings in
carriers of, 198–200, 199f
oculocutaneous, 185, 278
racial and ethnic concentration of, 197
tyrosinase activity/defect in, 175t, 185, 278
Albumin
in aqueous humor, 229, 233
in vitreous, 251–252
Albuterol, 308t
Alcaftadine, 338t, 339
Alcaine. See Proparacaine
Aldehyde dehydrogenase, in cornea, 224
Aldose reductase
in cataract formation, 247–248
in lens glucose/carbohydrate metabolism,
247–248, 247f
Alkaptonuria, 175t
All-trans-retinol/all-trans-retinaldehyde, 259, 259f,
274–275, 275f
Allele-specific marking (genetic imprinting), 138,
153–154
Alleles, 131, 184–185
null, gene therapy and, 169
Allelic, definition of, 131
Allelic association. See Linkage disequilibrium
Allelic heterogeneity, 132
Allergic conjunctivitis, drugs for, 337–339, 338t

Allergic reactions/allergies
drugs for
corticosteroids, 329, 333–334, 333t, 337, 338, 339
mast-cell stabilizers and antihistamines,
337–339, 338t
to penicillin/cephalosporin, 343
Alocril. See Nedocromil
Alomide. See Lodoxamide
Alpha (α)-actinin, in retinal pigment epithelium, 273
Alpha (α)-adrenergic agents, 308t, 317–321, 318t, 320f
agonists, 308t, 317–320, 318t, 320f
direct-acting, 317–318
for glaucoma, 318–319, 318t
indirect-acting, 320, 320f
antagonists, 308t, 321
Alpha (α)-adrenergic receptors (adrenoceptors),
308t, 316t
drugs affecting, 308t, 317–321, 318t, 320f. See also
Alpha (α)-adrenergic agents
effects mediated by, 316, 317f
ocular decongestant mechanism of action and, 342
signal transduction and, 316t
in tear secretion, 218, 218f
Alpha$_1$ (α$_1$)-antitrypsin, in aqueous humor, 234
Alpha (α)-blockers, 321
Alpha (α)-crystallins, 64, 244
Alpha (α)-galactosidase, defective/deficiency of, 175t
Alpha (α)-L-iduronidase, defective/deficiency of,
175t, 184
Alpha$_2$ (α$_2$)-macroglobulin, in aqueous humor, 231,
233, 234
Alpha (α)-mannosidase, defective/deficiency of, 175t
Alpha (α)-melanocyte-stimulating hormone (α-MSH),
in tear secretion, 219
Alphagan. See Brimonidine
Alport syndrome, pleiotropism in, 196
Alrex. See Loteprednol
Altafrin. See Phenylephrine
Alternative splicing, 148, 152–153
Alu repeat sequence, 150
Amacrine cells, 71f, 257, 258f, 266, 267
Amaurosis, Leber congenital
genetic heterogeneity in, 183, 183f
guanylate cyclase mutations causing, 263
RPE65 gene defects causing, 264
American Academy of Ophthalmology
on genetic testing, 171, 207–208
on intravitreal medication sources, 306–307
Amethocaine. See Tetracaine
Amikacin, 344t, 351
Amino acids
in tear film, 233
translation and, 151, 151f, 152
Aminocaproic acid/ε-aminocaproic acid, 369, 370
Aminoglycosides, 351–352
ototoxicity of, mitochondrial DNA mutations
and, 157
Amniocentesis, 206–207
Amoxicillin, 345
Amphotericin B, 354, 355t
Ampicillin, 344t, 345
intravenous administration of, 301
Amplifying cells, transient, in corneal epithelium, 40

Anaerobic glycolysis, in glucose/carbohydrate
    metabolism
  in cornea, 224
  in lens, 246
Anaphase, 149, 149f
Anaphylactoid reactions, penicillin/cephalosporin
    causing, 343
Anaphylaxis, penicillin/cephalosporin allergy
    causing, 343
Ancobon. See Flucytosine
Androgens, in tear secretion, 219–220
Anemia, aplastic
  carbonic anhydrase inhibitors causing, 326
  chloramphenicol causing, 351
Anestacaine. See Lidocaine
Anesthesia (anesthetics), local (topical/regional),
    362–366, 362t, 363t
  for anterior segment surgery, 365–366
  cholinesterase inhibitor use and, 312, 363
Aneuploidy, 132, 189. See also specific disorder
  of autosomes, 189–190
  of sex chromosomes, 189
Aneurysms, cranial nerve III (oculomotor) affected
    by, 94, 95
Angelman syndrome, imprinting abnormalities
    causing, 138, 154
Angiogenesis, vitreous as inhibitor of, 253–254
Angiotensin/angiotensinogen, in aqueous humor,
    231, 234
Angular artery
  eyelids supplied by, 25, 26f
  orbit supplied by, 33f
Angular vein, 35f
Aniridia, 193
  short arm 11 deletion syndrome/PAX6 gene
      mutations and, 152, 177, 193
Annulus of Zinn, 8, 9f, 13f, 14f, 16–17, 87
Antagonist (drug), 304
Antazoline, 337
Antazoline/naphazoline, 338t
Anterior banded zone, of Descemet membrane, 41, 42f
Anterior border/pigmented layer, of iris, 54–55, 55, 56f
Anterior cerebral artery, 90, 107f
  cranial nerve relationship and, 85f
Anterior chamber, 37, 37f, 45–48, 45f, 46f, 47f
  depth of, 45–46
  development of, 121f, 123f
Anterior chamber angle, 37f, 45, 45f, 46f, 47f, 49f
  development of, 116t
  topography of, 37f
Anterior ciliary arteries, 17, 30, 32–35
Anterior clinoid process, 8f, 84f, 105f
Anterior communicating artery, 90
  cranial nerve relationship and, 84f, 85f
Anterior conjunctival artery, 30
Anterior ethmoidal foramen, 6f, 7
Anterior inferior cerebellar artery, cranial nerve
    relationship and, 102
Anterior lacrimal crest, 5, 6f
Anterior pole, 38, 65f, 242f
Anterior segment
  development of, 65f, 117–122, 120f, 121f
  topical anesthetics for surgery on, 365–366

Anterior uveitis, corticosteroid route of administration
    in, 333t
Antibacterial drugs, 343–354, 344t, 347t, 348t. See also
    Antibiotics
Antibiotics, 343–354, 344t, 347t, 348t
  for Acanthamoeba keratitis, 361
  in combination preparations, 347t
    with anti-inflammatory drugs, 348t
  intravenous administration of, 301
  intravitreal administration of, 300t
  resistance to, 343, 346, 351, 352, 353
Anticholinergic agents, 308, 308t, 315, 315t. See also
    Antimuscarinic agents
Anticipation (genetic), 132, 144, 195
Antidepressants, apraclonidine/brimonidine
    interactions and, 319
Antifibrinolytic agents, 369–370
Antifibrotic agents, 340–341
Antifungal drugs, 354–356, 355t
Antigen-presenting cells, in cornea, 40
Antiglaucoma drugs
  adrenergic agonists
    α-adrenergic agonists, 318–319, 318t
    β-adrenergic agonists, 321
  β-blockers, 230, 318t, 321–323, 322t
  carbonic anhydrase inhibitors, 230, 323–326, 324f, 325t
  ciliary body as target for, 237
  combined preparations, 328
  cycloplegics, 313, 314t
  hyperosmotic/osmotic drugs, 328–329, 329t
  miotics, 311, 318t
  muscarinic drugs, 311
  as prodrugs, 302
  prostaglandins/prostaglandin analogues, 237–238,
      318t, 327–328, 327t
  receptors in mode of action of, 318t
Antihistamines, 337–338, 338t
Anti-inflammatory drugs, 329–341, 330t, 333t, 335t,
    338t. See also Corticosteroids; Nonsteroidal anti-
    inflammatory drugs
  arachidonic acid release affected by, 238f, 239,
      331, 336
  in combination preparations with antibiotics, 348t
  for dry eye/keratoconjunctivitis sicca, 221–222, 221f
Antimetabolites, 340
Antimicrobial therapy, 343–361
Antimuscarinic agents, 308t, 313–314, 314t
  adverse effects of, 313–314
Antioncogene. See Tumor-suppressor genes
Antioxidants
  in lens, 284, 284–285, 284f
  in retina and retinal pigment epithelium, 286,
      286–288, 289f
  supplemental, 285, 370
Antiproliferative drugs, 340
Antiretroviral therapy (ART), 361
Antisense DNA, 132
  in gene therapy, 170
Antisense oligonucleotides, in gene therapy, 169–170, 170f
α₁-Antitrypsin, in aqueous humor, 234
Anti–vascular endothelial growth factor (anti-VEGF)
    drugs, 372
  intravitreal administration of, 300t, 372

Anti-VEGF drugs. *See* Anti–vascular endothelial growth factor (anti-VEGF) drugs
Antiviral drugs, 356–361, 357–358*t*
    for herpetic eye disease, 356–361, 357–358*t*
    interferons, 370–371
    resistance to, 358, 360
    systemic, 357–358*t*, 358–361
    topical, 356–358, 357–358*t*
Aplastic anemia
    carbonic anhydrase inhibitors causing, 326
    chloramphenicol causing, 351
Apocrine glands of eyelid, 19, 22*f*, 23*t*
Apolipoprotein D, in aqueous humor, 231, 233
Aponeurosis, levator, 20*f*, 24, 216
Apoptosis, 132, 155
    in DNA repair, 154, 155
Apraclonidine, 308*t*, 318–319, 318*t*, 319
Aquaporin (major intrinsic protein/MIP), 242, 245
Aqueous humor, 46, 229–236
    biochemistry and metabolism of, 229–236
    carbohydrates in, 232
    carbon dioxide in, 236
    composition of, 230–236, 231*t*
    dynamics of, 229–230, 323–324, 324*f*
    formation of, 323–324, 324*f*
        suppression of, 318*t*
            carbonic anhydrase inhibitors in, 230, 323–324
    functions of, 229
    glutathione in, 232–233
    growth modulatory factors in, 229, 234–235
    inorganic ions in, 232
    intraocular pressure and, 230
    organic anions in, 232
    oxygen in, 235–236
    proteins in, 229, 233–234
    separation of, from blood. *See* Blood–aqueous barrier
    sodium transport and, 230–231, 323, 324*f*
    urea in, 233
    vascular endothelial growth factor (VEGF) in, 234, 235
Aqueous layer (component) of tear film, 38, 213*f*, 215–217
Aqueous tear deficiency, 220, 221–222, 221*f*
Aqueous veins, 51, 52*f*
Arachidonic acid (arachidonate)
    in eicosanoid synthesis, 237, 238, 238*f*
    NSAID derivation and, 334–335
    NSAIDs affecting, 239
    release of, 237, 238, 238*f*
        anti-inflammatory drugs affecting, 238*f*, 239, 331, 336
    in retinal pigment epithelium, 274
Arachnoid mater, optic nerve, 87–89, 88*f*, 89*f*
Area centralis, 75. *See also* Macula
AREDS (Age-Related Eye Disease Study), 285, 370
Arrestin, 260*f*, 261
    mutations in, 161, 263
ARRP. *See* Autosomal recessive retinitis pigmentosa
ART. *See* Antiretroviral therapy
Arterial circles, 34*f*, 35, 45*f*, 52*f*, 54*f*, 55, 55*f*
    ciliary body, 58
Arteritis, temporal, corticosteroid route of administration in, 333*t*
Artificial insemination, genetic counseling and, 206
Artificial tears, 220, 221, 341, 342
Arylsulfatase A, defective/deficiency of, 175*t*

Ascorbate. *See* Ascorbic acid
Ascorbic acid (vitamin C)
    antioxidant effect of, 285, 288
        in lens, 283, 285
        in retina and retinal pigment epithelium, 288
    in aqueous humor, 231*t*, 232
    oral supplements and, 285
    in tear film, 214
    in vitreous, 231*t*
Asian eyelid, 19, 21*f*
Aspirin, 335–336, 335*t*
    prostaglandin synthesis affected by, 239, 335
    Reye syndrome and, 335–336
Association (genetic), allelic. *See* Linkage disequilibrium
Assortative mating, 132
Astrocytes
    optic nerve, 86, 87, 88*f*
    retinal, 73, 268
Ataxia
    intermittent, 175*t*
    with neuropathy and retinitis pigmentosa (NARP), 158–159
        mitochondrial DNA mutations and, 157, 158–159
Ataxia-telangiectasia (Louis-Bar syndrome), *ATM* (ataxia-telangiectasia mutated) gene in, 154
Ataxia-telangiectasia mutated *(ATM)* gene, 154
Atenolol, 317*f*
ATM (ataxia-telangiectasia mutated) gene, 154
ATP binding cassette (ABC) transporters, 261
    mutations in, 263
ATP production
    in lens, 246
    in rod outer segments, 261
ATPase-6 gene, in neuropathy with ataxia and retinitis pigmentosa, 158–159
Atrial natriuretic peptide, in aqueous humor, 231
Atrophy, gyrate, 175*t*
    ornithine aminotransferase defects causing, 175*t*, 265
    retinal pigment epithelium in, 279
Atropine, 308*t*, 313, 314, 314*t*, 315*t*
    adverse effects of, 313
    in Down syndrome, pharmacogenetics and, 201
    for edrophonium adverse effects, 315
    systemic absorption of, 296
Atropine-Care. *See* Atropine
Autologous serum drops, for dry eye, 342
Autonomic pathways, cholinergic drug action and, 307, 307*f*
Auto-oxidation, 282–283
    in lens, 283
    vitamin E affecting, 283
Autosomal dominant inheritance, 177–178, 178*t*
    gene therapy for diseases related to, 169–170, 170*f*
Autosomal dominant retinitis pigmentosa, 177
    peripherin/*RDS* gene mutations in, 161, 264
    rhodopsin mutations causing, 161, 263
Autosomal recessive inheritance, 174–177, 175*t*, 177*t*
Autosomal recessive retinitis pigmentosa
    retinal pigment epithelium defects causing, 278
    rhodopsin mutations causing, 263
    rod cGMP-gated channel mutations causing, 161, 263
    rod cGMP phosphodiesterase mutations causing, 161, 263

Autosomes, 132, 184, 189f
  aneuploidy of, 189–190. *See also specific disorder*
Axenfeld loop/Axenfeld nerve loop, 44
AzaSite. *See* Azithromycin
Azelastine, 337–338, 338t, 339
Azithromycin, 347t, 353
Azlocillin, 345
Azopt. *See* Brinzolamide

B-type natriuretic peptide (BNP), in aqueous
    humor, 231
BAC (bacterial artificial chromosome), 145
Bacampicillin, 345
Bacitracin, 344t, 347t, 353
  in combination preparations, 347t, 348t, 353
Bacterial artificial chromosome (BAC), 145
Bacteriophage, λ, as vector, 145
BAL (British antilewisite), for Wilson disease, 203
Balanced salt solution
  intracameral administration of, 300t
  vancomycin in, 352
Bardet-Biedl syndrome, pleiotropism in, 196
Baroreceptors, phenylephrine affecting, 318
Barr body, 132, 197. *See also* Lyonization
Basal lamina (basal cell layer)
  ciliary body, 57, 58f
  corneal, 39–40, 40f, 41, 42f, 223f. *See also* Descemet
      membrane/layer
    development of, 120–122, 121f
  lens. *See* Lens capsule
  retinal blood vessel, 73
  retinal pigment epithelium, 68
Base pair, 132
  mutations in, 155, 156
    conserved, 156
Basement membrane, corneal, 41, 120–121, 223f, 227.
    See also Descemet membrane/layer
Basic fibroblast growth factor. *See also* Fibroblast growth
    factor
  in aqueous humor, 234
Basic secretors, 217
Basilar artery, 105–107, 107f
  cranial nerve relationship and, 84f
Bassen-Kornzweig syndrome, microsomal triglyceride
    transfer protein (MTP) defects causing, 265
Batson venous plexus, 102
BAX gene, in DNA repair, 154
Bcl-2 proteins, apoptosis and, 154
Beaded filaments, 245
Benoxinate, with fluorescein, 363t, 365
Benzalkonium
  absorption affected by, 298
  in artificial tears, 341
  in irrigating solutions, 367
  toxic reactions to, 294, 341
Bepotastine, 338t
Bepreve. *See* Bepotastine
Bergmeister papilla, 80
Besifloxacin, 346, 347–349, 347t
Besivance. *See* Besifloxacin
Best disease (vitelliform macular dystrophy)
  bestrophin defect causing, 265
  identification of carriers for, 178, 196
  retinal pigment epithelium in, 278

Bestrophin, mutations in, 265
Beta (β)-adrenergic agents, 308t, 321–323, 322t
  agonists, 308t, 318t, 321
  antagonists, 308t, 321–323, 322t
  for glaucoma, 230, 318t, 321–323, 322t
Beta (β)-adrenergic receptors (adrenoceptors), 308t, 316t
  drugs affecting, 308t, 321–323, 322t. *See also* Beta
      (β)-adrenergic agents
  effects mediated by, 316, 317f
  locations of, 321
  signal transduction and, 316t
  in tear secretion, 219, 219f
Beta (β)-blockers, 230, 321–323, 322t
  aqueous humor suppression and, 230, 321, 323
  for glaucoma, 230, 318t, 321–323, 322t
Beta (β) carotene
  antioxidant effect of, 285, 288
  oral supplements and, 285
  in retina, 288
Beta (β)-crystallins, 64, 244
Beta (β)-galactosidase, defective/deficiency of, 175t
Beta (β)-lactam antibiotics, 343–346, 344t
Beta (β)-lactamases, 343, 345, 346
Betagamma (β,γ)-crystallins, 244
Betagan. *See* Levobunolol
Betaxolol, 308t, 321, 322t, 323
Bethanechol, 309f
Betimol. *See* Timolol
Betoptic. *See* Betaxolol
Bevacizumab, 372
  intravitreal administration of, 300t
    endophthalmitis and, 306
  off-label use of, 306
bFGF. *See* Basic fibroblast growth factor
Bicarbonate
  in aqueous humor, 231t, 232
  in tear film, 214t, 216
  in vitreous, 231t
Biguanides, for *Acanthamoeba* keratitis, 361
Bimatoprost, 237, 302, 327, 327t
  in combination preparations, 327t
Bioavailability, 293
Biomicroscopy, ultrasound, 47, 47f
Bipolar cells, 71f, 257, 258f, 266
  cone, 257, 266, 266f
  rod, 257, 258f
Blastocyst, 112f
Bleph-10. *See* Sulfacetamide
Blephamide. *See* Prednisolone, in combination
    preparations
Blepharitis, corticosteroid route of administration
    in, 333t
Blessig-Iwanoff cysts, 78, 79f
Blinking (blink reflex)
  medication absorption and, 296
  tear secretion and, 220
Bloch-Sulzberger syndrome (incontinentia
    pigmenti), 180
Blood–aqueous barrier, 229, 230, 233
  clinical implications of breakdown of, 236
Blood–ocular barriers, 229–230. *See also specific type*
  systemic drug administration and, 300, 301
Blood pressure, phenylephrine affecting, 317, 318
Blood–retina barrier, 73, 229

Blood vessels. *See* Vascular system
Blue-cone monochromatism, 264
    ocular findings in carriers of, 199*t*
Blue-light hazard, 286
Blunt trauma, optic neuropathy caused by, 89
Bony orbit. *See* Orbit
Border tissue of Elschnig, 88*f*
Botulinum toxin/botulinum toxin type A, 366
    intramuscular administration of, 301
    periocular injection of, 299, 366
    for strabismus, 366
Bow zone/region, 242, 242*f*
Bowman layer/membrane, 40, 40*f*, 45*f*, 223*f*, 225
    anatomy of, 40, 40*f*, 45*f*, 223*f*
    biochemistry and metabolism of, 225
    development of, 120
    refractive surgery and, 225
bp. *See* Base pair
Brain natriuretic peptide (BNP), in aqueous humor, 231
Branch chain decarboxylase, defective/deficiency of, 175*t*
Brimonidine, 318*t*, 319
    in combination preparations, 318*t*, 322*t*
Brinzolamide, 324–325, 325*t*
British antilewisite (BAL), for Wilson disease, 203
Broad-spectrum penicillins, 345
Bromday. *See* Bromfenac
Bromfenac, 330*t*
Bruch membrane, 60–61, 61*f*, 70*f*, 71*f*, 271–272, 272*f*
    development of, 116*t*, 122–124
Buccal nerve, 104
Bulbar conjunctiva, 25, 26*f*, 30
Bupivacaine, 362*t*, 364, 365
Butoxamine, 308*t*
Butyrylcholinesterase, 312

C4 complement, in aqueous humor, 231, 233
Ca²⁺/protein kinase C–dependent pathway, in tear
    secretion, 218, 218*f*
CAIs. *See* Carbonic anhydrase inhibitors
Calcitonin gene-related peptide (CGRP), 316*t*
    outflow facility affected by, 48
    in signal transduction, 316*t*
    in tear secretion, 216
Calcium
    in aqueous humor, 232
    in tear film, 214*t*
    in tear secretion, 218, 218*f*
Calcium channels, L-type, mutations in, 264
Calcium (Ca²⁺)/protein kinase C–dependent pathway,
    in tear secretion, 218, 218*f*
CALT. *See* Conjunctiva-associated lymphoid tissue
cAMP (cyclic adenosine monophosphate), 321
    in signal transduction, 316*t*
    in tear secretion, 218, 219*f*
Canaliculi, lacrimal, 23*f*, 29, 30
Cancer
    genetic and familial factors in, 156–157
    loss of telomeric DNA and, 150
Cancer genes, 156–157
Candidate gene screening, 161
    positional, 161
Canthal tendons, lateral/medial, 17*f*
Canthus, lateral/medial, 18*f*
CAP. *See* Chromosome arm painting

Capillary-free zone (foveal avascular zone), 74*f*, 77, 78*f*
Capillary plexus, of ciliary process, 57
Capsulopalpebral muscle, 20*f*
Carbachol, 309*f*, 311, 311*t*
    intracameral administration of, 300*t*, 309, 310
Carbamates, 312
Carbenicillin, 344*t*, 345
    gentamicin incompatibility and, 351
Carbocaine. *See* Mepivacaine
Carbohydrate ("sugar") cataracts, 246–248
    aldose reductase in development of, 247–248, 247*f*
Carbohydrates
    in aqueous humor, 232
    metabolism of
        in cornea, 224
        in lens, 246
        in retinal pigment epithelium, 273
Carbon dioxide, in aqueous humor, 236
Carbonic anhydrase
    aqueous humor dynamics and, 230, 323–324, 324*f*
    retinal pigment epithelial transport and, 277
Carbonic anhydrase inhibitors (CAIs), 230, 323–326,
    324*f*, 325*t*
    adverse effects of, 326
    aspirin use and, 336
    for glaucoma/suppression of aqueous formation, 230,
        323–326, 324*f*, 325*t*
Carboxymethylcellulose, in artificial tears, 341
Carboxypeptidase E, in aqueous humor, 231
Carcinogenesis, loss of telomeric DNA and, 150
Carotenoids (xanthophylls)
    antioxidant effects of, 284*f*, 288
    in lens, 285
    in retina, 77, 286, 288, 289*f*
Carotid artery, internal, 90
    cranial nerve relationship and, 84*f*, 85*f*
    optic nerve supplied by, 84*f*, 85*f*, 90, 91
Carotid plexus, 102, 104
Carrier (genetic), 132, 176, 197–200
    identification of, 205, 206
    ocular findings in, 198–200, 198–199*f*, 199*t*
Carteolol, 321, 322*t*, 323
Caruncle, 18*f*, 27
Catalase, 282*f*, 284, 288
    in lens, 284
    in retina and retinal pigment epithelium, 273, 288
Cataract
    carbohydrate ("sugar"), 246–248
        aldose reductase in development of, 247–248, 247*f*
    free radicals/antioxidants and, 284
    muscarinic therapy and, 311
Cathepsin D, in aqueous humor, 231, 233–234
Cathepsin O, in aqueous humor, 231, 233, 234
Cavernous sinus, 35*f*, 105, 105*f*, 106*f*
    cranial nerve V₁ (ophthalmic) in, 100
cDNA, 133
    sequencing, 161
cDNA library, 138
Cefadroxil, 345
Cefamandole, 345
Cefazolin, 344*t*, 345
Cefepime, 346
Cefoperazone, 346
Cefotaxime, 346

Cefoxitin, 345
Cefpirome, 346
Ceftazidime, 344t, 346
Ceftizoxime, 346
Ceftriaxone, 344t
Cefuroxime, 345
Celecoxib, 335t
    cardiovascular toxicity and, 239
Cell adhesion molecules, neural, in retinal pigment
        epithelium, 273
Cell cycle, 148–150, 149f
Cell death, programmed (PCD/apoptosis), 132, 154, 155
    in DNA repair, 154, 155
Cellular retinaldehyde-binding protein/cytoplasmic
        retinal-binding protein (CRALBP)
    in aqueous humor, 231
    mutations in, 265
Cellulose, in artificial tears, 341
Centimorgan, 132, 150
Central cornea, 38–39, 39f
Central dogma of genetics, 151–154, 151f
Central retinal artery, 73, 88f, 90, 91, 91f, 92f
Central retinal vein, 35f, 88f, 91f, 92f
Central supporting connective strand, 88f
Central zone, of lens epithelium, 64, 242
Centromere, 132
CEP290 gene, in Leber congenital amaurosis, 183f
Cephalexin, 345
Cephalosporins, 343, 344t, 345–346
    allergic reaction to, 343
Cephalothin, 345
Cephradine, 345
Ceramide trihexosidase, defective/deficiency of, 175t
Ceramide trihexoside, in Fabry disease, 203
Cerebellar arteries
    anterior inferior, cranial nerve relationship and, 102
    superior, cranial nerve relationship and, 94, 95f, 97
Cerebellopontine angle, 101, 103
Cerebral artery
    anterior, 90, 107f
        cranial nerve relationship and, 85f
    middle, 107f
        cranial nerve relationship and, 84f, 85f
    posterior, 93, 107f
        cranial nerve relationship and, 84f
Cerebroside α-galactosidase, defective/deficiency
        of, 175t
Ceruloplasmin, in Wilson disease, 203
Cervical ganglia, superior, 11
    dilator muscle innervation and, 56
Cervicofacial division, of cranial nerve VII (facial), 104
cGMP (cyclic guanosine monophosphate)
    in cone phototransduction, 261
    mutations in, 161
    in rod phototransduction, 259, 260f, 261
cGMP (cyclic guanosine monophosphate)-gated channel
    cone, 261
        mutations in, 264
    rod, 259, 260f, 261
        mutations in, 161, 263
CGRP. See Calcitonin gene-related peptide
Chamber angle. See Anterior chamber angle
Chelation therapy, for Wilson disease, 203
Chiasm (optic), 85f, 90, 92–93

Children, drug toxicity and, 294
    muscarinic antagonists, 313
Chloramphenicol, 347t, 350–351
    intravenous administration of, 301
Chlorhexidine, for Acanthamoeba keratitis, 361
Chloride
    in aqueous humor, 231t, 232
    in tear film, 214t, 216
    in vitreous, 231t, 252
Chlortetracycline, 350
Cholinergic drugs, 307–315, 307f, 308t, 309f, 310f,
        311t, 314t, 315t. See also Muscarinic drugs;
        Nicotinic agents
    agonists, 308t, 309f
        direct-acting, 308, 308–312, 309f, 310f, 311t
        indirect-acting, 308, 309f, 312–313, 314–315
    antagonists, 308, 308t, 315, 315t
    ciliary muscle affected by, 59
    as miotics, 308–313, 308t, 311t
Cholinergic receptors, 308, 308t
    drugs affecting, 307–315, 307f, 308t, 309f, 310f, 311t,
        314t, 315t. See also Cholinergic drugs
    signal transduction and, 316t
Cholinesterase inhibitors, 312–313
    miotic action of, 311t, 312–313
Chondroitin sulfate
    in cornea, 226
    as viscoelastic, 368
Chondroitinase, for enzymatic vitreolysis, 255
Chorda tympani, 101f, 103, 104
Choriocapillaris, 59, 60f, 61–62, 61f, 62f, 70f
Chorionic villus sampling, 132, 206–207
Choroid, 37f, 59–62, 60f, 61f, 62f
    anatomy of, 37f, 59–62, 60f, 61f, 62f
    development of, 122
    gyrate atrophy of, 175t
    vasculature of, 59–60, 60f, 61–62, 61f, 62f
        development of, 116t
Choroidal artery, 62
    optic nerve supplied by, 91
Choroidal capillaries, 59, 60f, 61–62, 61f, 62f
Choroidal fissure. See Embryonic fissure
Choroideremia
    ocular findings in carriers of, 198f, 199t
    REP-1 (Rab escort protein 1) gene in, 265
    retinal pigment epithelium in, 279
Chromatid, 133
Chromatin, 133
Chromosomal aneuploidy, 132, 189. See also specific
        disorder
    autosome, 189–190
    sex chromosome, 189
Chromosome arm painting, 188, 189f
Chromosomes, 147, 148f, 184–187
    abnormalities of. See also specific type
        identification of, 187–193, 189f, 191t
        incidence of, 188
        ophthalmically important, 192–193
    analysis of, 187–193, 189f, 191t
    bacterial artificial (BAC), 145
    homologous, 137, 184
    sex, 147. See also X chromosome; Y chromosome
        aneuploidy of, 189
        mosaicism and, 191–192

translocation of, 144
  Down syndrome caused by, 190
variant (as genetic markers), 159
yeast artificial (YAC), 145
Chronic progressive external ophthalmoplegia
  (CPEO), 158
  mitochondrial DNA defects and, 157, 158
Chronic progressive external ophthalmoplegia
  (CPEO)-plus syndromes, 158
Cidofovir, 357t, 360–361
Cilia (eyelashes), 19, 22f, 24
  misdirection of. See Trichiasis
Ciliary arteries, 17f, 32–35, 33f
  anterior, 17, 30, 32–35
  choroid supplied by, 60
  conjunctiva supplied by, 30
  extraocular muscles supplied by, 17
  posterior, 17f, 32, 33f, 34f, 90, 91, 91f, 92f
Ciliary body, 17f, 37f, 46f, 57–59, 58f, 59f, 236–240
  anatomy of, 17f, 37f, 46f, 57–59, 58f, 59f
  biochemistry and metabolism of, 236–240
  development of, 116t, 122
  epithelium of. See Ciliary epithelium
  smooth muscle in, 58–59, 59f, 237
  stroma of, 57–58, 58f
  uveal portion of, 58
Ciliary epithelium, 57–58, 58f
  aqueous humor formation/dynamics and, 229, 230,
    231, 323, 324, 324f
  nonpigmented, 57, 58f, 229, 230
  pigmented, 57, 58f, 230
Ciliary ganglion, 11–12, 12f
  branches of, 11–12
Ciliary muscle, 58–59, 59f
  in accommodation, 63
  innervation of, 94, 95
  miotic/muscarinic agents affecting, 308, 308–309,
    311–312
  mydriatic/muscarinic agents affecting, 313
Ciliary nerves, 59
  long, 12, 32, 100, 223–224
    dilator muscle supplied by, 100
  posterior, 32, 223–224
  short, 12, 12f, 100
    ciliary muscle supplied by, 95
    posterior, 32
    sphincter muscle supplied by, 56
Ciliary processes, 47f, 57, 59f
  development of, 116t
Ciliary sulcus, 47f
Cilioretinal artery, 73, 91
Cilium, photoreceptor, 69, 72f
Ciloxan. See Ciprofloxacin
Ciprofloxacin, 346, 347–349, 347t
Circle of Willis, 90, 90f, 105–107, 107f
Circle of Zinn-Haller (circle of Haller and Zinn/circle of
  Zinn), 88f, 91
11-cis-retinol/retinaldehyde, 274, 275, 275f
11-cis-retinol dehydrogenase, mutations in, 265
Citrate, in tear film, 216
Cl. See Chloride
Clarithromycin, 353
CLIA (Clinical Laboratory Improvement
  Amendments), 133

Clindamycin, 344t
Clinical heterogeneity, 133
Clinical Laboratory Improvement Amendments
  (CLIA), 133
Clinical trials, for new drug, 305
Clinoid process
  anterior, 8f, 84f, 105f
  posterior, 84f, 95, 102
Clivus, 102
Cloquet canal, 80
Clostridium botulinum, toxin derived from, 366
Cloxacillin, 344
cM. See Centimorgan
Cocaine, 320
  norepinephrine uptake affected by, 320, 320f
  as topical anesthetic, 363t, 364, 365
Codominance (codominant inheritance/alleles),
  133, 173
Codon, 133, 147
  stop/termination, 144
  frameshift mutation and, 135, 155
Cohesive viscoelastics, 368
Colistimethate, 344t
Collagen
  in choroid, 62
  in ciliary muscle, 59
  corneal, 40–41, 225–226
  in lens capsule, 64, 120, 241
  mutations in, in hereditary hyaloideoretinopathy, 255
  scleral, 44
  stromal, 40–41, 225–226
  in vitreous, 78–79, 79f, 249–250, 250f, 251f
    liquefaction and, 253
Collagen cornea shields, for drug administration, 303
Collagenase, for enzymatic vitreolysis, 255
Collarette (iris), 54f, 55
Collector channels, 51, 52f
Colliculus, facial, 101, 103
Colobomas
  embryonic fissure closure and, 117, 119f
  optic nerve/optic disc, 152
Color vision, 262–263
  defects in, 262–263, 264
    blue-cone monochromatism, 264
    genetic basis of, 262–263, 264
    ocular findings in carriers of, 199t
  trivariant, 262–263
Combigan. See Brimonidine, in combination
  preparations
Communicating arteries
  anterior, 90
    cranial nerve relationship and, 84f, 85f
  posterior, 107f
    cranial nerve relationship and, 84f, 85f
Compartment syndrome, visual loss after trauma
  and, 90
Complement, in aqueous humor, 231, 233
Complementary DNA (cDNA), 133
  sequencing, 161
Complementary DNA library (cDNA library), 138
Complex genetic disorder (multigene disorder), 133,
  200–201
Compound heterozygote, 133
Compounding pharmaceuticals, 306

Cone inner segments, 70, 72f. *See also* Cones
Cone outer segments, 69, 70, 72f. *See also* Cones
   shed, retinal pigment epithelium phagocytosis
     of, 276–277, 276f
Cone response, 262, 269, 269f
Cones, 69, 71f, 72f, 77, 88f, 257, 258f. *See also* Cone
   outer segments
   amacrine cells for, 267
   bipolar cells for, 257, 266, 266f
   development of, 116t
   electrophysiologic responses of, 269, 269f
   extrafoveal, 70
   foveal, 70, 77
   gene defects in, 264
   horizontal cells for, 258f, 262, 266–267, 266f
   phototransduction in, 261–263
Congenital, definition of, 133, 181. *See also* Genetics
Congenital stationary night blindness, with myopia,
   ocular findings in carriers of, 199t
Conjunctiva, 20f, 25, 26f, 30–31
   anatomy of, 20f, 25, 26f, 30–31
   blood supply of, 30
   bulbar, 25, 26f, 30
   drug absorption and, 297
   epithelium of, 30–31, 215f, 216
     tear secretion and, 215f, 216, 217
   forniceal, 25, 26f, 30
   innervation of, 30, 216
   lymphoid tissue associated with (CALT), 30
   palpebral, 25, 26f, 30
Conjunctiva-associated lymphoid tissue (CALT/
   conjunctival MALT), 30
Conjunctival arteries, anterior and posterior, 30
Conjunctival sac, 213
Conjunctivitis
   allergic, drugs for, 337–339, 338t
   corticosteroid route of administration in, 333t
Connective tissue
   eyelid, 21
   pericanalicular, 49–50, 50f
Connexins, in lens gap junctions, 246
Consanguinity, 133, 172, 172f, 176, 205
Consensus DNA sequence, 142
Conservation (genetic), 133
Conserved base-pair mutations, 156
Contact lens drug-delivery systems, 303
Contact lenses, *Acanthamoeba* keratitis associated
   with, 361
Contig map, 163f
Contiguous gene deletion syndrome, 193
Contraceptives, oral, tetracycline use and, 350
Convergence, near reflex and, 96
Copper
   in aqueous humor, 232
   in free-radical formation, 282, 283
   in Wilson disease, 203
Copy number variation (indels), 133–134, 148
Cornea
   anatomy of, 37, 37f, 38, 38–43, 39f, 40f, 42f, 43f
   basal lamina of, 39–40, 40f, 41, 42f
   biochemistry and metabolism of, 223–227, 223f
   Bowman layer/membrane of, 40, 40f, 45f, 223f, 225.
     See also Bowman layer/membrane
   central, 38–39, 39f

Descemet membrane of, 41, 42f, 223f, 227. *See also*
   Descemet membrane/layer
   development of, 118, 120–122, 121f
   drug absorption and, 296–297
   endothelium of, 41–43, 42f, 43f, 223f, 227
     anatomy of, 41–43, 42f, 43f, 223f
     biochemistry and metabolism of, 227
     development of, 118, 120, 121f, 122
     dysfunction of, 43
     glucose metabolism in, 224
   epithelium of, 39–40, 40f, 215f, 223f, 224–225
     anatomy of, 39–40, 40f, 223f
     biochemistry and metabolism of, 224–225
     development of, 118, 120, 121f
     glucose metabolism in, 224
     tear secretion and, 215f, 217
   guttae, 41
     central, 41
     in Fuchs endothelial dystrophy, 43f
   innervation of, 216, 223–224
   layers of, 223, 223f
   nonepithelial cells in, 40
   peripheral, 38–39, 39f
   size of, 38, 39
   stroma of, 40–41, 42f, 223f, 225–226
     anatomy of, 40–41, 42f, 223f
     biochemistry and metabolism of, 225–226
     development of, 118, 120, 121f
   topography of, 37, 37f, 38
Cornea shields, collagen, for drug administration, 303
Corneal dystrophies, Fuchs endothelial, 43f
Corneal nerves, 223–224
Corneoscleral junction, 44–45, 47f
Corneoscleral meshwork, 48, 49, 50f
Cortex, lens, 64, 242–243, 242f
Cortical–nuclear barrier, in lens, 285
Corticosteroids (steroids), 329–334, 330t, 333t
   adverse effects of, 331–333
   anti-inflammatory effects/potency of, 332, 333t
   for dry eye, 221
   intraocular pressure affected by, 299, 332,
     332–333, 333t
   intravitreal administration of, 300t, 334
   for ocular allergies/inflammation, 329, 337,
     338, 339
     route of administration of, 329, 333–334, 333t
   in tear secretion, 219–220
Cortisporin. *See* Hydrocortisone, in combination
   preparations
Cosmid vector, 145
Cosopt. *See* Timolol, in combination preparations
Counseling, genetic. *See* Genetic testing/counseling
COX-1/COX-2. *See* Cyclooxygenase
COX-2 inhibitors, 239, 336
CPEO. *See* Chronic progressive external
   ophthalmoplegia
CPEO-plus syndromes. *See* Chronic progressive
   external ophthalmoplegia (CPEO)-plus syndromes
CRA. *See* Central retinal artery
CRALBP. *See* Cellular retinaldehyde-binding protein/
   cytoplasmic retinal-binding protein
Cranial dysinnervation disorders, congenital, 124
Cranial nerve I (olfactory nerve), 83, 84f, 85f
Cranial nerve II. *See* Optic nerve

Cranial nerve III (oculomotor nerve), 9f, 93–96, 94f, 95f
  aneurysms affecting, 94, 95
  extraocular muscles innervated by, 15f, 17, 93–96, 94f
  motor root of, 11, 12f
  palsy of, 95
Cranial nerve IV (trochlear nerve), 9f, 96–97
  extraocular muscles innervated by, 17
Cranial nerve V (trigeminal nerve), 9f, 10, 97–101, 98f,
    99f, 101f
  divisions of, 98f, 99f, 100–101, 101f
    V₁ (ophthalmic nerve), 9f, 98f, 99f, 100, 101f
      sensory root of, 11, 12f
    V₂ (maxillary nerve), 9f, 10, 98f, 99f, 100, 101f
    V₃ (mandibular nerve), 98f, 99f, 101, 101f
Cranial nerve VI (abducens nerve), 9f, 101–102, 102f
  extraocular muscles innervated by, 17
Cranial nerve VII (facial nerve), 101f, 102–104, 102f
  cervicofacial division of, 104
  labyrinthine segment of, 103
  mastoid segment of, 103
  temporofacial division of, 104
  tympanic segment of, 103
Cranial nerve VIII (auditory nerve), 101f, 103
Cranial nerves, 11, 83–107, 84f. See also specific nerve
  extraocular muscles supplied by, 15f
Crest cells. See Neural crest cells
Cribriform plate, 10f, 11. See also Lamina cribrosa
Crigler-Najjar syndrome, 175t
Crolom. See Cromolyn
Cromolyn, 337, 338t
Crossing over (genetic), 134, 150, 187
  unequal, 145
Crouzon syndrome, 177
CRV. See Central retinal vein
Crystalline lens. See Lens
Crystallins, 64, 241, 243–244
  α, 64, 244
  β, 64, 244
  β,γ, 244
  γ, 64, 244
  taxon-specific, 244
Cu-Zn SOD (superoxide dismutase), 287
Cupping of optic disc, 86
CVS. See Chorionic villus sampling
Cyclic adenosine monophosphate (cAMP), 321
  in signal transduction, 316t
  in tear secretion, 218, 219f
Cyclic guanosine monophosphate (cGMP)
  in cone phototransduction, 261
  mutations in, 161
  in rod phototransduction, 259, 260f, 261
Cyclic guanosine monophosphate (cGMP)-gated channel
  cone, 261
    mutations in, 264
  rod, 259, 260f, 261
    mutations in, 161, 263
Cyclogyl. See Cyclopentolate
Cyclomydril. See Cyclopentolate, with phenylephrine
Cyclooxygenase (COX-1/COX-2), 239
  aspirin affecting, 335
  in eicosanoid synthesis, 238–239, 238f
  NSAIDs and, 239, 334
  in prostaglandin synthesis, 238–239, 238f, 334

Cyclooxygenase-2 (COX-2) inhibitors, 239, 336
Cyclopentolate, 313, 314t
  with phenylephrine, 314t
Cycloplegia/cycloplegics, 313, 314t
Cyclosporine/cyclosporine A, 337
  for dry eye, 221–222, 221f, 337, 342
  off-label use of, 306
  topical, 337
Cylate. See Cyclopentolate
Cystathionine synthase, abnormality of in
    homocystinuria, 175t
Cystinosis, renal transplant for, 203
Cystoid macular edema
  carbonic anhydrase inhibitors for, 324
  corticosteroid route of administration in, 333t
Cytochrome oxidase complex, 281, 282f, 286
Cytochrome P450, drug toxicity and, 294
Cytogenetics, 187–193, 189f, 191t
  indications for, 188, 189f
  markers in, 159
Cytokines, in tear film, 217
Cytokinesis, 148, 149f
Cytomegalovirus (CMV) retinitis
  cidofovir for, 357t, 360–361
  foscarnet for, 357t, 360
  ganciclovir for, 357t, 358t, 359–360
Cytoplasmic retinal-binding protein/cellular
    retinaldehyde-binding protein (CRALBP)
  in aqueous humor, 231
  mutations in, 265
Cytoskeletal lens proteins, 245
Cytovene. See Ganciclovir

ᴅ-penicillamine, for Wilson disease, 203
Dacryocystorhinostomy, angular artery as landmark
    in, 25
DAG. See Diacylglycerol
Dapiprazole, 308t, 321
Daranide. See Dichlorphenamide
Database of Genotypes and Phenotypes
    (dbGaP), 134
Deafness (hearing loss), mitochondrial DNA mutations
    and, 157
Decamethonium, 315
Decongestants, ocular, 342–343
Decussation
  cranial nerve III (oculomotor), 94
  cranial nerve IV (trochlear), 96
Deep petrosal nerve, 101f, 104
Defensins, in tear film, 216
Degeneracy, of genetic code, 134
Degenerations, retinal
  gene defects causing, 265–266
  retinal pigment epithelium defects and, 278–279
Deletions, 145, 148, 150, 153–154, 155, 159
  mitochondrial DNA, disorders caused by, 157
Demecarium, 312, 313
Demeclocycline, 350
Demulcents, 341
Denaturing gradient gel electrophoresis (DGGE), 162
Deoxyribonucleic acid. See DNA
Depolarizing neuromuscular blocking agents, 315
Dermatan sulfate, in cornea, 226

Descemet membrane/layer, 41, 42f, 223f, 227
  anatomy of, 41, 42f, 223f
  biochemistry and metabolism of, 227
  development of, 41, 116t, 120–121, 121f
  guttae in, 41
    in Fuchs endothelial dystrophy, 43f
Desmosomes, in corneal epithelium, 40
Deutan defects, ocular findings in carriers of, 199t
Dexacidin. See Dexamethasone, in combination
    preparations
Dexamethasone, 300t, 302, 330t
  anti-inflammatory potency of, 333t
  in combination preparations, 348t
  intravenous administration of, 301
  pressure-elevating potency of, 332, 333t
Dexamethasone implant, 300t, 302
Dexasporin. See Dexamethasone, in combination
    preparations
Dextran, in artificial tears, 341
DFP. See Diisopropyl phosphorofluoridate
DGGE. See Denaturing gradient gel electrophoresis
DHA. See Docosahexaenoic acid
Diabetes insipidus, diabetes mellitus, optic atrophy,
    and neural deafness (DIDMOAD) syndrome,
    pleiotropism in, 196
Diabetes mellitus
  aqueous humor glucose and, 232
  cataracts associated with, 232, 246–247
    carbohydrate ("sugar"), 246–248
      aldose reductase in development of, 247–248, 247f
  type 2 (non–insulin-dependent/NIDDM/adult-
    onset), mitochondrial DNA mutations and, 157
Diabetic macular edema, corticosteroid route of
    administration in, 333t
Diacylglycerol (DAG), in tear secretion, 218, 218f
Diagnostic agents, 367–368
Diamox. See Acetazolamide
Dibromopropamidine, for Acanthamoeba keratitis, 361
Dichlorphenamide, 326
Diclofenac, 330t, 335t, 336
Dicloxacillin, 344
DIDMOAD (diabetes insipidus, diabetes mellitus,
    optic atrophy, and neural deafness) syndrome,
    pleiotropism in, 196
Diet/diet therapy, in inborn errors of metabolism, 203
Diffusion, in aqueous humor dynamics/formation, 230
Diflucan. See Fluconazole
Diflunisal, 335t
Difluprednate, 330t
Digenic inheritance, 134
Digital polymerase chain reaction (dPCR), 141
Diisopropyl phosphorofluoridate (DFP), 312, 313
Dilator muscle (iris), 53f, 55–56
  α-adrenergic agents affecting, 55, 317–318, 320
  development of, 55, 116t, 122
  muscarinic agents affecting, 313
Dinucleotide repeats, 139
Dipivefrin (dipivalyl epinephrine), 318t
Diploid/diploid number, 134, 149
Diquafosol, 342
Direct sequencing, 161–162, 162f, 163f, 164f, 165f, 166f
Direct-to-consumer genetic testing, 134
Discontinuity, lamellar/optic zones of, 64

Disodium ethylenediaminetetraacetic acid (EDTA)
  in artificial tears, 341
  for band keratopathy, 306
  in irrigating solutions, 367
  off-label use of, 306
Disomy, uniparental, 145, 154
Dispase, for enzymatic vitreolysis, 255
Dispersive viscoelastics, 368
Distichiasis, 24
DNA
  amplification of, in polymerase chain reaction, 141–142
  antisense, 132
    in gene therapy, 170
  complementary (cDNA), 133
    sequencing, 161
  damage to, 154
  encyclopedia of elements of (ENCODE), 135
  methylation of, 139, 151, 153
  mitochondrial (mtDNA), 147, 148f
    diseases associated with deletions/mutations
      of, 157–159
      chronic progressive external
        ophthalmoplegia, 157, 158
      Leber hereditary optic neuropathy, 157, 158
      maternal inheritance/transmission and, 157, 181
      MELAS and MIDD, 159
      NARP (neuropathy/ataxia/retinitis pigmentosa)
        syndrome, 157, 158–159
    replicative segregation and, 143, 157
  noncoding (junk), 150, 151
  recombinant, 143
  repair of, 154. See also Mutation
  replication of, 143
    segregation and, 143
    slippage and, 143
  satellite, 150
  sequencing of, 161–162, 162f, 163f, 164f, 165f, 166f
    next-generation (NGS/massively parallel), 140,
      142, 161, 163f, 164f, 165f, 166f
  structure of, 147, 148f
  telomeric (telomeres), 144, 150
DNA code, 134
DNA library, 138
  cDNA, 138
  genomic, 138
Docosahexaenoic acid, in retina/retinal pigment
    epithelium, 274
  oxidative damage and, 285
Dominant inheritance (dominant gene/trait), 134,
    173–174, 177
  autosomal, 177–178, 178t
  disorders associated with, 134
    gene therapy for, 169–170, 170f
    X-linked, 180–181
  X-linked, 179–180, 181t
Dominant negative mutation/dominant-negative
    effect, 134
  gene therapy for disorders caused by, 169
Dopamine, outer-segment disc shedding and, 277
Dopamine-β-hydroxylase, defective/deficiency of, 175t
Dorello canal, 102
Dorzolamide, 324–325, 325t
  in combination preparations, 322t, 325, 325t

Double helix, DNA, 147, 148*f*
Double heterozygotes, 185
Down syndrome (trisomy 21), 189–190, 191*t*
  mosaicism in, 191
  pharmacogenetics and, 201
Doxycycline, 350
  for dry eye, 221
  off-label use of, 306
Doyne honeycombed dystrophy, EFEMP1 defects
      causing, 265
dPCR. *See* Digital polymerase chain reaction
Drug resistance. *See also specific agent*
  antibiotic, 343, 346, 351, 352, 353
  antiviral, 358, 360
Drugs
  allergic reaction to, penicillins/cephalosporins, 343
  drug penetration and, 298
  genetics affecting (pharmacogenetics), 141, 201–202
  metabolism of
    age-related changes in, 294, 295
    toxicity and, 294, 295
  ocular
    absorption of, 294, 295–297, 296*f*
    adrenergic, 316–323, 316*t*, 317*f*, 318*t*, 320*f*, 322*t*
    antibiotic, 343–354, 344*t*, 347*t*, 348*t*
    antifibrinolytic, 369–370
    antifungal, 354–356, 355*t*
    anti-inflammatory, 329–341, 330*t*, 333*t*, 335*t*, 338*t*
    antimicrobial, 343–361
    antioxidant/vitamin supplements, 370
    antiviral, 356–361, 357–358*t*
    carbonic anhydrase inhibitors, 230, 323–326,
        324*f*, 325*t*
    cholinergic, 307–315, 307*f*, 308*t*, 309*f*, 310*f*, 311*t*,
        314*t*, 315*t*
    combined medications, 328
    compounded, 306–307
    concentration of, absorption affected by, 297
    decongestants, 342–343
    diagnostic agents, 367–368
    for dry eye, 221–222, 221*f*, 341–342
    in eyedrops, 295–298, 296*f*
    fibrinolytic, 369
    growth factors, 371–372
    hyperosmolar, 366
    interferons, 370–371
    intraocular injection of, 299, 300*t*
    intravenous administration of, 301
    investigational, 305
    for irrigation, 367
    legal aspects of use of, 205–207
    local administration of, 299, 300*t*
    local anesthetics, 362–366, 362*t*, 363*t*
    mechanisms of action of, 293, 304
    methods of design and delivery of, 301–304
        new technologies and, 303–304
    new, clinical testing of, 305
    off-label usage of, 305, 306
    in ointments, 298–299
    osmotic drugs, 328–329, 329*t*
    partition coefficients of, 298
    periocular injection of, 299
    pharmacodynamics of, 293, 304
        age-related changes in, 295

    pharmacokinetics of, 293, 295–304, 296*f*, 300*t*
        age-related changes in, 295
    pharmacologic principles and, 293–304
    pharmacotherapeutics of, 293, 294
    prostaglandin analogues, 302, 327–328, 327*t*
    purified neurotoxin complex, 366
    receptor interactions and, 304
    solubility of, absorption affected by, 297, 297–298
    sustained-release preparations
        oral, 301
        topical, 302
    systemic absorption of, 294, 296
    systemic administration and, 300–301
    thrombin, 369
    tissue binding of, 298
    topical, 295–299, 296*f. See also* Eyedrops
        sustained-release devices for, 302
    toxicity of, 294
        age/aging and, 294, 295
        tissue binding and, 298
    viscoelastic agents, 368
    viscosity of, absorption affected by, 297
    vitamin/antioxidant supplements, 370
Drusen, 69
Dry eye
  drugs for, 21–222, 221*f*, 341–342
  surface inflammation and, 221–222, 221*f*
  tear-film abnormalities and, 220, 221–222, 221*f*
Dulcitol, in lens glucose/carbohydrate metabolism, 247*f*
DuoTrav. *See* Travoprost, in combination preparations
Duplications, 145, 150, 155, 159
Dura mater, optic nerve, 88*f*, 89, 89*f*
Durezol. *See* Difluprednate
Dysautonomia, familial (Riley-Day syndrome), 175*t*
  racial and ethnic concentration of, 197
Dystrophin, 153

Echothiophate, 311*t*, 312, 313
  in Down syndrome, pharmacogenetics and, 201
  local anesthetic use and, 312
Econopred. *See* Prednisolone
Ectoderm, 111, 112*f*, 113*f*, 114*f*
  ocular structures derived from, 115*t*
    cornea, 120–121, 121*f*
    lens, 117–122, 120*f*
Ectropion, 55
  uveae, 55
Edetate disodium (salt of EDTA)
  in artificial tears, 341
  for band keratopathy, 306
  in irrigating solutions, 367
  off-label use of, 306
Edinger-Westphal nucleus, 56, 94, 94*f*, 96
Edrophonium, 309*f*, 312, 314–315
  intravenous administration of, 301
  in myasthenia gravis diagnosis, 301, 315
EDTA
  in artificial tears, 341
  for band keratopathy, 306
  in irrigating solutions, 367
  off-label use of, 306
EFEMP1 gene/EFEMP1 protein (EGF-containing
      fibrillin-like extracellular matrix gene/protein)
  mutations, 265

Efferent fibers, visceral, 103
Efferent pupillary pathway, 96
EGF-containing fibrillin-like extracellular matrix gene/
    protein (*EFEMP1*/EFEMP1) mutations, 265
Ehlers-Danlos syndrome, 175*t*
Eicosanoids, 237–240, 238*f*
    synthesis of, 238–239, 238*f*
Eighth cranial nerve. *See* Cranial nerve VIII
Elderly patients
    carbonic anhydrase inhibitor use and, 326
    corticosteroid use and, 332
    pharmacologic principles in, 295
Electrolytes, in tear film, 214*t*, 216
Electro-oculogram, trans-RPE potential as basis for, 277
Electrophoresis, denaturing gradient gel (DGGE), 162
Electrophysiologic testing, of retina, 268–269, 269*f*
Electroretinogram (ERG), 269
Elestat. *See* Epinastine
Elevated intraocular pressure
    corticosteroids causing, 299, 332, 332–333, 333*t*
    cycloplegics causing, 313
    drugs for. *See* Antiglaucoma agents
11p13 syndrome (short arm 11 deletion syndrome/
    PAX6 gene mutation), 193
    in aniridia, 152, 177, 193
Ellipsoid
    of cone, 70, 72*f*
    of rod, 69, 72*f*
ELM. *See* External limiting membrane
Elschnig, border tissue of, 88*f*
Emadine. *See* Emedastine
Embryogenesis, 111, 112*f*
Embryology. *See* Eye, development of
Embryonic fissure, 117*f*, 118*f*
    closure of, 116*t*, 118*f*, 119*f*
        colobomas and, 117, 119*f*
Embryonic lens nucleus, 65*f*
Emedastine, 337, 338*t*
Emissaria, scleral, 44
Emollients, ocular, 341
En grappe nerve endings, for tonic (slow twitch) fibers, 18
En plaque nerve endings
    for fast twitch fibers, 18
    neuromuscular blocking agents affecting, 315
Encapsulated-cell technology, for drug delivery, 303
Encephalopathy, Leigh necrotizing (Leigh syndrome),
    159, 175*t*
    mitochondrial DNA mutation and, 159
ENCODE (ENCyclopedia Of DNA Elements), 135
Endoderm, 111, 112*f*, 113*f*, 114*f*
Endonucleases, 135
Endophthalmitis
    compounded bevacizumab causing, 306
    corticosteroid route of administration in, 333*t*
Endothelial dystrophies, Fuchs, 43*f*
Endothelial meshwork, 49–50
Endothelin (ET)
    in aqueous humor, 234
    receptors for, 316*t*
        in signal transduction, 316*t*
Endothelium, corneal, 41–43, 42*f*, 43*f*, 223*f*, 227
    anatomy of, 41–43, 42*f*, 43*f*, 223*f*
    biochemistry and metabolism of, 227
    development of, 118, 120, 121*f*, 122

dysfunction of, 43
glucose metabolism in, 224
Energy production
    in lens, 246
    in retinal pigment epithelium, 273, 274
Enhancer (of transcription rate), 135
Enzymatic (Sanger) method, for DNA sequencing, 143,
    161, 162, 162*f*
Enzymatic vitreolysis, 255
Enzyme defects, disorders associated with, 174, 175*t*
    management of, 203–204
Enzymes, in aqueous humor, 229, 234
EOMs. *See* Extraocular muscles
Epiblast, 112*f*
Epidermal growth factor, 371–372
    in tear film, 217
Epidermal growth factor–containing fibrillin-like
    extracellular matrix gene/protein (*EFEMP1*/
    EFEMP1) mutations, 265
Epifrin. *See* Epinephrine
Epigenetics/epigenomics, 135, 151
Epinastine, 338*t*, 339
Epinephrine, 318*t*, 321
    adrenergic receptor response and, 316, 321
    dipivalyl. *See* Dipivefrin
    intracameral administration of, 300*t*
    with local anesthetic, 363–364
Episclera, 44
Episcleral plexus, 51, 52*f*
Episcleritis, corticosteroid route of administration
    in, 333*t*
Epithelium
    ciliary, 57–58, 58*f*
        aqueous humor formation/dynamics and, 229, 230,
            231, 323, 324, 324*f*
        nonpigmented, 57, 58*f*, 229, 230
        pigmented, 57, 58*f*, 230
    conjunctival, 30–31, 215*f*, 216
        tear secretion and, 215*f*, 216, 217
    corneal. *See* Cornea, epithelium of
    lens, 63*f*, 64, 65*f*, 120, 242, 242*f*
Equator (lens), 63, 63*f*, 65*f*, 242, 242*f*
ERG. *See* Electroretinogram
Erythromycin, 344*t*, 347*t*, 352–353
    intravenous administration of, 301
Esotropia, accommodative, muscarinic antagonists for
    management of, 313
EST. *See* Expressed sequence tags
Esterase D, retinoblastoma and, 159
ET. *See* Endothelin
Ethmoid/ethmoidal bone (lamina papyracea), 6, 6*f*
Ethmoidal arteries, 33*f*, 34*f*
Ethmoidal foramina, anterior/posterior, 6*f*, 7–8
Ethmoidal sinuses, 10–11, 10*f*, 17*f*
Ethnic background, genetic disorders and, 196–197
Ethylenediaminetetraacetic acid (EDTA)
    in artificial tears, 341
    for band keratopathy, 306
    in irrigating solutions, 367
    off-label use of, 306
Etodolac, 335*t*
Euchromatin, 133
Eukaryotes, 135, 147
Excision repair, 154

Excretory lacrimal system, 29–30, 29*f*
Exome sequencing, 135
Exon, 135, 147, 148, 148*f*, 151, 152
Exon shuffling, 148
Expressed sequence tags (EST), 135
Expressivity (genetic), 135, 196. *See also* Transcription
  (gene)
External limiting membrane (ELM), 71*f*, 72*f*, 74, 76*f*,
  88*f*, 258*f*
Extrafoveal cones, 70
Extraocular muscles, 13–18, 13*f*, 14*f*, 15*t*, 16*f*, 17*f*. *See
  also specific muscle*
  anatomy of, 13–18, 13*f*, 14*f*, 15*t*, 16*f*, 17*f*
  blood supply/arterial system of, 15*t*, 17
  development of, 124–125
  fiber types in, 18
  fine structure of, 18
  innervation of, 12*f*, 17, 93–96, 94*f*
  insertions of, 13–15, 14*f*, 15*t*
  orbital relationships of, 14*f*, 15–16, 16*f*, 17*f*
  origins of, 15*t*, 16–17
Eye
  anatomy of, 37–81. *See also specific structure*
  development of, 115–126. *See also specific structure*
    chronology of, 115–117, 116*t*, 117*f*, 118*f*, 119*f*
    general principles and, 111, 112*f*, 113*f*, 114*f*, 115*t*
    genetic cascades and morphogenic gradients
      and, 111, 126–128
    homeobox genes and, 126
    neural crest cells and, 111, 113*f*, 114*f*, 115*t*
  dimensions of, 37
  glands of, 23*t*
Eye movements, extraocular muscles in control of, 18
Eyeball. *See* Globe
Eyedrops (topical medications), 295–298, 296*f*
  in examination/diagnosis and, 367–368
  sustained-release devices for, 302
Eyelashes (cilia), 19, 22*f*, 24
  misdirection of. *See* Trichiasis
Eyelid–globe incongruity, in tear deficiency, 220
Eyelids, 18–27, 18*f*
  accessory structures of, 18*f*, 27
  anatomy of, 18*f*, 19–25, 20*f*, 21*f*, 22*f*, 23*f*, 23*t*, 25*f*, 26*f*
    racial variations in, 19, 21*f*
  conjunctiva of, 20*f*, 25, 26*f*. *See also* Conjunctiva
  connective tissue structures of, 21
  development of, 116*t*, 125, 125*f*
  lower
    anatomy of, 20*f*, 21, 22*f*, 25*f*
    development of, 125, 125*f*
  lymphatics of, 27, 27*f*
  margin of, 19, 22*f*, 23*t*, 25*f*
  movement of, in tear film renewal and
    distribution, 220
  orbital fat and, 20*f*, 23
  orbital septum and, 20*f*, 22–23
  skin of, 19, 20*f*, 21*f*
  subcutaneous tissue of, 20*f*, 21
  tarsus of, 20*f*, 24, 25*f*
  upper
    anatomy of, 18–19, 19–25, 20*f*, 21*f*, 22*f*, 23*f*, 25*f*
    development of, 125, 125*f*
  vascular supply of, 25–26, 26*f*
  venous drainage of, 26

Fabry disease, 175*t*
  enzyme replacement therapy for, 203
  ocular findings in carriers of, 199*t*
Facial artery
  eyelids supplied by, 25, 26*f*
  orbit supplied by, 33*f*
Facial bones, aging and, 7
Facial colliculus, 101, 103
Facial nerve. *See* Cranial nerve VII
Facial vein, 35*f*
Fallopian canal, 103
Famciclovir, 302, 357*t*, 359
Familial, definition of, 181. *See also* Genetics
Familial dysautonomia (Riley-Day syndrome), 175*t*
  racial and ethnic concentration of, 197
Family history/familial factors, 171
  genetic counseling and, 204
  pedigree analysis and, 171, 172–173, 172*f*
Family planning, genetic counseling and, 206
Famvir. *See* Famciclovir
Fanconi syndrome, tetracyclines causing, 350
Fascia bulbi (Tenon capsule), 31–32, 31*f*, 32*f*, 43
Fascicles
  cranial nerve IV (trochlear), 96
  optic nerve, 86, 88*f*
Fast twitch fibers, 18
Fat, orbital, 20*f*, 23
Fatty acids
  oxidation of, 281, 282–283
    in retina, 285
  in retinal pigment epithelium, 274
FAZ. *See* Foveal avascular zone
FDA (Food and Drug Administration), 305
Fenoprofen, 335*t*
Fetal fissure. *See* Embryonic fissure
FGF. *See* Fibroblast growth factor
FGFR2 gene, in Crouzon syndrome, 177
Fibril-associated proteins, in vitreous, 251–252
Fibrillar opacities, 253
Fibrillin, 66, 252
  defects in, in Marfan syndrome, 66, 252
Fibrin sealant, 369
  off-label use of, 306, 369
Fibrinolytic agents, 369
Fibroblast growth factor (FGF), 371–372
  in aqueous humor, 234
  gene expression/ocular development and, 127
  in tear film, 217
Fibroblast growth factor receptor *(FGFR)* genes, in
  Crouzon syndrome, 177
Fibronectin, in vitreous, 249, 250, 251*f*
Fibrous astrocytes, 73
Fibulin-1, in vitreous, 249
Fifth cranial nerve. *See* Cranial nerve V
Filensin, 245
First cranial nerve. *See* Cranial nerve I
First-degree relatives, 143
First-order neuron, dilator muscle innervation
  and, 56
FISH. *See* Fluorescence in situ hybridization
Fissures
  embryonic, 117*f*, 118*f*
    closure of, 116*t*, 118*f*, 119*f*
      colobomas and, 117, 119*f*

orbital, 6f, 8–10, 8f, 9f
   inferior, 6f, 8–10
   superior, 6f, 8, 8f, 9f, 14f
   palpebral, 18–19, 18f, 25f
5′ untranslated region, 145
Flarex. See Fluorometholone
Flicker fusion frequency, 262
Floxacillin, 344
Flucaine. See Fluorescein, with proparacaine
Fluconazole, 355t, 356
Flucytosine/5-fluorocytosine, 355t, 356
Fluocinolone implant, 300t, 302, 334
Fluor-Op. See Fluorometholone
Fluorescein, 367
   with benoxinate, 363t, 365
   intravenous administration of, 301, 367. See also
      Fluorescein angiography
   with proparacaine, 363t
Fluorescein angiography, 367
Fluorescence in situ hybridization (FISH), 188
Fluorocaine. See Fluorescein, with proparacaine
5-Fluorocytosine. See Flucytosine
Fluorometholone, 330t
   anti-inflammatory/pressure-elevating potency
      of, 333t
   in combination preparations, 348t
Fluoroquinolones, 346–349, 347t
Fluorouracil, 339
   off-label use of, 306
Flurbiprofen, 330t, 335t, 336
Fluress. See Fluorescein, with benoxinate
Flurox. See Fluorescein, with benoxinate
FML. See Fluorometholone
Fodrin, in retinal pigment epithelium, 273
Folinic acid, 349
Food and Drug Administration (FDA), 305
Foramen (foramina)
   ethmoidal, anterior/posterior, 6f, 7–8
   infraorbital, 7
   optic, 7
   orbital, 7–8
   rotundum, 100
   supraorbital, 5, 7
   zygomatic, 8
Forniceal conjunctiva, 25, 26f, 30
Fornices, 25, 26f, 30
Foscarnet, 357t, 360
Foscavir. See Foscarnet
Fossae
   lacrimal, 5–6, 6, 6f
   trochlear, 6
454 next-generation sequencing method, 164f. See also
   Next-generation sequencing
Fourth cranial nerve. See Cranial nerve IV
Fovea, 67, 70f, 74f, 75, 77
   development of, 116t
Fovea ethmoidalis, 10f, 11
Fovea externa, 77
Foveal avascular zone (FAZ), 74f, 77, 78f
Foveal cones, 70, 77
Foveal fibers, 86
Foveola, 68, 75, 77
Fragile sites, in chromatids, 135
Fragile X syndrome, 135

Frameshift mutation (framing error/frameshift), 135, 155
Free radicals (oxygen radicals), 281–286
   cellular sources of, 281–282, 282f
   detoxification of, 281–282, 282f
   lens damage and, 283–285, 284f
   lipid peroxidation and, 281, 282–283
   retinal damage and, 285–286
Frontal bone, 5, 6, 6f
Frontal nerve, 9f, 100, 101f, 104
Frontal sinuses, 10–11, 10f
Frontalis muscle, 20f
Frontoethmoidal suture, 6, 6f
5-FU. See Fluorouracil
Fuchs crypts, 54–55, 54f
Fuchs endothelial corneal dystrophy, 43f
Fundus
   albipunctus, 11-cis-retinol dehydrogenase defects
      causing, 265
   oculi, 67
Fungizone. See Amphotericin B

G_0 phase, cell cycle, 148, 149f
G_1 phase, cell cycle, 148, 149, 149f
G_2 phase, cell cycle, 148, 149f
G6PD deficiency. See Glucose-6-phosphate
   dehydrogenase deficiency
G38D mutation, 263
G-protein–linked/coupled receptors
   prostaglandin, 239–240, 316t
   in tear secretion, 217–218, 218f, 219, 219f
G proteins, in tear secretion, 217–218, 218f, 219, 219f
GABA (gamma [γ]-aminobutyric acid), horizontal cell
   release/cone phototransduction and, 262, 266, 267
GAGs. See Glycosaminoglycans
Gain of function mutations, 156
Galactokinase, defective/deficiency of, 175t
   galactosemia/cataract formation and, 247
Galactose
   in cataract formation, 247
   in lens glucose/carbohydrate metabolism, 247, 247f
Galactose-free diet, 203
Galactose-1-phosphate uridyltransferase, galactosemia
   caused by defects in, 175t
Galactosemia, 175t
   cataracts in, 246, 247
   dietary therapy for, 203
α-Galactosidase, defective/deficiency of, 175t
β-Galactosidase, defective/deficiency of, 175t
Galanin, in aqueous humor, 231
Gallamine, 315, 315t
Gametes, 186
Gamma (γ)-aminobutyric acid (GABA), horizontal cell
   release/cone phototransduction and, 262, 266, 267
Gamma (γ)-crystallins, 64, 244
Ganciclovir, 300t, 302, 357t, 358, 358t, 359–360
Ganciclovir sustained-release intraocular device/
   implant, 300t, 302, 357t, 360
Ganfort. See Bimatoprost, in combination preparations
Ganglion-blocking drugs, 315
Ganglion cells, retinal, 70, 70f, 71f, 74, 74f, 76f, 88f, 257,
   258f, 267, 267f, 268f
   development/differentiation of, 116t, 119f, 122
Ganglionic neurons, dilator muscle innervation and, 56
Gangliosidoses. See specific type under GM

Gap junctions, in lens, 246
Garamycin. *See* Gentamicin
Gases, intraocular, 300*t*
Gasserian ganglion (semilunar/trigeminal ganglion), 9*f*,
    98*f*, 99, 99*f*, 101*f*
Gastrulation, 111, 112*f*, 113*f*
Gatifloxacin, 346, 347–349, 347*t*
Gaucher disease, racial and ethnic concentration of, 197
GCAPs. *See* Guanylate cyclase–assisting proteins
GCL (ganglion cell layer). *See* Ganglion cells
Gel electrophoresis, denaturing gradient(DGGE), 162
Gelatinase (MMP-2), in vitreous, 249
Gene, 136, 184–187
    cancer, 156–157
    candidate, 161
    defective copy of (pseudogene), 142
    expression of. *See* Gene transcription
    structure of, 147–148, 148*f*
Gene assignments, 160
Gene dosage, 159
Gene duplication. *See* DNA, replication of
Gene linkage, 138, 150, 160, 184, 187
Gene mapping, 160, 184
Gene replacement therapy, 169
Gene therapy, 169–170, 170*f*, 204
Gene transcription, 144, 147, 151, 151*f*, 152
    embryogenesis and, 111
    reverse, 143
Gene translation, 144, 147, 151, 151*f*, 152
    gene product changes/modification after
        (posttranslational modification), 142
    of lens proteins, 245
Generalized gangliosidosis (GM₁ gangliosidosis
    type I), 175*t*
Genetic, definition of, 181
Genetic cascades, 111, 126
    in neural retinal development, 122
Genetic code, degeneracy of, 134
Genetic heterogeneity, 137, 183, 183*f*, 185
Genetic imprinting, 138, 153–154
Genetic Information Nondiscrimination Act
    (GINA), 136
Genetic map, 160, 184
Genetic markers, 159. *See also specific type*
Genetic testing/counseling, 171, 204–208
    accurate diagnosis and, 202, 204
    autosomal dominant disorders and, 178
    direct-to-consumer, 134
    disease process explanation and, 202
    family history/pedigree analysis and, 171, 204
    issues in, 205
    polygenic and multifactorial inheritance and, 140,
        141, 200
    prenatal diagnosis and, 188, 206–207
    recommendations for, 207–208
    reproductive issues and, 206–207
    support group referral and, 207
Genetics
    clinical, 171–208. *See also specific disorder*
        chromosomal analysis and, 187–193, 189*f*, 191*t*
        disease management and, 202–204
        genes and chromosomes and, 184–187, 186*f*
        genetic counseling and, 202, 204–208

importance of accurate diagnosis and, 202, 204
inheritance patterns and, 173–181. *See also
    specific type*
lyonization (X-chromosome inactivation) and, 132,
    139, 197–200, 198–199*f*, 199*t*
mutations and, 193–196
pedigree analysis in, 172–173, 172*f*
pharmacogenetics and, 141, 201–202
polygenic and multifactorial inheritance and, 140,
    141, 200–201
racial and ethnic concentration of disorders
    and, 196–197
terminology used in, 181–183, 182*f*, 183*f*
    introduction to, 131–145
    molecular, 147–170
        cell cycle and, 148–150, 149*f*
        correlation of genes with specific diseases
            and, 159–161
        DNA damage/repair and, 154–155
        gene structure and, 147–148, 148*f*
        gene therapy and, 169–170, 170*f*
        independent assortment and, 150
        linkage and, 138, 150, 160
        lyonization (X-chromosome inactivation) and, 132,
            139, 153
        mitochondrial disease and, 157–159
        mutations/disease and, 140, 155–157
            screening and, 161–167, 162*f*, 163*f*, 164*f*, 165*f*,
                166*f*, 167*f*, 168*f*
        noncoding (junk) DNA and, 150, 151
        transcription and translation (central dogma)
            and, 151–154, 151*f*
    personalized, 141
    terms used in, 131–145
Geniculate body/nucleus/ganglion, 101*f*, 103
    lateral, 90, 90*f*, 93, 267
Geniculocalcarine pathways (optic radiations), 90,
    90*f*, 93
Genome, 136, 181, 194
    reference, 143
Genome-wide association studies (GWAS), 136,
    163–167, 166*f*, 167*f*, 168*f*
Genomic DNA library, 138
Genomics, 136
Genoptic. *See* Gentamicin
Genotype, 136, 194
    database of, 134
Gentak. *See* Gentamicin
Gentamicin, 344*t*, 347*t*, 351
    in combination preparations, 348*t*
Gentasol. *See* Gentamicin
Germ layers, formation of, 111
Germinal mosaicism, 136
Germinative zone, of lens epithelium, 64, 242, 242*f*
Giant vacuoles, in Schlemm canal, 50–51, 50*f*, 51*f*
Gillespie syndrome (OMIM 206700), aniridia in, 193
GINA (Genetic Information Nondiscrimination
    Act), 136
Glands of Krause, 20*f*, 22*f*, 23*t*, 29, 216
Glands of Moll, 19, 22*f*, 23*t*
Glands of Wolfring, 20*f*, 22*f*, 23*t*, 29, 216
Glands of Zeis, 19, 22*f*, 23*t*, 215
    in tear-film lipids/tear production, 215

Glaucoma
    corticosteroid-induced, 334
    drugs for. *See* Antiglaucoma drugs
    genetic/hereditary factors in, 200
        genome-wide association studies (GWAS)
            and, 164, 166*f*, 168*f*
    ocular receptors and, 318*t*
Glial cells
    optic nerve, 86, 88*f*
    retinal, 73, 266
Globe, topographic features of, 37–38, 37*f*
Glucocorticoids, 329–334, 330*t*, 333*t*. *See also*
    Corticosteroids
Glucose
    in aqueous humor, 231*t*, 232
    in cataract formation, 247
    metabolism of
        in cornea, 224
        in lens, 246, 247, 247*f*
        in retinal pigment epithelium, 273
    in tear film, 216
    in vitreous, 231*t*
Glucose-6-phosphate, in lens glucose/carbohydrate
    metabolism, 246
Glucose-6-phosphate dehydrogenase deficiency,
    pharmacogenetics and, 201
Glucuronide transferase, defective/deficiency of, 175*t*
Glutamate
    in cone phototransduction, 266, 267
    in rod phototransduction, 259, 261
Glutathione
    in aqueous humor, 232–233
    in lens, 246, 284–285
        oxidative changes and, 283, 284–285
    in retina and retinal pigment epithelium, 251, 273, 287
Glutathione disulfide (GSSG), 283, 284
Glutathione peroxidase
    in aqueous humor, 231
    in lens, 284
    in retina and retinal pigment epithelium, 287
Glutathione redox cycle, 284, 285
Glutathione-S-transferase (GSH-S-Ts), in retina and
    retinal pigment epithelium, 287
Glycerin, 329, 329*t*
    in artificial tears, 341
Glycine cell transport, defective, 175*t*
Glycocalyx, corneal epithelium, 224
Glycolysis, in glucose/carbohydrate metabolism
    in cornea, 224
    in lens, 246
    in rod outer segments, 261
Glycoproteins
    corneal, 224–225
    in vitreous, 252
Glycosaminoglycans (GAGs), stromal, 41, 226
GM₁ gangliosidosis type I (generalized), 175*t*
GM₂ gangliosidosis type I (Tay-Sachs disease), 175*t*
    racial and ethnic concentration of, 197
GM₂ gangliosidosis type II (Sandhoff disease), 175*t*
Goblet cells, 22*f*, 23*t*, 30, 215*f*
    mucin tear secretion by, 22*f*, 215*f*, 217
Gramicidin, with polymyxin B and neomycin, 347*t*
    for *Acanthamoeba* keratitis, 361

Gray line (intermarginal sulcus), 19, 22*f*, 215
Greater superficial petrosal nerve, 101*f*, 103, 104
Ground substance, of cornea, 41
Growth factors, 127, 371–372
    in aqueous humor, 229, 234–235
    in ocular development, 111, 127
    in tear film, 217
Gruber (petroclinoid) ligament, 102
GSH. *See* Glutathione
GSH-Px. *See* Selenium-dependent glutathione peroxidase
GSH-S-Ts. *See* Glutathione-S-transferase
GSSG. *See* Glutathione disulfide
Guanylate cyclase
    mutations in, 263
    in rod phototransduction, 260*f*, 261
Guanylate cyclase–assisting proteins (GCAPs), 260*f*, 261
Gustatory nucleus, 103
GWAS (genome-wide association studies), 136, 163–167,
    166*f*, 167*f*, 168*f*
Gyrate atrophy, 175*t*
    ornithine aminotransferase defects causing, 175*t*, 265
    retinal pigment epithelium in, 279
Gyrus rectus, 83, 85*f*

Haller and Zinn, circle of (circle of Zinn), 88*f*, 91
Haploid/haploid number, 136, 149, 186
Haploid insufficiency (haploinsufficiency), 136
    in aniridia/*PAX6* gene disorders, 136, 193
    gene therapy for disorders caused by, 169
Haplotype, 136
HapMap, 136, 163
Hassall-Henle warts, 41
HCO₃. *See* Bicarbonate
Healon/Healon-GV/Healon-5, 368
Hearing loss (deafness), mitochondrial DNA mutations
    and, 157
Hedgehog family, gene expression/ocular development
    and, 127
Helicases, 154
Hemidesmosomes, 39, 40*f*
Hemizygote/hemizygous alleles, 137
    X-linked recessive inheritance and, 179
Hemoglobin, sickle cell, 184
Hemoglobinopathies, sickle cell. *See* Sickle cell disease
Hemorrhages, vitreous, 254
Henle, lacrimal gland of, 215*f*, 217
Henle fiber layer, 74, 74*f*
Heparan sulfate sulfatase, defective/deficiency of, 175*t*
Hepatolenticular degeneration (Wilson disease), 203
Hereditary, definition of, 137, 181. *See also* Genetics
Hereditary optic neuropathy, Leber, 158
    mitochondrial DNA mutations and, 157, 158
Heritable/heritability, definition of, 137, 182, 182*f*
Hermansky-Pudlak syndrome (HPS), racial and ethnic
    concentration of, 197
Herpes simplex virus, antiviral drugs for, 356–361,
    357–358*t*
    acyclovir, 357*t*, 358
Herpes zoster
    acyclovir for, 357*t*, 359
    famciclovir for, 357*t*, 359
    valacyclovir for, 357*t*, 359
Heterochromatin, 133

Heterogeneity, 137
  allelic, 132
  clinical, 133
  genetic, 137, 183, 183f, 185
  locus, 138
Heteroplasmy, 137, 147
  mitochondrial disease and, 157
Heterozygosity, loss of, 157
Heterozygote/heterozygous alleles, 137, 184. See also
    Carrier (genetic)
  carrier, 176
  compound, 133
  double, 185
  X-linked recessive inheritance and, 179
Hexokinase, in lens glucose/carbohydrate
    metabolism, 246
Hexosaminidase, defective/deficiency of, in
    gangliosidoses, 175t
Hexose monophosphate shunt, in glucose/carbohydrate
    metabolism
  in cornea, 224
  in lens, 246
  in rod outer segments, 261
Hexosidase, defective, 175t
HGP. See Human Genome Project
Hiatus semilunaris, 10f
Histamine, 337
  in tear film, 216
Histones, 148f, 151
History, family, 171
  genetic counseling and, 204
  pedigree analysis and, 171, 172–173, 172f
HMP shunt. See Hexose monophosphate shunt
HMS. See Medrysone
Holes, macular, vitreous in formation of, 254–255
Homatropine, 313, 314t
Homeobox, 137. See also Homeobox genes
Homeobox gene program, 126
Homeobox genes/homeotic selector genes, 126, 137, 152
  in ocular development, 126
Homeodomain, 126
Homeotic genes/homeotic selector genes. See
    Homeobox genes
Homocystinuria, 175t
  vitamin B₆ replacement therapy for, 203
Homogentisic acid/homogentisic acid oxidase,
    alkaptonuria and, 175t
Homologous chromosomes, 137, 184
Homoplasmy, 137
  replicative segregation and, 143, 157
Homotropaire. See Homatropine
Homozygote/homozygous alleles, 137, 184
Horizontal cells, 71f, 257, 258f, 266, 266–267, 266f
  in cone phototransduction, 262
Horner muscle, 21
Horner syndrome, dilator muscle and, 56
HOX genes, 126, 137
Hox (homeobox) gene program, in ocular
    development, 126
HPMC. See Hydroxypropyl methylcellulose
HPS. See Hermansky-Pudlak syndrome
Human gene mapping, 160, 184
Human Genome Project (HGP), 137, 160

Hunter syndrome, 175t
Hurler-Scheie syndrome, 185
Hurler syndrome, 175t, 184–185
Hyalocytes, 78–79
Hyaloid artery/system, development/regression of, 116t,
    118f, 119f, 122, 123f
Hyaloid (Cloquet) canal, 80
Hyaloideoretinopathies, hereditary, collagen chain
    mutations and, 255
Hyaluronan/hyaluronic acid
  off-label use of, 306
  in vitreous, 79, 79f, 249, 250–251
Hyaluronate/sodium hyaluronate, as viscoelastic, 306
Hyaluronidase
  for enzymatic vitreolysis, 255
  with local anesthetics, 364–365
  in vitreous, 249
Hybridization, 137–138
  fluorescence in situ (FISH), 188
Hydrocortisone
  anti-inflammatory/pressure-elevating potency
    of, 333t
  in combination preparations, 348t
Hydrogen peroxide, 281–282, 282, 282f, 287, 288. See
    also Free radicals
Hydroperoxides (ROOH), 283
Hydroxyamphetamine, 314t, 320
  with tropicamide, 314t
Hydroxyethylcellulose, in artificial tears, 341
Hydroxyl/hydroxy radicals, 281, 282, 282f, 283. See also
    Free radicals
9-2-Hydroxypropoxymethylguanine. See Ganciclovir
Hydroxypropyl methylcellulose (HPMC)
  in artificial tears, 341
  as viscoelastic, 368
Hyperglycemia, cataract formation and. See Diabetes
    mellitus, cataracts associated with
Hyperglycinemia, 175t
Hyperosmolar agents, 366
Hyperosmotic/osmotic agents, 328–329, 329t
Hypertension, phenylephrine causing, 317, 318
Hypoblast, 112f
Hypokalemia, carbonic anhydrase inhibitors
    causing, 326

Ibuprofen, 335t
ICA. See Internal carotid artery
ICSI. See Intracytoplasmic sperm injection
Idoxuridine, 356, 357t
α-L-Iduronidase, defective/deficiency of, 175t, 184
Ig. See under Immunoglobulin
IGF. See Insulin-like growth factors
IGFBPs. See Insulin-like growth factor binding proteins
Ihh factor, gene expression/ocular development
    and, 127
ILM. See Internal limiting membrane
Imidazoles, 355t, 356
  for Acanthamoeba keratitis, 361
Imipenem-cilastin, 344t
Immune response (immunity), glucocorticoids
    affecting, 331
Immunoglobulin A (IgA)/secretory immunoglobulin A
    (sIGA), in tear film, 216

Immunoglobulin D (IgD), in tear film, 216
Immunoglobulin E (IgE), in tear film, 216
Immunoglobulin G (IgG), in tear film, 216
Immunoglobulin M (IgM), in tear film, 216
Immunomodulatory therapy, 333
Imprinting (genetic), 138, 153–154
IMT. *See* Immunomodulatory therapy
In situ hybridization, fluorescence (FISH), 188
In vitro fertilization (IVF), genetic counseling
    and, 206, 207
Inborn errors of metabolism
    dietary therapy in, 203
    enzyme defect in, 174, 175*t*
    ocular findings in, 175*t*
Incest, pedigree analysis and, 172, 172*f*, 205
Incomplete penetrance (skipped generation), 177
Incontinentia pigmenti (Bloch-Sulzberger syndrome), 180
Indels, 133–134, 148
Independent assortment, 150, 187
Index case (proband), 142, 172
Indirect traumatic optic neuropathy, 89
Indocyanine green, 367, 367–368
    intravenous administration of, 301, 367. *See also*
        Indocyanine green angiography
Indocyanine green angiography, 367
Indomethacin, 335*t*, 336
    prostaglandin synthesis affected by, 239
Infantile, 181
Infantile Refsum disease, 175*t*
    gene defects causing, 265, 266
Inferior meatus, 6, 8
Inferior oblique muscle, 7, 13, 13*f*, 14*f*, 15*t*, 20*f*
    blood supply of, 15*t*, 33*f*, 34*f*
    innervation of, 17, 94*f*, 95
    insertions of, 14*f*, 15, 15*t*
    origins of, 15*t*, 17
Inferior oblique tendon, 14*f*
Inferior orbital fissure, 6*f*, 8–10
Inferior petrosal nerve, 103
Inferior petrosal sinus, 106*f*
Inferior punctum, 29
Inferior rectus muscle, 9*f*, 13, 13*f*, 14*f*, 15*t*, 16*f*, 20*f*
    blood supply of, 15*t*, 17, 33*f*, 34*f*
    innervation of, 17, 94*f*, 95
    insertions of, 13–15, 14*f*, 15*t*
    origins of, 15*t*, 17
Inferior rectus tendon, 13*f*, 14*f*
Inflamase Forte. *See* Prednisolone
Inflammation (ocular)
    treatment of. *See* Anti-inflammatory drugs
    vitreal, 254
Inflammatory mediators. *See* Mediators (inflammatory)
Infraorbital artery
    extraocular muscles supplied by, 17
    orbit supplied by, 33*f*
Infraorbital canal, 6*f*, 8, 16*f*
Infraorbital foramen, 7
Infraorbital groove, 7
Infraorbital nerve, 8, 100
Infraorbital vein, 9*f*, 35*f*
Inheritance. *See also* Genetics
    codominant, 133
    digenic, 134

    dominant, 134, 173–174, 177
        autosomal, 177–178, 178*t*
        disorders associated with, 134
            gene therapy for, 169–170, 170*f*
            X-linked, 180–181
        X-linked, 179–180, 181*t*
    maternal, 157, 181
    multifactorial/polygenic, 140, 141, 200–201
    patterns of, 173–181
    recessive, 142, 173–174
        autosomal, 174–177, 175*t*, 177*t*
        disorders associated with, 142, 174–177, 175*t*
        gene therapy for, 169
        X-linked, 179, 180*t*
    sex-linked, 143
    X-linked, 145, 178–181
        disorders associated with, 180–181
        gene therapy for, 169
    Y-linked, 145
Inhibitors (drugs), 304
INL. *See* Inner nuclear layer
Inner nuclear layer (INL), 70*f*, 71*f*, 74, 74*f*, 76*f*, 88*f*, 258*f*,
    266–268, 266*f*, 267*f*, 268*f*
Inner plexiform layer (IPL), 70*f*, 71*f*, 74, 74*f*, 88*f*
Inner segments, photoreceptor, 69, 70, 70*f*, 72*f*, 74*f*. *See
    also* Cone inner segments; Rod inner segments
    free-radical leakage from, 285
Inositol, in aqueous humor, 232
Inositol-1,4,5-triphosphate (IP$_3$), in tear
    secretion, 218, 218*f*
Insertions, mitochondrial DNA, disorders caused by, 157
Insulin-like growth factor binding proteins, in aqueous
    humor, 234, 235
Insulin-like growth factors, 371–372
    in aqueous humor, 234, 235
Intercavernous sinus, 106*f*
Interferons, 370–371
    in tear film, 216–217
Interleukin-1α, in tear film, 217
Interleukin-1β, in tear film, 217
Intermarginal sulcus (gray line), 19, 22*f*, 215
Intermediate zone, of lens epithelium, 64, 65*f*
Intermediated filaments, 245
Intermittent ataxia, 175*t*
Intermuscular septum, 31
Internal carotid artery, 90, 105
    cranial nerve relationship and, 84*f*, 85*f*
    optic nerve supplied by, 84*f*, 85*f*, 90, 91
Internal limiting membrane (ILM), 70*f*, 71*f*, 75, 88*f*, 258*f*
    optic disc, 86, 88*f*
    vitreous detachment and, 253
Internal scleral sulcus, 48
Interphase, 149
Interphotoreceptor matrix (IPM), 273, 275*f*
    retinal pigment epithelium in maintenance of, 273
Interphotoreceptor retinoid-binding protein (IRBP),
    275, 275*f*
Intersexes, 192
Intervening sequence. *See* Intron
Intracameral injections, 299, 300*t*
    acetylcholine, 300*t*, 309, 310
    carbachol, 300*t*, 309, 310
    lidocaine, 300*t*, 365–366

Intracanalicular region of optic nerve, 83, 85*t*, 89–90
  blood supply of, 85*t*, 89, 91
Intracranial region of optic nerve, 83, 85*t*, 90, 90*f*
  blood supply of, 85*t*, 90, 91, 92*f*
Intracytoplasmic sperm injection (ICSI), 207
Intramuscular circle of iris, 34*f*, 35
Intramuscular drugs, in ocular pharmacology, 301
Intramuscular plexus, ciliary body, 58
Intraocular medications, 299, 300*t*
Intraocular pressure
  aqueous humor dynamics and, 230
  corticosteroids affecting, 299, 332, 332–333, 333*t*
  cycloplegics affecting, 313
  drugs for lowering. *See* Antiglaucoma drugs
Intraocular region of optic nerve, 83, 85, 85*t*, 86–87, 88*f*
  blood supply of, 85*t*
Intraorbital region of optic nerve, 83, 85, 85*t*, 87–89
  blood supply of, 85*t*, 91, 91*f*
Intravenous drug administration, in ocular
    pharmacology, 301
Intravitreal medications, 299, 300*t*
  compounded, 306–307
Intron, 138, 147, 148, 148*f*, 151
  excision of, 152. *See also* Splicing
Iodine, 354
Ionic charge, of ocular medication, absorption affected
    by, 298
Ionizing radiation
  DNA repair after, 154
  in free-radical generation, 282, 283
Iontophoresis, for drug delivery, 304
Iopidine. *See* Apraclonidine
IP₃. *See* Inositol-1,4,5-triphosphate
IPL. *See* Inner plexiform layer
IPM. *See* Interphotoreceptor matrix
IRBP. *See* Interphotoreceptor retinoid-binding protein
Irides. *See* Iris
Iridocyclitis, muscarinic antagonists for, 313
Iris, 37*f*, 46*f*, 47*f*, 53–56, 53*f*, 54*f*, 56*f*, 236–240
  absence of/rudimentary (aniridia), 193
    short arm 11 deletion syndrome/*PAX6* gene
        mutations and, 152, 177, 193
  anatomy of, 37*f*, 46*f*, 47*f*, 53–56, 53*f*, 54*f*, 56*f*
  anterior border/pigmented layer of, 54–55, 55, 56*f*
  biochemistry and metabolism of, 236–240
  collarette of, 54*f*, 55
  cysts of, muscarinic therapy and, 311
  development of, 116*t*, 122
  innervation of, 55
  intramuscular circle of, 34*f*, 35
  pigmentation of, 53, 54, 55, 56*f*, 236
    prostaglandin analogues/latanoprost affecting, 327
  posterior pigmented layer of, 53*f*, 55, 56*f*
  smooth muscle in, 237
  stroma of, 54–55, 56*f*
    development of, 122
  topography of, 37*f*
  vessels of, 35, 54*f*, 55
Iris diaphragm, 53
Iris dilator. *See* Dilator muscle
Iris pigment epithelium, 53*f*, 55, 56*f*
Iris processes, 46*f*
Iris sphincter. *See* Sphincter muscle
Iritis, mydriatic/muscarinic antagonists for, 313

Iron
  in aqueous humor, 232
  in free-radical formation, 281–282, 283
Irreversible cholinesterase inhibitors, 312
Irrigation, solutions for, 367
Ismotic. *See* Isosorbide
Isoflurophate, 309*f*
Isoforms, 152
Isolated (simplex) case/genetic disease, 143, 182
Isoniazid, pharmacogenetics of, 201
Isoproterenol, 308*t*
Isopto Atropine. *See* Atropine
Isopto Carbachol. *See* Carbachol
Isopto Carpine. *See* Pilocarpine
Isopto Homatropine. *See* Homatropine
Isopto Hyoscine. *See* Scopolamine
Isosorbide, 329
Istalol. *See* Timolol
Itraconazole, 355*t*, 356
IVF. *See* In vitro fertilization

Junctional complexes
  in corneal endothelium, 43, 227
  in retinal pigment epithelium, 68, 272
Junk (noncoding) DNA, 150, 151
Juxtacanalicular tissue, 48

K. *See* Potassium
Kanamycin, 344*t*, 351
Karyotype/karyotyping, 138, 188, 189*f*
kb. *See* Kilobase
KCS. *See* Keratoconjunctivitis sicca
Kearns-Sayre syndrome, 158
  mitochondrial DNA defects and, 157, 158
Keratan sulfate, in cornea, 41, 226
Keratectomy, photorefractive (PRK), Bowman layer
    and, 225
Keratitis
  Acanthamoeba, treatment of, 361
  corticosteroid route of administration in, 333*t*
  herpes simplex, antiviral drugs for, 356–361,
    357–358*t*
Keratoconjunctivitis sicca (dry eye syndrome), tear
    dysfunction in, 220, 221–222, 221*f*
Keratocytes, 41, 225
  glucose/carbohydrate metabolism in, 224
Ketoconazole, 355*t*, 356
Ketoprofen, 335*t*
Ketorolac, 330*t*, 335*t*, 336, 338*t*
Ketotifen, 238, 338*t*, 339
Kidney transplantation, for cystinosis, 203
KIF21A gene mutations, congenital extraocular muscle
    disorders and, 124
Kilobase, 138
Krabbe leukodystrophy, 175*t*
Krause, glands of, 20*f*, 22*f*, 23*t*, 29, 216

L-cone opsin genes, 262
  mutations in, 262, 264
L cones, 262
  bipolar cells for, 266
  horizontal cells for, 266
  retinal ganglion cells for, 267, 267*f*, 268*f*
L-type calcium channels, mutations in, 264

Labyrinthine segment, of cranial nerve VII (facial), 103
Lacrimal artery, 28–29, 33f, 34f
    extraocular muscles supplied by, 17
Lacrimal bone, 5, 6, 6f
Lacrimal canaliculi, 23f, 29, 30
Lacrimal crests, anterior and posterior, 5, 6f
Lacrimal drainage system, 29–30, 29f
Lacrimal ducts, 22f, 28
Lacrimal glands, 9f, 22f, 23t, 28–29, 28f, 101f, 215f, 216
    accessory, 22f, 23t, 29, 215f, 216
    aqueous component/tears produced by, 22f, 215f, 216,
        217–220, 218f, 219f
    development of, 125–126
    of Henle and Manz, 215f, 217
    orbital, 28, 216
    palpebral, 28, 216
    parasympathetic innervation of, 100, 101f, 104, 216
Lacrimal nerve, 9f, 100, 101f
Lacrimal nucleus, 103, 104
Lacrimal papillae, 29
Lacrimal pump, ocular medication absorption affected
        by, 296
Lacrimal puncta, 18f, 22f, 29
Lacrimal reflex arc, 101f
Lacrimal sac (tear sac), 29
Lacrimal system. See also specific structure
    excretory apparatus of, 29–30, 29f
    secretory apparatus/function of, 22f, 28–29, 28f,
        217–220, 218f, 219f. See also Lacrimal glands
Lactate/lactic acid
    in aqueous humor, 232
    in cornea, glucose metabolism and, 224
    in tear film, 216
Lactoferrin, in tear film, 216
Lambda (λ)-bacteriophage, as vector, 145
Lamellae, corneal, 40–41, 225–226
Lamina cribrosa, 87, 88f
    blood supply of, 91, 91f, 92f
    development of, 116t
Lamina fusca, 44
Lamina papyracea (ethmoid/ethmoidal bone), 6, 6f
Laminar area of optic nerve, 85t, 86, 87
    blood supply of, 91
Laminin, 64, 250, 251f
Langerhans cells, 40
LASEK (laser subepithelial keratomileusis), Bowman
    layer and, 225
LASIK (laser in situ keratomileusis), Bowman layer
    and, 225
Lastacaft. See Alcaftadine
Latanoprost, 237, 302, 327, 327t
    in combination preparations, 327t
Lateral canthal tendon, 17f
Lateral geniculate body/nucleus, 90, 90f, 93, 267
Lateral orbital tubercle of Whitnall, 7
Lateral orbital wall, 7
Lateral pontine cistern, 103
Lateral rectus muscle, 9f, 13, 14f, 15t, 16f, 17f
    blood supply of, 15t, 17, 34f
    innervation of, 17
    insertions of, 13–15, 14f, 15t
    origins of, 15t, 17
Lateral rectus tendon, 13f, 14f

Leber congenital amaurosis
    genetic heterogeneity in, 183, 183f
    guanylate cyclase mutations causing, 263
    RPE65 gene defects causing, 264
Leber hereditary optic neuropathy, 158
    mitochondrial DNA mutations and, 157, 158
Leigh syndrome (Leigh necrotizing encephalopathy),
        159, 175t
    mitochondrial DNA mutations and, 159
Lens (crystalline), 17f, 37f, 63–67, 63f, 65f, 77f,
        241–248
    anatomy of, 17f, 37f, 63–67, 63f, 65f, 77f, 241–243, 242f
    antioxidants in, 284f
    biochemistry and metabolism of, 241–248
        carbohydrate ("sugar") cataracts and, 246–248
    capsule of. See Lens capsule
    carbohydrate metabolism in, 246
    changing shape of. See Accommodation
    chemical composition of, 243–245
    cortex of, 64, 242–243, 242f
    development/embryology of, 65f, 117–122, 120f
    energy production in, 246
    epithelium of, 63f, 64, 65f, 242, 242f
    free radicals affecting, 283–285, 284f
    in Marfan syndrome, 66
    membranes of, 243
    nucleus of, 64, 242–243, 242f
        embryonic, 64, 65f
    oxidative damage to, 283–285, 284f
    physiology of, 245–246
    size of, 63
    sutures of, 64, 65f
    topography of, 37f
    zonular fibers/zonules of, 37f, 46f, 63f, 65f, 66–67, 241
        development of, 120, 120f
Lens capsule, 37f, 63, 63f, 64, 65f, 241, 242f
    anatomy of, 37f, 63, 63f, 64, 65f, 241, 242f
    development of, 118–120, 119f
Lens crystallins, 64, 241, 243–244. See also Crystallins
Lens-fiber plasma membranes, 243, 245
Lens fibers, 63f, 64, 65f, 66f, 242–243, 242f
    development of, 120f
    zonular (zonules of Zinn), 37f, 46f, 63f, 65f, 66–67, 241
        development of, 120, 120f
Lens pit, 117–118, 117f
Lens placode, 115, 116t, 117f
Lens plate, 117
Lens proteins, 243–245
    crystallins, 64, 241, 243–244. See also Crystallins
    cytoskeletal and membrane, 245
    posttranslational modification of, 245
Lens vesicle, 117f, 118, 120f
Leucine zipper, neural retinal (Nrl), in retinal
        development, 122
Leukodystrophy
    Krabbe, 175t
    metachromatic, 175t
Leukotrienes, 237, 334
    synthesis of, 238f
Levator aponeurosis, 20f, 24, 216
Levator muscle (levator palpebrae superioris), 9f, 13,
        13f, 14f, 16f, 20f, 23–24
    innervation of, 17, 94f, 95
    origins of, 17

Levobunolol, 321, 322*t*, 323
Levocabastine, 337, 338*t*
Levofloxacin, 346, 347–349, 347*t*
LHON. *See* Leber hereditary optic neuropathy
Library, DNA, 138
    cDNA, 138
    genomic, 138
Lid margin. *See* Eyelids, margin of
Lidocaine, 362*t*, 363*t*, 364, 365, 365–366
    intracameral administration of, 300*t*, 364, 365, 365–366
Lifitegrast, 342
Ligands, 111, 127
    optic nerve development and, 124
Light
    cone opsin changes caused by, 261
    eye injury caused by, 283, 286
    photo-oxidative processes triggered by, 283
        in retina, 286
    pupillary response to. *See* Pupillary light reflex
    retinal changes caused by, 283, 286
    retinal pigment epithelial transport systems affected
        by, 277
    rhodopsin changes caused by, 258, 259, 259*f*
Light adaptation, 262
Light–near dissociation, 96
Light reflex, pathways for, 96
Light toxicity/photic damage/phototoxicity
    free-radical damage and, 283, 286
    retinal, 286
Likelihood ratio, 160
    logarithm of (LOD score), 138–139, 160
Limbal stem cells, deficiency of, 40
Limbus, 44–45, 45*f*
Limiting membranes
    external (ELM), 71*f*, 72*f*, 74, 76*f*, 88*f*, 258*f*
    internal (ILM), 70*f*, 71*f*, 75, 88*f*, 258*f*
        optic disc, 86, 88*f*
        vitreous detachment and, 253
    middle, 258*f*
LINEs. *See* Long interspersed elements
Lingual nerve, 101*f*
Link protein, in vitreous, 249
Linkage (gene), 138, 150, 160, 184, 187
Linkage disequilibrium (allelic association), 138, 150
Lipid layer of tear film, 38, 213*f*, 214–215, 215*f*
Lipid peroxidation, 281, 283
    mechanisms of, 282–283
    retinal vulnerability and, 285
Lipid strip, 214
Lipids
    in retinal pigment epithelium, 274
    solubility of, medication absorption affected
        by, 297–298, 300
    in tear film. *See* Lipid layer of tear film
Lipocalins, in tear film, 216
Lipofuscin granules (wear-and-tear pigment), 69
    in retinal pigment epithelium phagocytosis, 276, 276*f*
Liposomes, for drug delivery, 303–304
Lipoxygenase, in eicosanoid synthesis, 238–239, 238*f*,
    334
Lissamine green, 367
Local anesthesia, 362–366, 362*t*, 363*t*
    for anterior segment surgery, 365–366
    cholinesterase inhibitor use and, 312, 363

Lockwood, suspensory ligament of (Lockwood
    ligament), 32, 32*f*
Locus (gene), 138, 184. *See also* Gene
Locus heterogeneity, 138
LOD score, 138–139, 160
Lodoxamide, 337, 338*t*
Logarithm of *odds*/logarithm of the likelihood ratio
    (LOD score), 138–139, 160
Long (q) arm, 142, 148*f*
Long arm 13 deletion (13q14) syndrome, 192
Long ciliary nerves, 12, 32, 100, 223–224
Long interspersed elements (LINEs), 150
Longitudinal fasciculus, medial, 101–102, 102*f*
Loop of Meyer, 90*f*, 93
Loss of function mutations, 156
Loss of heterozygosity, 157
Lotemax. *See* Loteprednol
Loteprednol, 330*t*, 334, 338*t*, 339
    with tobramycin, 334, 348*t*
Louis-Bar syndrome (ataxia-telangiectasia), *ATM*
    (ataxia-telangiectasia mutated) gene in, 154
Low-molecular-weight solutes, in vitreous, 252
Lowe syndrome, ocular findings in carriers of, 199*t*, 200
LOXL1, in exfoliation syndrome, 167, 168*f*
Lumigan. *See* Bimatoprost
Lutein, 77
    antioxidant effect of, 286, 288
    in retina, 267, 288
Lymphatics (afferent lymphatic channels), eyelid, 27, 27*f*
Lymphoid tissues, mucosa-associated (MALT), of
    conjunctiva (conjunctiva-associated/CALT), 30
Lyonization (X-chromosome inactivation/Barr body),
    132, 139, 153, 197–200
    ocular findings in carrier states and, 197–200, 198*f*,
        199*t*
Lysozyme, in tear film, 216
Lysyl hydroxylase, in Ehlers-Danlos syndrome, 175*t*

M-cone opsin genes, 262
    mutations in, 262, 264
M cones, 262
    bipolar cells for, 266
    horizontal cells for, 266
    retinal ganglion cells for, 267, 267*f*, 268*f*
M phase, cell cycle, 148, 148–149, 149*f*
Macroglia, retinal, 268
α_2-Macroglobulin, in aqueous humor, 231, 233, 234
Macrolides, 352–353
    polyene, 354, 355*t*
Macugen. *See* Pegaptanib
Macula/macula lutea, 67, 68*f*, 75–77, 75*f*, 76*f*
    anatomy of, 67, 68*f*
Macular dystrophies
    Sorsby
        retinal pigment epithelium in, 278
        TIMP3 defects causing, 161, 265
    vitelliform (Best disease)
        bestrophin defect causing, 265
        identification of carriers for, 178, 196
        retinal pigment epithelium in, 278
Macular edema
    cystoid, corticosteroid route of administration in, 333*t*
    diabetic, corticosteroid route of administration
        in, 333*t*

Macular fibers/projections, 92–93
Macular holes, vitreous in formation of, 254–255
Magnesium
    in aqueous humor, 232
    in tear film, 214t
Main sensory nucleus, of cranial nerve V (trigeminal),
    97, 98f, 101f
Major (greater) arterial circle, 34f, 35, 45f, 55
    ciliary body, 58
Major intrinsic protein (MIP/aquaporin), 242, 245
MAK-associated retinitis pigmentosa, racial and ethnic
    concentration of, 197
Malattia leventinese
    EFEMP1 defects causing, 265
    retinal pigment epithelium in, 279
MALT. See Mucosa-associated lymphoid tissue
Mandibular nerve. See Cranial nerve V (trigeminal
    nerve), V₃
Manhattan plot, 139, 164, 166f, 167f
Mannitol, 233, 328–329, 329t
α-Mannosidase, defective/deficiency of, 175t
Mannosidosis, 175t
Manz, lacrimal gland of, 215f, 217
Maple syrup urine disease, 175t
Marcaine. See Bupivacaine
Marfan syndrome
    fibrillin defects in, 66, 252
    pleiotropism and, 196
Margin, lid. See Eyelids, margin of
Marginal arterial arcades
    conjunctiva supplied by, 30
    eyelids supplied by, 25, 26f
Marginal mandibular nerve, 104
Marginal tear strip (tear meniscus), 213
Markers (gene), 159. See also specific type
Marshall syndrome, vitreous collapse in, 255
Massively parallel DNA sequencing (next-generation
    sequencing/NGS), 140, 142, 161, 163f, 164f, 165f, 166f
Mast-cell stabilizers, 337, 338, 338t
Mast cells, 337
Mastoid segment, of cranial nerve VII (facial), 103
Maternal age, Down syndrome incidence and, 190
Maternal inheritance, 157, 181. See also
    Mitochondrial DNA
Maternally inherited diabetes and deafness (MIDD),
    mitochondrial DNA mutation and, 159
Mating, assortative, 132
Matrix metalloproteinases (MMPs)
    in cornea, 226
    for dry eye, 221, 221f
    in vitreous, 249
Maxidex. See Dexamethasone
Maxilla/maxillary bone, 5, 6, 6f
Maxillary artery, 33f
Maxillary nerve. See Cranial nerve V (trigeminal
    nerve), V₂
Maxillary sinuses, 10–11, 10f
Maxitrol. See Dexamethasone, in combination
    preparations
Mecamylamine, 315t
Meckel cave, 99
Medial canthal tendon, 17f
Medial longitudinal fasciculus, 101–102, 102f
Medial orbital wall, 6

Medial rectus muscle, 9f, 13, 14f, 15t, 16f, 17f
    blood supply of, 15t, 17, 33f, 34f
    innervation of, 17, 94, 94f, 95
    insertions of, 13–15, 14f, 15t
    optic nerve and, 87
    origins of, 15t, 17
Medial rectus tendon, 13f, 14f
Mediators (inflammatory), 337
Medications. See Drugs
Medrysone, 330t
    anti-inflammatory/pressure-elevating potency
        of, 333t
Meibomian (tarsal) glands, 20f, 22f, 23t, 24, 25f,
    214–215, 215f
    dysfunction of, 220
    in tear-film lipids/tear production, 24, 214–215,
        214f, 217
Meiosis, 139, 149–150, 186, 186f
    nondisjunction during, 186f, 189. See also
        Nondisjunction
Melanin
    defective synthesis of, in albinism, 174, 278
    photoprotective function of, 278, 286
    in retinal pigment epithelium, 272, 277–278
α-Melanocyte-stimulating hormone (α-MSH), in tear
    secretion, 219
Melanocytes
    choroidal, 60f, 62
    in iris stroma, 54
Melanogenesis, 277–278
    latanoprost and, 327
Melanosomes
    in choroid, 62
    in ciliary body epithelium, 57
    in iris dilator muscle, 55
    in retinal pigment epithelium, 68–69
MELAS (mitochondrial myopathy with encephalopathy/
    lactic acidosis/strokelike episodes) syndrome,
    mitochondrial DNA mutation and, 157, 159
Meloxicam, 335t
Membrane lens proteins, 245
Membrane sacs, in rods, 257
Membranes
    Bowman, 40, 40f, 45f, 223f, 225. See also Bowman
        layer/membrane
    Bruch, 60–61, 61f, 70f, 71f, 271–272, 272f. See also
        Bruch membrane
    Descemet, 41, 42f, 223f, 227. See also Descemet
        membrane/layer
    limiting membranes, 70f, 71f, 72f, 74, 75, 76f, 88f,
        258f. See also Limiting membranes
    retrocorneal fibrous, 227
Mendelian disorder (single-gene disorder), 139, 194
Meninges, optic nerve, 87–89, 89f
Mepivacaine, 362t, 364
MERRF. See Myoclonic epilepsy with ragged red fibers
Mesencephalic nucleus, of cranial nerve V (trigeminal),
    97, 98f, 101f
Mesencephalon, cranial nerve III (oculomotor) arising
    from, 94
Mesoderm, 111, 112f, 113f, 114f
    ocular structures derived from, 115t
Messenger RNA (mRNA), 147, 151, 151f, 152
    precursor, 148, 151f, 152

Metabolic acidosis, carbonic anhydrase inhibitors
  causing, 325–326
  aspirin interactions and, 336
Metabolic disorders, enzyme defects/ocular signs
  in, 175t
Metabolomics, 136
Metachromatic leukodystrophy, 175t
Metalloproteinases, matrix
  in cornea, 226
  for dry eye, 221, 221f
  in vitreous, 249
Metaphase, 149, 149f
Metarhodopsin II, 259
Methazolamide, 324, 325, 325t, 326
Methicillin, 344, 344t
Methylation, DNA, 139, 151, 153
Methylcellulose, 297
  in artificial tears, 341
  hydroxypropyl (HPMC)
    in artificial tears, 341
    as viscoelastic, 368
Methylene blue, intracameral administration of, 300t
Methylprednisolone, 329
Metipranolol, 321, 322t, 323
Metoprolol, 317f
Meyer loop, 90f, 93
Mezlocillin, 345
Miconazole, 355t, 356
  for Acanthamoeba keratitis, 361
Microglia, retinal, 73, 268
Microperoxisomes, in retinal pigment epithelium, 273
Microplicae, in corneal epithelium, 39–40, 40f, 224
MicroRNA (miRNA), 139
Microsatellites, 139, 150
Microsomal triglyceride transfer protein (MTP)
  mutations, 265
Microtubules, 245
Microvilli, in corneal epithelium, 39–40, 40f, 224
Midbrain, cranial nerve III (oculomotor) arising
  from, 94
MIDD (maternally inherited diabetes and deafness),
  mitochondrial DNA mutation and, 159
Middle cerebral artery, 107f
  cranial nerve relationship and, 84f, 85f
Middle limiting membrane, 258f
Minocycline, 350
Minor (lesser) arterial circle, 54f, 55
Miochol. See Acetylcholine
Miosis/miotic drugs, 308, 308t, 309, 310, 311, 311t
  adrenergic antagonists, 321
  direct-acting muscarinic agonists, 308–312, 308t, 311t
  for glaucoma, 311, 318t
  indirect-acting muscarinic agonists (cholinesterase
    inhibitors), 311t, 312–313
MIP. See Major intrinsic protein
miRNA. See MicroRNA
Mismatch repair, 154
Missense mutation, 140, 155
  of mitochondrial DNA, 157
Mitochondria, 147, 148f
Mitochondrial DNA (mtDNA), 147, 148f
  diseases associated with deletions/mutations
    of, 157–159

Leber hereditary optic neuropathy, 157, 158
  maternal inheritance/transmission and, 157, 181
  MELAS and MIDD, 159
  NARP (neuropathy/ataxia/retinitis pigmentosa)
    syndrome, 157, 158–159
  replicative segregation and, 143, 157
Mitochondrial myopathy, with encephalopathy/
  lactic acidosis/strokelike episodes (MELAS),
  mitochondrial DNA mutation and, 157, 159
Mitomycin/mitomycin C, 339
  off-label use of, 306
Mitosis, 140, 148, 149f, 185
  nondisjunction during, 191. See also Nondisjunction
Mittendorf dot, 80, 81f
MMP. See Matrix metalloproteinases
MMP-2, in vitreous, 249
MMP-2 proenzyme, in cornea, 226
Mn SOD (superoxide dismutase), 287
Molecular genetics. See Genetics, molecular
Moll, glands of, 19, 22f, 23t
Monoamine oxidase inhibitors, apraclonidine/
  brimonidine interactions and, 319
Monochromatism/achromatopsia
  blue-cone, 264
    ocular findings in carriers of, 199t
  gene defects causing, 264
  with myopia, racial and ethnic concentration of, 197
  rod, 264
Monogenic (mendelian) disorder, 139
Monosomy, 189
Morphogenic gradients, 127
Morphogens, 127
Morula, 112f
Mosaicism (mosaic), 140, 190–192
  germinal, 136
  sex chromosome, 191–192
  trisomy 21, 191
Motor nucleus
  of cranial nerve III (oculomotor), 94, 94f
  of cranial nerve IV (trochlear), 96
  of cranial nerve V (trigeminal), 97, 98f, 99
  of cranial nerve VI (abducens), 101, 102f
  of cranial nerve VII (facial), 102f, 103
Motor root
  of cranial nerve III (oculomotor), 11, 12f
  of cranial nerve V (trigeminal), 99
  of cranial nerve VII (facial), 102
Moxeza. See Moxifloxacin
Moxifloxacin, 346, 347–349, 347t
Moxisylyte. See Thymoxamine
mRNA. See Messenger RNA
α-MSH (α-melanocyte-stimulating hormone), in tear
  secretion, 219
mtDNA. See Mitochondrial DNA
MTP (microsomal triglyceride transfer protein)
  mutations, 265
Mucins, tear film, 38, 213f, 217, 224
  deficiency/dysfunction and, 217, 220
  secretion of, 217
Mucoceles, 10
Mucomyst. See Acetylcysteine
Mucopolysaccharidosis I H (Hurler syndrome), 175t,
  184–185

Mucopolysaccharidosis I S (Scheie syndrome), 175*t*, 184
Mucopolysaccharidosis II (Hunter syndrome), 175*t*
Mucopolysaccharidosis III (Sanfilippo syndrome), 175*t*
Mucosa-associated lymphoid tissue (MALT), of
    conjunctiva (conjunctiva-associated/CALT), 30
Müller cells/fibers
    optic nerve, 86, 88*f*
    retinal, 71*f*, 73, 258*f*, 266, 268
Müller muscle (superior tarsal muscle), 20*f*, 24
Multifactorial/polygenic inheritance, 140, 141, 200–201
Multigene disorder (complex genetic disorder), 133,
    200–201
Mural cells, retinal blood vessel, 73
Muscarine, 308, 308*t*
Muscarinic drugs, 308*t*, 311*t*
    agonists, 308*t*
        direct-acting, 308–312, 310*f*, 311*t*
        indirect-acting, 312–313
    antagonists, 308*t*, 313–314, 314*t*
        adverse effects of, 313–314
Muscarinic receptors, 308, 308*t*
    drugs affecting, 308*t*, 311*t*, 315*t*. See also Muscarinic
        drugs
    signal transduction and, 316*t*
    in tear secretion, 218, 218*f*
Muscle of Riolan, 21
Muscles, extraocular. See Extraocular muscles
Mutagens, 194
Mutation, 140, 155–157, 193–196. See also specific type
    base pair, 155, 156
        conserved, 156
    carrier of, 132, 176, 197–200
        identification of, 205, 206
        ocular findings in, 198–200, 198–199*f*, 199*t*
    dominant negative, 134
    frameshift (framing error/frameshift), 135, 155
    gain/loss of function, 156
    missense, 140, 155
        of mitochondrial DNA, 157
    nonsense, 140, 155
        of mitochondrial DNA, 157
    null, 155
    point, 193
        mitochondrial DNA, 157
        screening for, 161, 163*f*, 164*f*, 165*f*, 166*f*
    polymorphism and, 155, 156, 194
    repair and, 154
    screening for, 161–167, 162*f*, 163*f*, 164*f*, 165*f*, 166*f*,
        167*f*, 168*f*
Myasthenia gravis, 315
    diagnosis of, 301, 315
Mydfrin. See Phenylephrine
Mydral. See Tropicamide
Mydriacyl. See Tropicamide
Mydriasis/mydriatics, 314*t*
    adrenergic agents, 314*t*, 317–318
    muscarinic antagonists, 313–314, 314*t*
Myocilin gene, in glaucoma, 200
Myoclonic epilepsy with ragged red fibers (MERRF),
    mitochondrial DNA mutations and, 157
Myoepithelial cells
    iris, 55, 56*f*
    lacrimal gland, 28, 28*f*

Myoid
    of cone, 70, 72*f*
    of rod, 69, 72*f*
Myopathies, mitochondrial, with encephalopathy/
    lactic acidosis/strokelike episodes (MELAS),
    mitochondrial DNA mutation and, 157, 159
Myopia
    with achromatopsia, racial and ethnic concentration
        of, 197
    Bruch membrane affected in, 61
    congenital stationary night blindness with, ocular
        findings in carriers of, 199*t*
    muscarinic agents causing, 311
    vitreous changes and, 252, 253
Myosin, in retinal pigment epithelium, 273
Myosin VIIA gene mutations, 264

Na. See Sodium
Na⁺,K⁺-ATPase (sodium-potassium pump)
    in aqueous humor secretion/suppression, 230, 323
    in lens ionic balance, 246
    in retinal pigment epithelium, 273, 277
    in rods, 259
Na⁺,K⁺-Ca exchanger (sodium-potassium-calcium
    exchanger), in rods, 259
Nabumetone, 335*t*
NADH dehydrogenase, mutations in gene for, in Leber
    hereditary optic neuropathy, 158
NADPH
    in free-radical generation, 282
    in lens glucose/carbohydrate metabolism, 246
        glutathione redox cycle and, 284, 284*f*
Nafcillin, 344
Nalidixic acid, 346
Nanopore sequencing technology, in next-generation
    sequencing, 166*f*. See also Next-generation
    sequencing
Nanotechnology, for drug delivery, 304
Naphazoline, 337, 338*t*, 342
Naphazoline/antazoline, 338*t*
Naphazoline/pheniramine, 337, 338*t*
Naphcon-A. See Naphazoline/pheniramine
Naproxen, 335*t*
NARP (neuropathy/ataxia/retinitis pigmentosa)
    syndrome, 158–159
    mitochondrial DNA mutations and, 157, 158–159
Nasal artery, 26*f*, 33*f*
Nasal vein, 35*f*
Nasociliary nerve, 9*f*, 100
Nasofrontal vein, 35*f*
Nasolacrimal canal, 6
Nasolacrimal duct, 8, 29–30
    occlusion of, ocular medication absorption and,
        296, 296*f*
Natacyn. See Natamycin
Natamycin, 354, 355*t*
    for *Acanthamoeba* keratitis, 361
Natriuretic peptides, in aqueous humor, 231, 234
NCAM-140, in retinal pigment epithelium, 273
ND-1/ND-4/ND-6 genes, in Leber hereditary optic
    neuropathy, 158
NDP (Norrie disease) gene, 183
Near reflex, pathways for, 96

Necrotizing encephalopathy, Leigh (Leigh syndrome), 159, 175*t*
  mitochondrial DNA mutations and, 159
Nedocromil, 338*t*, 339
Neofrin. *See* Phenylephrine
Neomycin, 351
  for *Acanthamoeba* keratitis, 361
  in combination preparations, 347*t*, 348*t*
Neonates, drug toxicity and, 294
Neosporin. *See* Gramicidin, with polymyxin B and neomycin
Neostigmine, 309*f*, 312
  in myasthenia gravis diagnosis, 301, 315
Neo-Synephrine. *See* Phenylephrine
Nepafenac, 330*t*, 336
Nephrotoxicity, of aminoglycosides, 352
Nerve block, local anesthetics for, 363, 365
Nerve endings
  en grappe, 18
  en plaque, 18
    neuromuscular blocking agents affecting, 315
  in scleral spur, 48
Nerve fiber layer, 70*f*, 71*f*, 74–75, 74*f*, 88*f*
  development of, 117*f*
  optic nerve/disc, 86, 88*f*
    blood supply of, 91, 91*f*, 92*f*
Nerve loop (Axenfeld loop), 44
Nerve of pterygoid canal, 101*f*, 104
Nervus intermedius, 101*f*, 102–103, 102*f*, 103
Nettleship-Falls X-linked ocular albinism, ocular findings in carriers of, 198–200, 199*f*
Neural cell adhesion molecules, in retinal pigment epithelium, 273
Neural crest cells, 111, 113*f*, 114*f*, 116*t*, 119*f*
  ocular structures derived from, 111, 115*t*, 119*f*
    cornea, 41, 120, 121*f*
    optic nerve, 124
    orbit and extraocular muscles, 124–126
    sclera, 124
    uvea, 122
Neural folds, 113*f*
Neural plate, 112*f*, 113*f*, 114*f*
Neural retinal leucine zipper (Nrl), in retinal development, 122
Neural tube, 111, 112*f*, 113*f*, 114*f*, 118*f*
Neuritis, optic. *See* Optic neuritis
Neuroectoderm (neural ectoderm), 111, 112*f*
  ocular structures derived from, 115*t*
Neuroendocrine peptides, in aqueous humor, 231, 234
Neurofibromatosis, von Recklinghausen (type 1), expressivity in, 196
Neuroglia, 268
Neuromuscular blocking agents, 315
Neuropathy
  with ataxia and retinitis pigmentosa (NARP), 158–159
    mitochondrial DNA mutations and, 157, 158–159
  optic. *See* Optic neuropathy
Neuropeptide-processing enzymes, in aqueous humor, 231
Neuropeptide Y (NPY), in tear secretion, 214, 216
Neurosensory retina, 69–75, 70–71*f*, 72*f*, 73*f*, 74*f*, 257–266, 258*f*. *See also* Retina
  anatomy of, 69–75, 70–71*f*, 72*f*, 73*f*, 74*f*, 258*f*

biochemistry and metabolism of, 257
development of, 115, 116*t*, 117*f*, 119*f*, 122
glial elements of, 73
neuronal elements of, 69–73, 72*f*, 73*f*
stratification of, 70–71*f*, 74–75, 74*f*
vascular elements of, 73–74. *See also* Retinal blood vessels
  development of, 116*t*
Neurotensin, in aqueous humor, 231, 234
Neurotoxin complex, purified, 366
Neurotransmitters
  cholinergic action and, 307, 307*f*, 309*f*, 310*f*
  in tear secretion, 216, 217–218
Neurotrophic proteins, in aqueous humor, 234
Neutrophil elastase inhibitor, in vitreous, 252
Nevanac. *See* Nepafenac
Next-generation sequencing (NGS/massively parallel DNA sequencing), 140, 142, 161, 163*f*, 164*f*, 165*f*, 166*f*
NFL. *See* Nerve fiber layer
NGS. *See* Next-generation sequencing
Nicotinamide adenine dinucleotide phosphate (NADPH)
  in free-radical generation, 282
  in lens glucose/carbohydrate metabolism, 246
    glutathione redox cycle and, 284, 284*f*
Nicotine, 308, 308*t*, 315*t*. *See also* Nicotinic drugs
Nicotinic drugs, 308*t*, 314–315
  antagonists, 315, 315*t*
  indirect-acting agonists, 314–315
Nicotinic receptors, 308, 308*t*
Nidogen-1, in vitreous, 249
Niemann-Pick disease, 175*t*
  racial and ethnic concentration of, 197
Night blindness, congenital stationary, with myopia, ocular findings in carriers of, 199*t*
Nizoral. *See* Ketoconazole
Nonallelic, definition of, 131
Noncoding (junk) DNA, 132, 148*f*, 150, 151
Noncoding strand of DNA (antisense DNA), 132
  in gene therapy, 170
Nondepolarizing neuromuscular blocking agents, 315
Nondisjunction, 140
  aneuploidy and, 189
  in Down syndrome, 190
  meiotic, 186*f*, 189
  mitotic, 191
  in mosaicism, 191
Nonhomologous chromosomes, independent assortment and, 187
Nonpenetrance/nonpenetrant gene, 141, 195, 205
Nonpigmented ciliary epithelium (NPE), 57, 58*f*
  in aqueous dynamics, 229, 230, 231, 323, 324, 324*f*
Nonsense mutation, 140, 155
  of mitochondrial DNA, 157
Nonsteroidal anti-inflammatory drugs (NSAIDs), 330*t*, 334–337, 335*t*
  COX-1/COX-2 inhibition by, 239, 335
  prostaglandins affected by, 239
Norepinephrine, 308*t*
  adrenergic receptor response and, 316, 317*f*. *See also* Adrenergic drugs
  synthesis and release of, 320, 320*f*
  in tear secretion, 216, 218, 218*f*, 219, 219*f*

Norfloxacin, 349
Norrie disease *(NDP)* gene, 183
Nose, inferior meatus of, 6, 8
Notochord, 112f, 114f
Nougaret disease, rod transducin mutation causing, 263
Novocain. *See* Procaine
NPE. *See* Nonpigmented ciliary epithelium
NPY. *See* Neuropeptide Y
Nrl (neural retinal leucine zipper), in retinal development, 122
NSAIDs. *See* Nonsteroidal anti-inflammatory drugs
Nuclear layer
    inner (INL), 70f, 71f, 74, 74f, 76f, 88f, 258f, 266–268, 266f, 267f, 268f
    outer (ONL), 70f, 71f, 72f, 74f, 76f, 88f
Nucleic acids, in retinal pigment epithelium, 274
Nucleoside, 140
Nucleosome, 140
Nucleotides, 140, 147, 148f
Nucleus, lens. *See* Lens (crystalline), nucleus of
Null allele, gene therapy and, 169
Null mutations, 155
Nyctalopia, rod-specific mutations causing, 263, 264

OAT (ornithine aminotransferase) gene, in gyrate atrophy, 175t, 265
Oblique muscles, 7, 9f, 13, 13f, 14f, 15t, 16f, 20f
    anatomy of, 7, 9f, 13, 13f, 14f, 15t, 16f, 20f
    blood supply of, 15t, 33f, 34f
    innervation of, 17, 94f, 95
    insertions of, 14f, 15, 15t
    origins of, 15t, 17
OCA1 (albinism), 278
OCA2 (albinism), 278
Occipital association cortex, near reflex initiated in, 96
Occipital sinus, 106f
Ocriplasmin, for enzymatic vitreolysis, 255
Ocucoat, 368
Ocufen. *See* Flurbiprofen
Ocuflox. *See* Ofloxacin
Ocular adnexa. *See also specific structure*
    anatomy of, 5–11, 6f, 8f, 9f, 10f
    glands of, 23t
Ocular albinism
    ocular findings in carriers of, 198–200, 199f, 199t
    X-linked (Nettleship-Falls), ocular findings in carriers of, 198–200, 199f
Ocular development, 111–128
    general principles and, 111, 112f, 113f, 114f, 115t
    genetic cascades and morphogenic gradients and, 111, 126–128
Ocular inflammation, treatment of. *See* Anti-inflammatory drugs
Ocular motility, extraocular muscles in control of, 18
Ocular pharmacology. *See also* Drugs, ocular
    legal aspects of, 205–207
    principles of, 293–304
Ocular receptors. *See* Receptors
Oculocardiac reflex, 99
    atropine affecting, 314
Oculocutaneous albinism, 185, 278
    racial and ethnic concentration of, 197
Oculomotor nerve. *See* Cranial nerve III

Ocupress. *See* Carteolol
Ocusert delivery system, 302. *See also* Pilocarpine
Off-bipolar cells, 257, 266, 266f
Off-label uses, of drug, 305, 306
Off retinal ganglion cells, 267, 267f, 268f
Ofloxacin, 346, 347–349, 347t
Oguchi disease
    arrestin mutation causing, 161, 263
    racial and ethnic concentration of, 197
    rhodopsin kinase mutations causing, 263
Ointments, ocular, 298–299
    for dry eye, 341
Oleic acid, in pigment retinal epithelium, 276
Olfactory bulb, 83, 85f, 106f
Olfactory nerve. *See* Cranial nerve I
Olfactory tract, 83, 85f
Oligodendrocytes, 88f
Oligodendroglia
    optic nerve, 87
    retinal, 257, 268
Oligonucleotides, in gene therapy, 169–170, 170f
Olopatadine, 238, 338t, 339
Omega-3 fatty acid supplements, for dry eye, 370
OMIM (Online Mendelian Inheritance in Man), 140, 160
Omnipred. *See* Prednisolone
On-bipolar cells, 257, 266, 266f
On retinal ganglion cells, 267, 267f, 268f
Oncogenes/oncogenesis, 140
1000 Genomes Project, 144
ONL. *See* Outer nuclear layer
Online Mendelian Inheritance in Man (OMIM), 140, 160
Opacities, vitreous, fibrillar, 253
Opcon-A. *See* Naphazoline/pheniramine
Open-angle glaucoma
    cycloplegic use in, 313, 314t
    genetic/hereditary factors in, 200
    primary (POAG), intraocular pressure–lowering drugs for, 311
Open reading frame, 141, 147
Ophthalmia, sympathetic, corticosteroid route of administration in, 333t
Ophthalmic artery, 9f, 16f, 17f, 33f, 34f, 90
    extraocular muscles supplied by, 17
    eyelids supplied by, 25
    optic nerve supplied by, 84f, 89, 90, 91
    orbit supplied by, 33f, 34f
Ophthalmic irrigants, 367
Ophthalmic nerve. *See* Cranial nerve V (trigeminal nerve), V₁
Ophthalmic vein, 9f, 16f, 35f
Ophthalmoplegia, chronic progressive external, 158
    mitochondrial DNA defects and, 157, 158
    syndromes associated with, 158
Ophthetic. *See* Proparacaine
OPL. *See* Outer plexiform layer
Opsins
    cone, 261
        genes for, 262, 264
    rod. *See* Rhodopsin
Optic canal, 6f, 17f, 87, 88f. *See also* Intracanalicular region of optic nerve
Optic chiasm. *See* Chiasm

Optic cup, 86
    development of, 115, 117, 117*f*, 118*f*, 119*f*
    enlargement of, 86
    extraocular muscle development and, 124
    retinal development and, 117*f*
Optic disc (optic nerve head), 37*f*, 67, 85, 85*t*, 86–87, 88*f*
    anatomy of, 37*f*, 67, 85, 85*t*, 86–87, 88*f*
    blood supply of, 85*t*, 89, 90, 90–91, 91*f*, 92*f*
    coloboma of, 152
Optic disc topography, 37*f*
Optic foramen, 7
Optic nerve (cranial nerve II). *See also* Optic disc
    anatomy of, 9*f*, 16*f*, 37*f*, 70–71, 83–93, 84*f*, 85*f*, 85*t*,
        88*f*, 89*f*, 90*f*, 91*f*, 92*f*
    blood supply of, 85*t*, 89, 90, 90–91, 91*f*, 92*f*
    coloboma of, 152
    development of, 119*f*, 124
    intracanalicular region of, 83, 85*t*, 89–90
        blood supply of, 85*t*, 89, 91
    intracranial region of, 83, 85*t*, 90, 90*f*
        blood supply of, 85*t*, 90, 91, 92*f*
    intraocular region of, 83, 85, 85*t*, 86–89, 88*f*, 89*f*
        blood supply of, 85*t*
    intraorbital region of, 83, 85, 85*t*, 87–89
        blood supply of, 85*t*, 91, 91*f*
    laminar area of, 85*t*, 86, 87
        blood supply of, 91
    prelaminar area of, 85*t*, 86. *See also* Optic disc
        blood supply of, 85*t*, 91, 91*f*, 92*f*
    regional differences in, 83–85, 85*t*
    retrolaminar area of, 86, 87
        blood supply of, 90–91, 92*f*
    topography of, 37*f*
Optic nerve head. *See* Optic disc
Optic neuritis, corticosteroid route of administration
    in, 333*t*
Optic neuropathy
    indirect traumatic, 89
    Leber hereditary, 158
        mitochondrial DNA mutations and, 157, 158
Optic radiations (geniculocalcarine pathways), 90, 90*f*, 93
Optic stalk, 117*f*, 118*f*, 124
Optic strut, 6*f*, 9*f*
Optic tract, 90, 90*f*, 93
Optic vesicle, 115, 116*t*, 117*f*, 118*f*
    lens development and, 118
Opticin, in vitreous, 249, 252
    angiogenesis suppression and, 254
OptiPranolol. *See* Metipranolol
Optivar. *See* Azelastine
Ora serrata, 37*f*, 67, 78, 79*f*
    muscle insertion relationships and, 15
Oral contraceptives, tetracycline use and, 350
Oral medication, sustained-release preparations of, 301
Orbicularis oculi muscle, 20*f*, 21, 23*f*
Orbit
    anatomy of, 5–11, 6*f*, 8*f*, 9*f*, 10*f*
        vascular
            arterial supply, 32–35, 33*f*, 34*f*
            venous drainage, 35, 35*f*
    bony, 5
    development of, 124–126
    fissures in, 6*f*, 8–10, 8*f*, 9*f*

floor of, 6–7
foramina in, 7–8
lateral wall of, 7
margin of, 5
medial wall of, 6
optic nerve in, 83, 85, 85*t*, 87–89
    blood supply of, 85*t*, 91, 91*f*
roof of, 5–6
septum of, 20*f*, 22–23
vascular system of, anatomy of, 32–35, 33*f*, 34*f*, 35*f*
volume of, 5
walls of
    lateral, 7
    medial, 6
Orbital fat, 20*f*, 23
Orbital fissures, 6*f*, 8–10, 8*f*, 9*f*
    inferior, 6*f*, 8–10
    superior, 6*f*, 8, 8*f*, 9*f*, 14*f*
Orbital lacrimal gland, 28, 216
ORF. *See* Open reading frame
Organophosphates, 312
Ornithine aminotransferase *(OAT)* gene, in gyrate
    atrophy, 175*t*, 265
Osmitrol. *See* Mannitol
Osmolarity, tear-film, 214*t*
    dysfunctions and, 220
Osmotic/hyperosmotic drugs, 328–329, 329*t*
Osmotic hypothesis, of carbohydrate ("sugar") cataract
    formation, 247
Ototoxicity, mitochondrial DNA mutations and, 157
Outer nuclear layer (ONL), 70*f*, 71*f*, 72*f*, 74*f*, 76*f*, 88*f*
Outer plexiform layer (OPL), 70*f*, 71*f*, 72*f*, 74, 74*f*, 88*f*
Outer segments, photoreceptor, 69, 70, 70*f*, 72*f*, 74*f*. *See
    also* Cone outer segments; Rod outer segments
    development of, 116*t*
    oxidative damage and, 285
Ovum, 186
Oxacillin, 344
Oxaprozin, 335*t*
Oxidoreductases, taxon-specific crystallins as, 244
Oxy radicals, 282, 282*f*, 283. *See also* Free radicals
Oxybuprocaine (benoxinate with fluorescein), 363*t*, 365
Oxychloro complex, as ocular medication preservative, 294
Oxygen
    in aqueous humor, 235–236
    corneal supply of, 224
    metabolism of, 281, 282*f*
    singlet, 281, 283
    vitrectomy affecting movement of, 254
Oxygen radicals. *See* Free radicals
Oxygen tension
    in lens, energy production and, 246
    in retina, oxidative damage and, 285–286
Oxymetazoline, 342
Oxyradicals. *See* Free radicals
Oxytetracycline, 350
    with polymyxin B, 347*t*

P2Y$_2$ receptors, diquafosal mechanism of action
    and, 342
P23H rhodopsin mutation, 263
p53 gene, in DNA repair, 154
p arm, 141, 148*f*

P gene, in albinism, 185
PABA. *See Para*-aminobenzoic acid
PAHX gene, Refsum disease caused by mutations in, 266
Paired box genes, 152
Palatine air cells, 10
Palatine bone, 5, 6*f*
Palmitic acid, in retinal pigment epithelium, 274, 275
Palpebral arteries, 26*f*, 33*f*
Palpebral conjunctiva, 25, 26*f*, 30
Palpebral fissures, 18–19, 18*f*, 25*f*
Palpebral lacrimal gland, 28, 216
2-PAM. *See* Pralidoxime
Pancuronium, 315*t*
Papilla, Bergmeister, 80
Papillomacular bundle/fibers, 68, 68*f*, 71
Para-aminobenzoic acid (PABA), sulfonamides derived from, 349
Para-aminoclonidine. *See* Apraclonidine
Parafovea, 77
Paramedian pontine reticular formation, 102, 102*f*
Paranasal sinuses, 10–11, 10*f*
Parasympathetic ganglia/nerves
    cholinergic drug action and, 307, 307*f*, 308
    in ciliary ganglion, 11–12, 12*f*, 95
    ciliary muscle innervation and, 59, 100
    cranial nerve III (oculomotor) and, 94, 95
    cranial nerve VII (facial) and, 103, 104
    dilator muscle innervation and, 55
    sphincter muscle innervation and, 56, 94, 95, 100
    in tear secretion, 214, 216, 217–218, 218*f*, 219, 219*f*
Parcaine. *See* Proparacaine
Paredrine. *See* Hydroxyamphetamine
Paremyd. *See* Hydroxyamphetamine, with tropicamide
Parental age, chromosomal abnormalities/Down syndrome and, 190
Pars plana, 57
Pars plicata, 54*f*, 57
Partition coefficient, drug lipid solubility and, 298
Passive transport, in aqueous humor dynamics, 230
Pataday. *See* Olopatadine
Patanol. *See* Olopatadine
PAX genes, 126, 137, 152
    in aniridia, 152, 177, 193
PAX2 gene, 126
    mutation in, 152
PAX3 gene, mutation in, 152, 177
PAX6 gene, 126, 152, 193
    mutation in, 152, 193
    in aniridia, 152, 177, 193
PCAB (Pharmacy Compounding Accreditation Board), 306
PCD. *See* Programmed cell death
PCR. *See* Polymerase chain reaction
PDE. *See* Phosphodiesterase
Pearson marrow-pancreas syndrome, 158
    mitochondrial DNA defects and, 157, 158
Pedicle, of cone, 70, 73*f*
Pedigree analysis, 172–173, 172*f*
Pegaptanib, 372
Pemirolast, 238, 337, 338*t*
Penciclovir, 302, 359
Penetrance/penetrant gene, 141, 195–196, 205
    incomplete (skipped generation), 177

Penicillamine, for Wilson disease, 203
Penicillin G, 343, 344*t*
Penicillin V, 343
Penicillinase (β-lactamase), 343, 345, 346
Penicillinase-resistant penicillins, 344
Penicillins, 343, 343–345, 344*t*
    allergic reaction to, 343
    broad-spectrum, 345
    penicillinase-resistant, 344
Pentolair. *See* Cyclopentolate
Pentose phosphate pathway (hexose monophosphate shunt), in glucose/carbohydrate metabolism
    in cornea, 224
    in lens, 246
    in rod outer segments, 261
Peptide hormones
    in aqueous humor, 231
    in tear secretion, 219–220
Peptidyl-glycine-α-amidating monooxygenase, in aqueous humor, 231
Perfluorocarbon, intravitreal administration of, 300*t*
Pericanalicular connective tissue, 49–50, 50*f*
Pericytes
    choriocapillaris, 61, 62*f*
    retinal blood vessel, 73
Perifovea, 77
Periocular drug administration, 299
Periorbital sinuses, 10–11, 10*f*
Peripapillary fibers, 86
Peripheral arterial arcade, eyelids supplied by, 25–26, 26*f*
Peripheral zone, of lens epithelium, 64
Peripherin, 261
Peripherin/*RDS* gene mutations, 161, 264
Peroxidase, 282*f*, 287
    in retina and retinal pigment epithelium, 273
Peroxidation, lipid, 281, 282–283
Peroxyl/peroxy radicals, 281, 283. *See also* Free radicals
Personalized genetics, 141
Pes anserinus, 104
Peters anomaly, 152
Petroclinoid (Gruber) ligament, 102
Petrosal nerve
    deep, 101*f*, 104
    greater superficial, 101*f*, 103, 104
    inferior, 103
Petrosal sinuses, inferior/superior, 105, 106*f*
PEX1 gene, Refsum disease caused by mutations in, 265
PG. *See* Prostaglandins; Proteoglycans
PG analogues. *See* Prostaglandin analogues
PG synthetase (prostaglandin synthetase). *See* Cyclooxygenase
PGD. *See* Preimplantation genetic diagnosis
PGI$_2$. *See* Prostacyclin; Prostaglandin I$_2$
pH
    of ocular medication, absorption affected by, 298
    of tear film, 214*t*
Phagocytosis, by retinal pigment epithelium, 276–277, 276*f*
Phagosomes, in retinal pigment epithelium, 69, 272
Phakinin, 245
Pharmacodynamics, 293, 304
    age-related changes in, 295

Pharmacogenetics/pharmacogenomics, 141, 201–202
Pharmacokinetics, 293, 295–304, 296f, 300t
  age-related changes in, 295
Pharmacology, ocular. See also Drugs, ocular
  legal aspects of, 205–207
  principles of, 293–304
Pharmacotherapeutics, 293, 294, 305–372. See also
    Drugs, ocular
  legal aspects of, 205–207
  principles of, 293–304
Pharmacy Compounding Accreditation Board
    (PCAB), 306
Phasic cells, 267, 268f
Phenethicillin, 343
Pheniramine, 337
Pheniramine/naphazoline, 337, 338t
Phenocopy, 141, 194, 205
Phenotype, 141, 194
  alleles and, 184, 185
  database of, 134
Phenoxybenzamine, 308t
Phentolamine, 308t
Phenylephrine, 308t, 314t, 317–318, 342
  with cyclopentolate, 314t
  drug interactions and, 317
PHMB. See Polyhexamethylene biguanide
Phosphate, in aqueous humor, 232
Phosphatidylcholine, in retinal pigment
    epithelium, 274
Phosphatidylethanolamine, in retinal pigment
    epithelium, 274
Phosphocreatine shuttle, in rod outer segments, 261
Phosphodiesterase, rod (rod PDE), 259–261, 260f
  mutations in, 161, 263
Phospholine. See Echothiophate
Phospholipase A₂
  in eicosanoid synthesis, 237, 238f
  NSAID derivation and, 334
  in tear film, 216
Phospholipase C, in tear secretion, 218, 218f
Phospholipids
  oxidation of, 281, 285
  in retina/retinal pigment epithelium, 274
    oxidative damage and, 285
  in tear film, 215. See also Lipid layer of tear film
Phosphonoformic acid. See Foscarnet
Photo-oxidation, 283
  in retina, 286
Photoreceptor inner segments, 69, 70, 70f, 72f, 74f. See
    also Cone inner segments; Rod inner segments
Photoreceptor outer segments, 69, 70, 70f, 72f, 74f. See
    also Cone outer segments; Rod outer segments
  development of, 116t
  shed, retinal pigment epithelium phagocytosis
    of, 276–277, 276f
Photoreceptors, 69–70, 70f, 71f, 72f, 77, 257–266, 258f.
    See also Cones; Rods
  biochemistry and metabolism of, 257
  blue-light damage to, 286
  development of, 116t, 122
  oxidative damage to, 285–286
Photorefractive keratectomy (PRK), Bowman layer
    and, 225

Phototransduction
  cone, 261–263
  rod, 257–261, 259f, 260f
PHOX2A gene disorders, congenital extraocular muscle
    disorders and, 124
Physiologic cup, 86. See also Optic cup
Physostigmine, 309f, 311t, 312, 313
  for muscarinic antagonist adverse effects, 314
Phytanic acid oxidase, defective/deficiency of, 175t. See
    also Refsum disease
Pia mater, optic nerve, 87, 88f, 89f
"Pie in the sky" defect, 93
Pigment epithelium. See Ciliary epithelium, pigmented;
    Iris pigment epithelium; Retinal pigment epithelium
Pigment epithelium–derived factor
  in aqueous humor, 231
  in vitreous, 253
Pigment granules, in retinal pigment
    epithelium, 277–278
Pigment ruff, iris, 54f, 55
Pigmentations/pigment deposits
  iris, 53, 54, 55, 56f, 236
    prostaglandin analogues/latanoprost and, 327
  retinal/retinal pigment epithelium, 277–278
Pigments, visual, retinal pigment epithelium in
    regeneration of, 274–276, 275f
Pilocarpine, 309f, 310, 311, 311t
  sustained-release gel for administration of, 302
Pilopine. See Pilocarpine
Pink-eyed dilution gene defects, in albinism, 278
Piperacillin, 345
Piroxicam, 335t
PitX2 gene, 126
PLA₂. See Phospholipase A₂
Placental-like growth factor, in aqueous humor, 235
Placode, lens, 115, 116t, 117f
Plasma proteins. See also Proteins
  in aqueous humor, 231, 233
  drug-binding by, systemic administration
    and, 300–301
  in retinal pigment epithelium, 273, 277
Plasmid-liposome complexes, in gene therapy, 169
Plasmin
  in aqueous humor, 234
  for enzymatic vitreolysis, 255
Plasminogen
  antifibrinolytic agents affecting, 369
  in aqueous humor, 234
Plasminogen activator
  in aqueous humor, 234
  tissue. See Tissue plasminogen activator
Platelet-derived growth factors, 371
Platelets, aspirin affecting, 335, 336
Pleiotropism, 141, 196
Plexiform layer
  inner (IPL), 70f, 71f, 74, 74f, 88f
  outer (OPL), 70f, 71f, 72f, 74, 74f, 88f
PlGF. See Placental-like growth factor
Plica semilunaris, 18f, 27
PND. See Prenatal diagnosis
POAG. See Primary open-angle glaucoma
Point mutations, 193. See also Mutation
  screening for, 161, 163f, 164f, 165f, 166f

Poly-Dex. *See* Dexamethasone, in combination preparations
Poly-Pred. *See* Neomycin, in combination preparations
Polyacrylamide, as viscoelastic, 368
Polyallelism, 184
Polycin-B. *See* Polymyxin B, in combination preparations
Polyenes, 354, 355t
Polyethylene glycol (PEG)-400, in artificial tears, 341
Polygenic/multifactorial inheritance, 140, 141, 200–201
Polyhexamethylene biguanide (PHMB), for *Acanthamoeba* keratitis, 361
Polyinosinic acid–polycytidylic acid, 370
Polymerase chain reaction (PCR), 141–142
Polymorphisms, 142, 155, 156, 194
    restriction fragment length (RFLP), 162
    single-nucleotide (SNP), 144, 194
        in genome-wide association studies (GWAS), 163–168, 168f, 194
    single-stranded conformational (SSCP), 162
Polymyxin B, 344t, 353
    for *Acanthamoeba* keratitis, 361
    in combination preparations, 347t, 348t, 353
Polyol (sorbitol) pathway
    in cataract formation, 247–248
    in lens glucose/carbohydrate metabolism, 247–248, 247f
Polypropylene glycol, in artificial tears, 341
Polyquaternium-1, as ocular medication preservative, 294
Polysorbate, in artificial tears, 341
Polytrim. *See* Trimethoprim, with polymyxin B
Polyvinyl alcohol (PVA), 297
    in artificial tears, 341
Pontine cistern, lateral, 103
Pontine paramedian reticular formation, 102, 102f
Pontomedullary junction, 102, 103
Positional candidate gene screening, 161
Posterior cerebral artery, 93, 107f
    cranial nerve relationship and, 84f
Posterior chamber, 37, 37f, 47f
Posterior ciliary arteries, 17f, 32, 33f, 34f, 90, 91, 91f, 92f
Posterior ciliary nerves, 32, 223–224
Posterior clinoid process, 84f, 95, 102
Posterior communicating artery, 107f
    cranial nerve relationship and, 84f, 85f
Posterior conjunctival arteries, 30
Posterior ethmoidal foramen, 6f, 7–8
Posterior lacrimal crest, 5, 6f
Posterior nonbanded zone, of Descemet membrane, 41, 42f
Posterior pigmented layer, of iris, 53f, 55, 56f
Posterior pole, 65f, 75, 242f. *See also* Macula
Posterior segment, development of, 122–124, 123f
Posterior synechiae, mydriasis in prevention of, 313
Posterior uveitis, corticosteroid route of administration in, 333t
Posterior vitreous detachment (PVD), 80, 80f, 81f, 252–253
Postganglionic nerves/neurons
    cholinergic drug action and, 308
    dilator muscle innervation and, 56
    sphincter muscle innervation and, 56
Posttranslational modification, 142
    of lens proteins, 245

Potassium
    in aqueous humor, 232
    in lens, 245–246
    in tear film, 214t, 216
    in vitreous, 252
Potassium channels, in lens, 246
Povidone, in artificial tears, 341
Povidone-iodine, 353–354
Prader-Willi syndrome, imprinting abnormalities causing, 138, 153–154
Pralidoxime (2-PAM), 309f, 312
Prazosin, 308t
Precorneal tear film, 38, 213–214, 213f. *See also* Tear film (tears)
    dysfunction of, 220–222
Precursor messenger RNA, 15, 148, 151f
Pred Forte/Pred Mild. *See* Prednisolone
Pred-G. *See* Prednisolone, in combination preparations
Prednisol. *See* Prednisolone
Prednisolone, 330t
    anti-inflammatory potency of, 333t
    in combination preparations, 348t
    off-label use of, 306
    pressure-elevating potency of, 332, 333t
Preganglionic autonomic nerves, cholinergic drug action and, 307, 307f
Preganglionic neurons, dilator muscle innervation and, 56
Pregnancy
    antifibrinolytic use contraindicated in, 370
    carbonic anhydrase use during, 326
Preimplantation genetic diagnosis (PGD), genetic counseling and, 206, 207
Prelaminar nerve/prelaminar area of optic nerve, 85t, 86. *See also* Optic disc
    blood supply of, 85t, 91, 91f, 92f
Premelanosomes, in retinal pigment epithelium, 69
Prenatal diagnosis (PND), 188, 206–207
Presbyopia, 58, 63
Preservatives, in ocular medications
    allergic/adverse reactions to, 294
    demulcents, 341, 342
    irrigating solutions, 367
Pretectal nuclei, 96
Primary lens fibers, development of, 118
Primary open-angle glaucoma, pilocarpine for, 311
Primary visual cortex, 90, 93
Primary vitreous, 122, 123f
Primers, in polymerase chain reaction, 141
Primitive streak, 112f
Proband, 142, 172
Procaine, 362t
    cholinesterase inhibitor use and, 312
Prodrugs, 302
    for β-blockers, 323
Profenal. *See* Suprofen
Programmed cell death (PCD/apoptosis), 132, 154, 155
    in DNA repair, 154, 155
Progressive (chronic progressive) external ophthalmoplegia, 158
    mitochondrial DNA defects and, 157, 158
    syndromes associated with, 158
Prolensa. *See* Bromfenac

Promoter, 142, 151
in alternative splicing, 152–153
Propamidine, for *Acanthamoeba* keratitis, 361
Proparacaine, 363t, 365
with fluorescein, 363t
Prophase, 148, 149f
Propine. *See* Dipivefrin
Proposita/propositus, 142
Propranolol, 308t, 317f
Propylene glycol, in artificial tears, 341
Prostacyclin, 237, 334
Prostaglandin analogues, 302, 327–328, 327t
for glaucoma, 237–238, 318t, 327–328, 327t
Prostaglandin I₂, 237
Prostaglandins, 237, 327–328, 334
anti-inflammatory drugs and, 239, 331
receptors for, 239–240, 316t
in signal transduction, 316t
Prostigmin. *See* Neostigmine
Protan defects (protanopia), ocular findings in carriers
of, 199t
Protein kinase C/Ca²⁺–dependent pathways, in tear
secretion, 218, 218f
Proteinase inhibitors
in aqueous humor, 234
in cornea, 226
Proteinases, in aqueous humor, 231, 233–234
Proteins
in aqueous humor, 229, 233–234
breakdown of blood–aqueous barrier and, 236
corneal, 224
drug-binding by, systemic administration
and, 300–301
lens. *See* Lens proteins
in retinal pigment epithelium, 273, 277
in rod outer segments ("rim" proteins), 261
in tear film, 216
vitreous, 251–252
Proteoglycans, corneal, 41, 226
Proteomics, 136
Proto-oncogene, 156
Protoplasmic astrocytes, 73
Pseudocholinesterase, 312
defective, succinylcholine effects and, 201–202
Pseudodominance, 142, 177
Pseudogene, 142
Pseudohermaphrodites, 192
Pseudoxanthoma elasticum, Bruch membrane affected
in, 61
Pterygoid canal, nerve of, 101f, 104
Pterygoid venous plexus, 35f
Pterygopalatine ganglion/nerves, 101f, 104
Pulley system, 31, 31f
Punctal occlusion/plugs
drug-delivery systems using, 303
for dry eye, 220
Punctum (puncta), 18f, 22f, 29
Pupil. *See* Pupils
Pupillary light reflex (pupillary response to light)
indirect-acting adrenergic agonists in evaluation
of, 320
pathways for, 96
Pupillary membrane, development and, 116t, 121f, 123f

Pupils
Adie tonic, pharmacologic testing for, 310
constriction of, in near and light reflexes, 96
Purified neurotoxin complex, 366
Purine nucleotides/purines, 140
Purite. *See* Oxychloro complex
PVA. *See* Polyvinyl alcohol
PVD. *See* Posterior vitreous detachment
Pyridoxine (vitamin B₆), for homocystinuria, 203
Pyrimethamine, 349
Pyrimidine nucleotides/pyrimidines, 140
fluorinated, 355t
Pyruvate carboxylase, defective/deficiency of, 175t
Pyruvate dicarboxylase, defective/deficiency of, 175t

q arm, 142, 148f
qPCR. *See* Quantitative polymerase chain reaction
Quantitative polymerase chain reaction (qPCR),
141–142
Quixin. *See* Levofloxacin

RA. *See* Retinoic acid
Rab escort protein 1 *(REP-1)* gene, mutation in, 265
Race
genetic disorders and, 196–197
pharmacogenetics and, 201
Radiation
DNA repair after, 154
in free-radical generation, 282, 283
Ranibizumab, 372
intravitreal administration of, 300t
ras oncogene, 156
Rathke pouch, 113f
Rb locus, 192
RCFM. *See* Retrocorneal fibrous membrane
RDS/peripherin gene mutations, 161, 264
Reactive oxygen intermediates, 281. *See also* Free
radicals
Real-time polymerase chain reaction (PCR), 141–142
Rebamipide, 342
Receptor agonist, 304
Receptor antagonist, 304
Receptors, 240
ocular drug interactions and, 304
in signal transduction, 316t
Recessive inheritance (recessive gene/trait), 142,
173–174
autosomal, 174–177, 175t, 177t
disorders associated with, 142, 174–177, 175t
gene therapy for, 169
X-linked, 179, 180t
Recessive tumor-suppressor gene, Rb locus as, 192
Recombinant, definition of, 142
Recombinant DNA, 143
Recombination, 134, 143
Recombination frequency, 160
Recoverin, 260f, 261
Rectus muscles, 9f, 13, 13f, 14f, 15t, 16f, 20f
blood supply of, 15t, 17, 33f, 34f
innervation of, 17, 94, 94f, 95
insertions of, 13–15, 14f, 15t
optic nerve and, 87
origins of, 15t, 16–17

Red-green color vision, 262
  defects in
    gene defects causing, 262–263
    ocular findings in carriers of, 199t
"Red-man syndrome," 352
Reduction division, in meiosis, 139
Reference genomes, 143
Reflex secretors, 217
Reflex tear arc, 101f
Reflex tearing, 104, 217
  absorption of ocular medication affected by, 295, 298
  initiation of, 126, 217
Refsum disease, 175t
  gene defects causing, 265, 266
Regional anesthesia, 362–366, 362t
  for anterior segment surgery, 365–366
  cholinesterase inhibitor use and, 312, 363
Relatives, first-degree/second-degree, 143
Renal disease, vancomycin dose adjustments in, 352
Renal metabolic acidosis, carbonic anhydrase inhibitors
    causing, 325–326
  aspirin interactions and, 336
Renal transplantation, for cystinosis, 203
REP-1 (Rab escort protein 1) gene, mutation in, 265
Repeat element/sequence, Alu, 150
Replication, DNA, 143
Replication slippage, 143
Replicative segregation, 143, 157
Reproductive issues, genetic counseling and, 206–207
Rescula. See Unoprostone
Residence time (of medication), 295
Resistance (drug). See also specific drug
  antibiotic, 343, 346, 351, 352, 353
  antiviral, 358, 360
Restriction endonucleases, 135
Restriction fragment length polymorphisms (RFLPs), 162
Reticular formation, paramedian pontine, 102, 102f
Retina, 37f, 38, 67–75, 257–269. See also under Retinal
  anatomy of, 37f, 38, 67–75, 68f, 70f, 71f, 72f, 74f, 76f,
      257, 258f
  antioxidants in, 286, 286–288, 289f
  biochemistry and metabolism of, 257–269
  blood supply of. See Retinal blood vessels
  detachment of. See Retinal detachment
  development of, 115, 116t, 117f, 119f, 122–124, 123f, 257
    melanin in, 278
  electrophysiology of, 268–269, 269f
  free radicals affecting, 285–286
  gyrate atrophy of, 175t
  neurosensory, 69–75, 257–266, 258f
    anatomy of, 69–75, 70–71f, 72f, 73f, 74f, 258f
    biochemistry and metabolism of, 257–266
    development of, 115, 116t, 117f, 119f, 122
    glial elements of, 73
    neuronal elements of, 69–73, 72f, 73f
    stratification of, 70–71f, 74–75, 74f
    vascular elements of, 70f, 73–74. See also Retinal
        blood vessels
      development of, 116t
  pigment epithelium of. See Retinal pigment
      epithelium
  regional differences in, 68, 68f
  topography of, 37f, 38

Retinal adhesion, retinal pigment epithelium in
    maintenance of, 278
Retinal artery, central, 73, 88f, 90, 91, 91f, 92f
Retinal blood vessels, 70f, 73–74. See also specific vessel
  development of, 116t, 119f
Retinal degenerations
  gene defects causing, 265–266
  retinal pigment epithelium and, 278–279
Retinal detachment, 68
  posterior vitreous detachment and, 80, 80f, 81f, 253
  retinal pigment epithelial maintenance of adhesion
      and, 278
Retinal pigment epithelium (RPE), 60, 61f, 67–69, 68f,
      70f, 71f, 74f, 88f, 271–279, 271f
  anatomy of, 60, 61f, 67–69, 68f, 71f, 271–273, 271f, 272f
  antioxidants in, 286, 286–288, 289f
  biochemistry and metabolism of, 271–279
  composition of, 273–274
  detachment of, 68. See also Retinal detachment
  development of, 115, 116t, 117f, 119f, 122–124, 271
  in disease, 278–279
  gene defects affecting, 264–265
  lipids in, 274
  nucleic acids in, 274
  phagocytosis by, 276–277, 276f
  physiologic roles of, 274–278, 275f, 276f
  pigment granules in, 277–278
  proteins in, 273, 277
  regional differences in, 68, 68f
  retinal adhesion and, 278
  subretinal space maintenance and, 277
  transport functions of, 273, 277
  visual pigment regeneration and, 274–276, 275f
Retinal pigment epithelium–specific protein 65 kDa.
    See RPE65
Retinal tears, in posterior vitreous detachment, 81f, 253
Retinal vein, central, 35f, 88f, 91f, 92f
Retinaldehyde, in retinal pigment epithelium, 274–275
Retinitis, cytomegalovirus
  cidofovir for, 357t, 360–361
  foscarnet for, 357t, 360
  ganciclovir for, 357t, 358t, 359–360
Retinitis pigmentosa
  autosomal dominant, 177
    peripherin/RDS gene mutations causing, 161, 264
    rhodopsin mutations causing, 161, 263
  autosomal recessive
    retinal pigment epithelium defects in, 278
    rhodopsin mutations causing, 263
    rod cGMP-gated channel mutations causing, 161, 263
    rod cGMP phosphodiesterase mutations
        causing, 161, 263
  congenital/infantile/childhood (Leber congenital
      amaurosis)
    genetic heterogeneity in, 183, 183f
    guanylate cyclase mutations causing, 263
    RPE65 gene defects causing, 264
  MAK-associated, racial and ethnic concentration
      of, 197
  with neuropathy and ataxia (NARP), 158–159
    mitochondrial DNA mutations and, 157, 158–159
  retinal pigment epithelium in, 278
  ROM1 gene mutations in, 264

X-linked
  ocular findings in carriers of, 198f, 199t
  retinal pigment epithelium in, 278
Retinitis punctata albescens, CRALBP defects causing, 265
Retinoblastoma, 193
  long arm 13 deletion syndrome and, 192
Retinoblastoma gene, 159, 192
Retinoic acid, gene expression/ocular development
    and, 127
Retinoid-binding proteins, 275–276
  interphotoreceptor (IRBP), 275, 275f
Retinol, 275, 275f, 276
Retinyl ester, 275, 275f, 276
Retrobulbar anesthesia, drugs for, 363
Retrobulbar drug administration, 299
Retrocorneal fibrous membrane (RCFM), 227
Retrolaminar nerve/retrolaminar area of optic nerve,
    86, 87
  blood supply of, 90–91, 92f
Retro-orbital plexus, 101f
Retrovir. See Zidovudine
Reverse transcription, 143
Reversible cholinesterase inhibitors, 312
Reye syndrome, aspirin use and, 335–336
RFLPs (restriction fragment length polymorphisms), 162
Rhodopsin, 258–259, 259f, 260f, 261
  gene for, mutations in, in retinitis pigmentosa, 161, 263
  light affecting, 258, 259, 259f, 261
  phosphorylation of, 258, 259f, 261
  regeneration of, retinal pigment epithelium
    in, 274–276, 275f
Rhodopsin kinase, 260f, 261
  mutations in, 263
Ribonucleic acid. See RNA
Ribosomal RNA (rRNA), mitochondrial DNA-encoded,
    mutations of, 157
Ribosomes, 147, 148f, 151f, 152
Riley-Day syndrome (familial dysautonomia), 175t
  racial and ethnic concentration of, 197
"Rim" proteins, 261. See also specific type
Rimexolone, 330t, 334
Riolan, muscle of, 21
RNA
  amplification of, in polymerase chain reaction, 141–142
  messenger (mRNA), 147, 151, 151f, 152
    precursor, 148, 151f, 152
  micro (miRNA), 139
  in retinal pigment epithelium, 274
  ribosomal (rRNA), mitochondrial DNA-encoded,
    mutations of, 157
  short interfering (small interference) (siRNA), 143
    in gene therapy, 170
  splicing of, 144, 152
    alternative, 148, 152–153
  transfer (tRNA), mitochondrial DNA-encoded,
    mutations of, 157
Rod cGMP-gated channel, 259, 260f, 261
  mutations in, 161, 263
Rod cGMP phosphodiesterase (rod PDE), 259–261, 260f
  mutations in, 161, 263
Rod inner segments, 69, 72f. See also Rods
  free-radical leakage from, 285
Rod monochromatism, 264

Rod outer segment protein 1 (ROM1), 261
  mutations in, 264
Rod outer segments, 69, 70, 72f, 257–258, 258f. See also
    Rods
  antioxidants in, 288, 289f
  energy metabolism in, 261
  oxidative damage to, 285
  phototransduction in, 257–261, 259f, 260f
  shed, retinal pigment epithelium phagocytosis
    of, 276–277, 276f
Rod PDE. See Rod phosphodiesterase
Rod phosphodiesterase (rod PDE), 259–261, 260f
  mutations in, 161, 263
Rod response, 262, 269, 269f
Rod transducin, 259, 260f, 261
  mutations in, 263
Rods, 69, 71f, 72f, 88f, 257, 258f. See also Rod outer
    segments
  amacrine cells for, 267
  bipolar cells for, 257, 258f
  development of, 116t, 122
  electrophysiologic responses of, 269, 269f
  gene defects in, 263, 264
  phototransduction in, 257–261, 259f, 260f
Rofecoxib, cardiovascular toxicity and, 239
ROIs. See Reactive oxygen intermediates
ROM1 (rod outer segment) gene/protein, 261
  mutations in, 264
Romycin. See Erythromycin
ROOH. See Hydroperoxides
Rose bengal stain, 367
RPE. See Retinal pigment epithelium
RPE65 gene/RPE65 protein, 273, 275, 275f
  mutations in, 264
    gene therapy and, 169
rRNA. See Ribosomal RNA
RX gene, 126

S cones, 262
  horizontal cells for, 266
  retinal ganglion cells for, 267, 267f
S phase, cell cycle, 148, 149, 149f
Sagittal sinus, superior, 105, 106f
Salivatory (salivary) nucleus, 101f, 103, 104
Sandhoff disease (GM$_2$ gangliosidosis type II), 175t
Sandimmune. See Cyclosporine/cyclosporine A
Sanfilippo syndrome, 175t
Sanger sequencing, 143, 161, 162, 162f
Satellite DNA, 150
Scheie syndrome, 175t, 184
Schlemm canal, 45f, 46f, 50–51, 50f, 51f, 52f, 59f
  development of, 116t
Schwalbe line, 38, 44, 45f, 46f, 54f
Schwann cells, retinal, 38
Sclera, 17f, 37f, 38, 43–44, 46f
  anatomy of, 17f, 37f, 38, 43–44, 46f
  development of, 116t, 124
  rupture of, 43–44
  stroma of, 44
Scleral spur, 45f, 46f, 47f, 48
Scleral spur cells, 48
Scleral sulcus, internal, 48
Scleritis, corticosteroid route of administration in, 333t

Scopolamine, 313, 314t, 315t
Sebaceous glands of eyelid, 19, 24
    glands of Zeis, 19, 22f, 23t, 215
    meibomian glands, 20f, 22f, 23t, 24, 25f
Second cranial nerve. See Optic nerve
Second-degree relatives, 143
Second-order neuron, dilator muscle innervation and, 56
Secondary vitreous, 122, 123f
Secretogranin II, in aqueous humor, 231
Secretory IgA, in tear film, 216
Secretory lacrimal apparatus, 22f, 28–29, 28f, 217–220,
    218f, 219f. See also Lacrimal glands
Segregation (genetic), 143, 184, 186–187
    replicative, 143, 157
Selenium, in retina and retinal pigment epithelium,
    287, 289f
Selenium-dependent glutathione peroxidase
    (GSH-Px), 287
Selenoprotein P, in aqueous humor, 231, 233
Semilunar ganglion (gasserian/trigeminal ganglion), 9f,
    98f, 99, 99f, 101f
Sensorcaine. See Bupivacaine
Sensory nucleus
    of cranial nerve V (trigeminal), 97, 98f, 99, 99f, 101f
    of cranial nerve VII (facial), 103
Sensory root
    of cranial nerve V (trigeminal), 97
    of cranial nerve V₁ (ophthalmic), 11, 12f
    of cranial nerve VII (facial), 102–103
Sequencing, DNA, 161–162, 162f, 163f, 164f, 165f, 166f
    next-generation (NGS/massively parallel), 140, 142,
        161, 163f, 164f, 165f, 166f
Serum drops, for dry eye, 342
Seventh cranial nerve. See Cranial nerve VII
Sex chromosomes, 147, 184, 189f
    aneuploidy of, 189
    mosaicism and, 191–192
Sex-determining region Y (SRY/testis-determining
    factor/TDF), 179
Sex-linked inheritance (sex-linked genes), 143, 178. See
    also X-linked inheritance; Y-linked inheritance
Shh factor, gene expression/ocular development
    and, 127
Short (p) arm, 141, 148f
Short arm 11 deletion syndrome (11p13 syndrome/
    PAX6 gene mutation), 193
    in aniridia, 152, 177, 193
Short ciliary nerves, 12, 12f, 100
    ciliary muscle supplied by, 95
    posterior, 32
    sphincter muscle supplied by, 56
Short interfering (small interference) RNA (siRNA), 143
    in gene therapy, 170
Short interspersed elements (SINEs), 150
Shotgun sequencing, whole-genome, 163f
Sickle cell disease
    mutations causing, 184
    racial and ethnic concentration of, 197
sIgA. See Secretory IgA
Sigmoid sinus, 105, 106f
Signal transduction
    mechanisms of, 316t
    in tear secretion, 217–219, 218f, 219f

Silicone oil, intravitreal administration of, 300t
Simplex case/genetic disease, 143, 182
SINEs. See Short interspersed elements
Single-gene disorder (mendelian disorder), 139, 194
Single-nucleotide polymorphism (SNP), 144, 194
    in genome-wide association studies (GWAS),
        163–168, 168f, 194
Single-stranded conformational polymorphism
    (SSCP), 162
Singlet oxygen, 281, 283
Sinus thrombosis, 105
Sinuses
    paranasal, 10–11, 10f
    periorbital, 10–11, 10f
siRNA. See Short interfering (small interference) RNA
Sister chromatids, 133
Sixth cranial nerve. See Cranial nerve VI
Skin, eyelid, 19, 20f, 21f
Skipped generation (incomplete penetrance), 177
Slow inactivators, isoniazid use in, 201
Slow-reacting substance of anaphylaxis, 335. See also
    Leukotrienes
Slow twitch (tonic) fibers, 18
Small interference (short interfering) RNA
    (siRNA), 143
    in gene therapy, 170
Small nuclear ribonucleoprotein polypeptide N
    (SNRPN) gene, imprinting of, 153, 154
SMAS. See Superficial musculoaponeurotic system
"Snowflake" cataract, 247
SNP. See Single-nucleotide polymorphism
SNRPN (small nuclear ribonucleoprotein polypeptide N)
    gene, imprinting of, 153, 154
SOD. See Superoxide dismutase
Sodium
    in aqueous humor, 231t, 232
    in lens, 245–246
    in tear film, 214t, 216
    transport of
        aqueous humor composition/secretion and,
            230–231, 323, 324f
        carbonic anhydrase inhibitors affecting, 323–324
    in vitreous, 231t, 252
Sodium chloride, for ocular edema, 366
Sodium hyaluronate, as viscoelastic, 368
Sodium perborate, as ocular medication
    preservative, 294
Sodium-potassium-calcium exchanger (Na⁺,K⁺-Ca
    exchanger), in rods, 259
Sodium-potassium pump (Na⁺,K⁺-ATPase)
    in aqueous humor secretion/suppression, 230, 323
    in lens ionic balance, 246
    in retinal pigment epithelium, 273, 277
    in rods, 259
Solexa technology, in next-generation sequencing, 165f.
    See also Next-generation sequencing
Somatic afferent fibers, 103
Somatic motor nerves, cholinergic drug action and,
    307, 307f
Sondermann channels, 52f
Sorbitol/sorbitol pathway
    in cataract formation, 247–248
    in lens glucose/carbohydrate metabolism, 247–248, 247f

Sorsby macular dystrophy
retinal pigment epithelium in, 278
TIMP3 defects causing, 161, 265
Sperm, 186
Sphenoid bone, 5, 6, 6*f*, 7
Sphenoid sinuses, 10–11, 10*f*, 17*f*
Sphenoid wings, 5, 6, 6*f*, 7
Sphenoparietal sinus, 106*f*
Spherule, of rod, 69, 73*f*
Sphincter muscle (iris), 53*f*, 54*f*, 56
development of, 56, 116*t*, 122
innervation of, 56, 94, 95
miotic/muscarinic drugs affecting, 308
mydriatics affecting, 313
Sphingomyelinase, defective/deficiency of, 175*t*
Spinal nucleus and tract, of cranial nerve V (trigeminal), 97, 97–99, 99*f*, 101*f*
Spiral of Tillaux, 13, 14*f*
Splice junction site, 144
Spliceosome, 144, 152
Splicing, 144, 152
alternative, 148, 152–153
Sporadic, definition of, 144
Sporanox. *See* Itraconazole
SRY. *See* Sex-determining region Y
SSCP. *See* Single-stranded conformational polymorphism
Stapedial/stapedius nerve, 101*f*, 103
Stargardt disease
ABC transporter mutations causing, 263
retinal pigment epithelium in, 279
Stationary night blindness, congenital, with myopia, ocular findings in carriers of, 199*t*
Stationary nyctalopia, rod-specific mutations causing, 263, 264
Stearic acid, in retinal pigment epithelium, 274, 276
Stellate ganglion, dilator muscle innervation and, 56
Stem cell transplantation, 203
Stem cells, 127
corneal, 40
Steroids. *See* Corticosteroids
Stickler syndrome, vitreous collapse in, 255
Stomodeum, 113*f*
Stop codon (termination codon), 144
frameshift mutation and, 135, 155
Storage diseases. *See also* Enzyme defects, disorders associated with
enzyme defects/ocular signs in, 175*t*
Strabismus, botulinum toxin for, 366
Straight sinus, 105, 106*f*
Streptokinase, 369
Streptomycin, 351
Stroma
ciliary body, 57–58, 58*f*
corneal, 40–41, 42*f*, 223*f*, 225–226
anatomy of, 40–41, 42*f*, 223*f*
biochemistry and metabolism of, 225–226
development of, 118, 120, 121*f*
iris, 54–55, 56*f*
development of, 122
scleral, 44
Subarachnoid space, optic nerve in, 87–89
Subconjunctival drug administration, 299
for anesthetics, 365
Submandibular ganglion, 101*f*, 103, 104

Subretinal space, 70*f*, 257
retinal pigment epithelium in maintenance of, 277
Substance P, in tear secretion, 216
Substantia propria, corneal. *See* Stroma, corneal
Sub-Tenon drug administration, 299
local anesthetic, 365
Succinylcholine, 315, 315*t*
cholinesterase inhibitor use and, 312
pharmacogenetics and, 201–202
"Sugar" cataracts, 246–248
aldose reductase in development of, 247–248, 247*f*
Sulcus
intermarginal (gray line), 19, 22*f*, 215
internal scleral, 48
Sulfacetamide, 347*t*, 349
in combination preparations, 348*t*
Sulfadiazine, 349
Sulfite oxidase deficiency, 175*t*
Sulfoiduronate sulfatase, defective/deficiency of, 175*t*
Sulfonamides, 349
Sulindac, 335*t*
Superficial musculoaponeurotic system (SMAS), 104
Superficial petrosal nerve, greater, 101*f*, 103, 104
Superficial temporal artery, eyelids supplied by, 26, 26*f*
Superior cerebellar artery, cranial nerve relationship and, 94, 95*f*, 97
Superior cervical ganglion, 11
dilator muscle innervation and, 56
Superior oblique muscle, 9*f*, 13, 13*f*, 14*f*, 15*t*, 16*f*, 20*f*
blood supply of, 15*t*, 34*f*
innervation of, 17
insertions of, 14*f*, 15, 15*t*
origins of, 15*t*, 17
Superior oblique tendon, 13*f*, 14*f*
Superior orbital fissure, 6*f*, 8, 8*f*, 9*f*, 14*f*
Superior petrosal sinus, 106*f*
Superior punctum, 29
Superior rectus muscle, 9*f*, 13, 14*f*, 15*t*, 20*f*
blood supply of, 15*t*, 17, 34*f*
innervation of, 17, 94, 94*f*, 95
insertions of, 13–15, 14*f*
optic nerve and, 87
origins of, 15*t*, 16–17
Superior rectus tendon, 13*f*, 14*f*
Superior sagittal sinus, 105, 106*f*
Superior salivatory (salivary) nucleus, 101*f*, 103, 104
Superior tarsal muscle of Müller, 20*f*, 24
Superior transverse (Whitnall) ligament, 20*f*, 24
Superoxide, 281, 282, 287
Superoxide dismutase, 282*f*, 287
in lens, 284
in retina and retinal pigment epithelium, 273, 287
Support groups, genetic disorders and, 207
Supraorbital artery, 16*f*, 26*f*, 33*f*
Supraorbital foramen/notch, 5, 7
Supraorbital nerve, 7, 16*f*, 100
Supraorbital vein, 35*f*
Supratrochlear artery, 26*f*, 33*f*
Supratrochlear nerve, 100
Suprofen, 239
Surfactants
in eyedrops
absorption and, 298
toxicity and, 294

Suspensory ligament of Lockwood, 32, 32f
Suspensory ligaments of lens. See Zonular fibers
Sustained-release preparations
    oral, 301
    for topical administration, 302
Sutures (lens), 64, 65f
Sweat glands, of eyelid, 19, 22f, 23t
Sympathetic nerves/pathway
    in ciliary ganglion, 11, 12–13, 12f
    ciliary muscle innervation and, 59
    dilator muscle innervation and, 55
    sphincter muscle innervation and, 56
    in tear secretion, 214, 216, 218, 218f, 219, 219f
Sympathetic ophthalmia, corticosteroid route of
    administration in, 333t
Sympathetic root, in ciliary ganglion, 11, 12f
Synaptic body
    of cone (pedicle), 70, 73f
    of rod (spherule), 69, 73f
Synechiae, posterior, mydriasis in prevention of, 313
Synkinesis, near reflex and, 96
Syntenic traits, 187

Tafluprost, 237, 302, 327, 327t
Tandem repeats, variable/variable number of
    (microsatellites), 139, 150
Tarsal (meibomian) glands, 20f, 22f, 23t, 24, 25f,
    214–215, 215f
    dysfunction of, 220
    in tear-film lipids/tear production, 24, 214–215, 215f, 217
Tarsal muscles, superior (Müller), 20f, 24
Tarsal plates/tarsus, 20f, 24, 25f
TATA box, 142
Taxon-specific crystallins, 244
Tay-Sachs disease (GM₂ gangliosidosis type I), 175t
    racial and ethnic concentration of, 197
Tazolol, 308t
TCA cycle. See Tricarboxylic acid (TCA) cycle
TDF. See Testis-determining factor
Tear-deficiency states, 220–222, 221f
    aqueous, 220, 221–222, 221f
    mucin, 217, 220
Tear film (tears), 213–222, 213f, 214t, 215f
    aqueous layer of, 38, 213f, 215–217
        secretion of, 216–217
    biochemistry and metabolism of, 213–222
    drug absorption and, 295–296, 296f, 298
    dysfunction/alterations of, 220–222, 221f
    functions of, 213
    instability of, 220
    lipid layer of, 38, 213f, 214–215, 215f
    mucin layer of, 38, 213f, 217
    pH of, 214t
    precorneal, 38, 213–214, 213f
    preocular, 220
    secretion of, 214t, 217–220, 218f, 219f
    solutes in, 216
    thickness of, 213, 213f, 214t
Tear meniscus (marginal tear strip), 213
Tear pump, ocular medication absorption affected by, 296
Tear sac (lacrimal sac), 29
Tearing/epiphora, reflex, 104
    absorption of ocular medication affected by, 295, 298
    initiation of, 126

Tears (artificial), 220, 221, 341, 342
Telomeres/telomeric DNA, 144, 150
Telophase, 149, 149f
Temafloxacin, 346
Temporal arteritis, corticosteroid route of
    administration in, 333t
Temporal nerve, 104
Temporofacial division, of cranial nerve VII (facial), 104
Tenon capsule, 31–32, 31f, 32f, 43
Terak. See Oxytetracycline, with polymyxin B
Teratogens
    carbonic anhydrase inhibitors as, 326
    tetracyclines as, 350
Terminal web, 42–43, 42f
Termination codon (stop codon), 144
    frameshift mutation and, 135, 155
Tertiary vitreous, 123f
Testis-determining factor (TDF/sex-determining region
    Y/SRY), 179
Tetracaine, 363t, 365
Tetracyclines, 350
    intravenous administration of, 301
Tetrahydrotriamcinolone, anti-inflammatory/pressure-
    elevating potency of, 333t
Tetrahydrozoline, 342
Tetravisc. See Tetracaine
TFIIH, in DNA repair, 154
TGF-β. See Transforming growth factor βs
Thimerosal, allergic/sensitivity/toxic reactions and,
    294, 341
Third cranial nerve. See Cranial nerve III
Third nerve (oculomotor) palsy, pupil-sparing, 95
Third-order neurons, dilator muscle innervation and, 56
13q14 (long arm 13 deletion) syndrome, 192
Three cone opsins, 262. See also Color vision
3′ untranslated region, 145, 147
Threshold, genetic, 144
Thrombin, 369
Thrombospondin I, in vitreous, 253
Thromboxanes, 237, 334
    aspirin affecting, 335
Thymoxamine, 308t, 321
Ticarcillin, 344t, 345
Tight junctions (zonulae occludentes)
    in ciliary body epithelium, 57
    in corneal endothelium, 227
    in retinal pigment epithelium, 68, 272
Tillaux, spiral of, 13, 14f
Timolol, 308t, 321, 322t, 323
    in combination preparations, 318t, 322t, 325, 325t, 327t
    for glaucoma, 321, 322t, 325, 325t, 327t
Timoptic. See Timolol
TIMP3 gene/TIMP3 protein mutation, 161, 265
Tissue plasminogen activator (tPA), 369
    in aqueous, 369
    intracameral administration of, 300t
    off-label use of, 306, 369
    in vitreous, 252
Tobradex. See Tobramycin, in combination preparations
Tobramycin, 344t, 347t, 351
    in combination preparations, 334, 348t
Tobrasol. See Tobramycin
Tobrex. See Tobramycin
Tolmetin, 335t

Tonic cells, 267, 267*f*
Tonic (slow twitch) fibers, 18
Tonic pupil (Adie pupil), pharmacologic testing for, 310
Topical anesthesia, 362–366, 363*t*
  for anterior segment surgery, 365–366
  cholinesterase inhibitor use and, 312, 363
Topical medications, 295–299, 296*f. See also* Eyedrops
  sustained-release devices for, 302
Topography, 37–38, 37*f*
Toxicity (drug), 294
  age/aging and, 294, 295
  tissue binding and, 298
tPA. *See* Tissue plasminogen activator
Trabecular meshwork, 45*f*, 46*f*, 48–52, 49*f*, 50*f*
  corneoscleral, 48, 49, 50*f*
  endothelial, 49–50
  uveal, 48, 49
Trabecular outflow, drugs affecting, 318*t*
Trabeculectomy, antifibrotic drugs used with, 340
Trabeculocytes, 48
Trait, 173
Tranexamic acid, 369, 370
Transcribed strand of DNA (antisense DNA), 132
  in gene therapy, 170
Transcription (gene), 144, 147, 151, 151*f*, 152
  embryogenesis and, 111
  reverse, 143
Transcription factors, 152
Transcriptomics, 136
Transducin, rod, 259, 260*f*, 261
  mutations in, 263
Transfer RNA (tRNA), mitochondrial DNA-encoded,
  mutations of, 157
Transferrin
  in aqueous humor, 233, 234
  in vitreous, 252
Transforming growth factor βs, 371
  in aqueous humor, 234
  retinal pigment epithelial cell transformation and, 279
  in tear film, 217
Transient amplifying cells, in corneal epithelium, 40
Transketolase, in cornea, 224
Translation, 144, 147, 151, 151*f*, 152
  gene product changes/modification after
    (posttranslational modification), 142
  of lens proteins, 245
Translocation, chromosome, 144
  Down syndrome caused by, 190
Transplantation, organ, for enzyme deficiency
  disease, 203
Transport mechanisms, retinal pigment
  epithelium, 273, 277
Trans-RPE potential, electro-oculogram and, 277
Transverse ligament, superior (Whitnall), 20*f*, 24
Transverse sinus, 105, 106*f*
Trauma, optic neuropathy caused by, 89
Travatan. *See* Travoprost
Travoprost, 237, 302, 327, 327*t*
  in combination preparations, 327*t*
Triamcinolone
  intravitreal administration of, 300*t*, 334
  in macular hole repair, 367
Triazoles, 355*t*, 356
  for *Acanthamoeba* keratitis, 361

Tricarboxylic acid (TCA) cycle, in corneal glucose
  metabolism, 224
Trichiasis, 24
Tricyclic antidepressants, apraclonidine/brimonidine
  interactions and, 319
Trifluridine, 356, 357*t*
Trigeminal ganglion (gasserian/semilunar ganglion), 9*f*,
  98*f*, 99, 99*f*, 101*f*
Trigeminal nerve. *See* Cranial nerve V
Trimethaphan, 315*t*
Trimethoprim
  with polymyxin B, 347*t*, 353
  with sulfonamides, 349
Trinucleotide repeats, 139
  expansion/contraction of, 144–145
    anticipation and, 132, 144, 195
Trinucleotides, 147, 151
Triplets, 133
Trisomy, 189
Trisomy 21 (Down syndrome), 189–190, 191*t*
  mosaicism in, 191
  pharmacogenetics and, 201
Trisomy 21 mosaicism, 191
Trivariant color vision, 262–263. *See also* Color vision
tRNA. *See* Transfer RNA
Trochlea, 6, 13*f*, 14*f*
Trochlear fossa, 6
Trochlear nerve. *See* Cranial nerve IV
Tropicacyl. *See* Tropicamide
Tropicamide, 314*t*
  with hydroxyamphetamine, 314*t*
Trusopt. *See* Dorzolamide
Trypan blue, 367, 368
Tubocurarine, 308*t*, 315*t*
Tubulin, 245
Tumor necrosis factor α, in tear film, 217
Tumor-suppressor genes, 145, 154, 156–157. *See also*
  specific type
  in DNA repair, 154
  recessive, Rb locus as, 192
  Wilms tumor, imprinting of, 138, 153
Tunica vasculosa lentis, remnant of, Mittendorf dot, 80, 81*f*
Twin studies, 182, 182*f*
Twitch-type fibers, 18
2-hit hypothesis, 157
TXA. *See* Thromboxanes
Tympanic segment of cranial nerve VII (facial), 103
TYR (tyrosinase) gene mutations, in albinism, 185, 278
Tyrosinase activity, in albinism, 175*t*, 185
Tyrosinase *(TYR)* gene mutations, in albinism, 185, 278
Tyrosinase promoter, in melanogenesis, 277–278
Tyrosine aminotransferase, defective/deficiency of, 175*t*
Tyrosinemia, 175*t*
Tyrosinosis, 175*t*

Ultrafiltration, in aqueous humor dynamics/formation, 230
Ultrasound biomicroscopy, 47, 47*f*
Ultraviolet light/radiation, eye disorders/injury
  associated with, 283, 286
Unequal crossing over, 145
  color vision defects and, 262–263
Uniparental disomy, 145, 154
Unoprostone, 302, 327, 327*t*
Untranslated region (UTR), 145, 147

Upper eyelids. *See* Eyelids, upper
Urea
    in aqueous humor, 233
    as hyperosmotic agent, 233, 328–329, 329*t*
    in tear film, 216
Urinary tract stones, acetazolamide use and, 326
Urokinase, 369
Usher syndrome, 202, 204, 278
    myosin VIIA gene in, 264
    retinal pigment epithelium in, 278
UTR. *See* Untranslated region
Uvea (uveal tract), 38, 53–62, 236. *See also specific structure*
    development of, 122
Uveal meshwork, 48, 49
Uveitis, corticosteroid route of administration in, 333*t*
Uveoscleral drainage/outflow, 46
    drugs affecting, 318*t*

Valacyclovir, 302, 357*t*, 359
Valcyte. *See* Valganciclovir
Valdecoxib, cardiovascular toxicity and, 239
Valganciclovir, 357*t*, 360
Valtrex. *See* Valacyclovir
Vancomycin, 344*t*, 352
Variability, in genetic disease, 194–195
Variable/variable number of tandem repeats (microsatellite), 139, 150
Vascular endothelial growth factor (VEGF), 371–372
    alternative splicing and, 153
    in aqueous humor, 234, 235
    drugs inhibiting. *See* Anti–vascular endothelial growth factor (anti-VEGF) drugs
    in vitreous, 254
Vascular loops, 80
Vascular system
    of choroid, 59–60, 60*f*, 61–62, 61*f*, 62*f*
        development of, 116*t*
    of ciliary body, 57, 58*f*
    of extraocular muscles, 15*t*, 17
    of eyelids, 25–26, 26*f*
    of iris, 35, 54*f*, 55
    of orbit, anatomy of, 32–35, 33*f*, 34*f*, 35*f*
Vasculotropin. *See* Vascular endothelial growth factor
Vasoactive intestinal polypeptide (VIP)
    outflow facility affected by, 48
    in tear secretion, 214, 216, 219, 219*f*
Vasocidin. *See* Prednisolone, in combination preparations
Vasocon-A. *See* Naphazoline/antazoline
VECAT (Vitamin E, Cataract and Age-Related Maculopathy Trial), 285
Vector, 145
    cosmid, 145
    in gene therapy, 169
VEGF. *See* Vascular endothelial growth factor
VEGF gene, 372
Venous sinuses, 105, 106*f*
Versican, in vitreous, 249
Vertebral artery, 105
Vesicle
    lens, 117*f*, 118, 120*f*
    optic, 115, 116*t*, 117*f*, 118*f*
        lens development and, 118

Vexol. *See* Rimexolone
Vfend. *See* Voriconazole
Vidarabine, 356, 357*t*, 358
Vigamox. *See* Moxifloxacin
Vimentin, 245
Vinculin, in retinal pigment epithelium, 273
VIP. *See* Vasoactive intestinal polypeptide
Vira-A. *See* Vidarabine
Viroptic. *See* Trifluridine
Visceral afferent fibers, 103
Visceral efferent fibers, 103
Viscoat, 368
Viscoelastic agents, 368
    intracameral administration of, 300*t*
Viscosity, ocular medication absorption affected by, 297
Visine. *See* Naphazoline/pheniramine
Vistide. *See* Cidofovir
Visual cortex, 90, 93
Visual cycle, retinal pigment epithelium in, 274–276, 275*f*
Visual field defects, 90, 90*f*
Visual pathways, 90, 90*f*
Visual pigments, retinal pigment epithelium in regeneration of, 274–276, 275*f*
VIT1, in vitreous, 249, 252
Vitamin A
    for abetalipoproteinemia, 203
    in retinal pigment epithelium, 274, 275, 276
    in visual cycle, 274–276
Vitamin B$_6$ (pyridoxine), for homocystinuria, 203
Vitamin C (ascorbic acid)
    antioxidant effect of, 285, 288
        in lens, 283, 285
        in retina and retinal pigment epithelium, 288
    in aqueous humor, 231*t*, 232
    oral supplements and, 285
    in tear film, 214
    in vitreous, 231*t*
Vitamin E
    abetalipoproteinemia and, 203
    antioxidant effect of, 283, 284*f*, 285, 286, 287, 288
        in lens, 285
        oral supplements and, 285
        in retina and retinal pigment epithelium, 286, 287, 288, 289*f*
Vitamin E, Cataract and Age-Related Maculopathy Trial (VECAT), 285
Vitamin supplements, 370
    in genetic disorders, 203
Vitrasert. *See* Ganciclovir
Vitrectomy, physiologic changes after, 254
Vitreolysis, enzymatic, 255
Vitreous, 37–38, 37*f*, 78–81, 79*f*, 80*f*, 81*f*, 249–255
    aging affecting, 80, 252–255
    anatomy of, 37–38, 37*f*, 78–81, 79*f*, 80*f*, 81*f*
    as angiogenesis inhibitor, 253–254
    biochemistry and metabolism of, 249–255
    collagen in, 78–79, 79*f*, 249–250, 250*f*, 251*f*
        liquefaction and, 253
    composition of, 249–252, 250*f*, 251*f*
    detachment of, 80, 80*f*, 81*f*, 252–253
    development of, 122, 123*f*
    genetic disease involving, 255
    hyaluronan/hyaluronic acid in, 79, 79*f*, 250–251
    infection/inflammation of, 254

injury to, 254
liquefaction of, 252–253
    injury/hemorrhage/inflammation and, 254
low-molecular-weight solutes in, 252
macular hole formation and, 254–255
myopia caused by changes in, 252, 253
primary, 122, 123f
proteins in, 251–252
secondary, 122, 123f
tertiary, 123f
topography of, 37–38, 37f
zonular fibers in, 252
Vitreous base, 79
Vitreous detachment, posterior (PVD), 80, 80f, 81f, 252–253
Vitreous hemorrhage, 254
Vitreous opacities, fibrillar, 253
VNTRs. See Variable/variable number of tandem repeats
Voltaren. See Diclofenac
von Recklinghausen disease. See Neurofibromatosis, von Recklinghausen
Voriconazole, 355t, 356
Vortex veins, 34f, 35
    choroid drained by, 60
    development of, 116t
VTRs. See Variable/variable number of tandem repeats

Waardenburg syndrome, 152
WAGR syndrome, 193
Water-soluble lens proteins, 243, 245
Watershed zone, 91
Wear-and-tear pigment (lipofuscin granules), 69
    in retinal pigment epithelium phagocytosis, 276, 276f
Western blot analysis, 145
Whitnall ligament (superior transverse ligament), 20f, 24
Whitnall tubercle, 7
Whole-genome shotgun sequencing, 163f
Wilbrand knee, 92
Wild type, 145
Willis, circle of, 90, 90f, 105–107, 107f
Wilms tumor, aniridia and, 193
Wilms tumor–suppressor gene, imprinting of, 138, 153
Wilson disease (hepatolenticular degeneration), 203
"Wing" cells, 39, 40f, 223f, 224
Wnt (ligand), gene expression/ocular development and, 127
Wolfring, glands of, 20f, 22f, 23t, 29, 216

X chromosome, 147, 178, 179, 184, 189f
    genes for color vision on, 262–263
    inactivation of (lyonization/Barr body), 132, 139, 153, 197–200
        ocular findings in carrier states and, 197–200, 198–199f, 199t
    mosaicism and, 191–192
X-linked disorders, 180–181. See also specific disorder and X-linked inheritance
    albinism (Nettleship-Falls), ocular findings in carriers of, 198–200, 199f
    blue-cone monochromatism, 264
        ocular findings in carriers of, 199t
    dominant, 180–181
    gene therapy for, 169

ocular findings in carriers of, 197–200, 198–199f, 199t
    retinitis pigmentosa, ocular findings in carriers of, 198f, 199t
X-linked inheritance (X-linked genes), 145, 178–181. See also X-linked disorders
    dominant, 179–180, 181t
    recessive, 179, 180t
Xalacom. See Latanoprost, in combination preparations
Xalatan. See Latanoprost
Xanthophylls (carotenoids)
    antioxidant effects of, 284f, 288
    in lens, 285
    in retina, 77, 286, 288, 289f
Xeroderma pigmentosa/pigmentosum, 154
Xibrom. See Bromfenac
Xylocaine. See Lidocaine

Y chromosome, 147, 178, 179, 184, 189f
    mosaicism and, 192
Y-linked inheritance (Y-linked genes), 145
Y-sutures, lens, 64, 65f
Yeast artificial chromosome (YAC), 145
Yellow spot. See Macula/macula lutea
Yohimbine, 308t

Zaditor. See Ketotifen
Zeaxanthin, 77
    antioxidant effect of, 286, 288
    in retina, 286, 288
Zeis, glands of, 19, 22f, 23t, 215
    in tear-film lipids/tear production, 215
Zidovudine, 357t, 361
Zinc, in aqueous humor, 232
Zinn
    annulus of, 8, 9f, 13f, 14f, 16–17, 87
    circle of (circle of Zinn-Haller), 88f, 91
    zonules of (zonular fibers), 37f, 46f, 63f, 65f, 66–67, 241
        development of, 120, 120f
Zinn-Haller, circle of, 88f, 91
Zioptan. See Tafluprost
Zirgan. See Ganciclovir
Zone of discontinuity, 64
Zonulae adherentes, in retinal pigment epithelium, 68
Zonulae occludentes (tight junctions)
    in ciliary body epithelium, 57
    in corneal endothelium, 227
    in retinal pigment epithelium, 68, 272
Zonular apparatus, 252
Zonular fibers
    corneal epithelial, 39
    lens (zonules of Zinn), 37f, 46f, 63f, 65f, 66–67, 241
        development of, 120, 120f
    vitreous, 252
Zovirax. See Acyclovir
Zygomatic bone, 5, 6f, 7
Zygomatic foramen, 8
Zygomatic nerve, 104
Zygomaticofacial artery, 34f
Zygomaticotemporal artery, 34f
Zygote, 186
Zylet. See Loteprednol, with tobramycin
Zymar. See Gatifloxacin
Zymaxid. See Gatifloxacin